Managing Medical and Obstetric Emergencies and Trauma

Managing Medical and Obstetric Emergencies and Trauma

A Practical Approach

FOURTH EDITION

Advanced Life Support Group

EDITED BY

Rosamunde Burns

Kara Dent

WILEY Blackwell

ALSG Obstetric

ALSG Advanced Life Support Group

A charity dedicated to saving life by providing training

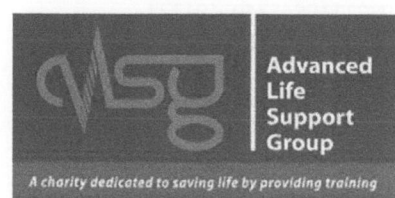

This fourth edition first published 2022

Edition History
Cambridge University Press (3e, 2014, 2e 2007, 1e 2002)

Registered Offices
John Wiley & Sons, Inc., 111 River Street, Hoboken, NJ 07030, USA
John Wiley & Sons Ltd, The Atrium, Southern Gate, Chichester, West Sussex, PO19 8SQ, UK

Editorial Office
9600 Garsington Road, Oxford, OX4 2DQ, UK

For details of our global editorial offices, customer services, and more information about Wiley products visit us at www.wiley.com.

Wiley also publishes its books in a variety of electronic formats and by print-on-demand. Some content that appears in standard print versions of this book may not be available in other formats.

Library of Congress Cataloging-in-Publication Data Applied for

Paperback ISBN: 9781119645740

Cover Design: Wiley
Cover Image: Courtesy of ALSG

Set in 10/12pt Myriad Light by Straive, Pondicherry, India
Printed and bound by CPI Group (UK) Ltd, Croydon, CR0 4YY

C9781119645740_191223

Dedication

Richard Johanson 1957–2002

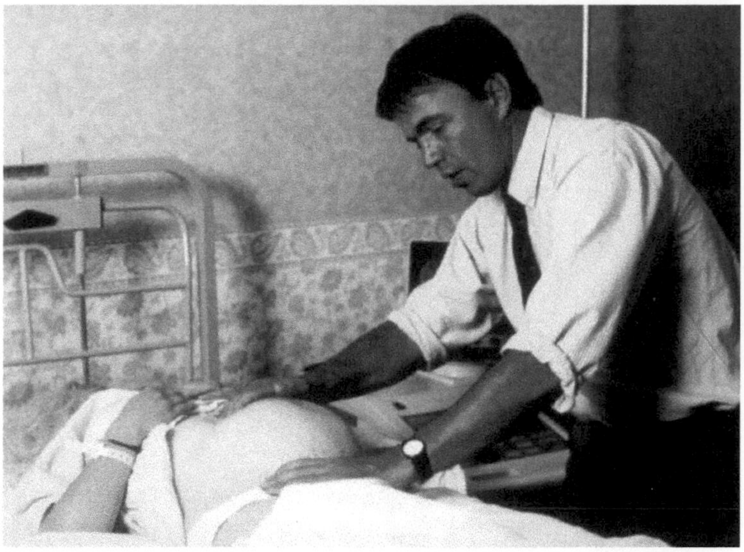

This book is dedicated to the memory of Richard Johanson, who died on 20 February 2002, before he could see this work come to fruition.

> ***'It's never too late to be what you might have been'***
>
> *George Eliot*

This quotation had meaning for Richard – it was posted on his study wall.

Richard had two major aims in obstetrics – to avoid unnecessary intervention but to apply urgent skilled intervention when needed, and he had a gift for both. He wanted interventions to be based on the best evidence available and for there to be good audit to check that the correct processes were being followed. His experience in Stoke and overseas had given him the skills to achieve these aims. His drive was for simple emergency protocols to save the lives of mothers and babies. This led to his leadership in practice and education in labour ward emergencies.

Initially he organised structured training for life-threatening obstetric emergencies in the West Midlands and in 1997 he and Charles Cox were the inspiration for developing the 'Managing Obstetric Emergencies and Trauma' (MOET) course, aimed at senior obstetricians and anaesthetists. A modified MOET course was taken overseas where he introduced ideas and protocols with tact and efficiency.

He worked closely with midwives in research and in the implementation of labour ward guidelines. He organised national meetings dealing with childbirth and worked with the National Childbirth Trust and Baby Lifeline, again to promote safer childbirth without overmedicalisation. The foundation of his research charity 'Childbirth without Fear' aims to continue to improve the care of women during childbirth.

Richard will be remembered by many, particularly by his trainees. His boundless enthusiasm and generosity with his time, ideas and academic work meant that there was a queue to work with him. The publication problem would be solved and the trainee would have a nationally respected mentor who continued to take an interest in their career.

Perhaps instinctively feeling that time was precious led him to achieve so much so quickly. Much of it was due to the intellectual sparking between him and his anaesthetist wife, Charlotte. They demonstrated the teamwork that is part of the philosophy of MOET.

> *'To see a human being reveal really exceptional qualities one must be able to observe his activities over many years. If these activities are completely unselfish; if the idea motivating them is unique in its magnanimity; if it is quite certain that they have never looked for any reward; and if in addition they have left visible traces on the world – then one may say, without fear of error, that one is in the presence of an unforgettable character.'*

Jean Giono, from a short story called *The Man Who Planted Trees*

Contents

Working group for fourth edition

Anita Banerjee FHEA FRCP, Obstetric Physician, Diabetes and Endocrinology and General Medicine Physician, Deputy Director of Medical Education, Guys and St Thomas' Hospitals NHS Foundation Trust; Honorary Reader in Obstetric Medicine, King's College London

Sam Bassett Lead Midwife for Education and Head of Department Midwifery, King's College London

Virginia A. Beckett BSc(Hons) MB BS FRCOG, Consultant Obstetrician and Gynaecologist, Bradford Teaching Hospitals NHS Foundation Trust

Janet Brennand MD FRCOG, Consultant in Maternal and Fetal Medicine, Queen Elizabeth University Hospital, Glasgow

Rosamunde Burns MBChB FRCA, Consultant Anaesthetist, Royal Infirmary of Edinburgh; Honorary Senior Lecturer, University of Edinburgh

Alastair Campbell BSc(Hons) MBChB FRCOG, Consultant Obstetrician and Gynaecologist, Royal Infirmary of Edinburgh; Associate Postgraduate Dean (Quality), NHS Education for Scotland

Janie Collie MB ChB FRCA, Consultant Anaesthetist, Assistant Director of Medical Education, University Hospital Crosshouse, Kilmarnock

Christina Cotzias MRCOG, Consultant Obstetrician and Gynaecologist, Chelsea and Westminster NHS Foundation Trust, West Middlesex Site

Kara Dent MBBS, FRCOG, Consultant in Fetal Maternal Medicine, University Hospitals of Derby and Burton Foundation Trust

R. John Elton FRCA, Consultant Obstetric Anaesthetist, University Hospitals of Coventry and Warwickshire NHS Trust, Coventry

Simon Grant DM FRCOG Consultant in Obstetrics and Fetal Medicine, North Bristol NHS Trust

Marie Hall RN RM MSc (critical care), Lead Midwife for Obstetric High Dependency, Queen Charlotte's and Chelsea Hospital, Imperial College Healthcare NHS Trust

Deborah Harrington FRCOG, Consultant in Maternal and Fetal Medicine, Deputy Director of Medical Education, Oxford University Hospitals NHS Foundation Trust; Head of School of Obstetrics and Gynaecology, Health Education England working across the Thames Valley

Brigid Hayden FRCOG PGCTLCC DMCC, Consultant Obstetrician and Gynaecologist and Labour Ward Lead, Princess Elizabeth Hospital and Medical Specialist Group, Guernsey

Kim Hinshaw FRCOG, Consultant Obstetrician and Gynaecologist, Sunderland Royal Hospital, South Tyneside and Sunderland NHS Foundation Trust; Visiting Professor, University of Sunderland

Alison Lansbury FRCA, Consultant Anaesthetist, Leeds General Infirmary

Douglas Mein FRCA FANZCA, Consultant Anaesthetist, Wellington Regional Hospital, New Zealand

Oliver Milling-Smith Consultant Obstetrician and Gynaecologist, Forth Valley Royal Hospital

Felicity Plaat BA MBBS FRCA, Consultant Anaesthetist, Queen Charlotte's and Hammersmith Hospitals, Imperial College Healthcare NHS Trust, London

Rahul Sen BA FRANZCOG Grad Dip Ec DTM&H MIPH, Consultant in Obstetrics and Gynaecology, Royal Hospital for Women, Conjoint Lecturer, University of New South Wales, Sydney

Farah Sethna BSc(Hons) MBBS MRCOG FRANZCOG, Consultant in Obstetrics and Maternal and Fetal Medicine Centenary Hospital for Women and Children, Canberra, Australia

Paul Sharpe FRCA, Consultant in Obstetric Anaesthesia, University Hospitals of Leicester NHS Trust

Anouk van der Knijff-van Dortmont MD, Consultant Anaesthetist, Erasmus MC, Sophia Children's Hospital University Medical Center Rotterdam, The Netherlands

Thierry van Dessel MD PhD, Consultant Obstetrics and Gynaecology, Elisabeth TweeSteden Hospital, Tilburg, The Netherlands

Darren Walter MPH FRCS FRCEM FIMC FAEMS, Senior Lecturer in Emergency Global Health, University of Manchester, Honorary Consultant in Emergency Medicine, Manchester University NHS Foundation Trust

Contributors to fourth edition

Claire Alexander MPhil FRCOG, Consultant Obstetrician and Maternal Medicine Lead, Royal Infirmary of Edinburgh; Associate Postgraduate Dean, NHS Education Scotland

Anita Banerjee FHEA FRCP, Obstetric Physician, Diabetes and Endocrinology and General Medicine Physician, Deputy Director of Medical Education, Guys and St Thomas' Hospitals NHS Foundation Trust; Honorary Reader in Obstetric Medicine, King's College London

Virginia A. Beckett BSc(Hons) MB BS FRCOG, Consultant Obstetrician and Gynaecologist, Bradford Teaching Hospitals NHS Foundation Trust

Janet Brennand MD FRCOG, Consultant in Maternal and Fetal Medicine, Queen Elizabeth University Hospital, Glasgow

Rosamunde Burns MBChB FRCA, Consultant Anaesthetist, Royal Infirmary of Edinburgh; Honorary Senior Lecturer, University of Edinburgh

Malcolm Cameron MBChB MRCPsych, Consultant Liaison Psychiatrist, Crosshouse Hospital, NHS Ayrshire and Arran

Alastair Campbell BSc(Hons) MBChB FRCOG, Consultant Obstetrician and Gynaecologist, Royal Infirmary of Edinburgh; Associate Postgraduate Dean (Quality), NHS Education for Scotland

Janie Collie MB ChB FRCA, Consultant Anaesthetist, Assistant Director of Medical Education, University Hospital Crosshouse, Kilmarnock

Christina Cotzias MRCOG, Consultant Obstetrician and Gynaecologist, Chelsea and Westminster NHS Foundation Trust, West Middlesex Site

Kara Dent MBBS, FRCOG, Consultant in Fetal Maternal Medicine, University Hospitals of Derby and Burton Foundation Trust

R. John Elton FRCA, Consultant Obstetric Anaesthetist, University Hospitals of Coventry and Warwickshire NHS Trust, Coventry

Peter-Marc Fortune FRCPCH FFICM, Consultant Paediatric Intensivist, Associate Medical Director, Royal Manchester Children's Hospital

Kyle Gibson MRCP FRCA FFICM, Specialty Trainee in Anaesthesia and Intensive Care Medicine, South East Scotland

Simon Grant DM FRCOG Consultant in Obstetrics and Fetal Medicine, North Bristol NHS Trust

Deborah Harrington FRCOG, Consultant in Maternal and Fetal Medicine, Deputy Director of Medical Education, Oxford University Hospitals NHS Foundation Trust; Head of School of Obstetrics and Gynaecology, Health Education England working across the Thames Valley

Brigid Hayden FRCOG PGCTLCC DMCC, Consultant Obstetrician and Gynaecologist, Labour Ward Lead, Princess Elizabeth Hospital and Medical Specialist Group, Guernsey

Bernhard Heidemann FRCA FFPMRCA, Consultant in Anaesthesia, Royal Infirmary of Edinburgh; Honorary Clinical Senior Lecturer, University of Edinburgh

Mark Hellaby MSc MEd PG Cert BSc(Hons) RODP FHEA, North West Simulation Education Network Manager, NHS Health Education England

Kim Hinshaw FRCOG, Consultant Obstetrician and Gynaecologist, Sunderland Royal Hospital, South Tyneside and Sunderland NHS Foundation Trust; Visiting Professor, University of Sunderland

Anjoke Huisjes Senior Consultant in Obstetrics and Gynaecology, Gelre ziekenhuizen, Apeldoorn, The Netherlands

Audrey Jeffrey FRCA, Consultant Anaesthetist, St John's Hospital, Livingston

Dean Kerslake FRCP FRCEM EDIC FFICM, Consultant in Emergency Medicine and Critical Care, Clinical Director for Major Trauma, Royal Infirmary of Edinburgh

Marian Knight	MA MBChB MPH DPhil FFPH FRCPE FRCOG, Professor of Maternal and Child Population Health, National Perinatal Epidemiology Unit (NPEU), Nuffield Department of Population Health, University of Oxford
Alison Lansbury	FRCA, Consultant Anaesthetist, Leeds General Infirmary
Douglas Mein	FRCA FANZCA, Consultant Anaesthetist, Wellington Regional Hospital, New Zealand
Judith Orme	MBChB MRCPCH, Consultant in Neonatal Medicine, NHS Lothian University Hospitals Division
Sara Paterson-Brown	FRCS FRCOG, Recently retired Obstetric Consultant, Queen Charlotte's Hospital, Imperial College NHS Trust, London
Felicity Plaat	BA MBBS FRCA, Consultant Anaesthetist, Queen Charlotte's and Hammersmith Hospitals, Imperial College Healthcare NHS Trust, London
Farah Sethna	BSc(Hons) MBBS MRCOG FRANZCOG, Consultant in Obstetrics and Maternal and Fetal Medicine, Centenary Hospital for Women and Children, Canberra, Australia
Gemma Sullivan	MBChB MRCPCH PhD, Clinical Senior Lecturer, University of Edinburgh; Honorary Consultant in Neonatal Medicine, Royal Infirmary of Edinburgh
Kate Theodosiou	MBChB FRCA, Consultant Anaesthetist and Airway Lead, Royal Infirmary of Edinburgh
Gill Tierney	FRCS DM, Consultant Colorectal Surgeon, University Hospitals of Derby and Burton Foundation Trust; Vice-President of the Association of Surgeons of Great Britain and Ireland
Thierry van Dessel	MD PhD, Consultant Obstetrics and Gynaecology, Elisabeth TweeSteden Hospital, Tilburg, The Netherlands
Darren Walter	MPH FRCS FRCEM FIMC FAEMS, Senior Lecturer in Emergency Global Health, University of Manchester; Honorary Consultant in Emergency Medicine, Manchester University NHS Foundation Trust
Arlene Wise	BSc (Hons) MBChB FRCA, Consultant Anaesthetist, Royal Infirmary of Edinburgh, NHS Lothian
Patrick H. Gibson	BMBCh MD FRCP, Consultant Cardiologist, Western General Hospital and Royal Infirmary of Edinburgh
Jennifer Service	MBChB FRCA FFICM, Consultant in Anaesthesia and Critical Care, NHS Lothian
Sarah L. Stobbs	BSc (hons), MBChB, MRCP, RCOA, Anaesthesia registrar, Royal Infirmary Edinburgh

Working group for third edition

Virginia Beckett

Alastair Campbell

Charles Cox

Johan Creemers

Kara Dent

R. John Elton

Diana Fothergill

Simon Grant

Brigid Hayden

Kim Hinshaw

Charlotte Howell

Shirin Irani

Geraldine Masson

Douglas Mein

Sara Paterson-Brown

Felicity Plaat

Bheemasenachar Prasad

Rahul Sen

Paul Sharpe

Contributors to previous editions

Contributors to third edition

Charles Cox	Consultant Obstetrician and Gynaecologist, Wolverhampton
Johan Creemers	Consultant Obstetrician and Gynaecologist, The Netherlands
James Drife	Professor of Obstetrics and Gynaecology, Leeds
R. John Elton	Consultant Anaesthetist, Coventry
Peter-Marc Fortune	Paediatric Intensive Care, Manchester
Diana Fothergill	Consultant Obstetrician and Gynaecologist, Sheffield
Simon Grant	Consultant Obstetrician and Gynaecologist, Bristol
Brigid Hayden	Consultant Obstetrician and Gynaecologist, Bolton
Carol Henshaw	Consultant in Perinatal Mental Health, Liverpool
Kim Hinshaw	Consultant Obstetrician and Gynaecologist, Sunderland
Charlotte Howell	Consultant Anaesthetist, Stoke-on-Trent
Shirin Irani	Consultant Obstetrician and Gynaecologist, Birmingham
Geraldine Masson	Consultant Obstetrician and Gynaecologist, Stoke-on-Trent
Douglas Mein	Consultant Anaesthetist, New Zealand
Jane Mooney	Medical Editor, ALSG, Manchester
Fidelma O'Mahoney	Consultant Obstetrician and Gynaecologist, Stoke-on-Trent
Sara Paterson-Brown	Consultant Obstetrician and Gynaecologist, London
Simon Paterson-Brown	Consultant General Surgeon, Edinburgh
Barbara Phillips	Medical Editor, ALSG, Manchester
Felicity Plaat	Consultant Anaesthetist, London
Bheemasenachar Prasad	Consultant Anaesthetist, Perth, Australia
Rahul Sen	Consultant Obstetrician and Gynaecologist, Australia
Paul Sharpe	Consultant Anaesthetist, Leicester
Abdul Sultan	Consultant Obstetrician and Gynaecologist, Croydon
Ranee Thaker	Consultant Obstetrician and Gynaecologist, Croydon
Derek Tuffnell	Consultant Obstetrician and Gynaecologist, Bradford
Sarah Vause	Consultant Obstetrician and Gynaecologist, Manchester
J. Wardrope	Consultant in Emergency Medicine, Sheffield
Sue Wieteska	CEO, ALSG, Manchester
Jonathan Wyllie	Consultant Neonatologist, Middlesbrough

Additional contributors to second edition

Kavita Goswami	Consultant Obstetrician and Gynaecologist, Coventry
Kate Grady	Consultant Anaesthetist, Manchester
Elaine Metcalfe	ALSG, Manchester
Margaret Oates	Consultant Perinatal Psychiatrist, Nottingham
Poonam Pradhan	Consultant Obstetrician and Gynaecologist, Birmingham
Abdul Sultan	Consultant Obstetrician and Gynaecologist, Croydon
Gargeswari Sunanda	Consultant Obstetrician and Gynaecologist, Birmingham
Ranee Thaker	Consultant Obstetrician and Gynaecologist, Croydon
Steve Walkinshaw	Consultant in Fetomaternal Medicine, Liverpool
Catherine Wykes	Consultant Obstetrician and Gynaecologist, Brighton

Additional contributors to first edition

The late Professor Richard Johanson

Nick Coleman	Consultant Anaesthetist, Stoke-on-Trent
David Griffiths	Consultant Obstetrician and Gynaecologist, Swindon
Mona Khadra	Specialist Registrar in Obstetrics, John Radcliffe Hospital, Oxford
Harmini Sidhu	Consultant Obstetrician and Gynaecologist, Craigavon
Peter Young	Consultant Obstetrician and Gynaecologist, Stoke-on-Trent

Foreword to fourth edition

There are few, if any, such polarised areas of clinical practice as obstetrics. The contrast between the magical beauty of normal pregnancy and childbirth and the often very rapidly progressive and terrifying emergency situation is extreme.

Being prepared for any eventuality is therefore the cornerstone of safe obstetric practice, and while this anticipation can help avoid a situation altogether, it can also enhance the likelihood of early recognition and damage limitation. In those absolutely unavoidable emergencies being well informed, prepared and practised can make the difference between life and death, or health and disability: this is reason enough for clinicians to go to every length to keep themselves informed, alert and vigilant.

This manual is a goldmine of information concerning the pathophysiology and management of emergencies concerning the pregnant (or recently pregnant) woman. It is practical, with useful tips and algorithms, as well as giving depth of knowledge with logical explanations to aid understanding. Whilst it forms part of the mMOET pre-course reading it also stands alone as an excellent text for all clinicians practicing in this specialty.

Don't be unprepared: read, learn, practice and teach what is here, expect the unexpected, and you will keep women and their babies safe.

Sara Paterson-Brown FRCS FRCOG

Preface to fourth edition

We have the honour of participating in the miracle of birth and sharing the experiences of families worldwide, but with that honour comes the responsibility of keeping our women and babies safe.

MOET was the brainchild of passionate Obstetricians and Anaesthetists who recognised that, whilst our specialty is very rewarding, it carries high risk for some of our women. By training and studying together, we can improve our practice and their outcomes. Since 1997, through MOET, we have trained over 8380 clinicians and we have around 720 instructors. We have shared our approach worldwide by taking the course overseas to Liberia, Switzerland, Australia, the Netherlands and Iran, to name but a few.

Over the last 24 years, the course has naturally evolved, as has our specialty. In recognition of this, acknowledging the recent national changes in trauma management, as well as the increasing number of medical complexities that we are all seeing in our local units, MOET wanted to change too. By developing the trauma aspect and maternal medicine content, we hope to improve care delivered by Obstetricians and Anaesthetists working on the front line with our Midwifery colleagues.

Teaching around pre-eclampsia and haemorrhage has been prioritised over the last few decades and maternal death from these causes has fallen accordingly. Now we need to address the new medical complications and emergencies that we are all experiencing in our day-to-day working lives. Recent MBRRACE-UK reports reveal that cardiac disease, thromboembolism and neurological disease are now the three leading causes of maternal deaths. Subsequently, MOET became mMOET to acknowledge that we are 'Managing Medical and Obstetric Emergencies and Trauma' and to address these challenges.

We have worked with our colleagues in the emergency services and thoroughly rejuvenated the trauma content of the course. Being called to your ED in the middle of the night to a pregnant trauma victim can be daunting. We hope that this manual will help prepare you, to understand what your role is within the attending Trauma team and give you the confidence to acknowledge how you can contribute to the vital emergency care that the patient requires with your very specialised knowledge. If we can help give you the tools needed to address the next emergency you have to tackle, then we will have achieved what we set out to do.

To all the current and future generations of Obstetricians and Anaesthetists, we hope this manual and the mMOET course will inspire you to keep learning, to do your very best in some of the most difficult situations and to give our women and their babies the highest quality of care.

Kara Dent and Rosamunde Burns
May 2022

Acknowledgements

A great many people have put a lot of hard work into the production of this book and the accompanying course. The editors would like to thank all the contributors for their efforts and all the mMOET providers and instructors who took the time to send their comments during the development of the text and the course.

Some of the material used in this text is from other Advanced Life Support Group (ALSG) publications, in particular from the books *Advanced Paediatric Life Support: The Practical Approach*, *Neonatal, Adult and Paediatric Safe Transfer and Retrieval: The Practical Approach* and *Major Incident Medical Management and Support: The Practical Approach in the Hospital*.

The chapters on resuscitation have been informed by the new international guidelines produced by an evidence-based process from the collaboration of many international experts under the umbrella of the International Liaison Committee on Resuscitation (ILCOR, 2020).

We would also like to thank members of our mMOET Trauma Review Group for all of their work in reviewing and updating the trauma section:

Rosamunde Burns	MBChB FRCA, Consultant Anaesthetist, Royal Infirmary of Edinburgh; Honorary Senior Lecturer, University of Edinburgh
R. John Elton	FRCA Consultant Obstetric Anaesthetist, University Hospitals of Coventry and Warwickshire NHS Trust, Coventry
Kyle Gibson	MRCP FRCA FFICM, Specialty Trainee in Anaesthesia and Intensive Care Medicine, South East Scotland
Brigid Hayden	FRCOG, PGCTLCC, DMCC Consultant Obstetrician and Gynaecologist, Labour Ward Lead, Princess Elizabeth Hospital and Medical Specialist Group, Guernsey
Audrey Jeffrey	FRCA Consultant Anaesthetist, St John's Hospital, Livingston
Dean Kerslake	FRCP FRCEM EDIC FFICM, Consultant in Emergency Medicine and Critical Care. Clinical Director for Major Trauma, Royal Infirmary of Edinburgh
Darren Walter	MPH FRCS FRCEM FIMC FAEMS Senior Lecturer in Emergency Global Health, University of Manchester, Honorary Consultant in Emergency Medicine, Manchester University NHS Foundation Trust
Arlene Wise	FRCA Anaesthetic Consultant, NHS Lothian

We would like to thank Catherine Giaquinto for the algorithm design, and Helen Carruthers and Kate Wieteska for their work on many of the line drawings within the text. We would also like to thank the following organisations for the shared use of their figures, tables and algorithms:

Alma Medical
American Journal of Obstetrics and Gynecology
Arrow
Association of Anaesthetists
COBIS
Difficult Airway Society (DAS)
Freelance Surgical
MBRRACE-UK
Northern Neonatal Network
Obstetric Anaesthetists' Association (OAA)
Omega Healthcare
Resuscitation Council UK
Royal College of Physicians
Scottish Patient Safety Programme Maternity and Children Quality Improvement Programme
The American Civil Defense Association (TACDA)
VBM
Victoria Health
Wiley
World Health Organization

We also thank the BMJ for the Trauma Timeline, Laura May for the TRAUMATIC mnemonic, Tim Nutbeam and Ron Daniels on behalf of the UK Sepsis Trust, and Gareth Owens on behalf of the 'Think Aorta' Campaign for kindly sharing their resources.

We would like to thank, in advance, those of you who will attend the Managing Medical Obstetric Emergencies and Trauma (mMOET) course and others using this text for your continued constructive comments regarding the future development of both the course and the manual.

Contact details and further information

ALSG: www.alsg.org

For details on ALSG courses visit the website or contact:

Advanced Life Support Group
ALSG Centre for Training and Development
29–31 Ellesmere Street
Swinton, Manchester
M27 0LA
Tel: +44 (0) 161 794 1999
Fax: +44 (0) 161 794 9111
Email: enquiries@alsg.org

Updates

The material contained within this book is updated on approximately a 4-yearly cycle. However, practice may change in the interim period. We will post any changes on the ALSG website, so we advise you to visit the website regularly to check for updates (www.alsg.org).

References

To access references visit the ALSG website www.alsg.org – references are on the course pages.

On-line feedback

It is important to ALSG that the contact with our providers continues after a course is completed. We now contact everyone 6 months after his or her course has taken place asking for on-line feedback on the course. This information is then used whenever the course is updated to ensure that the course provides optimum training to its participants.

How to use your textbook

The anytime, anywhere textbook

Wiley E-Text

Your textbook comes with free access to a **Wiley E-Text: Powered by VitalSource** version – a digital, interactive version of this textbook which you own as soon as you download it.

Your **Wiley E-Text** allows you to:

Search: Save time by finding terms and topics instantly in your book, your notes, even your whole library (once you've downloaded more textbooks)
Note and Highlight: Colour code, highlight and make digital notes right in the text so you can find them quickly and easily
Organise: Keep books, notes and class materials organised in folders inside the application
Share: Exchange notes and highlights with friends, classmates and study groups
Upgrade: Your textbook can be transferred when you need to change or upgrade computers
Link: Link directly from the page of your interactive textbook to all of the material contained on the companion website

The **Wiley E-Text** version will also allow you to copy and paste any photograph or illustration into assignments, presentations and your own notes.

To access your Wiley E-Text:

- Visit http://support.wiley.com to request a redemption code via the 'Contact Support' or 'Chat with an Expert' buttons (with proof of purchase).
- Go to https://online.vitalsource.co.uk and log in or create an account. Go to Redeem and enter your redemption code to add this book to your library.
- Or to download the Bookshelf application to your computer, tablet or mobile device go to www.vitalsource.com/ software/bookshelf/downloads.
- Open the Bookshelf application on your computer and register for an account.
- Follow the registration process and enter your redemption code to download your digital book.

The VitalSource Bookshelf can now be used to view your Wiley E-Text on iOS, Android and Kindle Fire!

- **For iOS:** Visit the app store to download the VitalSource Bookshelf: http://bit.ly/17ib3XS
- **For Android and Kindle Fire:** Visit the Google Play Market to download the VitalSource Bookshelf: http://bit.ly/BSAAGP

You can now sign in with the email address and password you used when you created your VitalSource Bookshelf Account. Full E-Text support for mobile devices is available at: http://support.vitalsource.com

We hope you enjoy using your new textbook. Good luck with your studies!

Abbreviations

95%CI	95% confidence interval
AAGA	accidental awareness during general anaesthesia
ABG	arterial blood gases
ACS	acute coronary syndrome
ACVPU	alert, new confusion, responds to voice, responds to pain, unconscious
AED	automated external defibrillator
AFE	amniotic fluid embolism
AIP	abnormally invasive placenta
ALSG	Advanced Life Support Group
ALSO	Advanced Life Support in Obstetrics
ALT	alanine aminotransferase
ARDS	acute respiratory distress syndrome
AST	aspartate aminotransferase
ATLS	Advanced Trauma Life Support
BMI	body mass index
BP	blood pressure
BSOTS	Birmingham Symptom-specific Obstetric Triage System
CEMACH	Confidential Enquiry into Maternal and Child Health
CEMD	Confidential Enquiry into Maternal Deaths
CESDI	Confidential Enquiry into Stillbirths and Deaths in Infancy
CGM	continuous glucose monitoring
CJD	Creutzfeldt–Jakob disease
CMACE	Centre for Maternal and Child Enquiries
CMDh	Coordination Group for Mutual and Decentralised Procedures – human
CNS	central nervous system
CO_2	carbon dioxide
CPAP	continuous positive airway pressure
CPD	cephalopelvic disproportion
CPR	cardiopulmonary resuscitation
CRP	C-reactive protein
CRT	capillary refill time
CS	caesarean section
CSE	combined spinal and epidural
CSF	cerebrospinal fluid
CT	computed tomography

CTG	cardiotocography
CTPA	computed tomography pulmonary angiography
CVP	central venous pressure
CVT	cerebral venous thrombosis
CXR	chest x-ray
DAS	Difficult Airway Society
DKA	diabetic ketoacidosis
DVT	deep vein thrombosis
EAS	external anal sphincter
ECG	electrocardiogram
ECMO	extracorporeal membrane oxygenation
ECV	external cephalic version
ED	emergency department
eFAST	extended focused assessment with sonography for trauma
ERCP	endoscopic retrograde cholangiopancreatography
FAST	focused assessment with sonography for trauma
FFP	fresh frozen plasma
FRC	functional residual capacity
GCS	Glasgow Coma Scale
GIC	Generic Instructor Course
GMC	General Medical Council
GP	general practioner
GTN	glyceryl trinitrate
hCG	human chorionic gonadotrophin
HDU	high dependency unit
HELLP	haemolysis, elevated liver enzymes, low platelet count (syndrome)
HIE	hypoxic ischaemic encephalopathy
IAS	internal anal sphincter
ICP	intracranial cerebrospinal pressure
IgE	immunoglobulin E
ILCOR	International Liaison Committee on Resuscitation
IO	intraosseous
ITU	intensive treatment unit
IV	intravenous
LDF	leucocyte depletion filter
LMA	laryngeal mask airway
LMWH	low molecular weight heparin
MBRRACE-UK	Mothers and Babies: Reducing Risk through Audits and Confidential Enquiries across the UK
MEOWS	modified early obstetric warning score
MEWS	maternity early warning scoring systems
MHRA	Medicines and Healthcare products Regulatory Agency
MIMMS	Major Incident Medical Management and Support
mMOET	Managing Medical and Obstetric Emergencies and Trauma
MMR	maternal mortality rate
MOH	major obstetric haemorrhage

MRI	magnetic resonance imaging
mRNA	messenger RNA
MRV	magnetic resonance venography
MSV	Mauriceau–Smellie–Veit
MTS	Manchester Triage System
MUD	manual uterine displacement
NACCS	Neuro Anaesthesia and Critical Care Society
NAP	National Audit Project
NAPSTaR	Neonatal, Adult and Paediatric Safe Transfer and Retrieval
NICE	National Institute for Health and Care Excellence
NICU	neonatal intensive care unit
NLS	newborn life support
NNT	number needed to treat
OAA	Obstetric Anaesthetists' Association
OASI	obstetric anal sphincter injury
ONS	Office for National Statistics
OR	odds ratio
OVD	operative vaginal delivery
PAST	posterior axillary sling traction
PCI	percutaneous coronary intervention
PDPH	postdural puncture headache
PDS	polydioxanone
PEA	pulseless electrical activity
PEEP	positive end-expiratory pressure
PEFR	peak expiratory flow rate
PET	pre-eclampsia toxaemia
PMCS	perimortem caesarean section
PND	postnatal depression
POCUS	point of care ultrasound
PPH	postpartum haemorrhage
PRES	posterior reversible encephalopathy syndrome
qSOFA	quick sequential organ failure assessment
RCoA	Royal College of Anaesthetists
RCOG	Royal College of Obstetricians and Gynaecologists
RCT	randomised controlled trial
RCVS	reversible cerebral vasoconstriction syndrome
Rh	rhesus
ROSC	return of spontaneous circulation
ROTEM®	rotational thromboelastometry
RR	respiratory rate
RR	risk ratio
SAD	supraglottic airway device
SAG-M	saline-adenine-glucose-mannitol
SALVO	Cell Salvage in Obstetrics (trial)
SAP	systolic arterial pressure

SBAR	situation, background, assessment and recommendation
SCAD	spontaneous coronary artery dissection
SHO	senior house officer
SSRI	selective serotonin reuptake inhibitor
STEMI	ST segment elevation myocardial infarction
SUDEP	sudden unexpected death in epilepsy
SVT	supraventricular tachycardia
tds	*ter die sumendum* (three times a day)
TEG®	thromboelastography
TFT	thyroid function test
TIVA	total intravenous anaesthesia
U&Es	urea and electrolytes
UK	United Kingdom
UKOSS	UK Obstetric Surveillance System
USA	United States of America
VAD	ventricular assist device
VF	ventricular fibrillation
V/Q	ventilation/perfusion
VT	ventricular tachycardia
VTE	venous thromboembolism
WHO	World Health Organization

PART 1

Introduction

CHAPTER 1
Introduction

Throughout both the developed and the developing world, maternal mortality continues to present a serious challenge. Globally, there is estimated to be one maternal death every minute. This course will provide you with a system for managing the seriously ill and seriously injured pregnant woman. The system is designed to be simple and easy to remember when life-threatening emergencies arise and is known as the structured approach.

The structured approach is based on the ABC of resuscitation and is practised throughout all areas of medicine and the emergency services. The concept is familiar to the lay person and known even to school children. This structured approach has led to the development of courses that attend to the resuscitation needs of all patients, from neonates to children, adults and women with the altered physiology and anatomy of pregnancy.

This manual, *Managing Medical and Obstetric Emergencies and Trauma* (mMOET), online material and the practical course are divided into sections that provide a structured revision in recognition, resuscitation and treatment of emergencies in pregnancy. This includes trauma, medical and surgical emergencies and obstetric emergencies and is aimed at obstetricians, anaesthetists, emergency and other physicians, and midwives. The structured approach is applied to resuscitation and is taught didactically as a drill. Subsequently, what has been learned is applied to both the recognition and management of the seriously ill and injured pregnant patient.

The physiological adjustments of pregnancy affect the response of the mother to illness and injury. These changes mean that resuscitation should be tailored to the pregnant patient and this manual, and the mMOET course, teaches how this is achieved.

The Managing Obstetric Emergencies and Trauma (MOET) course began in 2001 and runs under the auspices of the Advanced Life Support Group (ALSG). Its aim is to provide the knowledge, practical skills and procedures necessary to save the mother and fetus in life-threatening circumstances. The course runs in six countries and, since its inception, over 8380 providers and 720 instructors have been trained. Course information and links for candidates and faculty are available from the ALSG website (www.alsg.org).

Recent catastrophic traumatic events including terrorist attacks and major fires have heightened awareness of the need for expanding trauma education amongst the obstetric community. To date trauma management has not been widely taught to obstetricians, but when trauma does occur to pregnant women those in other specialties will consider the obstetrician the expert when managing them.

The importance of serious medical co-morbidities within the pregnant population contributing to maternal death and the need for early recognition of the seriously ill pregnant woman has been emphasised in confidential mortality reports,

Managing Medical and Obstetric Emergencies and Trauma: A Practical Approach, Fourth Edition. Edited by Rosamunde Burns and Kara Dent.

and this has resulted in a particular new focus for MOET teaching: we now call the course mMOET – managing Medical and Obstetric Emergencies and Trauma to reflect this.

This text is essential pre-course reading for the mMOET course and also provides a valuable reference for all healthcare workers involved in caring for pregnant women.

In more recent years, and in acknowledgement of the challenging study leave climate in the UK, a pre-course online learning component (Box 1.1) was devised, piloted and widely introduced to supplement the manual and the face-to-face material (www.alsg.org/vle). This continues to be updated and aims to reinforce the current text and provides an interactive method of delivering the knowledge components of the course. It prepares participants for the practical application of knowledge during the face-to-face course.

Box 1.1 Content of the mMOET online learning package

Structured approach
CPR, resuscitation and perimortem CS
Airway management and breathing
Trauma
Massive obstetric haemorrhage
Complications of delivery
Hypertensive disease of pregnancy
Neurological emergencies
Diabetic emergencies
Cardiac emergencies
Sepsis
Neonatal resuscitation
Local anaesthesia
Postnatal depression and vulnerabilities
Human factors

The face-to-face course offers participants the opportunity to further reinforce their pre-course learning and also to have hands-on practise of essential skills. Lectures, interactive sessions, demonstrations and workshops explore a variety of emergencies including obstetric and trauma, but increasingly focus on the acute medical emergencies identified as the leading causes of deaths of pregnant women in the confidential mortality reports by MBRRACE-UK (Mothers and Babies: Reducing Risk through Audit and Confidential Enquiries across the UK; previously Centre for Maternal and Child Enquiries (CMACE) or Confidential Enquiries into Maternal Deaths (CEMD)). Simulations, discussions and skills practise allow candidates to put knowledge and skills together and to practise and learn within a safe environment. In this, they are supported with structured debriefing by instructors and their fellow candidates. Continuous assessment indicates those candidates that have achieved the required standard to be a 'mMOET provider', a status which lasts for 4 years.

Those candidates who demonstrate the potential to be an instructor are invited to undertake a structured training programme. The Generic Instructor Course (GIC) prepares instructors to deliver lectures, skills teaching, small group discussions, simulations and also to carry out assessments. This is reinforced with support and assessment by experienced instructors when new instructors teach on mMOET courses on the first two occasions. Instructors then teach on three courses over each 2-year period to maintain their status.

As priorities for training change, the mMOET course is continually improved following feedback from course directors, instructors and candidates and from important trend information from major reports, for example MBRRACE and UK Obstetric Surveillance System (UKOSS). This ensures that it remains fit for purpose and focuses on the current leading causes of maternal mortality and morbidity.

CHAPTER 2
Saving mothers' lives: lessons from the Confidential Enquiries

2.1 Introduction

Much of the wisdom in this book has been learned the hard way, some of it in the hardest way of all. When a woman dies as a result of an obstetric complication, the only good thing that can come out of the tragedy is that appropriate lessons are learned. For over 60 years, England and Wales have had a system in place to analyse all maternal deaths, identify the causes and highlight avoidable factors, and over time this system has been expanded to include Scotland and Ireland.

The Confidential Enquiries into Maternal Deaths (CEMDs) have become so familiar to UK obstetricians and midwives that we can hardly imagine life without them. The UK, however, is one of only a few countries with a national system in which experienced clinicians scrutinise cases in detail to work out whether death could be prevented when a similar emergency happens again and, if so, how.

CEMD recommendations carry considerable weight at both political and clinical levels. This chapter will describe the system that produces these recommendations and will then focus on lessons relevant to emergencies and trauma – including those learned in the early years of the programme, which are all too easily forgotten.

2.2 How the enquiries work

England and Wales began collecting confidential data from maternal deaths in 1952 and published reports every 3 years from 1957 until 2008. Similar enquiries began in Northern Ireland in 1956 and in Scotland in 1965. Since 1985, the Confidential Enquiries covered the whole of the UK and, in 2003, it became part of the Confidential Enquiry into Maternal and Child Health (CEMACH), subsequently the Centre for Maternal and Child Enquiries (CMACE), and since 2012 (analysing deaths from 2009 onwards) it is part of the programme of MBRRACE-UK (Mothers and Babies: Reducing Risk through Audit and Confidential Enquiries across the UK), a collaboration based in the National Perinatal Epidemiology Unit in Oxford. Cases from the Republic of Ireland are now included as well.

From the outset, confidentiality was recognised to be essential if staff were to give an honest account of events without fear of litigation or disciplinary action. In this, and in other essentials, the approach initiated in the 1950s is still used today. The process summarised here applies to England, but is similar in the other UK countries.

Reporting

When a maternal death occurs, a form is sent to all the lead professionals involved to obtain anonymous factual information and reflective comments. The forms, along with a copy of the woman's medical records, are returned to the MBRRACE-UK office.

Managing Medical and Obstetric Emergencies and Trauma: A Practical Approach, Fourth Edition. Edited by Rosamunde Burns and Kara Dent.

Expert assessment

To ensure confidentiality, the information is kept under lock and key before digitising and storage on a secure server. All records are anonymised and reviewed by expert assessors, who are senior clinicians in obstetrics, midwifery, anaesthetics, pathology, perinatal psychiatry, medicine, cardiology, neurology, infectious diseases, emergency medicine, general practice and intensive care. They look for emerging patterns and lessons for clinical colleagues, managers and politicians. Public health messages are particularly important and denominator data are obtained from the Office for National Statistics (ONS) or equivalents in the devolved nations and Republic of Ireland.

Reports

A report is now published every year, which includes surveillance information as well as topic-specific chapters, each of which appears on a triennial basis. Chapters are drafted by a writing committee including expert assessors from the four UK countries and Republic of Ireland and other relevant experts in the topic area, and discussed by the whole editorial panel, which includes epidemiologists. Once the final report is sent to the printers, any information linked to the identity of the women concerned is destroyed. The published report is available to the public, a fact that surprises doctors in countries that have a less open approach.

A challenge for any report is to ensure that people read it. Recent confidential reports have been entitled *Saving Mothers' Lives, Improving Mothers' Care* (and before that *Why Mothers Die* with an emotive cover picture) and launched with a conference. They were bestsellers in the Royal College of Obstetricians and Gynaecologists (RCOG) bookshop, partly because examination candidates knew that they were essential reading. Reports are now available free to download from the MBRRACE-UK website, allowing for wider circulation; the link to the report is distributed through professional and voluntary organisations and the media on the day it is released. The report messages, however, increasingly need to be heard by other specialties and this is more difficult to achieve.

2.3 Lessons from the past

Effective intervention

Before the CEMDs started, maternal mortality had already dropped dramatically in the UK, from 400/100 000 in 1935 to 66/100 000 in 1952–1954 (in fact at this stage there were still problems with case ascertainment and a more realistic estimate was 90/100 000). The most rapid fall had occurred during the Second World War, contradicting the idea that social conditions are the major factor determining the safety of pregnancy. The reasons for the fall were the introduction of effective treatments as follows:

- Antibiotics: puerperal sepsis was the leading cause of maternal death in the 1930s, despite the widespread use of aseptic precautions; when sulphonamides were introduced in 1937 the effect on death rates was spectacular
- Blood transfusion became safe during the 1940s
- Ergometrine, for the treatment and prevention of postpartum haemorrhage, was introduced in the 1940s

In the 1930s, Britain had a well-developed medical infrastructure, so that when effective treatments finally became available their effects were rapidly felt.

Obstetric injury

In the first CEMD report, covering 1952–1954, obstetric injury was the second most common cause of death after hypertensive disease (Table 2.1). It did not, however, warrant its own chapter and Table 2.1 is drawn from the appendix to that report.

Table 2.1 Number of maternal deaths from obstetric injury, 1952–1954

Cause	Deaths (*n*)
Prolonged labour	63
Disproportion or malposition of the fetus	23
Other trauma	55
Other complications of childbirth	66
Total	207

Nowadays, we can hardly imagine a woman dying of prolonged labour and we can only guess at what the terms 'other trauma' and 'other complications' conceal (Table 2.1). In the 1950s, the caesarean section (CS) rate was less than 3% and maternity care was quite different from that of today. The 1955–1957 report included 33 women who died from a ruptured uterus, mostly due to intrauterine manipulations. In 1958–1960, there were 43 women who died from obstructed labour, of whom, according to the report for that triennium, 18 gave birth at home and 14 in a general practitioner maternity home. These reports are a useful corrective to the idea that the 1950s were a golden age of non-medicalised childbirth.

2.4 Recent lessons

Obstetric injury today

In 2006–2008 there were, for the first time, no deaths from genital tract trauma and the chapter dealing with these cases was discontinued. Nevertheless, the report commented that genital tract tears were implicated in two women who died of postpartum haemorrhage. The risk of trauma has not disappeared and, indeed, high vaginal tears have become more difficult to deal with because of the current prevalence of obesity. The CEMD recommended that a surgeon faced with life-threatening haemorrhage should routinely ask a colleague to come and help. Genital tract trauma is again featuring in maternal deaths and in the first MBRRACE-UK report covering deaths from 2009 to 2012 there were seven deaths due to haemorrhage following genital tract trauma. In 2013–2015 only one woman died from genital tract trauma but in 2016–2018 a further four women died of that cause. However, when the care of a random sample of 34 women who survived a major obstetric haemorrhage (transfusion of 8 or more units) was reviewed in the 2018 report, 11 women were noted to have had a haemorrhage caused by genital tract trauma, emphasising the substantial burden of morbidity that underlies the small number of deaths.

Who is at risk?

The Enquiry identifies groups at increased risk of complications and with increased awareness, death rates have fallen among, for example, those with a history of thromboembolism. Recognition of risk factors early in pregnancy is essential.

Age

Since the 2006–2008 CEMD report, the maternal mortality rate (MMR) has remained fairly constant up to age 34, but it doubles after age 35 and quadruples after 40 years of age. The same pattern is seen in the latest 2016–2018 report. The average age of childbearing in the UK has risen --in 2008 it was 29.3 years with 20% of births being to women aged 35 years or over, while in 2018 it was 30.6 years with 23% to women aged 35 years or over.

Obesity

This problem continues to grow. In the 2016–2018 report, 119 of 196 women who died whose body mass index (BMI) was known (i.e. 61%) were overweight compared with 49% in 2009–2012. Of these overweight women, 57 (29%) had a BMI of 25–29.9 and 62 (32%) were obese (with a BMI >30). This compares with 22% and 27%, respectively, in 2009–2012.

Socioeconomic classification

In 2016–2018, the MMR among women living in the most deprived areas was 15.3 compared with 5.7 for women living in the most affluent areas, a close to threefold difference. Attention should also be focused on women who book late or are poor attenders for antenatal care. In 2016–2018, 22% of women who died booked late, 61% did not receive the recommended level of antenatal care and 27% did not receive the minimum level of antenatal care as defined by National Institute for Health and Care Excellence (NICE) guidance.

Ethnicity

In the 2016–2018 report black women have more than fourfold higher MMRs than white women, a disparity which has been evident for many years and has been worsening more recently. The increase is less among other ethnic groups (Table 2.2), but is also significantly higher in women from Asian and mixed ethnic backgrounds. Women recently arrived from overseas often have communication difficulties and are at particular risk.

Table 2.2 Estimated maternal mortality rates by ethnic group, England 2016–2018

Ethnic group (England only)	Total maternities	Deaths (*n*)	Rate/100 000 (95%CI)	Relative risk (95%CI)
White (inc. not known)	1 486 428	117	7.87 (6.51–9.43)	1 (Ref.)
Asian	191 145	28	14.65 (9.73–21.17)	1.86 (1.19–2.83)
Black	81 704	28	34.27 (22.77–49.53)	4.35 (2.77–6.62)
Chinese/others	75 270	6	7.97 (2.93–17.35)	1.01 (0.36–2.27)
Mixed	31 823	8	25.14 (10.85–49.53)	3.19 (1.35–6.50)

2.5 Direct deaths

Hypertensive disease

The number of deaths from pre-eclampsia is a fraction of what it was in 1952–1954 (Table 2.3) and most recently has fallen dramatically from 19 in 2006–2008 to 10 deaths in 2009–2011, nine deaths in 2010–2012 and then six deaths in 2014–2016. This reduction is largely due to the introduction of guidelines on fluid management and none of the recent deaths have been due to pulmonary or cerebral oedema. However, there is a continuing problem with failure to control systolic hypertension, and preventing intracranial haemorrhage remains a challenge. Among the recent recommendations the following points are emphasised:

- Epigastric pain in the second half of pregnancy should be considered to be the result of pre-eclampsia until proved otherwise
- Keep blood pressure (BP) below 150/100, and very high systolic BP is a medical emergency with urgent treatment needed
- Neuroimaging should be performed if a woman with hypertension or pre-eclampsia has focal neurology, severe or atypical headache or incomplete recovery from a seizure
- Stabilising the mother including controlling her BP is vital prior to intubation
- New-onset hypertension or proteinuria needs prompt referral with clear communication between health professionals

Some of these recommendations are directed at non-obstetricians, and, unfortunately, maternity staff do not always recognise the need for effective control of BP.

Table 2.3 The changes in direct deaths reported to the CEMDs, 1952–2018

Cause	1952–1954 (England+Wales)	2006–2008 (UK)	2009–2011 (UK and Ireland)	2010–2012	2014–2016	2016–2018
Hypertensive disease	246	19	10	9	6	4
Obstetric injury	197	0	7	7	1	4
Haemorrhage	188	8	14	11	17	10
Early pregnancy/abortion	153	0	–	7	3	7
Thromboembolism	138	18	30	26	32	33
Anaesthesia	49	7	3	4	1	1
Genital tract sepsis	42	26	15	12	11*	12*

* Now reported as pregnancy-related sepsis, so now includes urinary tract infections.

Haemorrhage

Over the past 40 years, deaths from haemorrhage have fluctuated (Figure 2.1), which may represent relaxation and tightening of standards. For example, the peak in 1988–1990 included cases where doctors had ignored the recommendation that CS for placenta praevia should be carried out by a consultant.

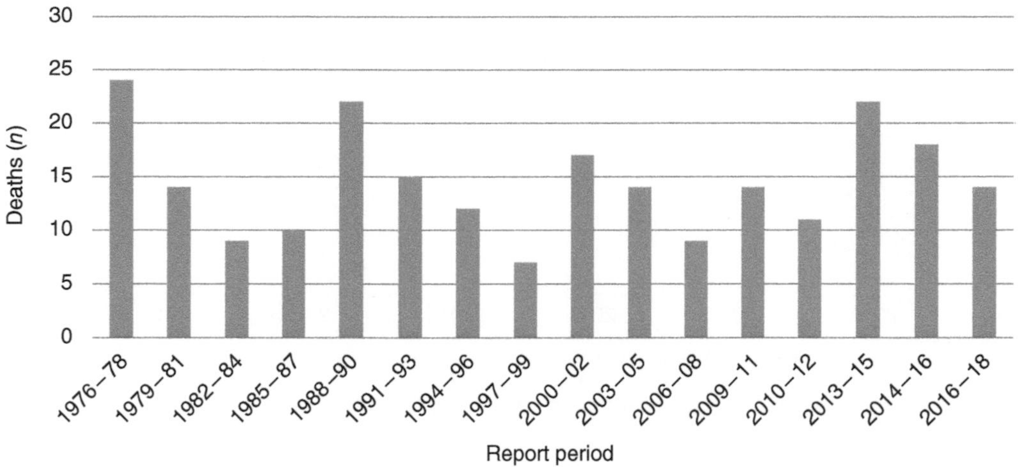

Figure 2.1 Deaths from haemorrhage reported to the CEMDs, 1976–2018

It is important, however, to see these numbers in context. Haemorrhage is by far the most common life-threatening complication of childbirth: surveys of severe morbidity show that haemorrhage of >2.5 litres occurs once in about 300 births. Therefore over a 3-year period with more than 2 million births in the UK, several thousand cases are treated successfully.

In 2016–2018, the total of 14 deaths due to haemorrhage included two cases of uterine atony, three of morbidly adherent placenta, three of abruption, two of uterine inversion and four of genital tract trauma. In 79% of cases there was room for improvements in care, and the main messages focused on:

- Ensuring a senior clinician takes a 'helicopter view' of the management of a woman with major obstetric haemorrhage to coordinate all aspects of care
- Early recognition (especially when haemorrhage is concealed) including awareness of the signs of uterine inversion
- Ensuring that the response to obstetric haemorrhage is tailored to the proportionate blood loss as a percentage of circulating blood volume based on a woman's body weight
- Early correction of coagulopathy
- Progressing to hysterectomy when bleeding is uncontrolled, particularly from a morbidly adherent placenta or uterine rupture

Every triennium, one or more deaths occur in women who refuse blood transfusion and guidelines have been issued about the management of such patients. Placenta praevia associated with a uterine scar is particularly dangerous and all women with a previous CS should have a scan for placental localisation in the second trimester and, if low lying, again at 32 weeks.

Thromboembolism

Thromboembolism has been the leading direct cause of maternal death in the UK since 1985, but while the number of deaths fell dramatically from 41 to 18 between 2003–2005 and 2006–2008, this improvement has not been sustained. In the 1990s, a previous fall occurred after the RCOG published recommendations on thromboprophylaxis at CS. Deaths during pregnancy and after vaginal delivery, however, continued to rise and these were targeted by a further RCOG guideline in 2004. These categories fell sharply in 2006–2008, the first full triennium after the new guideline was published. However deaths from thromboembolism have risen again and in 2016–2018 there were 33 (Figure 2.2).

The most important risk factor for thromboembolism is obesity and the current guidance includes weight-specific dosage advice on thromboprophylaxis. Risk assessment early in pregnancy is the key to reducing mortality further; this message needs to be heard in gynaecology wards and early pregnancy assessment units as well as in maternity units. However, a clear message from the 2020 report is that there remains confusion about risk assessment scores, which are done inaccurately in many of the cases reviewed.

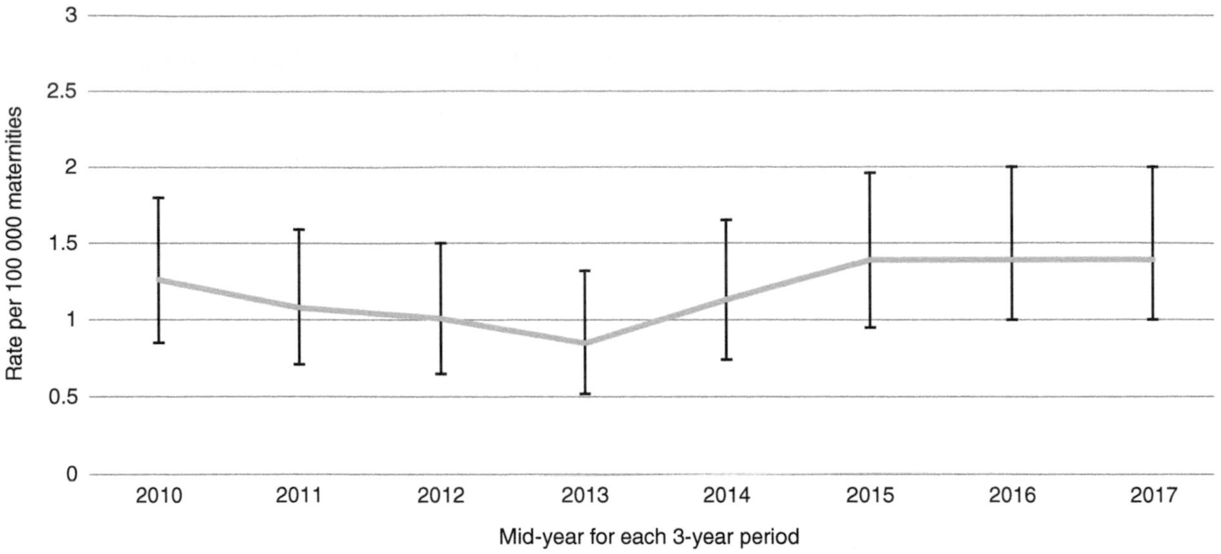

Figure 2.2 Maternal mortality from venous thromboembolism, 3-year rolling rates in the UK, 2010 to 2017

The value of individualised care also needs to be emphasised. The 2006–2008 report stresses that vulnerable women, for example those with a learning disability, may not be able to follow instructions about self-injection and will require particular care.

Chest symptoms (shortness of breath or discomfort/pain), 'panic attacks' or leg pains appearing for the first time in pregnancy or the puerperium need careful assessment, particularly in at-risk women. This lesson needs to get across to other specialties.

Ectopic pregnancy

Deaths from ectopic pregnancies still show no sign of falling. Atypical presentation is common and the CEMD has repeatedly drawn attention to gastrointestinal symptoms that may mimic food poisoning. The 2019 report recommended that all women of reproductive age presenting to an emergency department with collapse, dizziness, abdominal or pelvic pain or gastrointestinal symptoms (including vomiting and diarrhoea) should have a pregnancy test. Women from ethnic minorities are over-represented among deaths from ectopic pregnancy, possibly because of communication difficulties.

Abortion

The Abortion Act of 1967 eliminated deaths from criminal abortion, which in the 1950s caused about 30 deaths a year. In the 2019 report one woman died from complications associated with a self-induced termination of pregnancy. Previous deaths from termination have included women who received high doses of uterotonics in the presence of a CS scar and those who have developed sepsis, and hence prophylactic antibiotics are recommended in RCOG guidelines. Haemorrhage after spontaneous miscarriage has accounted for previous deaths, especially in the mid-trimester, and is associated with a placenta implanted over a CS scar. This again emphasises the importance of placental localisation.

Amniotic fluid embolism

The number of deaths from amniotic fluid embolism has remained constant for 30 years. The condition is not always fatal, and useful information may be gained when the woman survives. All cases, whether fatal or not, should be reported to the UK Obstetric Surveillance System (UKOSS) at the National Perinatal Epidemiology Unit in Oxford.

Most recently the CEMD has highlighted the dangers of hyperstimulation of the uterus as a cause of amniotic fluid embolism and in particular the excessive use of misoprostol for induction with intrauterine deaths. In terms of responding to collapse in the peripartum period (which is how women with this condition present), the take home messages, in addition to rapid response and resuscitation, are of anticipating the massive haemorrhage which will follow and putting out a major obstetric haemorrhage (MOH) call.

Sepsis

In 1982–1984, there were only nine deaths from this cause and none was due to puerperal sepsis. Deaths from sepsis subsequently rose steadily. In 2006–2008 it became the leading direct cause of maternal death with 26 deaths. Thirteen of these were due to the group A beta-haemolytic *Streptococcus* (*S. pyogenes*), compared with four in 2016–2018. Among a total of 10 women who died from genital tract sepsis in 2016–2018, six died after mid-trimester chorioamnionitis from *Escherichia coli*; three of these six women had preterm pre-labour rupture of the membranes. This highlights the high-risk nature of mid-trimester rupture of membranes, and the 2020 report emphasises the importance of early senior involvement in the care of women with extremely preterm pre-labour rupture of membranes and a full explanation of the risks and benefits of continuing the pregnancy.

Sepsis is often insidious in onset and can progress very quickly. If it is suspected, urgent referral to hospital is necessary. In hospital, high-dose broad-spectrum antibiotics should be started immediately, without waiting for the results of investigations. In 2012, in response to the rise in deaths, the RCOG published new guidelines on bacterial sepsis during and after pregnancy.

Sepsis due to respiratory causes remains a leading cause of death during or after pregnancy, as was evident in the 2009 AH1N1 influenza pandemic, and the covid-19 pandemic has highlighted this once again. Over the first wave of the covid-19 pandemic in the UK, 10 women died with SARS-CoV-2 infection, of whom eight died from complications of covid-19. A rapid report from MBRRACE-UK (*Saving Lifes, Improving Mothers' Care Rapid Report: Learning from SARS-CoV-2-related and associated maternal deaths in the UK March–May 2020*) noted that the severity of women's illnesses was often not recognised until they were in extremis, and emphasised the importance of multidisciplinary team care and obstetric leadership with daily review. This is essential in order to ensure timely recognition of deterioration, early assessment of the need for iatrogenic birth to help respiratory function and identification of postnatal complications.

It is also important to remember that deaths from influenza continue to occur despite widespread availability of vaccination. With immunisation rates in pregnancy at less than 50%, influenza remains a threat and influenza swabs should still be taken in women presenting with severe upper respiratory tract infections, with antiviral treatments commenced until results exclude it.

Anaesthesia

Deaths from anaesthesia fell steadily during the 1970s due to a move to regional anaesthesia and better training of anaesthetists. Since 1985, the number has been in single figures in each triennium and in view of the rising CS rate this represents an improvement. Failed tracheal intubation has been highlighted in recent years, together with anaphylaxis and aspiration causing difficult ventilation. The most recent report emphasised the crucial role of the anaesthetist in the resuscitation, management and postoperative care of women who have obstetric haemorrhage. Particular messages included: (i) the importance of ensuring adequate intravenous access to facilitate fluid resuscitation; (ii) the need to use appropriate rapid fluid warming devices during fluid resuscitation and transfusion; and (iii) the importance of ensuring that there is evidence that there has been adequate resuscitation of a woman who has had an obstetric haemorrhage and that the haemorrhage has ceased prior to extubation.

2.6 Indirect deaths

Indirect deaths have outnumbered direct deaths in the UK since 1994–1996 (Table 2.4). In that triennium, birth and death registrations were linked by the ONS, leading to better ascertainment.

Table 2.4 The rise in indirect deaths: maternal deaths notified to the CEMD, 1991–2018

	1991–1993	1994–1996	1997–1999	2000–2002	2003–2005	2006–2008	2009–2011	2010–2012	2016–2018
Direct	129	134	106	106	132	107	83	78	92*
Indirect	100	134	136	155	163	154	170	165	125
Total	229	268	242	261	295	261	253	243	217

* Suicides are included in the classification of direct maternal deaths after a change in World Health Organization guidance.

From 2000–2002 onwards, CEMACH regional managers were involved in collecting data and this improved ascertainment further. Better identification of cases, however, is only one reason for the rise in indirect deaths, the other being a rise in risk factors such as smoking, obesity and older age at childbearing.

Cardiac disease

Deaths from cardiac disease have been rising and this is now the leading cause of maternal death in the UK, with approximately 50 deaths in each triennium. In 2015–2017 only four were due to congenital heart disease. The leading causes were sudden adult death syndrome, myocardial infarction, dissection of the thoracic aorta and myocardial disease (including cardiomyopathies). Only a quarter of women who died from heart disease were known to have cardiac problems prior to pregnancy, and symptoms such as breathlessness were frequently misattributed to pregnancy. A third of the women who died from cardiac disease had a BMI of 30 or more. The main learning point from all these cases was that there must be a low threshold for investigation of pregnant or recently delivered women who complain of chest pain or breathlessness, especially if they have risk factors such as hypertension. Women with cardiac disease should be cared for by obstetricians, cardiologists and obstetric anaesthetists in a coordinated fashion, with combined clinics being the gold standard.

Mental health conditions

Mental health disorders are common in pregnancy and after delivery. However suicide, which causes the most deaths overall, most commonly occurs between 6 weeks and 1 year after delivery and because they occur more than 42 days after delivery are missed by the standard definition of maternal death. Suicide is usually by violent means. Most women who die by suicide have a history of an affective disorder, which has a high risk of recurrence after delivery. Previous psychiatric history must be identified in early pregnancy and the risk managed proactively. Psychiatric deaths were last analysed in the 2018 MBRRACE-UK report. This highlighted the huge variations in provision of mental health services around the UK and Ireland and the importance of 'red flag' symptoms such as new thoughts or acts of violent self-harm.

Other indirect deaths

Of the many other causes of indirect death, the leading category is central nervous system disease, including epilepsy, where women may stop taking their medication when they become pregnant. All medical diseases in pregnancy need careful supervision because of the effects of the disease on the pregnant woman and the effects of the pregnancy on the disease. This responsibility tends to be shared between the GP, midwife, obstetrician and physician, and they often work in isolation without appreciation of the full clinical picture and risks. Good communication among carers is essential, and if it cannot be done in joint clinics, there should at least be telephone discussions with a documented outcome. Communication should not be left to the patient or her handheld notes.

2.7 Coincidental deaths

The most common causes of coincidental death are road traffic accidents and murder. The 2006–2008 report recommended that all pregnant women should be advised to wear a three-point seat belt in a motor vehicle and the 2014–2016 report again recommended that routine enquiry about domestic abuse should be made at booking or during pregnancy. All women should be seen alone at least once in pregnancy. If an injury, like a black eye, is noticed, staff should ask sympathetically – but directly – how it was caused and should be prepared to offer support. All women who were murdered between 2014 and 2016 were murdered by a partner or former partner, and the rapid report into SARS-CoV-2-associated deaths also noted two deaths due to domestic violence. It remains important that women are given the opportunity to disclose domestic abuse, and that they are appropriately referred for support if they do.

2.8 Quality of care

The CEMD assessors try to be realistic when assessing the quality of care, and now focus attention on whether improvements in care could have been expected to affect the outcome, rather than grading care as substandard. The proportion of deaths where improvements in care could reasonably have been expected to affect outcome was 51% in the 2020 report, while 29% were considered to have good care. The main shortcomings remain: lack of clinical knowledge and failure to recognise high-risk clinical signs, and failure to identify very sick women with failure to escalate to senior support or sufficiently rapidly to other specialists.

In recent years, hospitals have undertaken their own investigations of 'serious untoward incidents' and these reports have been made available to the CEMD. The quality of these reports has been highly variable and a previous report commented that some were, 'Not worth the paper they were written on and a few [were] actually whitewashes or cover-ups for unacceptable situations.' Learning lessons from maternal deaths is not easy when they occur in your own hospital. MBRRACE-UK has made specific recommendations about these local reviews since 2015, including the recommendation that there are external panel members to ensure local review is robust and lessons are learned.

2.9 The international dimension

There are over 300 000 maternal deaths annually worldwide, of which 99% are in developing countries. The leading causes are shown in Table 2.5.

Table 2.5 Causes of maternal deaths worldwide

Cause	Percentage (%)
Haemorrhage	27
Sepsis	11
Unsafe abortion	8
Pre-eclampsia/eclampsia	14
Embolism	3
Other direct causes	10
Indirect causes	28

Source: Data from Maternal mortality, 2015, World Health Organization. https://data.unicef.org/topic/maternal-health/maternal-mortality/

The underlying problems include: lack of access to contraception, lack of primary care or transport facilities and inadequate equipment and staffing in district hospitals. The United Nations has made the reduction of maternal mortality one of its Millennium Development Goals. The worldwide proportion of births with a trained attendant has risen to 61%, but much remains to be done.

The UK Confidential Enquiries are globally respected as an example of good practice and several countries – for example South Africa, Moldova and Kazakhstan – have set up their own enquiries adapted from the UK model.

2.10 Summary

The common assumption that safe childbirth is a side effect of national prosperity is wrong: with prosperity we see increasing numbers of women with co-morbidities, an increase in age of the pregnant population, and most notably an increase in obesity. While complications such as thrombosis can often be prevented, this is not always the case. Other pathology such as haemorrhage (which can sometimes be prevented or minimised by prompt recognition and timely intervention) can still be catastrophic, and conditions such as pre-eclampsia cannot be prevented completely. In all these, and many more situations, prompt and effective treatment is saving lives routinely on a daily basis throughout the UK. When a death does occur, the public expects exhaustive analysis: sometimes this reinforces old lessons, but often new lessons emerge. One conclusion is clear from reviewing CEMD reports from the past 60 years: when vigilance is relaxed, people die.

2.11 Further reading

Knight M, Bunch K, Cairns A, et al. (eds), on behalf of MBRRACE-UK. *Saving Lives, Improving Mothers' Care Rapid Report: Learning from SARS-CoV-2-related and Associated Maternal Deaths in the UK March–May 2020.* Oxford: National Perinatal Epidemiology Unit, University of Oxford, 2020.

Knight M, Bunch K, Tuffnell D, et al. (eds), on behalf of MBRRACE-UK. *Saving Lives, Improving Mothers' Care – Lessons Learned to Inform Maternity Care from the UK and Ireland Confidential Enquiries into Maternal Deaths and Morbidity 2015–17.* Oxford: National Perinatal Epidemiology Unit, University of Oxford, 2019.

Knight M, Bunch K, Tuffnell D, et al. (eds), on behalf of MBRRACE-UK. *Saving Lives, Improving Mothers' Care – Lessons learned to Inform Maternity Care from the UK and Ireland Confidential Enquiries into Maternal Deaths and Morbidity 2016–18.* Oxford: National Perinatal Epidemiology Unit, University of Oxford, 2020.

Chapter 3: Structured approach to emergencies in the obstetric patient

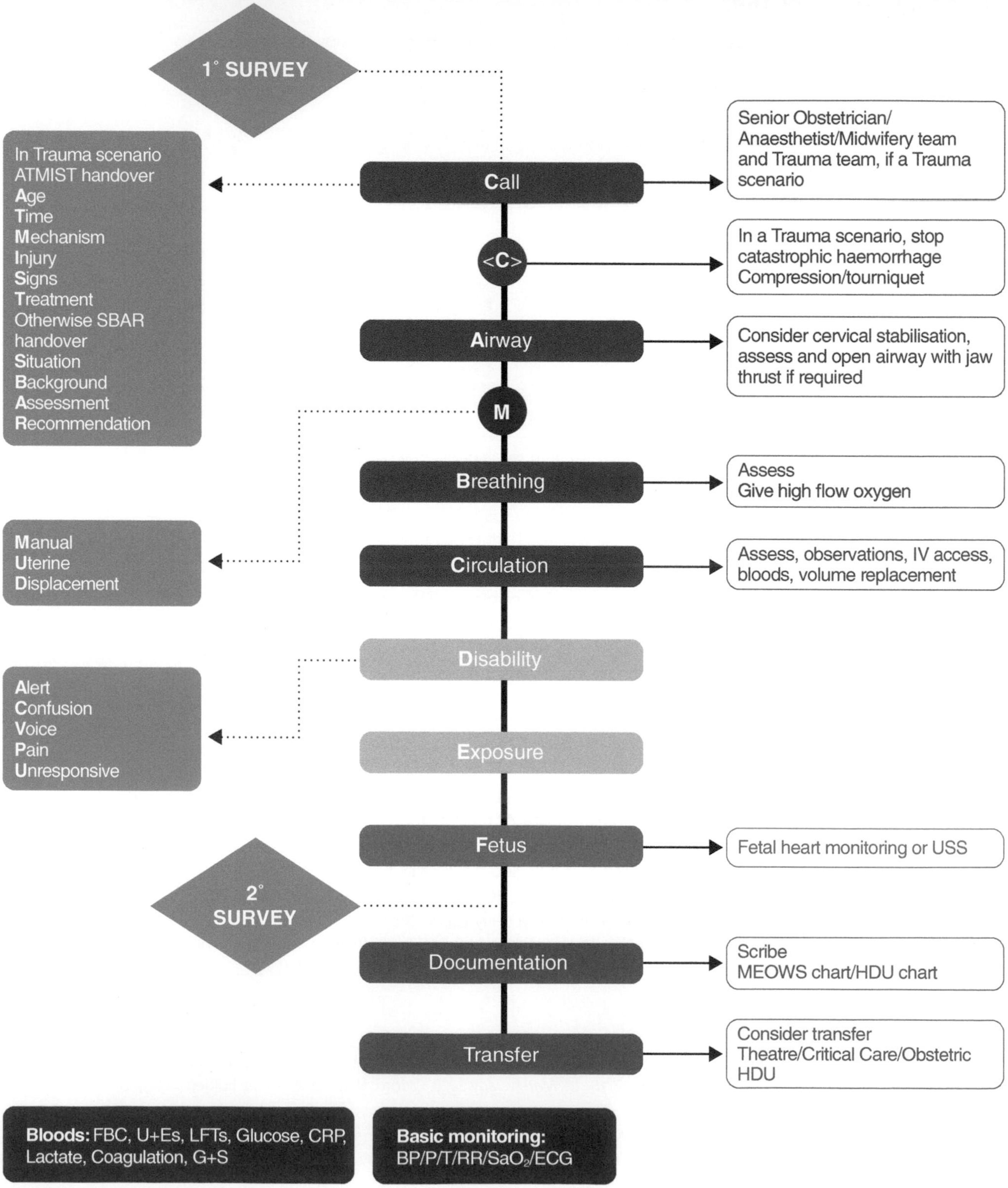

Algorithm 3.1 Structured approach to emergencies in the obstetric patient

CHAPTER 3

Structured approach to emergencies in the obstetric patient

Learning outcomes

After reading this chapter, you will be able to:

- Identify the correct sequence to be followed in assessing and managing seriously ill or seriously injured patients
- Outline the concept of the primary and secondary surveys

3.1 Introduction

The structured approach refers to the 'ABCDE' approach to life saving. The aim of the structured approach is to provide a system of assessment and management that is effective, and simple to remember, in the heat of an emergency. It can be applied to any patient with a threat to life, be that from illness or injury. Assessment is divided into primary survey and secondary survey. The approach is the same for all: adults, children, the elderly and pregnant women.

Primary survey

The system follows a simple ABCDE approach, with resuscitation taking place as problems are identified, i.e. a process of simultaneous evaluation and resuscitation.

The primary survey uncovers immediately life-threatening problems by priority, i.e. in the order in which they will most quickly kill. The medical sequence in the ABCDE approach is that an Airway problem will kill the patient more quickly than a Breathing problem, which in turn will kill a patient more quickly than a Circulation problem, which in turn will kill a patient more quickly than a Disability (neurological) problem.

Airway

Assess whether the airway is open by look, listen and feel. If not open, proceed to open the airway using simple manoeuvres, such as head tilt and chin lift, followed by more complex actions (as detailed in Chapter 10) where necessary. Manoeuvres to secure the patient's airway should not cause harm, or further harm, to the cervical spine. Therefore, if an injury to the cervical spine is suspected the cervical spine must be immobilised during airway care.

Managing Medical and Obstetric Emergencies and Trauma: A Practical Approach, Fourth Edition. Edited by Rosamunde Burns and Kara Dent.

Breathing

Look, listen and feel for respiration, using supplementary oxygen and ventilatory support as required.

Circulation

Assess the circulation by checking perfusion, heart rate and blood pressure. Volume replacement and haemorrhage control may be needed (see Chapters 6 and 8).

Disability

Assessment and support of the functioning of the neurological system including an assessment of conscious level (ACVPU), the pupils and a blood sugar.

Exposure

Adequately expose the patient to make a full assessment, taking care to avoid cooling and potential hypothermia by adjusting the environment.

3.2 Resuscitation

The resuscitation phase is carried out at the same time as the primary survey. Life-threatening conditions are managed as they are identified. Do not move on to the next stage of the primary survey until a problem, once found, has been corrected. If the patient's condition deteriorates, go back and reassess, starting again with ABCDE.

Secondary survey

The secondary survey is a comprehensive assessment, which takes place after life-threatening problems have been found and treated (primary survey) and uncovers problems that are not immediately life threatening. Ensure a full history is taken using AMPLE as an aide memoire:

A	Allergies
M	Medications
P	Past medical history, pregnancy issues
L	Last meal
E	Background to the illness/injury in terms of events and environment

The secondary survey is performed once the patient is stable. The secondary survey might not take place until after surgery, if surgery has been necessary as part of the resuscitation phase. The secondary survey is a top-to-toe and back-to-front process, as follows:

- Scalp and vault of skull
- Face and base of skull
- Neck and cervical spine
- Chest
- Abdomen
- Pelvis
- Remainder of spine and limbs
- Neurological examination
- Rectal and vaginal examinations, if indicated
- Examination of wounds caused by injury. Note: do not remove foreign objects from penetrating wounds, they may be tamponading a bleeding vessel

If the Glasgow Coma Score has not been evaluated in the primary survey it should be performed during the secondary survey (see Chapter 19).

Assessment of the collapsed patient using the ABC approach

First, speak loudly to the patient. To prompt manual uterine displacement (MUD) early in the process of resuscitation, remember:

'Hello, how are you Ms MUD?'

The response gives you several pieces of clinical information. To be able to respond verbally, the patient must have:

- Circulating oxygenated blood (i.e. has not had a cardiopulmonary arrest)
- A reasonably open airway
- A reasonable tidal volume to phonate
- Reasonable cerebral perfusion to comprehend and answer

If the patient does not respond then we cannot make the above assumptions.

Management of the apparently lifeless (unresponsive) patient

The approach to an apparently lifeless patient is the cardiopulmonary resuscitation (CPR) drill, which starts with opening the airway and assessing breathing, then proceeding to CPR as necessary (see Chapter 11 for details).

Management of the seriously injured pregnant patient

In the seriously injured patient who has signs of life, the following approach is taken.

If possible receive the ATMIST handover from the pre-hospital team and ensure left lateral tilt is ongoing or manually displace the uterus.

A	Age and gestational age
T	Time of injury
M	Mechanism of injury
I	Injuries sustained or suspected
S	Signs and symptoms
T	Treatment given so far

1. *Primary survey and resuscitation*: identify life-threatening problems and deal with these problems as they are identified. In a multiply injured patient **<C>** precedes ABCDE. **<C>** is control of **C**atastrophic haemorrhage such as applying a tourniquet and compression bandage to an amputated limb.
2. *Assess fetal well-being and viability*: may require delivery.
3. *Secondary survey*: top-to-toe, back-to-front examination.
4. *Definitive care*: specific management.

Continuous re-evaluation is very important to identify new life-threatening problems as they arise.

Monitoring (applied during primary survey)

- Pulse oximetry
- Heart rate/electrocardiogram (ECG)
- Blood pressure
- Respiratory rate
- End-tidal CO_2 monitoring is appropriate in an intubated patient
- Urine output: as a measure of adequate perfusion and fluid resuscitation
- Fetal heart monitoring will reflect the haemodynamic status of the mother until a circulation problem is addressed as part of the primary survey and as such provides information on the adequacy of maternal resuscitation in the primary survey

The pulse oximeter limitations are that the patient must be well perfused to obtain a reading. Ambient light and dyes, such as nail polish or circulating methaemoglobin, can cause erroneous readings. A fall in oxygen saturation is a late sign of an airway, breathing or circulation problem.

Adjuncts to assessment

- Blood tests (full blood count, blood group and save, venous blood gas, urea and electrolytes, thromboelastography, Kleihauer)
- Essential radiographs during the primary survey and resuscitation are chest and pelvis
- FAST (focused assessment with sonography for trauma) scan

Assess fetal well-being and viability

Use ultrasound to:

- Detect fetal heart and check rate
- Ascertain the number of fetuses and their positions
- Locate the position of the placenta and the amount of liquor
- Look for retroplacental bleeding and haematoma
- Detect an abnormal position of the fetus and free fluid in the abdominal cavity, suggesting rupture of the uterus
- Detect damage to other structures
- Check for free fluid and blood in the abdominal cavity

Adequately resuscitating the mother will improve the outcome for the fetus.

3.3 Definitive care

Definitive care takes place under the supervision of relevant specialists. It is of utmost importance to the patient's continued quality of life.

3.4 Summary

A systematic approach of primary survey (simultaneous assessment and resuscitation), fetal assessment, secondary survey and definitive care enables the clinician to give the best patient care possible in complex situations.

CHAPTER 4
Human factors

Learning outcomes

After reading this chapter, you will be able to:
- Describe how human factors affect the performance of individuals and teams in the healthcare environment

4.1 Introduction

The emphasis on the management of obstetric urgent or emergency care has traditionally concentrated on knowledge and application of the appropriate technical skills for the given situation. An often overlooked element is how in these high-pressure situations, maternity staff from several disciplines can come together to form an effective team that minimises error and works actively to prevent adverse events to minimise patient harm The maternity team in acute emergencies is made up of medical staff from different specialties and of varying seniority, midwives and ancillary staff (including healthcare assistants, operating department assistants, scrub nurses, etc.). The hospital-based maternity team also relies on close links with laboratory and imaging teams during emergencies, as well as support from administrative teams (ward clerks, hospital switchboard) and portering services. This is a complex system and requires knowledge of human factors and team working. The role of simulation and training as promoted within the mMOET course is vital in improving how individuals will work within their own teams during obstetric emergencies.

This chapter provides a brief introduction to some of the human factors that can affect the performance of individuals and teams in the healthcare environment. Human factors, also referred to as ergonomics, is an established scientific discipline and clinical human factors has been described as:

> *Enhancing clinical performance through an understanding of the effects of teamwork, tasks, equipment, workspace, culture and organisation on human behaviour and abilities and application of that knowledge in clinical settings* (Kohn et al., 2010).

4.2 Extent of healthcare error

In 2000 an influential report entitled *To Err is Human: Building a Safer Health System* (Kohn et al., 2010) suggested that across the USA somewhere between 44 000 and 98 000 deaths each year could be attributed to medical error. A pilot study in the UK demonstrated that approximately 1 in 10 patients admitted to healthcare experienced an adverse event.

Healthcare has been able to learn from a number of other high-risk industries including the nuclear, petrochemical, space exploration, military and aviation industries about how team issues have been managed. These lessons have been slowly adopted and translated to healthcare.

Managing Medical and Obstetric Emergencies and Trauma: A Practical Approach, Fourth Edition. Edited by Rosamunde Burns and Kara Dent.

Specialist working groups and national bodies have been instrumental in promoting awareness of the importance of human factors in healthcare. They aim to raise awareness and promote the principles and practices of human factors, identify current human factor activity, capability and barriers, and create conditions to support human factors being embedded at a local level. One such example of this in the UK is the Human Factors Clinical Working Group and the National Quality Board's concordat statement on human factors.

4.3 Causes of healthcare error

Consider this example of an adverse event:

A woman in labour needs to receive an infusion of a particular drug to manage severe hypertension. An error occurs and she receives an incorrect dose of the drug. What are the potential causes of this situation?

Potential causes of our example drug error	
Prescription error	Wrong drug prescribed
Preparation error	Correct drug prescribed but misread
Preparation error	Contents mislabelled during manufacture
Drawing up error	Incorrect drug selected
Administration error	Patient ID mix-up, drug given to wrong patient

Q. What one thing links all of these errors?
A. The humans involved – these are all examples of human errors.

Humans make mistakes. No amount of checks and procedures will mitigate this fact. In fact the only way to completely remove human error is to remove all the humans involved. It is vital therefore that we look to work in a way that, wherever possible, minimises the occurrence of mistakes and ensures that when they do occur the method minimises the chance of the error resulting in an adverse event.

4.4 Human error

It has been suggested that these human errors can be further categorised into: (i) those that occur at the sharp end of care by the treating team and individuals; and (ii) those that occur at the blunt or organisational level, typically through policies, procedures, staffing and culture. These errors can be further subdivided (Table 4.1).

Table 4.1 Types of errors

		Explanation	**Example**
Sharp errors that occur with the team/individuals treating the patient	Mistake	Lack or misapplication of knowledge	Not knowing the correct drug to prescribe
	Slip or lapse	Skills-based mistake	Knowing the correct drug but writing another one
	Violation	Deliberate action that may be routine or exceptional	Not attempting to get a drug second checked as there are no staff available
Blunt/organisational errors		Policies, procedures, infrastructure and building layout that has errors embedded	Different drugs used by different specialties and departments for same condition

It is typically found that the latent/organisational issues often coexist with the sharp errors; in fact it is rare for an isolated error to occur – often there is a chain of events that results in the adverse event. The 'Swiss cheese' model demonstrates how apparently random, unconnected events and organisational decisions can all make errors more likely (Figure 4.1). Conversely, a standardised system with good defences can capture these errors and prevent adverse events.

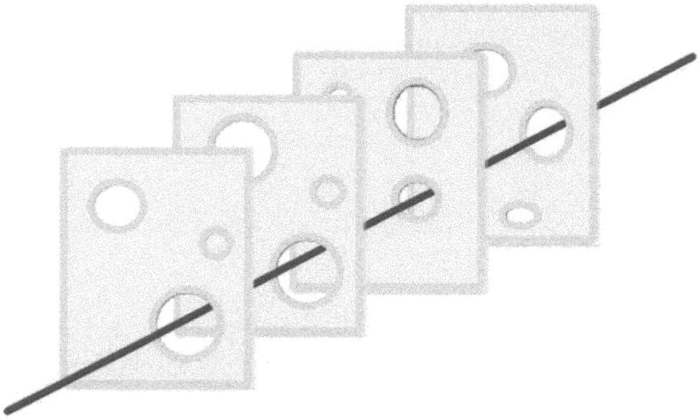

Figure 4.1 The 'Swiss cheese' model

Each of the slices of Swiss cheese represents barriers that, under ideal circumstances, would prevent or detect error. The holes represent weaknesses in these barriers; if the holes align the error passes through undetected with the potential to cause poor outcome and patient harm.

Reconsider the example of drug error using the Swiss cheese model. The first slice is the doctor writing the prescription, the second slice is the organisation's drug policy, the third is the midwife who draws up the drug and the fourth is the midwife who second checks the drug.

Now consider the following: What if the doctor is relatively new to the obstetric unit and unfamiliar with the specific drugs or doses used in this situation? – their 'slice of cheese' has larger holes. What if the organisation has failed to develop a robust drug policy that is fit for purpose and guidelines are out of date or not easily accessed? – this second slice is considerably weakened or may even be removed completely. What if the drug is drawn up by a midwife who has just returned from a career break who is not familiar with the particular antihypertensive drug used? – their 'slice' has also got larger holes. Labour wards are often chronically short of staff and the midwife who performs the second drug check is distracted as they are looking after two high-risk women in labour. Inadvertently their check is only cursory – this final slice (or barrier) is completely removed.

The end result is that multiple defences have been weakened or removed and error leading to unintentional harm is more likely. Also be aware of the different types of failure within the system: (i) latent failures include organisational error (e.g. no effective policy, out-of-date guidelines and inadequate staffing levels); and (ii) active failures (e.g. failure to escalate, drug errors, failure to monitor or act on deteriorating vital signs).

4.5 Learning from error

Historically, those making mistakes have been identified and singled out for punishment and/or retraining, in what is often referred to as a culture of blame. With our example drug error blame would most likely have fallen on the shoulders of the nurse administering and/or the doctor incorrectly prescribing. Does retraining these individuals make it safer for other or future patients? That clearly depends on the underlying reasons. If it was purely a knowledge gap, possibly, but does the same knowledge gap exist elsewhere? Potentially all the other issues remain unresolved. Moreover such punitive reactions make it less likely for individuals to admit mistakes and near misses in the future.

The focus is now on learning from error and, in shifting away from the individual, is much more focused on determining the system/organisational errors. Once robust systems, procedures and policies that work and are effective are in place, then errors can be captured. Of course issues will still need to be addressed where individuals have been reckless or lacked knowledge – but now reasons why the individuals felt the need to violate, or had not been given all the knowledge required, can be looked at.

For this to work health services need to learn from errors, adverse events and near misses. This requires engagement at both the individual level, by reporting errors, and the organisational level, investigating and feeding back the error using a systematic approach. It is also key that information is cascaded through the organisation and across the health service to raise awareness and prevent similar situations.

Violation may be indicative of the failure of systems, procedures or policies or other cultural issues. It is important that policies, procedures, roles and even our buildings and equipment are all designed proactively with human factors in mind so things do not have to be fixed retrospectively when adverse events occur. This means that all members of the organisation must be aware of human factors, not just the front-line clinical staff.

Improving team and individual performance

Having discussed the magnitude of the problem of healthcare error, the rest of this chapter will focus on how the performance of teams and individuals can be developed.

Raising awareness of the human factors and being able to practise these skills and behaviours within multiprofessional teams allows the development of effective teams in all situations. Simulation activity allows a team to explore these new ideas, practise them and develop them. To do this we need feedback on our performance within a safe environment where no patient is at risk and egos and personal interests can be set aside. Consider how you developed a clinical skill. It was something that needed to be practised again and again until eventually it started to become automatic and routine. The same applies for our human factor behaviours. In addition, recognising our inherent human limitations and the situations when errors are more likely to occur, we can all be hypervigilant when required.

4.6 Communication

Poor communication is the leading cause of adverse events. This is not surprising; to have an effective team there needs to be good communication. The leader needs to communicate with the followers, and followers communicate with leaders and other followers. Communication is not just saying something – it is ensuring that information is accurately passed on and received. We all want to ensure effective communication at all times. Remember there are multiple components to effective communication (Table 4.2).

Table 4.2 Elements of communication

Sender	Sender	Transmitted	Receiver	Receiver
Thinks of what to say	Communicates message	Face to face/phone/ email	Hears and confirms message	Considers and acts

When communicating face to face a lot of the information is transmitted non-verbally, which can make telephone or email conversations more challenging. Communication can be more difficult when talking across professional, specialty or hierarchal barriers as we do not always talk the same technical language, have the same levels of understanding, or even have a full awareness of the other person's role.

There are a variety of tools to aid communication, for example SBAR (situation, background, assessment and recommendation). SBAR is designed for acute clinical communications. It facilitates the sender to plan and organise the message, make it succinct and focused, and provide it in a logical and expected order. It is also an empowerment tool allowing the sender (who may be more junior) to request an action from a more senior individual. Find out what communication tool your organisation uses and practise using it; look out for other staff using it too. While these tools are useful, they tend to be reserved for certain situations, whereas we want to establish effective communication as the routine not the exception. One method to routinely improve communication is to incorporate a feedback loop.

Effective communication with a feedback loop

Errors can occur at any level or multiple levels. Consider a busy clinical situation and the team leader shouts *'We need four units of blood'* or *'Will someone order four units of blood'* while managing an ongoing postpartum haemorrhage (PPH) – what happens? The majority of times nothing – nobody goes to bring the blood! So how can this be improved? Avoid using instructions like the two examples above – remember – nobody is called 'someone'! Most obviously an individual can be identified to perform the task, by name: *'Michael can you please order four units of blood?'* If Michael says *'Yes'* effective communication might be assumed; but not always. What has Michael heard and what will he do? At the moment we do not really know what message has been received. Michael might dash over with a cup of tea as this is what he thought he heard. This may seem a slightly strange thing to happen; but how often in a clinical emergency have you asked for something and been presented with something else? People are less likely to ask questions in emergencies as everyone is busy. This could be the catalyst for an error or precipitate a missed task. So how do we find out what message Michael received? The easiest way is to use specific 'task allocation' incorporated within a formal 'feedback loop' (also known as 'closed loop communication').

Now the conversation goes:

Team leader (Liz):	'Michael, can you please order four units of blood?'
Michael:	'Okay, you'd like me to order four units of blood?'
Team leader:	'Correct'

The loop is finally closed when Michael returns to the room and confirms that the specific allocated task has been done:

Michael:	'Liz, the four units of blood are ordered and will be here in 5 minutes'
Team leader:	'Noted Michael – thanks'

We now know that the message has been transmitted and received correctly. For this process to work both parties (the sender and receiver) need to understand and expect it – again demonstrating the need for us to practise and train together. The phrase '*Will someone . . .*' is often used to avoid the embarrassment felt when you cannot remember someone's name. In emergency situations this must be avoided – use alternative ways of attracting attention: you may need to point or wave at the team member! This is never easy, but is absolutely vital if tasks are to be allocated and completed effectively.

4.7 Team working, leadership and followership

At a basic level a team is a group of individuals with a common cause. Historically we have tended to train individually or in professional silos; the risk here is that we are making a 'team of experts' rather than an 'expert team'. Often within healthcare our teams form at short notice and may arrive at different times. Much emphasis has previously been given to the role of the leader, but a leader cannot be a team on his or her own. Emphasis needs to be given to developing the other team members, the active followers. A good leader will be able to swap from the role of leader to follower as more senior staff arrive and agree to take over.

The leader

The leader's role is multifaceted and includes directing the team; assigning tasks and assessing performance; motivating and encouraging the team to work together; and planning and organising. All leadership skills and behaviours need to be developed and practised. There are different leadership styles and the leader needs to choose an appropriate style for that situation. Effective communication is key and should be reviewed and reflected upon regularly. Constructive feedback can both be given and sought in order to facilitate continuously improving performance.

Who is the leader?

It is vitally important to have a clearly identified leader. There can be times when people come and go, or different specialties arrive, creating a situation where it may not be clear who the leader is. In some situations or institutions individuals will wear tabards or other forms of identification to mitigate against this uncertainty. If there is a scribe recording events they should record who is leading and any changes to the leader.

Physical position of the leader

As soon as the leader becomes hands on, and task focused, they are primarily concentrating on the task at hand. This becomes the focus of their thoughts and they lose situation (or situational) awareness (i.e. their objective overview of the situation – see Section 4.8). The term 'situational leadership' is used to describe the fact that leadership can change as an emergency develops. If the leader is required to undertake a specific technical task, he/she must hand over leadership at that point. An example would be a situation where the consultant has assumed situational leadership during a shoulder dystocia. The midwife is unable to rotate the shoulders internally and asks the consultant to take over. As the consultant moves in to examine with the aim of removing the posterior arm, he/she must delegate 'situational leadership' to someone else – this will often be the senior midwife in the room.

The leader should be standing in an optimal position where they can gather all the information and ideally view the patient, the team members and the monitoring and diagnostic equipment. This enables them to recognise when a member is struggling with a task or procedure and support them appropriately.

Clear roles

Ideally the team should meet before the event and have the opportunity to introduce each other, and clarify roles and actions in emergencies. Sometimes this can be facilitated at the beginning of a shift but at other times it is impossible to predict or arrange. It is important, therefore, that individuals identify themselves to the leader as they arrive and roles are agreed, allocated and understood. A lot of the time their role may be determined purely in relation to the specific bleep the individual carries, but it is important that team members are flexible, for example if three airway providers are first on the scene we would expect other tasks to also be undertaken.

Followership

The followers have roles that are as mission critical as the leader. Followers are expected to work within their scope of practice but also take the initiative. No one would expect to turn up at a ward emergency and have a neat row of staff against the wall waiting for instructions. It is important to think about the level of communication required between the leader and followers. If it is obvious we are doing a task, this does not need to be communicated. There is a risk that followers can overwhelm the leader with verbal communications where, in fact, the key is to communicate concerns or abnormal things. In the Formula One pit lane during a tyre change, the crew communicate (visually) as tasks are completed; they also signal if they have a problem, they do not communicate verbally at every expected step.

Hierarchy

Within the team there needs to be a hierarchy. This is the 'power gradient'; the leader is at the top of this as the person coordinating, directing and making the decisions. However, this should not be absolute. There is much discussion in the literature about the degree of the hierarchical gradient. If it is too steep the leader has a massive position of power, his or her decisions are unquestionable and the followers blindly follow the orders. This is not safe because leaders are humans too and also make errors – their team is their safety net.

Safe practice is achieved where the followers feel they can raise concerns or question instructions. This must always be understood by the leaders as much as by the followers. One way to reduce the hierarchy gradient is for the leader to invite the team's thoughts and concerns, particularly around patient safety issues. It is also important for the follower to learn how to raise concerns appropriately. This is often referred to as 'flattening the hierarchial pyramid' – the leader is 'nearer' to his/her team, actively listening to concerns raised, whilst team members undertake allocated tasks effectively and feel empowered to 'challenge' or raise concerns.

One acronym that is sometimes used to raise concerns in a format which escalates appropriately is PACE (**p**robe, **a**lert, **c**hallenge and finally declare an **e**mergency). The probing question allows diplomacy and maintenance of the hierarchy whilst raising the relevant concern.

Stage		Level of concern
P	Probe	*'Do you know that . . .'*
A	Alert	*'I'm more concerned now . . .'*
C	Challenge	*'Please stop what you're doing and consider . . .'*
E	Emergency	*'I need you to stop immediately because . . .'*

These stages are described with examples below:

- **Probe** – this is used where a person notices something they think might be a problem. They verbalise the issue, often as a question. 'Have you noticed that this woman is bleeding excessively?'
- **Alert** – the observer strengthens and directs their statement and suggests a course of action. 'Dr Brown, I am concerned, the mother is still bleeding more than I'd expect – shall I give ergometrine?'

- **Challenge** – the situation requires urgent attention. One of the key protagonists needs to be directly engaged. If possible the speaker places him- or herself into the eye line of the person they wish to communicate with. 'Dr Brown, you must listen to me now, this patient needs more action now as the bleeding is not slowing down.'
- **Emergency** – this is used where all else has failed and/or the observer perceives a critical event is about to occur. Where possible a physical signal or physical barrier should be employed together with clear verbalisation. 'Dr Brown, you are not acting on this woman's significant ongoing bleeding. Please move aside and I will assess directly myself.'

The PACE structure can be commenced at any appropriate level and escalated until a satisfactory response is gained. If an adverse event is imminent then it may be relevant to start at the declaring 'emergency' stage, whereas a much lower level of concern may well start at a 'probing' question.

Some industries have also additionally adopted organisation-wide critical phrases that convey the importance of the situation, e.g. 'I am concerned', 'I am uncomfortable' or 'I am scared'. In an effective team where the leader actively listens to concerns raised by his/her team members, progressing beyond the 'P' or 'A' step should rarely be needed.

4.8 Situation (or situational) awareness

A key element of good team working and leadership is to be fully aware of what is happening; this is termed situation awareness. It not only involves seeing what is happening, but also captures how this is interpreted and understood, how decisions are made and ultimately involves planning ahead.

Typically, three levels of situation awareness are described:

Level 1 – What is going on? Collecting information

Level 2 – So what? Interpreting the information

Level 3 – Now what? Anticipating the future state

Level 1 – the basic level (What is going on? Collecting information)

We are prone to errors even at this level: the risk is that what is seen or heard is what is *expected* to be seen or heard, rather than what is actually occurring. Figure 4.2 shows the similar package design of two different medications, making errors more likely. It is important to really concentrate on seeing what is actually there.

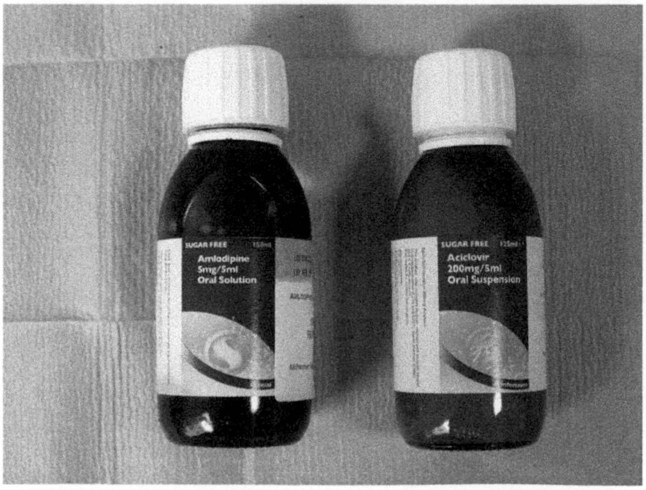

Figure 4.2 Similar package design of two different medications

Distraction

Within healthcare, distractions become the norm to such an extent individuals are often not even aware of them. The risk is that mistakes are made and information is missed. It is important to try to challenge interruptions when doing critical tasks, and when they do occur, restart the task from the beginning, rather than from where it is considered the interruption occurred. Some organisations are looking at specific quiet areas for critical tasks. Whatever the local set up, the key is to develop and maintain everyone's awareness of how distraction greatly increases the chance of error.

Level 2 (So what? Interpreting the information)

This encompasses how someone's understanding forms from what has been seen. To minimise level 2 errors consideration is needed as to how the human brain works, recognises things and makes decisions and choices. This level of detail is beyond the scope of this introductory chapter (for those who are interested in pursuing this further *Safety at the Sharp End* by Flin et al. (2008) is an excellent learning resource for the whole field of human factors in healthcare). Therefore this section will focus on a part of this – the decision making that leads into level 3.

On the face of it the practice of decision making is familiar to everyone. However, to understand the factors that can compromise this process it is important to understand the factors that will influence the decision made. To make a good decision a person needs to assess all aspects of a problem, identify the possible responses to the problem, consider the consequences of each of those responses and then weigh up the advantages and disadvantages in order to draw a conclusion. Having completed this, they then need to communicate their decision to their team.

Good situation awareness is a basic prerequisite of this process. To achieve this, the decision maker must ensure they have all the key information. In a well-functioning team everyone is on the alert for ambiguities, biases or conflicting information. Any inconsistent facts should be treated as a potential marker for faulty situation awareness. It is important not to brush them off as unimportant anomalies in the absence of evidence to support such a decision.

In many clinical situations there can be a significant pressure of time. Where this is not the case then no decision-making process should be concluded until the team is satisfied they have all the information and have considered all the options. Where time is a pressure, a certain amount of pragmatism must be employed. There is plenty of evidence to confirm that practice and experience can mitigate some of the negative effects of abbreviating a decision-making process. Those making decisions under such circumstances need to remain aware of the short-cuts they have taken and be ready to receive feedback from their team, particularly if any member of the team has significant concerns about the proposed course of action.

Level 3 (Now what? Anticipating the future state)

Having gathered information using all of our senses (level 1) we then need to interpret the information (level 2) before we plan forward using previous experience, seeking input from the team when required (level 3). Finally, we must decide the plan of action and communicate this to the team.

Team situation awareness

The individuals in the team may have a unique awareness of the situation depending on their previous experience, specialty, physical position, etc. The team's situation awareness will often be greater than that of any one individual. However this can only be exploited if the individual elements are effectively communicated clearly between team members. Effective leaders actively encourage this as it results in a 'shared mental model', a feature associated with effective teams.

The Royal College of Obstetricians and Gynaecologists (RCOG) is integrating human factors within the new UK postgraduate training curriculum and has developed learning resources within the 'Each Baby Counts' initiative: https://www.rcog.org.uk/en/guidelines-research-services/audit-quality-improvement/each-baby-counts/implementation/improving-human-factors/ (last accessed October 2020).

4.9 Improving team and individual performance

In addition to effective communication, team working, situation awareness, leadership and followership skills, there are a number of other ways that team and individual performance can be further developed and improved.

Awareness of situations when errors are more likely

If we are aware that an error is more likely we can be more proactive in detecting them. Alongside distractions, two common situations that make errors more likely are stress and fatigue. Stress is not only a source of error when we are overworked and overstimulated, but also, at the other end of the spectrum, when we are understimulated we become inattentive.

The acronym **HALT** has been used to describe situations when error is more likely:

H	Hungry
A	Angry
L	Late
T	Tired

Consider how many times in the last week you have been hungry, angry, late or tired and still worked in a setting where errors could have had significant implications. Unfortunately, in many work cultures these emotional and/or physical states are seen as inevitable.

I'M SAFE has been used as a checklist in the aviation industry, asking whether the individual may be affected by:

I	Illness
M	Medication
S	Stress
A	Alcohol
F	Fatigue
E	Eating

Ideally, individuals who are potentially compromised need to be supported appropriately, allowed time to recover and the team made aware. How this can be achieved in the middle of a night shift can be problematic.

Awareness of error traps

Humans are prone to several 'cognitive biases' (examples include normalcy, confirmation, conformity and fixation biases). *Normalcy bias* is the tendency to underestimate both the seriousness of a situation and the likelihood of a poor outcome – i.e. you rule out the worst-case scenario.

Confirmation bias is also common and is the tendency to only pay attention to information that fits in with your own 'mental model' of the situation in hand. There is a reluctance to change one's mind even in the presence of contradictory evidence. When this occurs, people favour information that confirms their preconceptions or hypotheses regardless of whether the information is true. This may be observed within the healthcare setting during the process of a referral or handover. An example of this might be a clinician receiving a phone call requesting them to attend the ward to review an acutely deteriorating postnatal woman. The clinician is advised that the woman has collapsed. On their way to the ward the clinician builds up a series of preconceived expectations around what they will find upon their arrival. They may even formulate a management plan whilst travelling to the scene, based upon their expectations. Once this 'mindset' is established it can be difficult to shift. On arrival, the clinician examines the systems affected by the presumed diagnosis. They seek to confirm their expectation of collapse due to PPH by focusing on palpating the uterine fundus at the expense of a thorough systematic assessment. They do not pick up the fact that the woman is having difficulty breathing and their preconceived ideas that this is due to PPH mean that the remainder of the assessment is completed without due attention and more as a rehearsed exercise rather than an open-minded exploration. In this case the eventual diagnosis was pulmonary embolism which was a very late consideration in the diagnostic pathway.

Apart from thorough history and clinical assessment, using the expertise within your team by carefully listening to alternative views or challenges can minimise the effects of these cognitive biases.

Cognitive aids: checklists, guidelines and protocols

Cognitive aids such as guidelines or checklists are important because the human memory is not infallible. They also confer team understanding through the use of a standardised response. This reduces stress. This is especially true where an uncommon emergency event occurs. The team may be unfamiliar with one another and each member will be trying to remember what to do, what treatments are required and in what order. A good team leader will use the available cognitive aids as a prompt and the team's members can use it as a resource so that they can plan ahead. Safe practice is promoted through the use of these tools in an emergency rather than relying on memory.

Calling for help early

Trainees in all disciplines are often reluctant to call for senior help, partly due to not recognising the severity of the situation and partly due to concerns about wasting the time of seniors. With all emergency events, and in particular with obstetric emergencies, escalation and appropriate help should be summoned as soon as possible. Remember, help will not arrive instantly.

Using all available resources

Team resources include staff, observations, equipment, cognitive aids and the facilities in the local area. It is the team leader's role to continually consider the appropriateness of utilising available, untasked staff or equipment to optimise the patient's care and prevent a bottleneck in the treatment pathway.

Debriefing

Wherever possible it helps to have a facilitated debrief following an adverse clinical event. It is best if the debrief is viewed as a normal part of the process of dealing with all obstetric emergencies rather than being reserved for catastrophic events. The aim of a debrief is to summarise any particular issues or problems that the team had, and reflect on how the team performed. Some organisations have set templates to facilitate this. It gives the opportunity for individuals, teams and organisations to continually develop.

Whilst a 'hot' debrief immediately after the event may be useful in certain situations, it is not always ideal. Some situations in obstetrics can be emotionally draining, especially when maternal or neonatal outcome is poor. A balance must be established whereby formal debrief and feedback to all involved team members occurs within a reasonably short timeframe. All team members must be aware of looking out for the emotional needs of colleagues who may have been particularly emotionally traumatised during an emergency situation.

4.10 Summary

In this chapter we have given a brief introduction to human factors and described how lack of awareness about the importance of communication, situation awareness, leadership, team working and decision making can lead to patient harm and adverse events. It is really important for you to use every opportunity to reflect on and develop your own performance and influence the development of others and the team. Appropriate debriefing is included in the scenarios for the mMOET course, which may be used to help you to incorporate this process into your own clinical practice.

4.11 Further reading

Bromiley M. *Just a Routine Operation*. https://vimeo.com/970665. Clinical Human Factors Group, www.chfg.co.uk (last accessed February 2022).

Flin R, O'Connor P, Crichton M. *Safety at the Sharp End: A Guide to Non-technical Skills*. Abingdon: CRC Press, 2008.

PART 2
Recognition

(a)

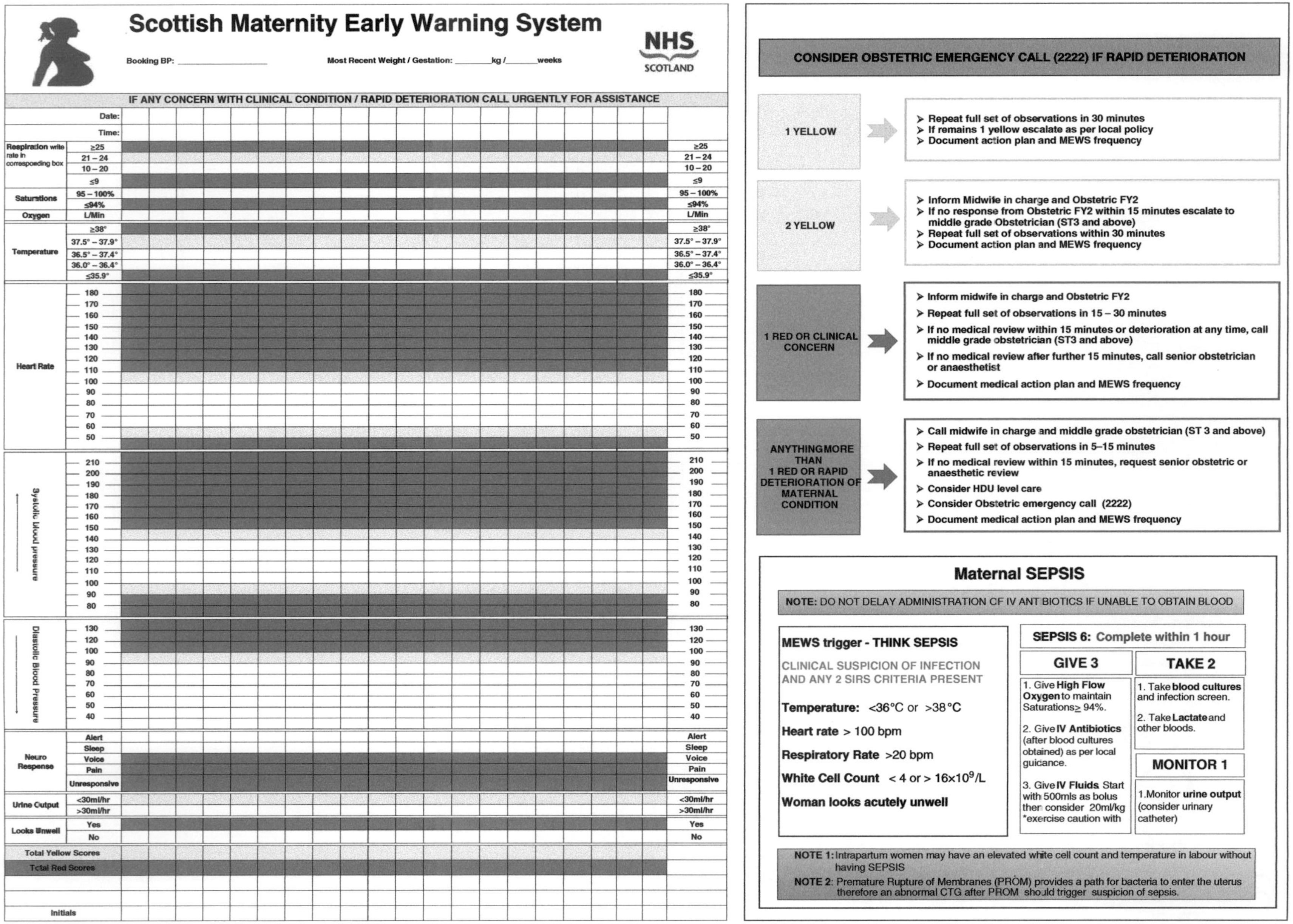

Continued on p. 32.

Algorithm 5.1 Scottish national MEWS chart: (a) front of MEWS chart

Source: Scottish patient safety programme, Maternity and Children quality Improvement programme. © The Improvement Hub

CHAPTER 5

Recognising the seriously sick patient

Learning outcomes

After reading this chapter, you will be able to:

- Identify the current causes of maternal mortality and morbidity and the issues with their detection and treatment
- Describe a systematic approach to monitoring using early warning charts to aid recognition of women at risk
- Recognise 'red flag' symptoms and their need for an urgent response by the obstetric team and other specialties

5.1 Introduction

Recurrent themes in mortality and morbidity reports identify that suboptimal care may have contributed to the deaths described in these reports. With more than two thirds of cases having pre-existing co-morbidities and indirect deaths exceeding direct, the importance of coordinated care across specialties is emphasised. Failure to recognise symptoms and signs of potentially life-threatening conditions, delay in acting on findings and delay seeking help from appropriate specialists are all of particular concern. Attention is therefore focused on ways to improve the recognition of, and timely response to, clinical signs of the deteriorating patient.

The diagnosis of a severe life-threatening condition in a pregnant or recently pregnant woman is challenging when the onset is insidious or atypical. This is compounded by the sick pregnant woman presenting to a non-obstetric area such as the emergency department where staff are not familiar with pregnancy physiology. The different response to impending critical illness through vital signs can be missed in these circumstances.

Not only 'high risk' women become critically ill. Often it is not possible to predict if or when this might happen to any obstetric patient. The relative rarity of life-threatening events in pregnancy reinforces the need for multiprofessional working and training involving emergency department staff and acute physicians.

The lessons that apply to all health professionals dealing with pregnant women can be summarised as follows:

- Understand the physiological adaptations of pregnancy in order to be able to recognise the pathological changes of serious illness – it is important to be able to distinguish between common discomforts of pregnancy and the signs of serious illness so that these signs are not missed (Table 5.1)
- Focus on getting things right the first time – high-quality history taking, physical examination, meticulous recording of basic observations and findings, and acting on those findings without delay
- Remember the red flags, including repeated presentation or readmission during pregnancy
- Ensuring good communication and timely, effective referrals between professionals

Managing Medical and Obstetric Emergencies and Trauma: A Practical Approach, Fourth Edition. Edited by Rosamunde Burns and Kara Dent.

(b)

The Scottish Maternity Early Warning Score (MEWS)

Physiological Parameters	Red	Yellow	Normal	Yellow	Red
Respiration rate	≤ 9		10–20	21–24	≥25
Oxygen saturation	≤94		95–100		
Temperature	≤35.9		36.0–37.4	37.5–37.9	≥38
Heart rate	≤ 50	50–60	61–99	100–109	≥110
Systolic BP	≤90	90–99	100–139	140–149	≥150
Diastolic BP			40–89	90–99	≥100
Neurological response – AVPU			A or S		V,P or U
Urine output (ml/hr)		<30	>30		
Looks unwell			No		Yes

ANY CONCERN WITH CLINICAL CONDITION /RAPID DETERIORATION CALL URGENTLY FOR ASSISTANCE

(c)

MEWS triggers, alert and review

Trigger	Alert	Review
1 yellow	Charge Midwife	Repeat observations in 30 minutes If unchanged escalate to FY2
2 yellow	Charge Midwife and FY2	Repeat full set of observations within 30 minutes.
1 red	Charge Midwife and FY2	Repeat full set of observations in 15–30 minutes
>1 red	Charge Midwife and ST3 or above. Consider Consultant Obstetrician and / or Anaesthetist review	Repeat full set of observations in 5–15 minutes Consider obsteric emergency call.Consider HDU level care

DOCUMENT ACTION PLAN FOR EACH MEWS TRIGGER INCLUDING MEWS FREQUENCY

Algorithm 5.1 ***(Continued)*** **Scottish national MEWS chart: (b, c) reverse of MEWS chart**
Source: Scottish patient safety programme, Maternity and Children quality Improvement programme. © The Improvement Hub

Table 5.1 Physiological changes and normal findings in pregnancy

Indicator	**What's normal in pregnancy?**
Heart rate	An increase of 10–20 beats per minute, particularly in third trimester
Blood pressure	Can decrease by 10–15 mmHg by 20 weeks, but returns to pre-pregnancy levels by term
Respiratory rate (RR)	Unaltered in pregnancy If RR >20 breaths per minute, consider a pathological cause
Oxygen saturation	Unchanged throughout pregnancy
Temperature	Unchanged throughout pregnancy
Full blood count	Ranges altered in pregnancy: Hb (105–140 g/l) WBC (6–16 × 10^9/l)
Renal function	Increased glomerular filtration rate Creatinine falls in first and second trimesters Normal urea reference range 2.5–4.0 mmol/l Normal creatinine <77 μmol/l
Liver tests	Raised alkaline phosphatase up to three- to fourfold of pre-pregnancy level is normal during pregnancy
Troponin	Not elevated during normal pregnancy May be elevated in pre-eclampsia, pulmonary embolism, myocarditis, arrhythmias and sepsis
D-dimer	Not recommended for use in pregnancy
Creatinine kinase	Normal range 5–40 IU/l, i.e. lower in pregnancy
Cholesterol	Up to five times elevated in pregnancy (therefore should not be checked routinely)
Thyroid function tests (TFTs)	Use local gestation-specific ranges
ECG	Sinus tachycardia 15° left axis deviation dueto diaphragmatic elevation T wave changes – commonlyT wave inversion in lead III and aVF Non-specific ST changes, e.g. depression, small Q waves
Holter monitor	Supraventricular and ventricular ectopics are more common
Chest X-ray (CXR)	Prominent vascular markings, raised diaphragm due to gravid uterus, flattened left hemidiaphragm
Peak expiratory flow rate (PEFR)	Unchanged in pregnancy
Arterial blood gas	Mild, fully compensated respiratory alkalosis is normal during pregnancy

Source: RCP (Royal College of Physicians). *Acute Care Toolkit 15: Managing Acute Medical Problems in Pregnancy*. London: RCP, 2019. © Royal College of Physicians

5.2 Modified early-warning systems

It is recognised that pregnancy and labour are normal physiological events but **'normality cannot be assumed without measurement'** (Knight et al., 2014). Maternity early warning score (MEWS) systems adapted for pregnancy are designed to detect when there is deviation from the normal. Regular observations of vital signs should be an integral part of care of *all* pregnant women. MEWS charts should be readily available and used in obstetric and non-obstetric areas of the hospital where pregnant woman may present.

There is a minimum dataset of observations suggested at each assessment which should be recorded on a MEWS chart (Algorithm 5.1). The minimum recommended frequency of observations as an inpatient is 12 hourly. Frequency of observations is determined by risk status, initial observations and working diagnosis. Women should retain the same MEWS chart when moving from one clinical area to another, so that physiological trends can be detected.

MEWS scores outside the normal range for pregnancy are recorded in the coloured zones of the chart and should immediately trigger communication using the SBAR (situation, background, assessment and recommendation) communication tool with appropriate medical staff asking for urgent review (Box 5.1). The clinician should undertake a full systematic review, resuscitate and treat as required and order appropriate investigations. It must be emphasised that just recording observations however regularly or meticulously is not enough: abnormal ones must be ***acted upon***. If the clinician who has been contacted is unable to attend within 10 minutes, options include contacting a more senior obstetrician or the anaesthetic team. Consider early obstetric consultant and anaesthetic consultant involvement. If a senior speciality trainee has deputised a more junior obstetrician to attend, then the midwife and charge midwife need to assess whether this is an appropriate level of clinician attending and consider escalation as outlined. It is important to care for the woman in the most appropriate clinical area. If this is not possible, then a delay in transfer must not delay immediate history taking, examination, investigations, treatment, note review and reassessment of ABCD. Contact the clinical manager on call for assistance if required.

Box 5.1 SBAR

Situation	Identify yourself, identify your patient and where you are calling from 'I am calling because . . .' be specific about your concern
Background	Set out the context of the admission, giving significant medical history, what operation/procedure has been had, any important blood results and recent observations. Outline her normal condition
Assessment	Give your assessment of the situation 'I think that she has suffered a . . .' 'I do not know what the problem is but I am very concerned about her deterioration . . .'
Recommendation	Here you need to be very specific in what you want the receiver to do 'I need you to come immediately . . .' 'I need you to come or in the next 10 minutes . . .' 'I would like to transfer her immediately to labour ward because . . .'

In non-obstetric areas such as the emergency department or acute medical unit there should be clear routes for effective communication with the obstetric team for ***all*** pregnant women. Routes for escalation should be clear to all staff should the woman's observations on the MEWS chart trigger a review or her condition clinically deteriorates. If a pregnant woman is triaged by the ambulance or emergency department staff to the emergency department resuscitation room a 2222 'obstetric emergency' call (or equivalent) should be activated to ensure a full team including a neonatologist is available.

Breathlessness

This common symptom can arise due to the normal respiratory adaptation to pregnancy, is gradual in onset and is usually noticed by the woman when she is talking or at rest. In normal pregnancy, there is a 40–50% increase in minute ventilation, mostly owing to an increase in tidal volume rather than respiratory rate and this leads to the subjective awareness of breathing. A mild, fully compensated respiratory alkalosis is therefore normal in pregnancy (see Table A5.1 in Appendix 5.1).

> ***However, in any pregnant woman complaining of breathlessness the 'red flag' features (Table 5.2) must be sought during history taking and acted upon.***

The differential diagnosis of breathlessness in pregnancy includes:

- Anaemia
- Respiratory causes: asthma, pneumonia, pneumothorax, pulmonary embolus, pulmonary oedema
- Cardiac causes: cardiomyopathy, pulmonary hypertension, valvular heart disease
- Amniotic fluid embolus
- Metabolic (e.g. diabetic ketoacidosis)
- Neuromuscular (e.g. myasthenia gravis)

Table 5.2 Red flag symptoms and signs

Breathlessness	Especially if: • of sudden onset • worse on lying flat • if associated with tachycardia, chest pain or syncope • respiratory rate >20 • SAO_2 <94% or falls to <94% on exertion
Headache	Especially if: • sudden onset/thunderclap or worst headache ever • headache that takes longer than usual to resolve or persists for more than 48 hours • there are associated fever, seizures, focal neurology, photophobia or diplopia • it requires opioids
Chest pain	Especially if: • pain severe enough to require opioids • radiates to arm, shoulder, back or jaw • sudden onset, tearing or exertional chest pain • associated with haemoptysis, breathlessness, syncope or abnormal neurology • associated with abnormal observations
Palpitations	Especially if: • the woman has a family history of sudden cardiac death • there is structural heart disease or previous cardiac surgery • associated with syncope • associated with chest pain • persistent severe tachycardia
Pyrexia >38°C	Absence of pyrexia does not exclude sepsis, as paracetamol and other antipyretics may temporarily suppress the pyrexia; equally, absence of pyrexia in the presence of sepsis is worrying
Abdominal pain	That requires opioids (excluding contractions) Associated with diarrhoea and/or vomiting
Reduced or absent fetal movements or fetal heart rate	
Uterine (excluding contractions) or renal angle pain or tenderness	
Generally unwell especially if distressed and anxious	Signs of a deteriorating condition

Source: Adapted from RCP (Royal College of Physicians). *Acute Care Toolkit 15: Managing Acute Medical Problems in Pregnancy.* London: RCP, 2019.

It is important also to remember that because respiratory rate does not increase in normal pregnancy, a ***rise in respiratory rate will often be the subtle first sign of impending critical illness in pregnancy*** and should prompt a systematic ABCDE clinical assessment.

Headache

This is a common problem in pregnancy. It is one of the most difficult symptoms to manage as it can not be seen, examined or measured. Most of the time it will have a benign cause, but there are a wide variety of serious conditions presenting with headache or confusion as the predominant feature (see Chapter 25). The red flag features should be sought in the history taking (Table 5.2).

Abdominal pain and diarrhoea

In early pregnancy it is essential to exclude ectopic pregnancy. Vaginal bleeding may be absent. Fainting and dizziness would not usually occur with gastroenteritis unless there is significant dehydration, but is seen with hypovolaemia from blood loss. A pregnancy test is essential to rule out pregnancy in women of childbearing age with abdominal pain.

Abdominal pain and diarrhoea can also be symptoms of intra-abdominal sepsis. See also Chapter 23 on abdominal emergencies.

5.3 Summary

- All pregnant women should have systematic measurements of vital signs, which should be plotted on a MEWS chart
- There should be an understanding of the triggering of escalation to senior medical review when vital signs are abnormal as deterioration can be rapid in pregnancy
- When a pregnant woman presents to a non-obstetric area of the hospital the obstetric team should be informed and a MEWS chart commenced
- Respiratory rate does not increase in normal pregnancy therefore tachypnoea should not be ignored
- Recognition of both significant red flag symptoms and often subtle clinical signs in pregnancy is essential to enable appropriate timely intervention to reduce maternal mortality and morbidity

5.4 Further reading

Knight M, Bunch K, Tuffnell D, et al. (eds), on behalf of MBRRACE-UK *Saving Lives, Improving Mothers' Care – Lessons Learned to Inform Maternity Care from the UK and Ireland Confidential Enquiries into Maternal Deaths and Morbidity 2015–17*. Oxford: National Perinatal Epidemiology Unit, University of Oxford, 2019.

Knight M, Bunch K, Tuffnell D, et al. (eds), on behalf of MBRRACE-UK. *Saving Lives, Improving Mothers' Care – Lessons Learned to Inform Maternity Care from the UK and Ireland Confidential Enquiries into Maternal Deaths and Morbidity 2016–18*. Oxford: National Perinatal Epidemiology Unit, University of Oxford, 2020.

RCP (Royal College of Physicians). *Acute Care Toolkit 15: Managing Acute Medical Problems in Pregnancy*. London: RCP, 2019.

Appendix 5.1 Blood gas interpretation

Lactate

Modern blood gas analysers are able to measure the blood lactate, a product of anaerobic metabolism and marker of the state of the microcirculation. In shock, elevated blood lactate levels can be used to predict mortality, and in septic shock raised lactate predicts the development of multiple organ failure more reliably than clinical observations. Failure of the lactate to fall with therapy is associated with higher mortality. Even haemodynamically stable patients with raised lactate levels, a condition referred to as compensated shock, are at increased risk of death. Lactate measurements >4 mmol/l can be taken as a marker of severe illness and used as a trigger to start resuscitation (see Chapter 7).

ABG interpretation

Normal values for both the non-pregnant and the pregnant state are given in Table 5A.1. To interpret a blood gas, review the following:

- Check PaO_2 (normal values 11–13 kPa **ON AIR**): if it is low, then the patient is hypoxaemic
- Check the pH value: to determine the direction of primary change (normal, acidosis or alkalosis); compensation is always incomplete
- Check $PaCO_2$, which is determined by breathing (alveolar ventilation): a low $PaCO_2$ (hyperventilation) indicates a respiratory alkalosis or respiratory compensation for a metabolic acidosis; a raised $PaCO_2$ (hypoventilation) indicates respiratory acidosis – note that $PaCO_2$ does not rise to compensate for a metabolic alkalosis
- Check standard bicarbonate (the bicarbonate value adjusted to what it would have been if the $PaCO_2$ were normal): if the standard bicarbonate is raised then there is either a metabolic alkalosis or metabolic compensation for a respiratory acidosis; if the standard bicarbonate is low then there is either a metabolic acidosis or metabolic compensation for a respiratory alkalosis
- Check base excess: if it is negative then there is a metabolic acidosis; if it is positive then there is a metabolic alkalosis

Table 5A.1 Blood gases in non-pregnant and pregnant women

	pH	$PaCO_2$	Standard bicarbonate	Base excess	
Normal values	7.34–7.44	4.7–6.0 kPa	21–27 mmol/l	−2 to +2 mmol/l	
Values in pregnancy	7.40–7.46	3.7–4.2 kPa	18–21 mmol/l	No change	
	Increased	**Decreased**	**Decreased**		
Respiratory acidosis	↓	↑	↑	+ve	Hypoventilation leading eventually to compensatory renal retention of bicarbonate
Respiratory alkalosis	↑	↓	↓	−ve	Hyperventilation leading to renal excretion of bicarbonate
Metabolic acidosis	↓	↓	↓	−ve	Excess metabolic acid leading to respiratory hyperventilation to compensate Raised lactate in most types of shock
Metabolic alkalosis	↑		↑	+ve	Excess metabolic alkali but no respiratory compensation compensation

Appendix 5.2 Radiology in the pregnant woman

Imaging using ionising radiation is often part of the management of seriously ill patients. Patients and healthcare workers are often concerned that the doses of radiation used may be harmful to the fetus (Table 5A.2). A chest X-ray confers a minimal amount of radiation to the fetus and is the equivalent of 1 week of background radiation in London. If a chest X-ray is clinically indicated as a first line investigation in chest pain or breathlessness it should be performed.

Table 5A.2 Safety of different imaging techniques

Investigation	Radiation dose (mGy)	First trimester	Breastfeeding
Chest X-ray	<0.01	Safe	Safe
CT head scan*		Safe	Avoid
MRI head scan*		Avoid	Safe
CTPA*	<0.13	Safe	Avoid
V/Q scan		Safe	Avoid
CT abdomen*		Safe	Avoid
Ultrasound		Safe	Safe

* Express and discard breastmilk for 24 hours if using contrast.

Ultrasound, computed tomography (CT) scans of the head and chest and magnetic resonance imaging (MRI) are safe throughout pregnancy. Gadolinium contrast should be avoided.

For women with suspected pulmonary embolism and a normal chest X-ray, a lung perfusion scan should be requested in preference to CT pulmonary angiography (CTPA) because the radiation dose to maternal lung and breast tissue is lower.

Chapter 6: Shock

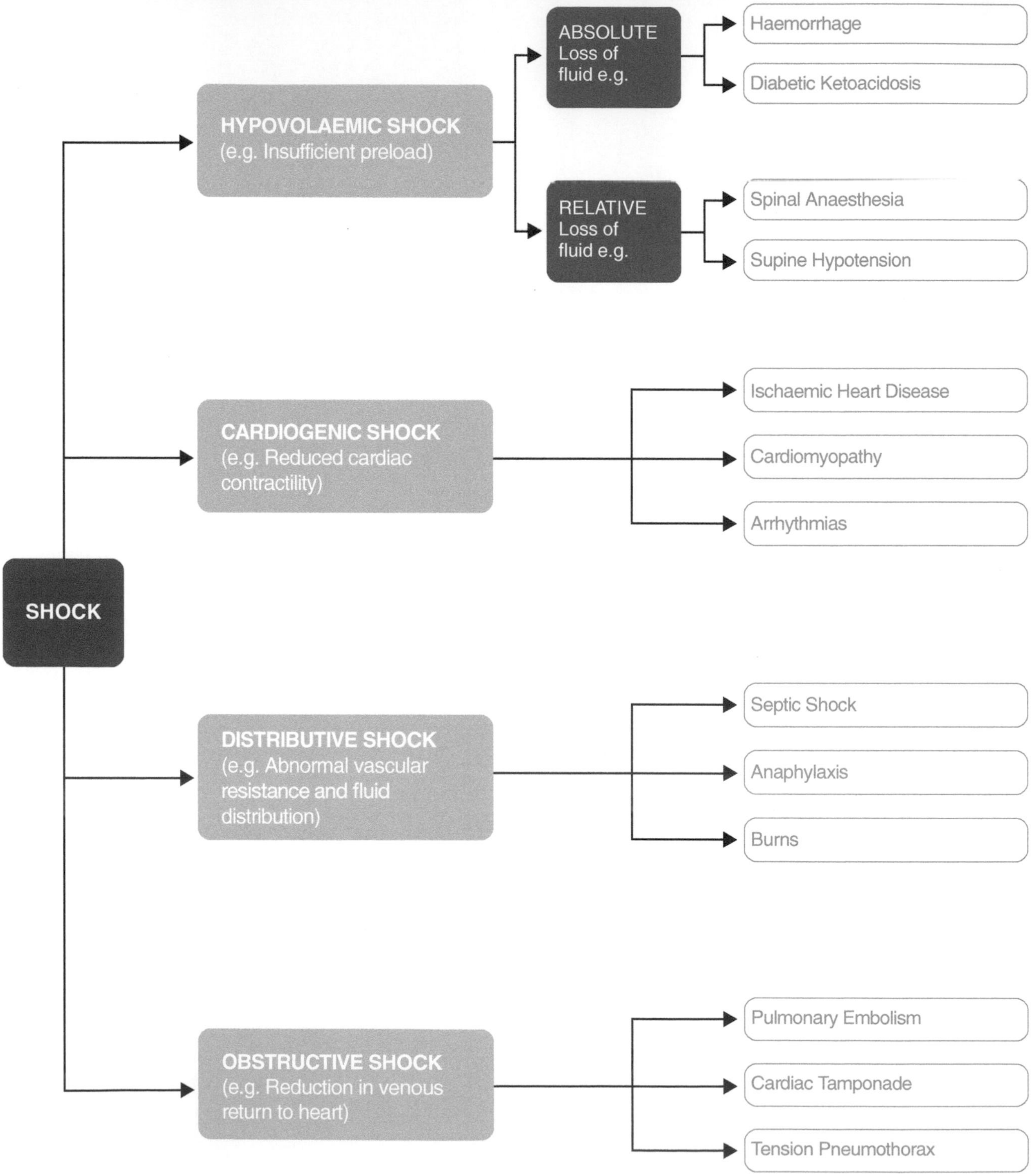

SHOCK
HYPOVOLAEMIC SHOCK (e.g. Insufficient preload)
ABSOLUTE Loss of fluid e.g.
Haemorrhage
Diabetic Ketoacidosis
RELATIVE Loss of fluid e.g.
Spinal Anaesthesia
Supine Hypotension
CARDIOGENIC SHOCK (e.g. Reduced cardiac contractility)
Ischaemic Heart Disease
Cardiomyopathy
Arrhythmias
DISTRIBUTIVE SHOCK (e.g. Abnormal vascular resistance and fluid distribution)
Septic Shock
Anaphylaxis
Burns
OBSTRUCTIVE SHOCK (e.g. Reduction in venous return to heart)
Pulmonary Embolism
Cardiac Tamponade
Tension Pneumothorax

Algorithm 6.1 Shock

CHAPTER 6
Shock

Learning outcomes

After reading this chapter, you will be able to:
- Define and recognise shock
- Discuss the principles of treatment of hypovolaemic shock
- Recognise the physiological changes to the cardiovascular system in pregnancy and how they affect the presentation of hypovolaemic shock
- Identify other shock syndromes and understand their management

6.1 Introduction

Shock is defined as a life-threatening failure of adequate oxygen delivery to the tissues. If left untreated, shock results in sustained multiple organ dysfunction, end-organ damage and death. It occurs when the cardiovascular response to systemic challenges such as blood loss or sepsis is inadequate.

Decreased blood perfusion of tissues, inadequate blood oxygen saturation or increased oxygen demand from the tissues result in failure of adequate oxygen delivery.

A reduction in cardiac output and a reduction in perfusion pressure will reduce the blood perfusion of tissues. Cardiac output is the product of stroke volume (the volume of blood pumped out of the heart with each beat) and heart rate.

Stroke volume is dependent on preload (filling status), cardiac contractility (pumping strength) and the afterload (vascular resistance – the resistance against which the myocardium has to pump). Shock may result if any of the these components are compromised.

During normal homeostasis, organ perfusion is regulated by local metabolic and microcirculatory factors within a set range of arterial pressures. This is called autoregulation. Beyond this range, blood flow to the organ is primarily determined by the pressure differential between the arterial and venous systems.

The blood supply to vital organs is maintained at lower blood pressures than that to non-vital organs. In shocked states, blood is preferentially supplied to the brain and the heart at the expense of perfusion elsewhere. Unfortunately for the fetus, the uterus does not count as one of the woman's vital organs, hence placental blood supply is not maintained in the presence of a life-threatening challenge to the mother. The resulting fetal compromise is an early and important indicator of maternal shock.

Managing Medical and Obstetric Emergencies and Trauma: A Practical Approach, Fourth Edition. Edited by Rosamunde Burns and Kara Dent.

6.2 Aortocaval compression and supine hypotension syndrome

In the pregnant woman in a supine position, the uterus compresses the vena cava, reducing venous return to the heart from 20 weeks' gestation. Vena caval obstruction and aortic compression can reduce cardiac output by up to 30%. The woman may experience symptoms such as nausea, vomiting or lightheadedness. This is known as supine hypotension syndrome. The reduction in venous return impacts on placental blood flow, which lacks autoregulation.

To prevent the effects of aortocaval compression, the pregnant woman should lie in the lateral position. Although a 15° tilt to the left (Figure 6.1b) is advocated there is evidence that the effects of compression still occur. Manual displacement of the uterus off the inferior vena cava up and to the left, relieves compression more effectively (Figure 6.1a). It is important to remember to relieve aortocaval compression in the initial management of the shocked woman to not exacerbate hypotension from other causes.

(a) (b)

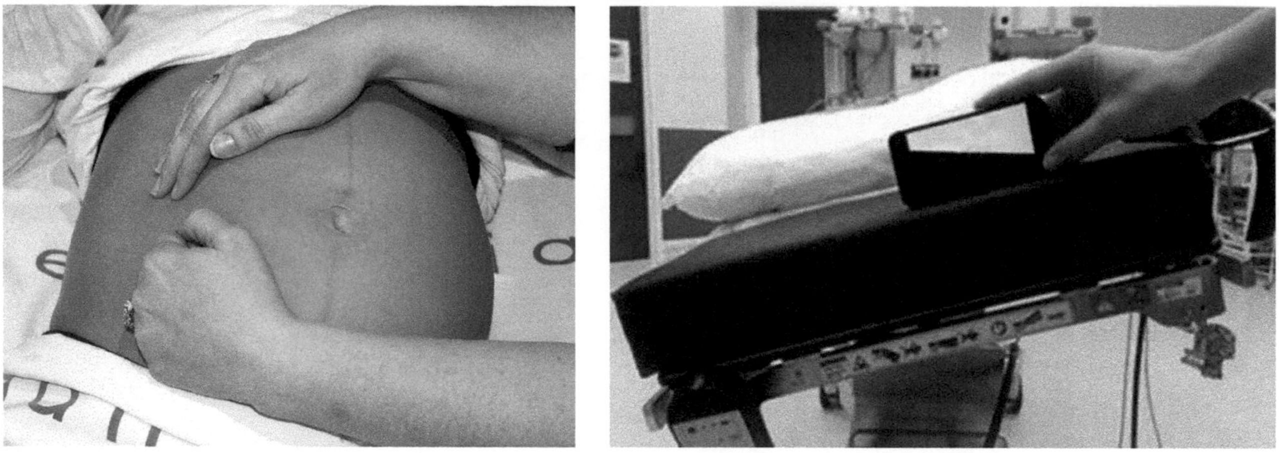

Figure 6.1 (a) Manual uterine displacement in the pregnant woman. (b) Fifteen degrees of left lateral tilt
Source: (a) Courtesy of Trauma Victoria – Obstetric Trauma guideline. http://trauma.reach.vic.gov.au/

To prompt manual uterine displacement (MUD) early in the process of resuscitation, remember:

> **'Hello. How are you Ms MUD?'**

6.3 Types of shock

Shock can be classified into four types:

- Hypovolaemic shock
- Cardiogenic shock
- Distributive shock
- Obstructive shock

In order to differentiate between these types of shock, clues can be gained from the history, examination, selected additional tests and the response to treatment.

Hypovolaemic shock: insufficient preload

- ***Absolute*** loss of fluid: e.g. haemorrhage
- ***Relative*** loss of fluid: vasodilatation, e.g. spinal/epidural anaesthesia

Absolute hypovolaemia – blood loss, fluid loss

This form of shock is due to a drop in the effective circulating volume resulting in a decrease in venous return. This causes a drop in stroke volume. There is usually a compensatory increase in heart rate to preserve cardiac output and also a compensatory increase in vascular resistance. This vasoconstriction, mediated by endogenous catecholamine release, increases the diastolic pressure without having the same effect on the systolic pressure thus there is a narrowed pulse pressure. Compensatory fluid shifts occur from the extravascular space into the vascular compartment, resulting in intracellular dehydration and a sensation of thirst.

Important implications of pregnancy physiology in haemorrhage

During pregnancy there is an increase in circulating blood volume of approximately 40% due to increases in both plasma and red cell volume. In a 70 kg woman, blood volume in pregnancy increases from 70 to 100 ml/kg (from 4900 to 7000 ml). This circulating volume enables the pregnant woman to lose 1200–1500 ml of blood before demonstrating any signs of hypovolaemia (35% of her circulating blood volume). This enhanced ability to compensate for blood loss increases our risk of underestimating the severity of blood loss, occasionally even until the point of maternal collapse.

Relative hypovolaemia – vasodilatation due to regional blockade

Intrathecal and to a lesser extent epidural local anaesthetics block the sympathetic nervous system, resulting in vasodilatation and hypotension. Usually there is a compensatory tachycardia associated with a fall in diastolic pressure. Subsequently, systolic blood pressure falls earlier than would occur during actual blood loss.

This sympathetic blockade exacerbates other simultaneous causes of hypotension such as haemorrhage and results in earlier decompensation.

A 'high' spinal will also affect the sympathetic nerves controlling the heart rate, causing a bradycardia and profound hypotension.

Cardiogenic shock – reduced cardiac contractility

Causes of cardiogenic shock include:

- Ischaemic heart disease
- Cardiomyopathy
- Arrhythmias

The distinguishing features of cardiogenic shock include orthopnoea and signs of pulmonary congestion, such as a raised jugular venous pressure, reduced oxygen saturation and basal pulmonary crackles. Symptoms and signs such as shortness of breath, chest pain, syncope, sweating, cool peripheries and tachycardia occur but are not specific to cardiogenic shock.

Distributive shock – abnormal vascular resistance and fluid distribution

The following pathologies can result in distributive shock:

- Sepsis
- Anaphylaxis
- Burns

Sepsis

In this form of shock (see Chapter 7), the patient will have signs and symptoms of systemic inflammation as well as those of the disease causing the sepsis. The pathological process is profound vasodilatation and hence these patients may have warm peripheries, particularly early in the process, despite being in shock. There is a compensatory tachycardia and increase in cardiac output to maintain perfusion pressure.

Varying degrees of organ dysfunction are seen, depending on the duration and degree of sepsis. In advanced stages of shock, the septic patient will become vasoconstricted, with cold extremities.

Anaphylaxis

Anaphylaxis is a severe, life-threatening, generalised, systemic hypersensitivity reaction to a trigger agent in which histamine, serotonin and other vasoactive substances are released. Anaphylactic reactions usually begin within 5–10 minutes of exposure to the trigger and the full reaction usually evolves within 30 minutes.

If anaphylaxis is suspected, samples for serial serum tryptase estimations should be taken. The enzyme tryptase is released from mast cells and it parallels histamine release. Peak concentrations well above 20 ng/ml indicate a true anaphylaxis/anaphylactic reaction. The peak value occurs anywhere between 30 minutes and 6 hours after exposure. Samples must be taken at the time of the acute event when the patient is stable, 1–2 hours later and a further sample at >24 hours.

Later investigation, after the acute event, involves skin testing to identify the presence of specific immunoglobulin E (IgE) antibodies. The value of skin tests, and especially the prick test, has been shown in extensive studies.

There are estimated to be 500 severe reactions in the UK each year. The estimated obstetric perioperative incidence of life-threatening allergic reactions is 3.4 per 100 000 anaesthetics (from the Royal College of Anaesthetists National Audit 6 published in 2017 (Kemp et al., 2017) or 1.2 per 100 000 maternities. This is significantly lower than the incidence in non-obstetric adult cases of 1 in 10 000 anaesthetics. The most frequent trigger agents perioperatively were antibiotics, neuromuscular blocking agents, chlorhexidine and patent blue dye. Anaphylaxis presented within 10 minutes of exposure to the triggering agent in 83% of cases; chlorhexidine and Patent Blue dye cases were slower to present. Hypotension was the presenting feature in 46% of the anaphylaxis cases and occurred during the reaction in all cases. Bronchospasm occurred in 49%. Urticaria and flushing were uncommon presenting features and skin signs were uncommon in the more severe reactions, sometimes only occurring after resuscitation. When the obstetric cases were examined the majority of patients were awake at the time of the reaction and complained of 'feeling unwell' before the onset of hypotension. Recognition of a critical event was prompt but recognition of anaphylaxis and starting anaphylaxis-specific treatment was slower than in non-obstetric cases. The report comments that this may have been because of the wider differential diagnosis for hypotension in the obstetric setting and that anaphylaxis was low on the list. Adrenaline was administered notably less often than in non-obstetric settings, which may have reflected the availability of phenylephrine in the obstetric setting. Maternal and neonatal outcomes were good however and there were no cardiac arrests.

Burns

The direct effect of the burn causes fluid loss from the body leading to hypovolaemic shock. In addition, inflammatory mediators are released causing a massive leak of fluid into the tissues, resulting in a problem of distribution. This topic is discussed further in Chapter 22.

Obstructive shock

Obstructive shock can result from the following:

- Massive pulmonary embolism (see Chapter 13)
- Cardiac tamponade (see Chapter 17)
- Tension pneumothorax (see Chapter 17)

This form of shock is due to a reduction in venous return to the heart. Patients, if conscious, are very dyspnoeic and struggle to sit upright, gasping for breath. Extreme tachycardia is a compensatory mechanism for compromised cardiac output. There will also be associated features of the pathology causing the obstruction of blood flow.

6.4 Symptoms and signs of shock

The signs and symptoms seen in the various forms of shock are primarily due to organ dysfunction resulting from inadequate tissue perfusion. The presentation is also partly influenced by the pathology causing the shock syndrome.

Hypovolaemic shock

This is the most common form of shock encountered on the labour ward. The signs of hypovolaemia are:

- Fetal heart rate abnormalities
- Increase in maternal heart rate
- Cold, pale, sweaty, cyanosed skin with delayed capillary refill
- Alteration of mental state
- Tachypnoea
- Fall in urine output
- Narrowed pulse pressure
- Hypotension (late sign)

Increase in heart rate

An increase in the heart rate occurs in compensation for hypovolaemia (1000–1500 ml blood loss) or vasodilatation, both of which can cause hypotension and shock. A maternal heart rate of more than 100 beats/min should be considered sinister, until proven otherwise. Most, but not all, women will become tachycardic if bleeding significantly, but paradoxical bradycardia also occurs. Vagal stimulation caused by cervical stimulation (e.g. products in the os) or peritoneal irritation can produce bradycardia profound enough to cause shock. Medications such a beta-blockers and labetalol (alpha- and beta-blocker) will prevent a tachycardic response to hypovolaemia and this may be falsely reassuring in the assessment of the bleeding patient.

Skin, capillary refill, mental state and urine output

The skin, kidneys and brain can be thought of as 'end organs' that reflect the adequacy of perfusion to tissues.

Capillary refill time (CRT)

This is an indication of skin perfusion. It can be assessed by compressing a fingernail, or pressing on the sternum, for 5 seconds. The test is normal if colour returns within 2 seconds of releasing compression (i.e. a CRT of less than 2 seconds – the time taken to say the words 'capillary refill'). If the patient is in a cold environment, CRT, especially peripherally, will be unreliable.

Mental state

If the woman is conscious and talking sensibly, she is not only breathing through an open airway, she is perfusing her cerebral cortex with sufficient oxygenated blood (50% of the normal cardiac output). Increasing hypovolaemia and subsequent cerebral hypoperfusion cause alterations in the level of consciousness. These alterations may begin with agitation and, if untreated, may proceed through confusion and aggression to eventual unresponsiveness and death.

Narrowed pulse pressure

This is caused by an increase in diastolic blood pressure, that reflects vasoconstriction occurring due to endogenous catecholamine release as a compensation for hypovolaemia.

Systolic hypotension

The sign most commonly referred to in the context of shock, hypotension, is a very late sign in the obstetric population, developing only when significant blood loss has occurred. A successful outcome for the patient depends on the early recognition of shock, restoration of volume and control of haemorrhage.

Recognition of hypovolaemia

Maternal blood loss can be categorised into four classes of severity, as shown in Table 6.1 and graphically in Figure 6.2.

To remember the different percentages in these classes of blood loss, think of the way of scoring in a tennis match!

Figure 6.2 illustrates the various clinical signs seen in ongoing acute blood loss suffered by a pregnant woman related to the volume lost. The point where the pulse rate is a higher number than the systolic blood pressure is a sign of significant decompensation.

Table 6.1 Severity of blood loss during maternal haemorrhage

Class	Loss of circulating volume (%)	Blood loss in a 70 kg pregnant woman (ml)	Signs and symptoms
I	0–15	<1000	Fully compensated due to blood diversion from the splanchnic pool. No symptoms. Minimal tachycardia is likely to be the only abnormal sign. No treatment needed in an otherwise healthy woman as long as the bleeding has stopped
II	15–30	1000–2000	Peripheral vasoconstriction maintains systolic blood pressure. The woman may be aware of increased heart rate and may display agitation or aggression. Narrowed pulse pressure and tachypnoea are the keys to early detection, as heart rate is only modestly increased and systolic blood pressure remains normal. Peripheral vasoconstriction maintains blood pressure. Requires crystalloid fluid replacement
III	30–40	2000–2700	Cardiovascular system shows signs of decompensation. The woman will look unwell. Tachycardia, tachypnoea, changes in mental status, fall in systolic blood pressure. Will require crystalloid and potential blood transfusion
IV	>40	>2700	Immediately life threatening. Tachycardia, fall in blood pressure, altered mental status, evidence of negligible urine output. Loss of >50% results in loss of consciousness, requiring immediate -surgery as well as massive transfusion

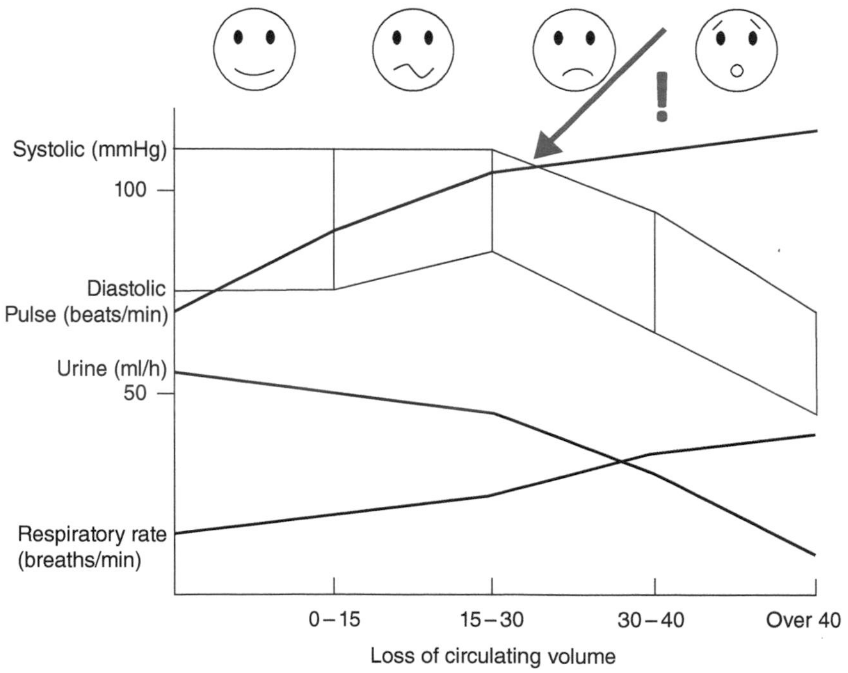

Figure 6.2 Clinical parameters following increasing blood loss in the pregnant and postpartum woman

Pitfalls in the recognition of shock in pregnancy

- Some pregnant women do not mount a tachycardia, or can even produce a bradycardia. This can be paradoxical, due to vagal stimulation [see above] or if the woman is taking beta-blocker medication
- Women with pacemakers have a fixed upper heart rate
- Athletes may have a very slow baseline heart rate
- Haemoglobin concentration is a useful measure of blood loss, only after there has been fluid resuscitation

During the acute phases of loss, the haemoglobin concentration will not change. Rapid movement of fluid from the extracellular to the intravascular compartment and intravenous clear fluids, will result in a fall in haematocrit. A falling haematocrit may be the only indicator of a slow steady bleed. A rapidly falling haematocrit associated with early signs of hypovolaemia is suggestive of severe loss.

6.5 Principles of treatment

Hypovolaemic shock

Primary survey and resuscitation should be carried out according to the ABC principles. See Chapter 10 for the management of A and B.

C: Circulation

A diagnosis of hypovolaemic shock must be promptly followed by:

- Restoration of adequate oxygen delivery to the tissues by restoration of adequate circulating volume and adequate oxygen carrying capacity (see Chapter 8 for intravenous fluids)
- Stopping the bleeding (see Chapter 28 for major obstetric haemorrhage)

Consider haemorrhage to be of two types:

- Compressible
- Non-compressible

Compressible haemorrhage is controllable by direct pressure, limb elevation, packing, by reduction and immobilisation of fractures or, in obstetric situations, compression of the uterus.

Non-compressible haemorrhage occurs in a body cavity (chest, abdomen, pelvis or retroperitoneum). See Chapters 17, 18 and 21 for haemorrhage in trauma.

Septic shock

Septic shock complicating delivery may be caused by infection from the genital tract, but can occur with any source of infection, for example a urinary tract or chest infection.

The development of shock is due to a dysregulated systemic inflammatory and immune response to microbial invasion that results in vasodilatation, hypotension and organ dysfunction. Septic patients have a metabolic acidosis with a raised lactate, detectable on sampling of arterial or venous blood.

In trauma patients, sepsis is unlikely to cause shock at presentation. It is most likely to develop later in patients with penetrating abdominal injuries and in whom the peritoneal cavity has been contaminated by intestinal contents.

The key to management is a high degree of suspicion, rapid diagnosis and urgent treatment, as perinatal sepsis is a rapidly progressive disease. Pregnant women with septic shock will require early referral to critical care. See Chapter 7 for further information on maternal septic shock.

Cardiogenic shock

Cardiogenic shock in pregnancy is a life-threatening condition due to failure of the ventricles to produce an adequate cardiac output. Ischaemic heart disease, valvular heart disease, arrhythmia, cardiomyopathy and pulmonary and amniotic fluid embolism are the main causes of cardiogenic shock in pregnancy.

In trauma, patients can develop cardiogenic shock due to penetrating injury, cardiac tamponade, tension pneumothorax and myocardial contusion.

There is a significant overlap in the signs and symptoms between these forms of shock and hypovolaemic shock. One distinguishing feature is the extreme air hunger and orthopnoea seen in patients suffering cardiogenic shock. Listening to the chest may give clues of congestion due to increased pressure in the pulmonary circulation causing pulmonary oedema.

Cardiogenic shock has a high mortality and mandates multidisciplinary consultant management with involvement from cardiology, cardiac surgery and critical care. Transfer to a centre able to offer complex invasive cardiac support may be required.

Anaphylactic shock

The diagnosis is made on clinical grounds and should be considered if the patient develops:

- Unexplained hypotension or bronchospasm
- Unexplained tachycardia or bradycardia
- Angioedema (often absent in severe cases)
- Unexplained cardiac arrest where other causes are excluded
- Cutaneous flushing in association with one or more of the above signs (often absent in severe cases)

Box 6.1 Management of anaphylactic shock

- Stop administration of drug(s)/blood product likely to have caused anaphylaxis
- Resuscitation as for any collapse following ABC principles with reassessment
- The key treatment therapies are *oxygen, adrenaline* and *fluids*. Adrenaline is very effective and should be given as early as possible
- Cardiopulmonary resuscitation (CPR) should be considered when systolic blood pressure is <50 mmHg or the patient is in cardiac arrest

Source: Adapted from AAGBI (Association of Anaesthetists of Great Britain and Ireland). *Quick Reference Handbook 3-1 Anaphylaxis*, 2019

Treatment of anaphylactic shock (Box 6.1) is as follows:

1. Call for help and note the time.
2. Call for cardiac arrest trolley, anaphylaxis treatment and investigation pack (should be in theatre recovery – familiarise where it is kept in your unit).
3. Remove all potential causative agents.
4. Manual uterine displacement.
5. Open and maintain airway. Give high-flow/100% oxygen and ensure adequate ventilation. Intubation may be required for severe stridor or cardiorespiratory collapse.
6. Elevate the legs if there is hypotension.
7. If systolic blood pressure is <50 mmHg or there is cardiac arrest start CPR.
8. Give drugs to treat hypotension:
   - **Adrenaline** 0.5 mg (0.5 ml of 1:1000) intramuscularly every 5 minutes until there is improvement in the pulse and blood pressure. Intravenous adrenaline may be used by experienced (anaesthetic) staff in a monitored patient in 50 microgram boluses (0.5 ml of 1:10 000) titrated against response.
     If intravenous access proves difficult obtain intraosseous access. ***Hypotension may be resistant and require prolonged treatment.***
     Consider starting an adrenaline infusion after three boluses: 5 mg in 500 ml dextrose (1:100 000) titrated to effect, or 3 mg in 50 ml 0.9% saline started at 3 ml/h (= 3 micrograms/min) titrated to maximum of 40 ml/h (40 micrograms/min).
   - **Glucagon** 1 mg repeated as necessary in beta-blocked patient unresponsive to adrenaline.
     If hypotension resistant give alternate vasopressor: metaraminol, noradrenaline or vasopressin.
9. Intravascular volume expansion with crystalloid 20 ml/kg: initial bolus repeated until hypotension is resolved.
10. Other drugs that can be given:
    - **Hydrocortisone** 200 mg intravenously.
    - **Chlorphenamine** 10 mg intravenously.
11. If there is persistent bronchospasm despite an adequate dose of adrenaline to stabilise the blood pressure, consider bronchodilators, e.g.:
    - **Salbutamol** 5 mg via oxygen-driven nebuliser, or 250 micrograms diluted intravenous slow bolus.
    - **Magnesium sulphate** 2 g intravenously over 20 minutes.
    - **Aminophylline** 5 mg/kg intravenously over 20 minutes if not already taking theophylline.

12. Check fetal heart and continuously monitor by cardiotocography. If in cardiac arrest, perform perimortem section. If not in cardiac arrest, consider timing and method of delivery once maternal status is stabilised.
13. Take a 5–10 ml clotted blood sample for serum tryptase as soon as the patient is stable. Plan for repeat sample at 1–2 hours and >24 hours.
14. Plan to insert arterial and central venous pressure lines and transfer the patient to a critical care area.
15. Prevent readministration of possible trigger agents (allergy band, update notes and drug chart, liaise with anaphylaxis lead regarding ongoing investigation and referral (www.bsaci.org) to identify causative agent). Inform the patient, obstetric consultant and GP and report to the Medicines and Healthcare products Regulatory Agency (MHRA, www.mhra.gov.uk/yellowcard).

6.6 Summary

- Hypovolaemia is the most common cause of shock in obstetric and trauma patients
- A high index of suspicion is essential during assessment to ensure early recognition and prompt resuscitation
- In haemorrhagic shock, management requires replacement of lost volume and oxygen carrying capacity, prevention of coagulopathy and immediate control of haemorrhage either by direct compression, splintage or, where necessary, by urgent surgery
- Other forms of shock require equal vigilance and early resuscitative measures to restore circulation and tissue perfusion

6.7 Further reading

Kemp HI, Cook TM, Harper NJN. UK anaesthetists' perspectives and experiences of severe perioperative anaphylaxis. *Br J Anaesth* 2017; 119: 132–9. (Gives details of the Sixth National Audit Project (NAP6).)

NAP (National Audit Projects). https://www.nationalauditprojects.org.uk/NAP6home (last accessed January 2022). (Gives resources for the management, investigation and communication required following life-threatening anaphylaxis.)

SEPSIS SCREENING TOOL - THE SEPSIS SIX

PREGNANT
OR UP TO 6 WEEKS POST-PREGNANCY

PATIENT DETAILS:

DATE:
NAME:
DESIGNATION:
SIGNATURE:

TIME:

COMPLETE ALL ACTIONS WITHIN ONE HOUR

01 ENSURE SENIOR CLINICIAN ATTENDS
NAME: GRADE:

TIME
☐☐:☐☐

02 OXYGEN IF REQUIRED
START IF O SATURATIONS LESS THAN 92% - AIM FOR O_2 SATURATIONS OF 94–98%
IF AT RISK OF HYPERCARBIA AIM FOR SATURATIONS OF 88–92%

TIME
☐☐:☐☐

03 OBTAIN IV ACCESS, TAKE BLOODS
BLOOD CULTURES, BLOOD GLUCOSE, LACTATE, FBC, U&Es, CRP AND CLOTTING
LUMBAR PUNCTURE IF INDICATED

TIME
☐☐:☐☐

04 GIVE IV ANTIBIOTICS
MAXIMUM DOSE BROAD SPECTRUM THERAPY
CONSIDER: LOCAL POLICY / ALLERGY STATUS / ANTIVIRALS

TIME
☐☐:☐☐

05 GIVE IV FLUIDS
GIVE FLUID BOLUS OF 20 ml/kg if age <16, 500 ml if 16+
NICE RECOMMENDS USING LACTATE TO GUIDE FURTHER FLUID THERAPY

TIME
☐☐:☐☐

06 MONITOR
USE NEWS-2. MEASURE URINARY OUTPUT: THIS MAY REQUIRE A URINARY CATHETER REPEAT LACTATE
AT LEAST ONCE PER HOUR IF INITIAL LACTATE ELEVATED OR IF CLINICAL CONDITION CHANGES

TIME
☐☐:☐☐

RED FLAGS AFTER ONE HOUR – ESCALATE TO CONSULTANT NOW

RECORD ADDITIONAL NOTES HERE:
e.g. allergy status, arrival of specialist teams, variance from Sepsis Six

THE UK
SEPSIS
TRUST

UKST 2019 1.2 PAGE 2 OF 2 / UKST, REGISTERED CHARITY 1158843

Algorithm 7.1 The Sepsis Six
Source: Nutbeam T, Daniels R on behalf of the UK Sepsis Trust. © 2019 UK Sepsis Trust

CHAPTER 7
Sepsis

Learning outcomes

After reading this chapter, you will be able to:
- Recognise the septic woman
- Commence emergency management
- Arrange appropriate investigations and referral

7.1 Introduction and definition

Worldwide sepsis causes 1 in 10 maternal deaths and is the third commonest cause of direct maternal death (Turner, 2019). To reduce *avoidable* deaths, women with sepsis need to be *recognised* so that treatment can be *initiated early*.

In 2017 the World Health Organization (WHO) defined maternal sepsis as **a life-threatening condition defined as organ dysfunction resulting from infection during pregnancy, childbirth, post-abortion, or postpartum period** (Figure 7.1).

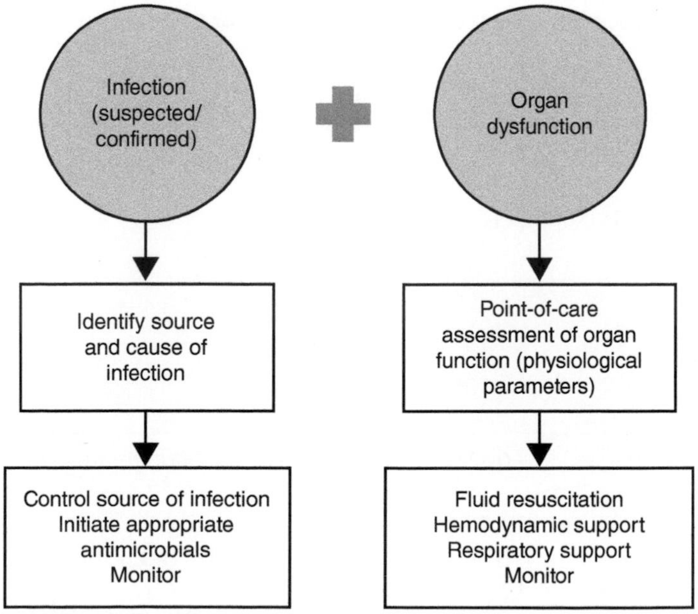

Figure 7.1 Approach for implementation of the new WHO definition of maternal sepsis
Source: Statement on maternal sepsis, WHO. © 2017 WHO

Managing Medical and Obstetric Emergencies and Trauma: A Practical Approach, Fourth Edition. Edited by Rosamunde Burns and Kara Dent.

The Third International Consensus (2016) definition of sepsis (SEPSIS-3) for the whole adult population is that **sepsis is a life-threatening organ dysfunction due to a dysregulated host response to infection.**

Septic shock is a life-threatening condition that is characterised by low blood pressure despite adequate fluid replacement, and organ dysfunction or failure. The Third International Consensus definition (SEPSIS-3) of septic shock is **persisting hypotension requiring vasopressors to maintain mean arterial pressure of 65 mmHg or more and having a serum lactate of greater than 2 mmol/l despite adequate volume resuscitation.**

These definitions depend on the identification of organ dysfunction in the presence of infection. In the general adult population, a brief bedside tool such as the quick SOFA (**s**equential **o**rgan **f**ailure **a**ssessment) or qSOFA score is used as described in SEPSIS-3. The qSOFA score evaluates the presence of three clinical criteria: systolic blood pressure ≤100 mmHg, respiratory rate ≥22 per minute and altered mental status. If two or more of these criteria are present *the patient is at increased risk* of a poor sepsis-related outcome and urgent action is prompted. An obstetric modified qSOFA has been produced by the Society of Obstetric Medicine Australia and New Zealand and modifies the systolic blood pressure to ≤90 mmHg, respiratory rate ≥25 per minute and altered mental state. Table 7.1 summarises the organ damage by system caused by sepsis.

Table 7.1 Organ damage caused by sepsis

Organ system	Clinical features
Central nervous system	Altered mental status
Cardiovascular system dysfunction	Hypotension from vasodilatation and third spacing; myocardial
Pulmonary system	Acute respiratory distress syndrome (ARDS)
Gastrointestinal	Paralytic Ileus
Hepatic system	Hepatic failure or abnormal transaminases
Urinary system	Oliguria or acute kidney injury
Haematological system	Thrombocytopenia or disseminated intravascular coagulation
Endocrine system	Adrenal dysfunction and increased insulin resistance

Source: Plant LA, Pacheco LD, Louis JM. Sepsis during pregnancy and the puerperium. SMFM Consult Series No. 47: *Am J Obstet Gynecol* 2019; 220(4): B2–B10. © 2019 Elsevier

Although people with sepsis may have an infection, *fever is not always present*. The signs and symptoms of sepsis can be non-specific and can be missed if clinicians do not think 'Could this be sepsis?'

The **key actions for the diagnosis and management of sepsis** (Knight et al., 2014, 2017) are:

- Timely recognition
- Fast administration of antibiotics
- Quick involvement of experts – senior review is essential

7.2 Sepsis in pregnancy

- Pregnant women have **increased susceptibility** to some infectious diseases, e.g. *Plasmodium falciparum* and *Listeria monoctogenes*
- In advanced pregnancy there are immunological changes that *decrease adaptive immunity* such that increased severity of infection is seen where cell-mediated immunity is important. Pregnant women are more **severely affected** by influenza virus, hepatitis E virus, herpes simplex virus and malaria parasites
- The physiological changes of pregnancy that reduce lung capacity and promote urinary stasis may promote more severe infection

The 2014 MBRRACE-UK report highlighted a substantial number of women who died following infection with influenza and the recommendation was made for influenza vaccination in pregnancy. The 2017 MBRRACE-UK report re-emphasised that pregnant women with influenza were dying from a **vaccine preventable disease** and that the messages around vaccination and treatment of influenza needed to be embedded to prevent deaths and to prepare for a future pandemic. Staff should **remain aware of the possibility of influenza infection** especially during peak seasonal periods. The Covid-19 pandemic has highlighted these messages once again.

Antepartum causes of sepsis are commonly non-pelvic in origin. Intrapartum and postpartum sepsis is more likely to be pelvic in origin. The classification of maternal infection is given in Box 7.1.

Box 7.1 Classification of maternal infection aligned with the WHO classification of maternal death

1. Pregnancy-specific infections:
   - Chorioamnionitis
   - Endometritis
   - Lactational mastitis
   - Site of perineal trauma
   - Surgical site, e.g. caesarean
2. Infections exacerbated by pregnancy, including:
   - Urinary tract infection
   - Influenza
   - Listeriosis
   - Hepatitis E
   - Herpes simplex virus
   - Malaria
3. Incidental infections, including:
   - Lower respiratory tract infections
   - Acute appendicitis
   - Acute cholecystitis
   - Acute pancreatitis
   - Necrotising fasciitis
   - Tuberculosis
   - Sexually transmitted diseases

Source: Turner MJ. Maternal sepsis is an evolving challenge. *Int J Gynecol Obstet* 2019: 146: 39–42. © 2019 John Wiley & Sons

7.3 Pathophysiology of sepsis

Once an infective agent enters the body it binds to the surface of immune cells such as macrophages and monocytes and initiates the immune and coagulation cascades. This involves the release of both pro- and anti-inflammatory cytokines along with pro-coagulant mediators which activate the extrinsic coagulation pathway and inhibit fibrinolysis. Infection becomes sepsis when the balance of pro- and anti-inflammatory mechanisms tips towards pro-inflammation.

The pro-inflammatory cytokines cause endothelial dysfunction and leaky capillaries resulting in vasodilatation and maldistribution of fluid. Activation of the extrinsic coagulation cascade and inhibition of fibrinolysis results in the formation of thrombi in the microcirculation. These thrombi then compromise organ perfusion, resulting in impaired delivery of oxygen to tissues and organs. If unchecked, this can lead to multiorgan failure and ultimately death.

Clinical manifestations of haemodynamic alterations

There is a decrease in arteriolar and venous tone. This causes venous pooling of blood and a drop in vascular resistance, resulting in hypotension. In the initial stages of sepsis, there is hypotension with reduced cardiac output and low filling pressures. With fluid resuscitation, cardiac output increases, resulting in a hyperdynamic circulation, but there is not much change in blood pressure owing to a reduced vascular resistance. There is an increase in pulmonary vascular resistance, resulting in raised pulmonary arterial pressures. The changes in the vascular tone differ in different vascular beds, resulting in the maldistribution of blood volume and flow. There is evidence to suggest that the ability of tissues to extract oxygen is impaired owing to mitochondrial dysfunction. This encourages anaerobic metabolism in tissues, promoting lactic acidosis.

7.4 Microbiology

A study of severe maternal sepsis in the UK (2011–2012) identified genital tract infection (31%) and the organisim *Escherichia coli* (21%) to be the most common causes, followed by group A *Streptococcus*, group B *Streptococcus*, other streptococci and *Staphylococcus*. Risk factors for severe sepsis were if the woman was black or of other ethnic minority, primiparous, had a pre-existing medical problem, had a febrile illness or were taking antibiotics in the 2 weeks preceding presentation, operative vaginal delivery or caesarean. Median time between delivery and sepsis was 3 days. Multiple pregnancy and group A *Streptococcus* were associated with progression to septic shock. *In the women with group A streptococcal infection the progression of sepsis was often rapid.* For each maternal sepsis death, 50 women had life-threatening morbidity from sepsis.

A study from Ireland (2005–2012) looking at maternal bacteraemia again found *E. coli* to be the predominant pathogen followed by group B *Streptococcus*. The source of infection was the genital tract in 61% of cases and the urinary tract in 25%; 17% of sepsis episodes occurred antenatally, 36% intrapartum and 47% postpartum. Sepsis was associated with preterm delivery and a high perinatal mortality rate. The most virulent organisms were group A streptococci associated with postpartum sepsis at term and *E. coli* sepsis preterm.

Group A *Streptococcus* is a common skin or throat commensal, carried asymptomatically by up to 30% of the population. It is easily spread and is responsible for streptococcal sore throat, a very common childhood condition. Worldwide, however, group A *Streptococcus* is still the most common cause of postpartum maternal death and can kill pregnant and recently pregnant women with devastating speed. The initial presentation can be vague and non-specific, thus delaying treatment. Primary symptoms include myalgia, fever, mild confusion, dizziness and abdominal pain.

Transmission in pregnant women is thought to be either through the blood stream with the throat as a portal of entry, or via the perineal route with translocation from colonisation in the vagina, even in the presence of an intact membrane, as bacteria can cross this apparent barrier. Translocation from the vagina may occur from nosocomial exposure at birth or via a caesarean section incision. Streptococcal infection has a seasonal rise in incidence between December and April in the northern hemisphere. The link between pregnant women and children with group A streptococcal sore throats is thought to be significant as a possible source of infection.

In the past, there was an emphasis on the transmission of infection from care-givers to women, much reduced since the advent of strict hygiene practices in hospitals. It is thought that raising public health awareness of the risks from family members and encouraging women to follow appropriate personal hygiene practices may be helpful in reducing transmission of infection; in particular, pregnant women should be encouraged **to handwash both before and after using the toilet** to avoid transmitting organisms from other household members.

7.5 Clinical issues and presentation

Minimising risk from infection in the antenatal period, by avoiding unnecessary vaginal examinations and paying attention to hygiene, may reduce the incidence of sepsis. Early recognition and increased surveillance of those at risk including careful assessment of postnatal mothers, especially those with prolonged rupture of membranes, ragged membranes or possible incomplete delivery of the placenta and women with uterine tenderness or enlargement, will help to identify women developing serious infection. Multiple presentations should be seen as a red flag and requires careful review with escalation to senior staff for assessment.

Symptoms of sepsis may include:

- Feeling unwell, anxious or distressed
- Shivery or feverish
- Sore throat, cough or influenza-like symptoms (pneumonia accounts for a significant number of admissions to the intensive care unit in pregnant women in the antenatal period)
- Rash (see Appendix 7.1 for weblink to assessment of pregnant woman reporting viral rash illness)
- Chest pain
- Vomiting and/or diarrhoea
- Abdominal pain, uterine and renal angle pain, and beware 'after pains' of a severity that is out of proportion to the known cause and not responding to usual analgesia
- Wound tenderness
- If pregnant may report reduced fetal movements
- Offensive vaginal discharge
- Persistent vaginal bleeding may be a sign of uterine sepsis
- Breast tenderness, suggesting mastitis
- Headache
- Unexplained physical symptoms

A high index of suspicion and close surveillance will help in identifying women with early sepsis. When assessing a woman who is unwell, revisit the history and consider her clinical condition in addition to the modified early obstetric warning score (MEOWS) and do not be reassured by a single set of observations on the MEOWS chart (Knight et al., 2017). *Chronic illness and immunosuppression* are risk factors for sepsis. Immunosuppression puts a woman at higher risk of rapid deterioration from sepsis, and sepsis should be considered a likely cause when they are unwell.

Serious clinical signs can be categorised as **red and amber flags**.

The Sepsis Trust UK Sepsis Screening Tool for Acute Assessment of the pregnant or up to 6 weeks' post-pregnancy woman is reproduced in Figure 7.2 and defines the red and amber flags.

SEPSIS SCREENING TOOL ACUTE ASSESSMENT

PREGNANT
OR UP TO 6 WEEKS POST-PREGNANCY

PATIENT DETAILS:

DATE: **TIME:**
NAME:
DESIGNATION:
SIGNATURE:

01 START THIS CHART IF THE PATIENT LOOKS UNWELL OR MEOWS HAS TRIGGERED

RISK FACTORS FOR SEPSIS INCLUDE:

- ☐ Impaired immunity (e.g. diabetes, steroids, chemotherapy)
- ☐ Recent trauma / surgery / invasive procedure
- ☐ Indwelling lines / IVDU / broken skin

YES

02 COULD THIS BE DUE TO AN INFECTION?

LIKELY SOURCE:

- ☐ Respiratory
- ☐ Breast abscess
- ☐ Urine
- ☐ Abdominal pain / distension
- ☐ Infected caesarean / perineal wound
- ☐ Chorioamnionitis / endometritis

NO → **SEPSIS UNLIKELY, CONSIDER OTHER DIAGNOSIS**

YES

03 ANY RED FLAG PRESENT?

- ☐ Objective evidence of new or altered mental state
- ☐ Systolic BP ≤ 90 mmHg (or drop of >40 from normal)
- ☐ Heart rate ≥ 130 per minute
- ☐ Respiratory rate ≥ 25 per minute
- ☐ Needs O_2 to keep SpO_2 ≥ 92%
- ☐ Non-blanching rash / mottled / ashen / cyanotic
- ☐ Lactate ≥ 2 mmol/l*
- ☐ Not passed urine in 18 hours (<0.5ml/kg/hr if catheterised)

*lactate may be raised in & immediately after normal delivery

YES → **RED FLAG SEPSIS**
START SEPSIS SIX

NO

04 ANY AMBER FLAG PRESENT?

- ☐ Acute deterioration in functional ability
- ☐ Respiratory rate 21 – 24
- ☐ Heart rate 100 – 129 or new dysrhythmia
- ☐ Systolic BP 91 – 100 mmHg
- ☐ Has had invasive procedure in last 6 weeks (e.g. CS, forceps delivery, ERPC, cerclage, CVs, miscarriage, termination)
- ☐ Temperature < 36°C
- ☐ Has diabetes or gestational diabetes
- ☐ Close contact with GAS
- ☐ Prolonged rupture of membranes
- ☐ Bleeding / wound infection
- ☐ Offensive vaginal discharge
- ☐ Non-reassuring CTG / fetal tachycardia >160
- ☐ Behavioural / mental status change

YES → **FURTHER REVIEW REQUIRED:**

- SEND BLOODS AND REVIEW RESULTS
- ENSURE SENIOR CLINICAL REVIEW within 1HR

TIME OF REVIEW: ■■ : ■■
ANTIBIOTICS REQUIRED:
■ Yes ■ No

NO AMBER FLAGS = ROUTINE CARE /CONSIDER OTHER DIAGNOSIS

THE UK SEPSIS TRUST

UKST 2019 1.2 PAGE 1 OF 2 / UKST, REGISTERED CHARITY 1158843

Figure 7.2 Sepsis Trust UK Sepsis Screening Tool for Acute Assessment
Source: Nutbeam T, Daniels R on behalf of the UK Sepsis Trust. © 2019 UK Sepsis Trust

7.6 Monitoring, investigations and urgent treatment

Monitor women who have red and amber flags with suspected sepsis continuously and record using a MEWS chart (NICE, 2016). The conscious level should also be monitored using **ACVPU** (**a**lert, new **c**onfusion, responds to **v**oice, responds to **p**ain, **u**nconscious). A **sepsis care bundle** must be applied in a structured and systemic way with **urgency.** The time to administration of antibiotics is a predictor of mortality in sepsis, **do not delay** and use local antibiotic prescribing guidance. Antiviral medication may also be appropriate. The woman must be continually reassessed and **senior review** is essential. Consider 'declaring sepsis', analogous to activation of the major obstetric haemorrhage protocol.

The UK Sepsis Trust recommends the Sepsis Six (Algorithm 7.1) **with all actions to be completed within 1 hour**.

> **You can think of it as:**
> **'3 in, 3 out": fluids, antibiotics and oxygen in / catheter, lactate and blood cultures out.**

Initial blood tests include **lactate** – either arterial if there is evidence of hypoxia or a venous sample. Any woman in whom sepsis is suspected, who has a lactate >2 mmol/l, needs to have resuscitation started immediately. Raised serum lactate is a marker for poor perfusion and tissue hypoxia from whatever cause and signifies severe illness.

Additional blood tests include blood cultures, full blood count, coagulation screen, urea and electrolytes, blood glucose, liver profile and C-reactive protein (CRP). Consider urinalysis, urine for culture, sputum culture, vaginal swabs, breast milk culture and throat swabs. Consider a chest x-ray in all with suspected sepsis. Consider imaging of the abdomen and pelvis if no likely source of infection is identified after clinical examination and initial tests.

Airway and breathing

Maintenance of adequate oxygenation is an important step in the resuscitation of women with sepsis. This includes a patent airway with adequate breathing and supplemental oxygen. Most patients in shock will ultimately need intubation and ventilation because of increased difficulty in breathing, development of acute respiratory distress syndrome (ARDS) or for primary underlying disease.

Fluids

Use 20 ml/kg crystalloid as an initial bolus of fluids over 30 minutes whilst looking for haemodynamic improvement. Hypovolaemia is demonstrated when elevation of the legs transiently improves blood pressure. Recording of accurate fluid balance is essential.

Fluid balance is difficult in septic shock, as there will be an inevitable tendency of fluid to leak into the lungs as a result of increased capillary permeability, myocardial dysfunction, renal impairment and a low plasma oncotic pressure. If there is no improvement in the blood pressure following the fluid bolus, **critical care referral is required**.

Vasopressors

In patients who remain hypotensive, despite adequate fluid resuscitation, early recourse to vasopressor therapy is recommended with invasive arterial and central venous pressure monitoring. The target blood pressure should be a mean arterial pressure of >65 mmHg.

Noradrenaline administered centrally is the vasopressor of choice but can be started peripherally if urgent, under guidance from the anaesthetic and critical care team. Adrenaline may be added if poorly responsive. Sensitivity to catecholamines is significantly altered in septic patients and they require much higher doses than in other clinical situations.

Early source identification and control of infection

On examination look for sources of infection that may require surgical drainage or surgical excision of infected tissue, and tailor the investigations to the history and examination findings. Mortality reports emphasize that the *recognition of the genital tract as the source of infection is often delayed* with over-reliance on antibiotics to control the infection. Imaging is often delayed in those cases of women who die from sepsis and there is a reluctance to undertake surgical measures.

- Identify source of infection as rapidly as possible; imaging and repeat imaging may be required
- Closed-space infections need surgical drainage, including evacuation of retained products of conception
- In women with endometritis not responding to antibiotics, a septic pelvic thrombosis should be considered; these patients will require anticoagulation together with antibiotics
- Women not responding may have myometrial necrosis and/or abscess formation, which continues to seed into the blood stream; in these cases, early surgical intervention, with possible recourse to hysterectomy, could save lives
- Necrotising fasciitis is another condition that requires early surgical intervention with fasciotomy and aggressive antibiotic therapy

Influenza A/H1N1

There has been a surge of deaths due to influenza in recent years. Pregnant women have been found to be seven times more likely to die from this illness than non-pregnant women in the same age group. Among this population:

- Minority ethnic groups were over-represented
- Clinical co-morbidities contributed, e.g. asthma, paraplegia, scoliosis
- None of the women who died had been vaccinated
- Presenting features were similar to any severe illness with tachycardia, tachypnoea and variable hypoxia
- CRP was unusually raised – which is not common with viral infections

Treatment

There were a number of delays documented in the women who died in recognising the illness, both in making the diagnosis and in administering oseltamivir. Women died from pneumonia or ARDS and some from complications of the extracorporeal membrane oxygen (ECMO) treatment used to try to maintain oxygenation.

Recommendations

- Maintain a high index of suspicion
- Ensure good multidisciplinary team working and planning
- Perform a basic check of O_2 saturation in all women presenting with respiratory symptoms
- Breathlessness as a symptom must be taken very seriously: remember it may be respiratory, cardiac or relate to a metabolic disturbance such as diabetic ketoacidosis
- Viral swabs should be taken and antivirals started immediately
- Antivirals can be started even if further imaging is planned
- Pay attention to infection control when the patient is admitted
- Give advice to pregnant women to be vaccinated with seasonal influenza vaccination

SARS-CoV-2

The common symptoms of Covid-19 in pregnancy are cough, fever, sore throat, shortness of breath, myalgia and loss of sense of taste. However, two-thirds of identified pregnant women with Covid-19 have no symptoms.

There is growing evidence that pregnant women may be at increased risk of severe illness from Covid-19 compared with non-pregnant women, especially in the third trimester. Risk factors for infection and hospitalisation in pregnancy include:

- Being unvaccinated
- Age >35 years
- Black, Asian and minority ethnic background

- BMI >25 kg/m^2
- Pre-pregnancy morbidity such as hypertension or diabetes

Maternal Covid-19 infection is associated with an approximately doubled risk of still birth and may be associated with small-for-gestational-age babies. The preterm birth rate (primarily iatrogenic) in women with symptomatic Covid-19 appears to be 2–3 times higher than the background rate.

Of the women who died during the first wave of the Covid-19 pandemic in the UK, severity of illness was often not recognised until the women were in extremis. The rapid report from MBRRACE-UK (see Chapter 2) learning from these deaths highlighted the importance of obstetric leadership of the multidisciplinary care team (MDT) and daily review allowing timely recognition of deterioration with planning for delivery to reduce respiratory work.

Treatment

Prevention is better than treatment and vaccination is safe at all stages of pregnancy and whilst breastfeeding. 98% of severe Covid-19 infections in pregnant women admitted to hospital were in unvaccinated women.

At the time of writing, detailed evidence-based treatment guidance is being regularly updated on the Royal College of Obstetricians and Gynaecologists website (rcog.org.uk).

Initial management of Covid-19 in pregnancy:

- Oxygen – titrate supplemental oxygen to keep SaO_2 >94%
- Thromboprophylaxis – prophylactic LMWH dose by weight for at least 10 days
- Corticosteroids – if oxygen dependent give for a total of 10 days or until discharge (oral prednisolone 40 mg OD or IV, hydrocortisone 80 mg BD)
- If steroids are required for fetal lung maturation use dexamethasone 12 mg IM for two doses followed by either of the above corticosteroids for 10 days
- Give tociluzimab (or sarilumab if unavailable) if hypoxic (oxygen requirement) and C-reactive protein >75
- If SARS-CoV-2 antibody negative and non-Omicron variant (anti-spike protein testing), consider 2.4 g Ronapreve® IV
- Chest imaging is essential for evaluation of the unwell pregnant woman with Covid-19 and should be performed if indicated
- Careful fluid balance

Clinical deterioration (increasing oxygen requirements, SaO_2 <93%, respiratory rate >22):

- Convene the MDT to consider the site and location of care, including an obstetrician, anaesthetist, neonatologist, intensivist and infectious disease physician
- Consider admission to critical care for respiratory support (invasive or non-invasive), proning and early discussion with ECMO centre

7.7 Summary

- Physiological and immune changes in pregnancy can increase the severity of some infections
- Awareness is need to recognise sepsis which can present with non-specific symptoms and signs
- Do not rely on temperature (either high or low)
- Altered mental state is a medical emergency
- Antibiotics, fluid resuscitation and senior review must all happen within 1 hour
- Puerperal sepsis can be insidious in onset and can progress rapidly to fulminating sepsis and death
- **Think sepsis; act quickly; assess and reassess; senior review; expert advice**

7.8 Further reading

Acosta CD, Kurinczuk JJ, Lucas DN, Tuffnell DJ, Sellars S, Knight M; United Kingdom Obstetric Surveillance System. Severe maternal sepsis in the UK, 2011–2012: a national case–control study. *PLoS Med* 2014; 11(7): e1001672.

Bonet M, Pileggi VN, Rijken MJ, et al. Towards a consensus definition of maternal sepsis: results of a systematic review and expert consultation. *Reprod Health* 2017; 14(1): 67.

Knight M, Bunch K, Tuffnell D, et al (eds) on behalf of MBRRACE-UK. *Saving Lives, Improving Mothers' Care – Lessons Learned to Inform Maternity Care from the UK and Ireland Confidential Enquiries into Maternal Deaths and Morbidity 2015–17*. Oxford: National Perinatal Epidemiology Unit, University of Oxford, 2019.

Knowles SJ, O'Sullivan NP, Meenan AM, Hanniffy R, Robson M. Maternal sepsis incidence, aetiology and outcome for mother and fetus: a prospective study. *BJOG* 2015; 122 (5): 663–71.

Kourtis AP, Read JS, Jamieson DJ. Pregnancy and infection. *N Engl J Med* 2014; 370: 2211–18.

NICE (National Institute for Health and Care Excellence). *Sepsis: Recognition, Diagnosis and Early Management*. NG51. London: NICE, 2016.

Singer M, Deutschman CS, Seymour CW, et al. The Third International Consensus Definitions for Sepsis and Septic Shock (Sepsis-3). *JAMA* 2016; 315(8): 801–10.

Surviving Sepsis campaign: http://www.survivingsepsis.org (last accessed January 2022).

Turner MJ. Maternal sepsis is an evolving challenge. *Int J Gynecol Obstet* 2019: 146: 39–42.

Appendix 7.1 Viral rash in pregnancy

Information on the investigation, diagnosis and management of a pregnant woman who has, or is exposed to, viral rash illness (including Zika virus) can be found at https://www.gov.uk/government/publications/viral-rash-in-pregnancy (updated in July 2019; last accessed January 2022).

CHAPTER 8

Intravenous access and fluid replacement

Learning outcomes

After reading this chapter, you will be able to:

- Identify the reasons behind the selection of cannula size and site
- Appreciate alternatives to peripheral cannula placement
- Define fluid, blood and clotting product administration

8.1 Intravenous access

Intravenous access is best achieved by inserting as large a cannula as possible into a large peripheral vein. Short, wide-bore cannulae deliver the fastest flow. The Hagen–Poiseuille equation describes the factors affecting the flow through a tube:

$$Q = \frac{\Delta p \pi r^4}{8 \eta l}$$

where $\boldsymbol{Q}$ is flow, $\boldsymbol{\Delta P}$ is pressure drop across the two ends of the tube, $\boldsymbol{r}$ is the radius of the tube, $\boldsymbol{\eta}$ is viscosity of the fluid and $\boldsymbol{l}$ is the length of the tube. The major variables we can control are $\boldsymbol{\Delta P}$, $\boldsymbol{r}$ and $\boldsymbol{l}$.

The effect of $\boldsymbol{\Delta P}$ can be demonstrated most simply by increasing the height of the infusion fluid above the patient. This will result in an observed increase in flow rate through the cannula. Simple pressure bags and more complex pneumatically controlled rapid infusion devices are available to maximise the effect on $\boldsymbol{\Delta P}$ and subsequently flow rate. Great care must be taken with these devices to ensure the vein does not become damaged by the high pressure, with subsequent extravasation of fluid into the extravascular tissues, as well as the risk of delivering too much fluid too rapidly causing circulatory overload.

Because $\boldsymbol{r}$ is affected by the power 4, relatively small increases in internal diameter will have major changes on achieved flow rates. Table 8.1 demonstrates the effect on flow rates of increasing the diameter of the cannula. The length of the cannula (l) should be short to optimise rapid fluid administration.

Veins in the forearm in the obstetric patient are often large and have the benefit of not traversing a joint and therefore being easier to protect from the effects of movement. Otherwise, large veins in the antecubital fossae may be good sites for the placement of peripheral intravenous cannulae for emergency fluid administration, with care taken to ensure an artery is not cannulated in error. Splinting and good fixation will be needed.

Managing Medical and Obstetric Emergencies and Trauma: A Practical Approach, Fourth Edition. Edited by Rosamunde Burns and Kara Dent.

Table 8.1 Typical flow rates under gravity through intravenous peripheral cannulae

Cannula gauge	Flow rate (ml/min)
22	36
20	61
18	96
16	196
14	343

8.2 Alternatives to peripheral venous access

Intraosseous access

In extreme situations, the placement of intravenous cannulae may not be possible. The intraosseous (IO) technique is quick and relatively simple (Figure 8.1). This skill is taught during the face-to-face element of the mMOET course.

Tibial	Humoral
Anterior surface, 2 cm below and slightly medial to the tibial tuberosity	Position arm with elbow close to side, with forearm flexed so hand is resting on abdomen Anterolateral surface, 1 cm above the greater tubercle (use only in patients where landmarks can be clearly identified)

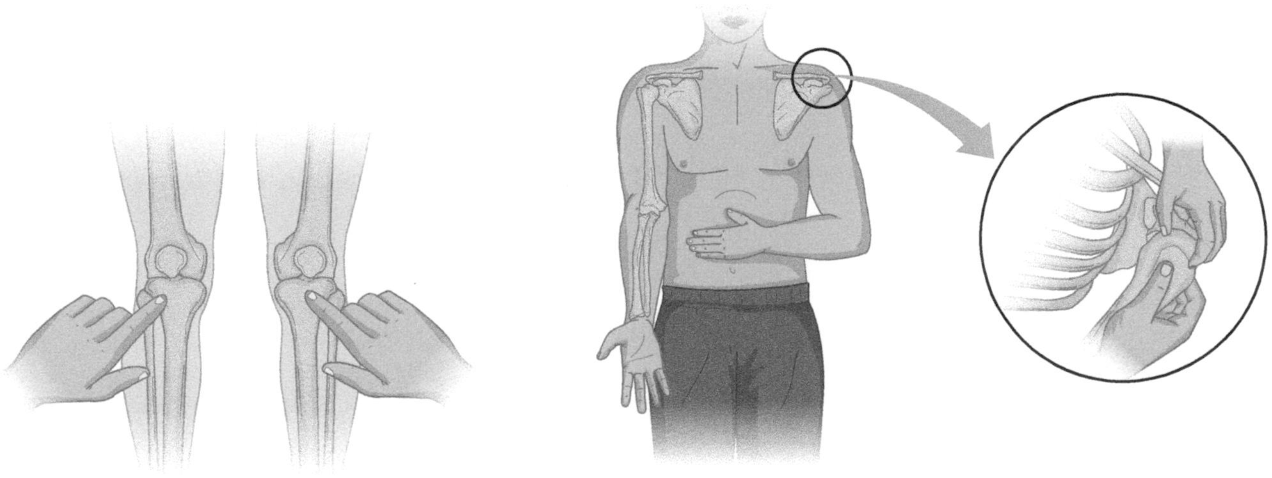

Figure 8.1 Sites for IO needle placement: tibial and humoral

Figure 8.1 shows the commonly used sites for access. The humerus has advantages in terms of flow rate and physical ease of access to the site. However, it may be covered with excessive tissue, making it impossible to establish IO access there. In this situation, it may be possible to gain access at the tibial site, where fat deposition is usually less marked. IO cannulae are available in 15, 25 and 45 mm lengths and should be chosen appropriately for the estimated amount of subcutaneous tissue to be punctured.

Uses for IO cannulae

- The administration of drugs
- The administration of fluid
- The aspiration of marrow, which can be used for crossmatching blood

It must be remembered that fluid will need to be administered under pressure, as gravity alone will not be sufficient to provide adequate flow through the IO cannula.

Contraindications to use of IO cannulae

- Fracture proximal or distal to insertion site
- Previous orthopaedic surgery at the site
- Infection at the puncture site
- Previous IO access within 24 hours at the same site should preclude the use of IO needles at that site
- The inability to palpate bony landmarks

Complications of insertion

- Cannula can become dislodged with subsequent high-volume infusion into the tissues
- Compartment syndrome as a result of the above
- Sinus formation
- Failure to deliver essential drugs and fluids
- Infection leading to osteomyelitis

The infection risk can be minimised by correct skin preparation, occlusive dressing and aseptic non-touch techniques when using the cannula.

While insertion of the IO cannula using the gun is relatively painless, running in the fluid can cause significant pain and local analgesia may be required.

CVP line access and monitoring

A central venous pressure (CVP) line may help to more accurately monitor the volume status of the patient and therefore avoid either under-transfusion or fluid overload. This requires the placement of an intravenous catheter into the central circulation. Placement is achieved most commonly by the internal jugular vein approach under ultrasound guidance where the tip of the catheter will sit just above the right atrium.

The pressure in the central veins is equated with the right ventricular end-diastolic pressure. The pressure measured depends on venous return, ability of the heart to respond, the state of filling of the circulation and venous tone. Normal values are 0–8 mmHg. Isolated measurements are of less value than the CVP *trend* in response to an intervention such as a fluid challenge. For example, in a fit hypovolaemic patient with vasoconstriction as a compensation mechanism for shock, CVP may be initially elevated. With a fluid challenge the CVP may decrease as cardiac output increases and vasodilatation occurs. In a patient with cardiac impairment, a fluid challenge produces a sustained increase in CVP as the heart does not have the ability to respond by increasing cardiac output.

The assumption is made monitoring the CVP that the right and left sides of the heart are functioning equally effectively and the right-sided filling pressure reflects the filling pressure on the left, or systemic, side of the circulation. For this to be true, we must assume that all of the interposed heart valves are functioning normally, that the resistance in the pulmonary vasculature is normal and the elasticity (compliance) of the ventricles is normal.

There are occasions when there is left ventricular dysfunction, so that the filling pressures on either side of the heart may not be equivalent. This makes interpretation of CVP readings difficult and critical care input will be required.

Conditions where CVP measurement may not be an accurate guide to fluid management are:

- Coexisting relevant disease, e.g. cardiac failure
- Coexisting severe sepsis
- Coexisting severe pre-eclampsia

Practical tips for the use of CVP lines

- The staff looking after them should receive training in their use
- The transducer should be zeroed at approximately the level of the heart
- The flush bag needs to be maintained at an adequate pressure, usually 300 mmHg pressure to avoid flow backtracking down the line; 300 mmHg is conventionally used and provides a steady infusion of 2–3 ml per hour via a flushing device
- Care needs to be taken to ensure all ports on the three-way taps used are capped to avoid an air embolus when the woman inhales

- Care should be taken on removal of the device to maintain closed caps, a head-down position and pressure over the site to avoid an air embolus
- Strict asepsis should be maintained when taking samples or giving drugs to avoid infected lines and subsequent bacteraemia
- Removal as soon as no longer needed to reduce risk of infection or venous thrombosis

Ultrasound-guided access

This is recommended practice for central line insertion and allows direct visualisation of the vein to be cannulated. The operator can observe puncture of the vein by real-time ultrasound guidance, thus reducing the risk of inadvertent arterial cannulation or failed venous access. In the absence of adequate peripheral intravenous access, for example with a past history of intravenous drug abuse, central venous access may be required.

In addition, ultrasound can be a very effective aid to site peripheral access cannulae in morbidly obese or oedematous women. Anatomical landmarks can be scanned to find veins, assess depth and observe direct puncture of veins that are not visible or palpable on the surface of the skin.

8.3 Intravenous fluid administration

Circulatory volumes

In obstetric practice, the commonest reason for urgent fluid administration is maternal haemorrhage. For that reason, the bulk of this section is written in the context of maternal bleeding unless otherwise commented on.

During pregnancy, there is an increase in circulating volume of approximately 40%. This means the volume increases from 70 to 100 ml/kg, or 4900 to 7000 ml in a 70 kg woman. It is this expansion in circulating volume that allows the woman to compensate so effectively for blood loss. It is also the reason why the severity of blood loss can be underestimated, leading to inadequate fluid resuscitation.

Maternal blood loss can be categorised into four classes of increasing severity (see Table 8.3). It is important to remember that absolute blood loss in a smaller woman reflects a larger percentage loss of her circulating volume.

Fluid warming and pressure devices

All intravenous fluids should be warmed prior to rapid administration in the context of major obstetric haemorrhage. Administration of large volumes of cold fluid will lead to significant hypothermia. Reduced maternal temperature will cause shivering in an attempt to raise body temperature, resulting in an increased oxygen demand. Failure to meet this demand will increase anaerobic metabolism and metabolic acidosis. Peripheral vasoconstriction, in an attempt to reduce any further heat loss from the periphery, will also lead to decreased oxygen delivery to the tissues, which will further add to metabolic acidosis. Significant drops in temperature will also have profound effects on the efficacy of the coagulation cascade and contribute to problems with clot formation.

High-pressure infusion devices are essential. Hand-inflated pressure bags are effective but labour intensive. Hazards of any high-pressure infusion include fluid overload and air embolism.

8.4 Types of intravenous fluid

Crystalloids

Crystalloids contain small molecules and therefore exert little oncotic pressure. As a result, these fluids distribute outside the intravascular compartment with ease, making their use in volume correction transient. They remain in the circulation for about 30 minutes, before passing into the extra- and intracellular spaces. They are useful for the immediate replacement of lost volume during haemorrhage before blood is available. It is important to remember that large volumes of crystalloid are undesirable in view of the relatively low oncotic pressure in pregnancy and can lead to pulmonary oedema.

Balanced salt solutions

These fluids have an isotonic composition closely matched with that of plasma and therefore are the crystalloid of choice; for example, Hartmann's solution (Ringer's lactate or compound sodium lactate) or Plasma-Lyte.

0.9% sodium chloride ('normal' saline)

The excessive use of solutions of sodium chloride can result in hyperchloraemic metabolic acidosis and clinicians should be aware of this, and avoid their use in large volume when possible.

Dextrose solutions

Dextrose within these fluids is rapidly metabolised by the body. The remaining fluid is therefore water, which is free to rapidly distribute into intracellular tissues. This increases the risk of cerebral and pulmonary oedema and hyponatraemia. The use of dextrose solutions should therefore be reserved for specific indications, e.g. intravenous insulin regimens.

Use of large volumes of hyponatraemic solutions can result in rapidly lowered serum and intracellular sodium levels which can result in seizures. However, actively restoring sodium levels may also be hazardous and expert advice must be sought urgently. The safest option may be to stop the hyponatraemic infusion, restrict fluid intake and allow levels to correct automatically.

Synthetic colloids

The administration of synthetic colloids is associated with a variety of adverse effects on coagulation. When large volumes are used in fluid resuscitation, these effects can be clinically significant; their use is not recommended over crystalloids by a recent Cochrane review.

It is generally agreed that an initial infusion of crystalloid is appropriate for emergency situations requiring volume resuscitation, but in the majority of haemorrhage situations blood products are likely to be required.

Blood products

Blood and blood product transfusions carry small risks, and anyone involved in their administration must be trained appropriately to understand the requirements for patient identification, product identification, storage and documentation (Table 8.2). National standards exist for blood transfusion and each hospital will have a training package that should be undertaken by practitioners and updated regularly as part of mandatory training.

Crossmatching blood

Full crossmatching of blood may take up to 1 hour. A woman's blood group and presence of abnormal red cell antibodies are usually established during pregnancy, which should facilitate the provision of blood when needed. The use of group-specific blood with antibody screening carries a risk of less than 0.1% of a haemolytic transfusion reaction, which rises to 1.0% if group-specific blood is used without antibody screening. In most circumstances, issuing of group- and rhesus (Rh)-compatible blood should be possible within 15 minutes.

Group O Rh-negative and Kell-negative blood should be kept on the delivery suite (or reliably available within 5 minutes) when immediate transfusion is required. Its use carries a small risk of sensitisation to the 'c' antigen with potential problems for future pregnancies.

The risk of viral transmission (e.g. hepatitis, cytomegalovirus) is extremely low in the UK due to screening by the blood transfusion services. In order to reduce the transmission of the Creutzfeldt–Jakob disease (CJD) prion, blood is leucodepleted before being issued from the blood bank.

Donor blood is an expensive and limited resource with some risks attached to its use. In the absence of significant co-morbidity, the laboratory trigger for red cell transfusion is a haemoglobin ≤70 g/l but other factors including the rate of fall of the woman's haemaglobin and presence or absence of cardiorespiratory compromise must be considered alongside the laboratory haemogloblobin. A higher transfusion threshold may be necessary when co-morbidities such as cardiac disease are present.

Even previously fit and well women can experience cardiac ischaemia, infarction and ultimately death in the face of extreme anaemia because haemoglobin is required to carry oxygen to maintain adequate tissue perfusion.

Table 8.2 Common blood components and their use in obstetrics

Component	Volume per unit	Dose	Number of donors	Storage	Need to defrost	Storage after defrosting	Time to transfusion	Filter required
Packed red cells	180–350 ml (mean 280 ml)	4 ml/kg equivalent to 1 unit will raise Hb by 1 g/dl	1	Designated temperature-controlled refrigerator at 4±2°C for 35 days	No	N/A	4 hours after removal from storage	Blood transfusion set with 170–200 micron filter
Fresh frozen plasma	240–300 ml (mean 273 ml)	10–15 ml/kg or 1:1 with RBC in major haemorrhage	1 donor per unit, 4 donors for a therapeutic dose of 4 units	Designated temperature controlled-freezer at −30°C for 24 months	Yes – takes 15–30 minutes	Can be stored in a blood fridge under controlled storage conditions for 24 hours	4 hours after removal from storage	As above
Platelets	200–300 ml	1 adult therapeutic dose increases platelet count by 20–40×10^9/l	Multiple	Temperature controlled at 22±2°C with continuous agitation for 7 days	No	N/A	As soon as possible over 30–60 minutes – they should not be put in the fridge	As above but not through giving set which has been used for other blood products
Cryoprecipitate	100–250 ml (mean 152 ml)	2×5 donor pools (equivalent to 10 single donor units) raise plasma fibrinogen by 1 g/l	Multiple	Designated temperature-controlled freezer at −30°C for 24 months	Yes – takes 15–30 minutes	Must be kept at ambient temperature for up to 4 hours	As soon as possible – it should not be put in the fridge	As above

Red cell concentrate

Concentrated red cells are the mainstay of treatment for the restoration of the oxygen carrying capacity of blood. Each pack contains approximately 220 ml of red cells and 80 ml of saline-adenine-glucose-mannitol (SAG-M) solution, and has a shelf-life of 35 days. The haematocrit varies from 55% to 70% so a plasma substitute needs to be given in appropriate amounts to provide the additional volume required in large volume transfusions.

Citrate anticoagulation

In massive and rapid transfusion there may be a requirement for calcium infusion because citrate anticoagulants are present in stored red blood cells and fresh frozen plasma (FFP). Citrate binds to ionised calcium, and may cause hypocalcaemia. This in turn contributes to coagulopathy and to a negative inotropic action on the heart. Both effects can be reversed by a slow (20 minute) infusion of calcium, e.g. 10 ml 10% calcium gluconate with subsequent checks of serum calcium on serial arterial blood gases.

Fresh frozen plasma

FFP contains naturally occurring clotting factors and anticoagulants that are further diluted by the addition of anticoagulants. Methylene blue-treated FFP is also available. This helps to inactivate the CJD prion and is used when required for administration to neonates, babies and children. It is much more expensive compared with the cost of untreated FFP.

Cryoprecipitate

Cryoprecipitate is another fraction of whole blood produced by further processing of FFP that is rich in fibrinogen and is therefore indicated in the presence of profound hypofibrinogenaemia, as may be seen in association with bleeding due to placental abruption. This means cryoprecipitate may be requested earlier in this type of haemorrhage than in a more straightforward bleed from an atonic uterus; see 'Decision making' section.

Platelets

Platelet packs have a limited shelf-life of around 5 days. They are rarely indicated above a platelet count of 50×10^9/litre but may be required to raise the level to 80–100 $\times 10^9$/litre if surgical intervention is planned.

Decision making to aid coagulation support in obstetric haemorrhage

It is important to maintain adequate coagulation in the face of obstetric haemorrhage to limit ongoing bleeding by enabling clot formation. Simple measures to prevent further coagulation dysfunction such as keeping the patient warm, giving tranexamic acid, maintaining normocalcaemia and avoiding metabolic acidosis are very important. Increasingly, the use of near patient testing of coagulation in obstetrics (rotational thromboelastometry (ROTEM®)/thromboelastography (TEG®)) has enabled more targeted use of blood products to support the coagulation.

Military and non-pregnant trauma experience has demonstrated increased survival when packed red cells and clotting products are administered in a ratio close to 1:1 during extreme blood loss. Multiple injury is rare in the pregnant population however, and the underlying pathophysiology of bleeding in multiple trauma is probably different to the common causes of obstetric bleeding. Pregnant women have the physiological adaptation that means they are able to maintain effective coagulation in the face of simple volume loss compared with the non-pregnant state. However, pregnant women with haemorrhage associated with a consumptive coagulopathy (abruption, amniotic fluid embolus) will require **much earlier** targeted support of the coagulation system.

During obstetric haemorrhage an early fall in fibrinogen level (<2 g/dl) is strongly associated with progression to major obstetric haemorrhage (MOH) with marked coagulopathy. Coagulation status should therefore be assessed as soon as possible, either by use of point-of-care measurements (ROTEM®/TEG®) or by laboratory tests where point of care is not available. Fibrinogen replacement should be directed to maintaining a fibrinogen level >2 g/dl. This can be achieved through use of fibrinogen concentrate or cryoprecipitate. Currently in the UK, fibrinogen concentrate is only licensed for use in congenital hypofibrinogenaemia, but can be used on a named patient basis in MOH under the advice of a haematologist. Protocols for the use of fibrinogen concentrate in MOH have been widely established in some parts of the UK. Typical doses of fibrinogen concentrate are 4–6 g, as guided by the fibrinogen level, and are repeated as required.

If conventional laboratory-based tests are available and the prothrombin time/activated partial thromboplastin time is >1.5 times normal, this suggests that a minimum of 4 units of FFP will be needed if fibrinogen concentrate and cryoprecipitate are not available.

Cell salvage

Increased cost, relative scarcity and concern over viral transmission have resulted in an increased use of autologous transfusion in modern surgical practice. Obstetrics was slow to follow this trend due to concern about amniotic fluid transmission and the potential for amniotic fluid embolism. Early use utilised a two sucker technique, one used prior to delivery and the second after the amniotic fluid had been removed. Recent practice, however, has only used one sucker as modern-day cell salvage machines clear amniotic fluid and the phenomenon of amniotic fluid embolism is better understood. The process of cell salvage involves anticoagulation, collection, filtration, washing and reinfusion of red cells at the time of surgery.

The National Institute for Health and Care Excellence (NICE) had approved its use in obstetrics but in 2017 the SALVO (Cell Salvage in Obstetrics) trial published. The results of this randomised controlled, multicentre UK trial demonstrated only modest evidence for routine prophylactic use of cell salvage during caesarean section and thought it was unlikely to be cost effective. The trial also found that its use was associated with a significant increase in feto-maternal transfusion.

This has implications for women who have RhD-negative blood groups. They must be screened and treated with appropriate levels of anti-D to avoid haemolytic complications in subsequent pregnancies. The SALVO authors were also unable to comment on the long-term antibody sensitisation effects to other red cell antibodies, potentially making crossmatching difficult in the future. This has led to a re-evaluation of the use of cell salvage. It should be noted that there was no subgroup benefit in women with abnormal placentation.

Cell salvage for Jehovah's witnesses

Many women who refuse blood products will accept cell salvage. However, it must be remembered and fully explained that the blood returned to the woman does not contain clotting factors: the risk of coagulation defects therefore remains as it does with homologous red cell transfusion. This is, in effect, a dilutional coagulopathy, as fluids returned gradually dilute the remaining pool of available natural clotting factors until eventually there is a catastrophic failure of the clotting mechanism. Although easily corrected in normal circumstances by the administration of clotting factors, it is particularly important to emphasise this very significant limitation of cell salvage to women who refuse blood products.

8.5 Clinical signs guiding fluid replacement

For the vast majority of situations, fluid administration in the otherwise healthy parturient will be guided by the maintenance or restoration of easily observed clinical variables. Raised heart rate is an early sign of absolute or relative (vasodilatatory) hypovolaemia. In general, a heart rate above 100 beats per minute should be considered sinister until proven otherwise (Table 8.3). A normal respiratory rate, normal capillary refill (less than 2 seconds) and normal pulse pressure (unless the patient is on beta-blockers) are also sensitive markers of a normal circulatory volume. It must be remembered that patients on beta-blockers have an impaired tachycardic response to hypovolaemia.

Table 8.3 Different classes of blood loss with resulting physiological indices

	Class I	Class II	Class III	Class IV
Blood loss:	15%	15–30%	30–40%	>40%
Non-pregnant (ml)	750	1000	1500	2000
Pregnant (ml)	<1000	1000–2000	2000–2700	>2700
Respiration rate (per minute)	14–20	20–30	30–40	>40
Heart rate (per minute):	<100	>100	>120	>140
Systolic	Normal	Normal	Decreased	Decreased
Diastolic	Normal	Increased	Decreased	Decreased
Mental state	Anxious	Anxious, confused	Confused, agitated	Lethargic
Urine (ml/h)	>30	20–30	<20	Negligible

Box 8.1 Response to resuscitation by intravenous fluids

Signs improve and remain improved
No further fluid challenge is required.

An initial but unsustained improvement in vital signs followed by regression to abnormal levels
Either:

- the fluid has been redistributed from the intravascular compartment to the extravascular compartments
- there is continued loss (as seen in continued haemorrhage)
- there is worsening of vasodilatation (sepsis/ anaphylaxis)

Further fluid challenge is required. Restoration of normal variables would imply there is no further fluid loss or worsening of vasodilatation.

Vital signs remain abnormal
If vital signs remain abnormal then this would be considered a type III response. In the face of haemorrhage, this implies significant ongoing losses and the patient requires urgent surgery. Patients with this response in the face of sepsis will almost certainly require vasoactive drug administration to reduce the degree of peripheral vasodilatation.

No response
This group show no response to rapid fluid administration of any type. In the face of haemorrhage, this patient requires immediate surgery (to 'turn off the tap') if she is to survive. Women with sepsis are likely to require continuous vasoactive infusion to support circulation and require immediate transfer to an intensive care unit.

A normal urine output (~1 ml/kg/h) is a measure of adequate renal perfusion. Box 8.1 is a guide to the response to fluid resuscitation and a guide to further action.

Use of acid–base status and lactate to guide resuscitation

Repeated measurement of acid–base status and lactate from blood gases should guide fluid therapy. Metabolic acidosis and a raised lactate indicate inadequate tissue perfusion and subsequent anaerobic metabolism. It is the acidosis that may be the driver for raised respiratory rate in shock. Adequate resuscitation and restoration of organ function is the best treatment. Alkalis such as bicarbonate are rarely required, and are for specialist use only.

8.6 Fluid administration in special circumstances

As already discussed, fluid administration in obstetric practice is most commonly in the face of haemorrhage, where adequate prompt fluid administration is the major aim. There are, however, situations within obstetric practice where a much more targeted administration of fluid must be considered.

Pre-eclampsia/eclampsia

Fluid management prior to delivery

The major concern is to avoid fluid overload. Intravenous input is limited to around 80 ml/h in most pre-eclampsia toxaemia (PET) protocols. If Syntocinon infusions are required, they should be given in high concentrations via a syringe driver to avoid the administration of further large volumes of fluid. The volume of this and any other infusion (magnesium, antihypertensives) should be included in the 80 ml/h total fluids.

If a fluid bolus is required, care should be taken to ensure that the volume given is not excessive by administration via a volumetric pump. If hypotension does occur it can usually be controlled with low-dose phenylephrine by bolus or infusion.

Fluid management post delivery

In the immediate post-delivery phase, women will often have a degree of oliguria before natural diuresis occurs. It is important not to risk fluid overload in the chase for adequate urine output. Total intravenous fluids (including drug infusions) should be limited and careful fluid balance charted. Numerous examples of fluid protocols exist around the UK; a suggested guide is shown in Chapter 27.

Sepsis

Hypovolaemia is present in almost all patients with septic shock and fluid resuscitation is vital. The volumes required can be very large as fluid is leaking rapidly into the interstitial tissues, due to capillary leak caused as part of the sepsis response. Initial crystalloid fluid resuscitation of 20 ml/kg for hypotension or a lactate >4 is recommended as part of the UK Sepsis Trust's Sepsis Six (see Chapter 7).

In patients who remain hypotensive despite adequate fluid resuscitation there should be early recourse to vasopressor therapy to maintain a mean arterial pressure of >65 mmHg and critical care involvement. Evidence supports the use of noradrenaline as the vasopressor of choice. Sensitivity to catecholamines is greatly reduced in sepsis and therefore patients may require exceedingly high doses. Vigilance, early recognition and regular reassessment remain vital to improve outcome.

Cardiac disease

Response to fluid administration can be extremely unpredictable in this group of patients. Central venous monitoring, or more advanced assessment of cardiac function, may be required to guide successful and safe fluid administration. These cases require senior clinician involvement across multidisciplinary teams.

8.7 Summary

- Intravenous access should be of large bore and short length
- Haemorrhage is likely to be the commonest indication for urgent fluid administration
- Advanced cardiovascular monitoring may be required in certain circumstances

8.8 Further reading

AAGBI (Association of Anaesthetists of Great Britain and Ireland). AAGBI guidelines: the use of blood components and their alternatives 2016. *Anaesthesia* 2016; 71: 829–42.

Cochrane Library. Colloids or crystalloids for fluid replacement in critically ill people. https://www.cochrane.org/CD000567/INJ_colloids-or-crystalloids-fluid-replacement-critically-people (last accessed January 2022).

Collis RE, Collins PW. Haemostatic management of obstetric haemorrhage. *Anaesthesia* 2015; 70 (Suppl 1): 78–86.

Khan KS, Moore PAS, Wilson MJ, et al. Cell salvage and donor blood transfusion during cesarean section: a pragmatic, multicentre randomized controlled trial (SALVO). *PLoS Med* 2017; 14912: e1002471.

Lewis SR, Pritchard MW, Evans DJW, et al. Colloids versus crystalloids for fluid resuscitation in critically ill people. *Cochrane Database of Syst Rev* 2018; Issue 8: CD000567.

NICE (National Institute for Health and Care Excellence). *Intravenous Fluid Therapy in Adults in Hospital.* CG174. London: NICE, 2017.

Robinson S, Harris A, Atkinson S, et al. The administration of blood components: a British Society for Haematology Guideline. *Transfus Med* 2018; 28(1): 3–21.

Sepsis Trust: https://sepsistrust.org (last accessed January 2022).

Chapter 9: Cardiac disease in pregnancy

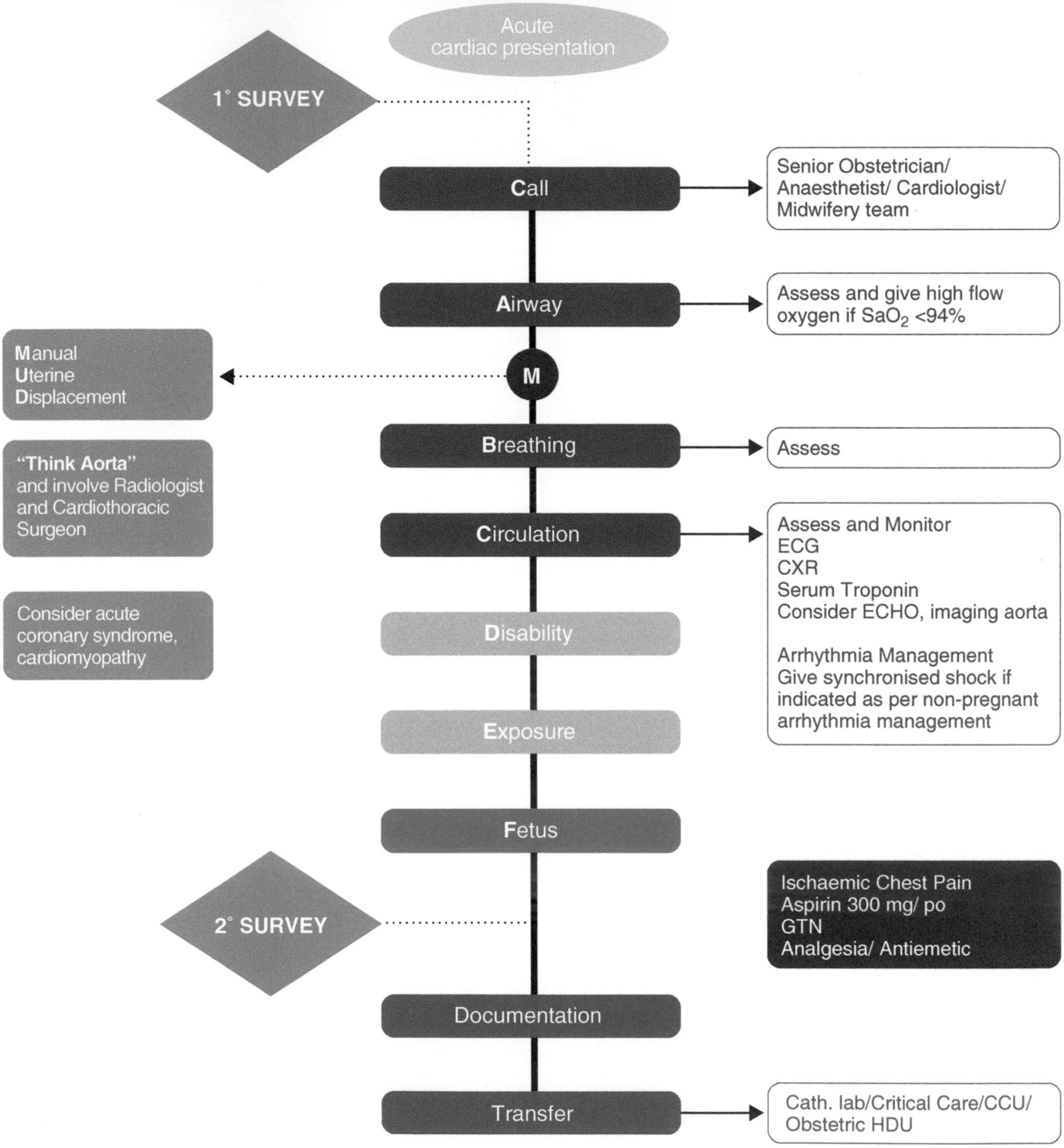

Algorithm 9.1 Cardiac disease in pregnancy.

CHAPTER 9

Acute cardiac disease in pregnancy

Learning outcomes

After reading this chapter, you will be able to:

- Describe the more common serious cardiac problems that can affect pregnant women
- Anticipate the health problems of pregnant women with pre-existing disease
- Appreciate the 'red flag' features heralding emergencies in pre-existing and new conditions
- Take part in the urgent multidisciplinary care of pregnant and puerperal women with acute cardiac presentation
- Understand important aspects of service provision for such women with complex disorders

9.1 Introduction

Medical problems in pregnancy are becoming more common as women are opting to delay childbirth to later in life, and are more likely to have coexisting medical problems at the time of conception. This is reflected by the increase in indirect maternal deaths reported worldwide. Cardiac conditions and other non-communicable diseases are the major causes of indirect maternal deaths in the UK and other high income countries (Figure 9.1). The 'obstetric transition' model developed by Souza suggests that with improvements in healthcare and a rise in maternal age, the causes of maternal death in low and middle income countries will also gradually shift from direct to indirect maternal deaths.

It is therefore necessary for all healthcare professionals to have an understanding and knowledge of the management of common medical emergencies that can present during pregnancy and in the postpartum period, to prevent indirect maternal deaths and work to provide coordinated multidisciplinary care.

In this chapter we will provide an overview of acute cardiac conditions and their presentation during pregnancy and the postpartum period. The emphasis is on positive decision making and the importance of identifying and considering an alternative diagnosis when required. Shared decision making facilitated by early referral to appropriate senior specialists and timely communication across the clinical team will optimise the care of a pregnant woman.

Managing Medical and Obstetric Emergencies and Trauma: A Practical Approach, Fourth Edition. Edited by Rosamunde Burns and Kara Dent.

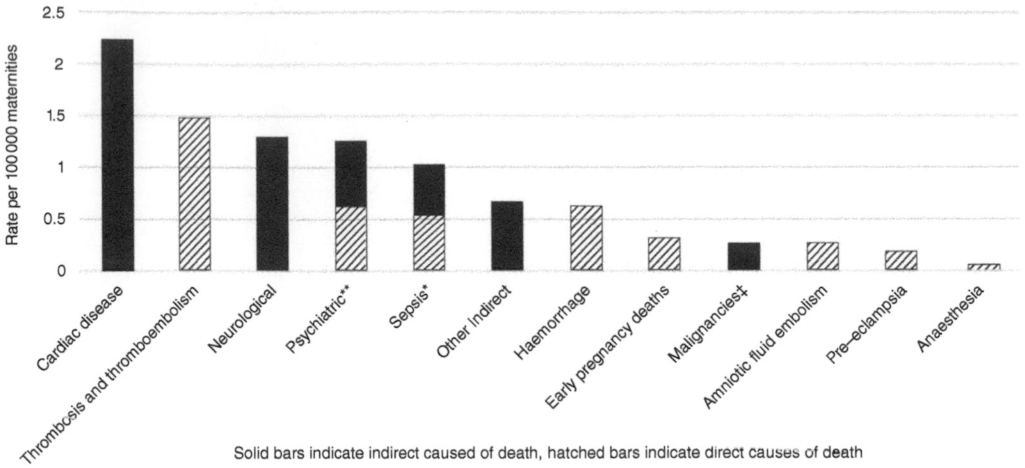

Figure 9.1 Causes of maternal death 2016–2018
Source: Knight M, Bunch K, Tuffnell D, et al. (eds), on behalf of MBRRACE-UK. *Saving Lives, Improving Mothers' Care – Lessons Learned to Inform Maternity Care from the UK and Ireland Confidential Enquiries into Maternal Deaths and Morbidity 2016–18*. Oxford: National Perinatal Epidemiology Unit, University of Oxford, 2020. © 2020 NPEU

9.2 Cardiac disease

The spectrum of cardiac disease encountered in maternity is shifting, with a rise in the prevalence of heart failure and ischaemic heart disease. With advancing maternal age, there is an increase in the prevalence of the traditional cardiovascular risk factors during pregnancy. Additionally, young women with repaired congenital heart disease, who are usually already known to the adult congenital heart clinic, are also pursuing pregnancy. Women with mechanical prosthetic heart valves are at a higher risk of complications in pregnancy, such as bleeding or thrombosis of the prosthetic valve.

Within the immigrant population or where there is limited access to healthcare, women may present during pregnancy with untreated rheumatic heart disease (particularly aortic and mitral stenosis) or unrepaired congenital heart disease. Women with pre-existing cardiac disease may exhibit decompensation of cardiac function due to the physiological demands of pregnancy. The common cardiac symptoms that women may present with during pregnancy are discussed below and include chest pain, shortness of breath and palpitation.

9.3 Chest pain

Chest pain can be challenging as there are many differential diagnoses to consider. The recognition of the 'red flags' (Box 9.1) including *recurrent presentation* with chest pain is critical but so is the importance of **not only excluding** a condition **but diagnosing** an alternative condition. There is more to a diagnosis of chest pain than simply ruling out myocardial infarction.

Box 9.1 Red flags in a pregnant patient presenting with chest pain

- Pain requiring opioids
- Pain radiating to arm, shoulder, back or jaw
- Sudden-onset, tearing or exertional chest pain
- Associated with haemoptysis, breathlessness, syncope or abnormal neurology
- Abnormal observations

Source: RCP (Royal College of Physicians). *Acute Care Toolkit 15: Managing Acute Medical Problems in Pregnancy*. London: RCP, 2019. © 2019 Royal College of Physicians

Causes of chest pain are manifold and a careful history is central to defining the origin. Aside from ischaemia, other cardiovascular causes include aortic dissection, myocarditis and pericarditis. Respiratory causes comprise pulmonary embolism, pneumonia, pneumothorax and pneumomediastinum – these commonly have a pleuritic component. Gastrointestinal problems may cause chest pain, such as gastro-oesophageal reflux, biliary colic or pancreatitis. Musculoskeletal chest pain is common and can sometimes be reproduced with movement or sternal pressure.

Clinically important differentials to consider early include myocardial infarction, aortic dissection and pulmonary embolism. Ischaemic chest pain is not always typical or classic but the presence of associated autonomic symptoms (sweating, nausea, light-headedness) should increase suspicion. A detailed history and complete physical examination is required. Where a cardiac aetiology for chest pain is suspected an ***electrocardiogram (ECG), chest x-ray (CXR) and troponin should be performed early*** as part of the diagnostic assessment. ECG changes may be subtle and can evolve so repetition with serial tracings can be very helpful, with prompt review from a cardiologist when there is any doubt.

Myocardial infarction/acute coronary syndrome

The acute coronary syndrome (ACS) comprises:

- Unstable angina
- Non-ST segment elevation myocardial infarction (non-STEMI)
- ST segment elevation myocardial infarction (STEMI)

Diagnosis is based on a combination of ischaemic symptoms, ECG changes and elevation in serum troponin. Typical ischaemic symptoms can include pressure or discomfort in the chest rather than 'pain' and these sensations can radiate into the jaw and/or arms. There is a 3–4-fold increased risk of ACS when pregnant, compared to an age-matched, non-pregnant population. Development of pregnancy-related ACS is most common during the third trimester and postpartum. The pathophysiology of ACS in the pregnant population may differ from that in the non-pregnant population. In contrast to the general population where atherosclerotic coronary heart disease is the major cause of ACS, during pregnancy and in the postpartum period, spontaneous coronary artery dissection (SCAD) and coronary thrombosis may occur more frequently due to specific physiological adaptations to pregnancy. These include a more hypercoagulable state, increase in stroke volume and increase in cardiac output.

Risk factors for development of atherosclerotic ACS in pregnancy include the more traditional risk factors such as pre-existing heart disease, obesity, advanced maternal age, hypertension, endocrine disorders, diabetes mellitus, smoking, dyslipidaemia and a family history of premature cardiovascular disease. Additional pregnancy-related risk factors include pre-eclampsia, thrombophilia, multiparity, postpartum haemorrhage, blood transfusion and infection.

Pharmacological agents that may predispose to coronary spasm include ergometrine and recreational drugs such as cocaine.

The initial management of suspected ACS aims to relieve symptoms, limit myocardial damage and reduce the risk of cardiac arrest:

1. Have a systematic ABCDE approach.
2. Relieve aortocaval compression if >20 weeks' gestation and supine by 15° of left lateral tilt or manual uterine displacement (MUD). Most patients with cardiac ischaemic chest pain will be more comfortable sitting up which is acceptable if they are not hypotensive.
3. Give oxygen if hypoxic (oxygen saturation <94% on air).
4. Perform initial investigations ECG, CXR and serum troponin.
5. **Give aspirin 300 mg orally**, crushed or chewed as soon as possible. In patients presenting with STEMI, additional antiplatelet medication (e.g. clopidogrel) and heparin should be administered prior to emergency coronary angioplasty (primary percutaneous coronary intervention (PCI)) following discussion with an interventional cardiologist.
6. Give sublingual glyceryl trinitrate (GTN) unless the patient is hypotensive or has uterine atony.
7. Analgesia with morphine/diamorphine should be titrated as required to control pain but avoiding sedation and respiratory depression. Give with an antiemetic.
8. Escalate early to senior clinicians including a consultant cardiologist for multidisciplinary decision making.
9. Early transfer to an appropriate high dependency unit location for consideration of invasive coronary angiography.

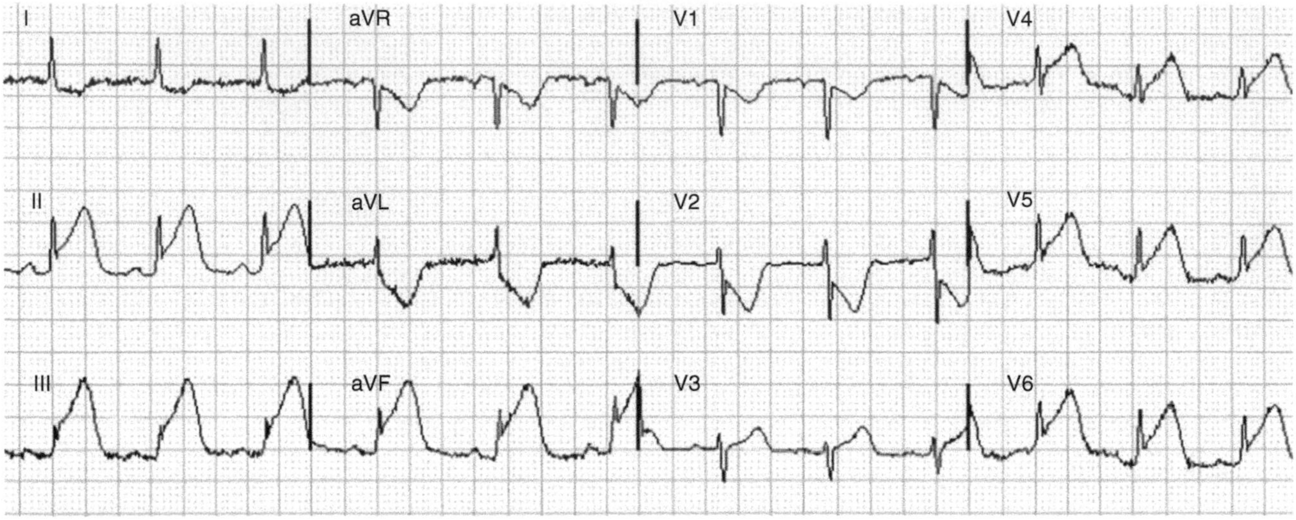

Figure 9.2 Inferior and lateral STEMI. There is ST elevation in leads II, III, aVF and V4–V6. Leads I and aVL show reciprocal ST depression. ST elevation in leads V1 and V2 represents lateral 'mirror-image' ST deviation
Source: Birnbaum Y, et al. ECG diagnosis and classification of acute coronary syndromes. *Ann Noninvasive Electrocardiol* 2014; 19(1): 4–14. With permission of John Wiley & Sons. https://doi.org/10.1111/anec.12130

For patients presenting with STEMI, the priority is to achieve coronary reperfusion as quickly as possible (Figure 9.2). **The management of choice is immediate referral to the nearest tertiary centre for coronary angiography, and consideration of emergency (primary) PCI without delay.** The aim is to restore blood flow to myocardium that has not yet been damaged irreversibly.

While thrombolysis is not contraindicated in pregnancy and does not cross the placenta it is not indicated for STEMI in pregnancy as the diagnosis may be SCAD. If the angiogram shows SCAD, medical management is preferred unless there is ongoing ischaemia, ECG change or haemodynamic instability.

The immediate treatment of ACS should not be delayed for delivery. Ideally, delivery should be postponed if feasible for at least 2 weeks after the cardiac event.

Invasive coronary angiography is preferably performed via the radial artery with local anaesthetic. Left lateral tilt should be used to avoid aortocaval compression. Consideration should be given to fetal radiation exposure, particularly in the first trimester. Angiography determines the presence and extent of coronary atherosclerosis, thrombotic occlusion and/or coronary artery dissection. A left ventriculogram can be helpful in assessing resulting wall motion abnormalities and left ventricular systolic function.

In the presence of coronary occlusion or flow-limiting stenosis, angioplasty with stenting may be performed (Figure 9.3). However, in some cases of suspected ACS the coronary arteries can appear normal, in which case alternative diagnoses must be considered. These include coronary vasospasm or transient coronary thromboembolism, myocarditis, acute stress-related 'takotsubo' cardiomyopathy and also a non-cardiac diagnosis such as pulmonary thromboembolism.

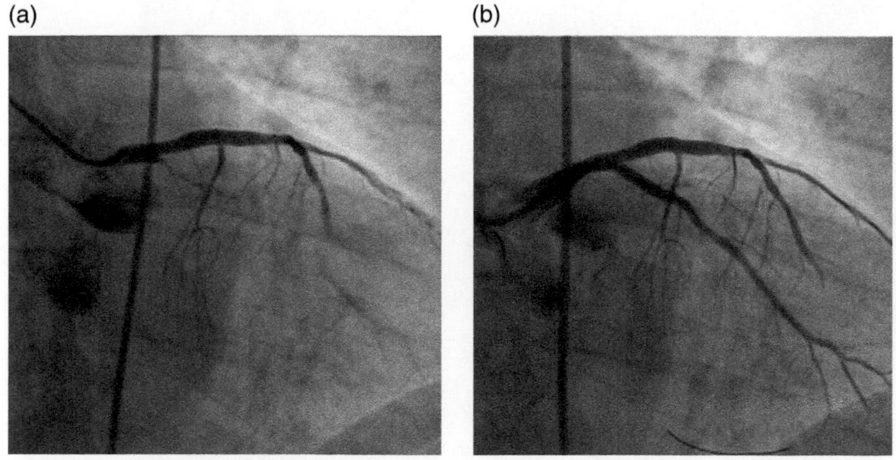

Figure 9.3 Total occlusion of the ostium of the circumflex artery (a), with flow restored following angioplasty (b)
Source: Nordkin I, et al. Complicated acute myocardial infarction with simultaneous occlusion of two coronary arteries. *Clin Case Rep* 2020;8(3): 449–52. With permission of John Wiley & Sons. https://doi.org/10.1002/ccr3.2685

Ongoing management of patients with ACS includes:

- Monitor for and identify potential complications – heart failure, cardiogenic shock, arrhythmias, bleeding or recurrent ischaemia
- Close monitoring of the mother and fetus is required in an appropriate critical care setting with a detailed plan agreed amongst the multidisciplinary team in case emergency delivery is required
- The preferred mode of delivery is a vaginal delivery. Syntocinon can be given as a slow infusion over 15–20 minutes at delivery to minimise tachycardia and hypotension. Ergometrine is contraindicated due to the risk of coronary vasospasm

Women with established coronary artery disease or ACS are at risk of serious morbidity and mortality during pregnancy. The risk is highest for those with atherosclerosis, with this risk having been previously reported in pregnancy as up to a 23% risk of maternal mortality.

A plan for contraception should be documented before discharge and the need for pre-pregnancy counselling communicated to the woman, cardiologist and GP.

Aortic dissection

Whilst rare, aortic dissection can be catastrophic for both mother and baby and accounts for 11% of maternal cardiac deaths (Knight et al., 2019). It is a condition that needs to be identified early, with prompt treatment, as the mortality rate increases by 1% each hour it is not treated. Recent UK Obstetric Surveillance System (UKOSS) data estimate its incidence at 0.8 per 100 000 maternities. Lessons from MBRRACE are a reminder that in patients presenting with red flag symptoms it is important not only to exclude a diagnosis such as pulmonary embolism, but also to continue on ***to make a diagnosis.***

Aortic dissection occurs most often in the last trimester of pregnancy (50%) but it should be remembered that the period of risk continues into the early postpartum period (33%). The classic presentation of aortic dissection is a sudden onset severe chest pain, felt between the shoulder blades, in the back, neck or abdomen, often tearing in nature. There may be neurological symptoms, haematuria or rectal bleeding depending on the organs affected by the dissection. Agitation, syncope and collapse can occur. Aortic dissection is underdiagnosed with tragic consequences. The Think Aorta campaign seeks to raise awareness of the diagnosis to aid early life-saving diagnosis (Figure 9.4).

The risk factors for the development of aortic dissection in pregnancy are multifactorial and include pre-existing conditions such as Marfan's syndrome, vascular Ehlers–Danlos, Loeys–Ditz syndrome, hypertension and aortopathy associated with a bicuspid aortic valve. There are also risk factors specific to pregnancy such as pre-eclampsia. There is a vasculopathy in pregnancy due to an increase in oestrogen and progesterone. This is thought to decrease the concentration of mucopolysaccharides and elastic fibres in the tunica media of the aorta, weakening the wall of the blood vessel. The pathophysiology begins with increased shear stress in the vascular lumen leading to a weakness in the wall. This can lead to bleeding into the media and the creation of a false lumen which may then extend to occlude aortic branches or cause a catastrophic haemorrhage.

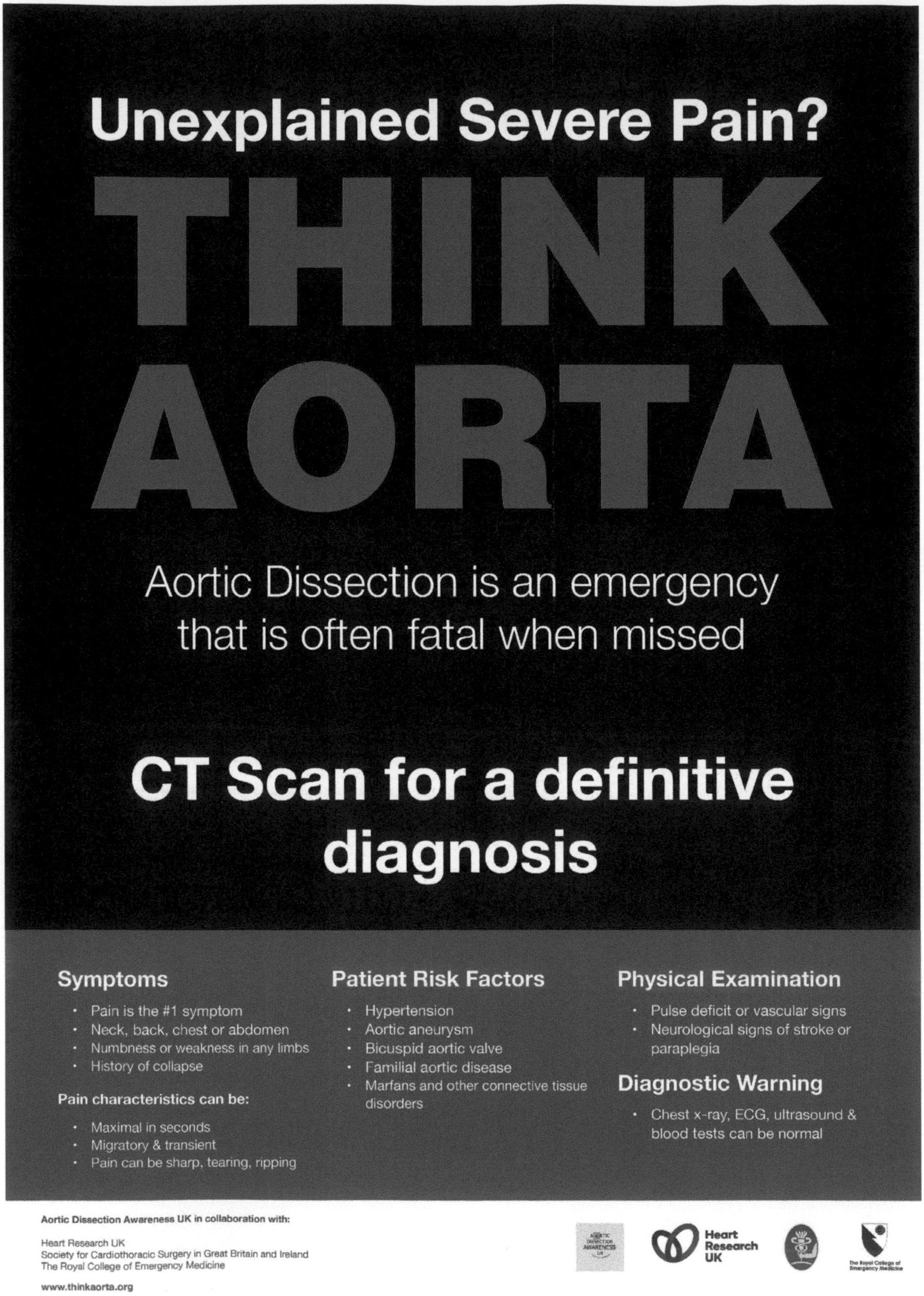

Unexplained Severe Pain?
THINK
AORTA
Aortic Dissection is an emergency that is often fatal when missed
CT Scan for a definitive diagnosis
Symptoms
• Pain is the #1 symptom
• Neck, back, chest or abdomen
• Numbness or weakness in any limbs
• History of collapse
Pain characteristics can be:
• Maximal in seconds
• Migratory & transient
• Pain can be sharp, tearing, ripping
Patient Risk Factors
• Hypertension
• Aortic aneurysm
• Bicuspid aortic valve
• Familial aortic disease
• Marfans and other connective tissue disorders
Physical Examination
• Pulse deficit or vascular signs
• Neurological signs of stroke or paraplegia
Diagnostic Warning
• Chest x-ray, ECG, ultrasound & blood tests can be normal
Aortic Dissection Awareness UK in collaboration with:
Heart Research UK
Society for Cardiothoracic Surgery in Great Britain and Ireland
The Royal College of Emergency Medicine
www.thinkaorta.org
Heart Research UK
The Royal College of Emergency Medicine

Figure 9.4 Think Aorta
Source: Think Aorta. thinkaorta.org. © Think Aorta

Aortic dissection can be classified into Stanford type A and type B. Stanford type A includes dissections that involve the ascending aorta (with or without extension to the arch and descending thoracic aorta), whilst Stanford type B describes dissection originating in the descending thoracic and abdominal aorta (Figure 9.5).

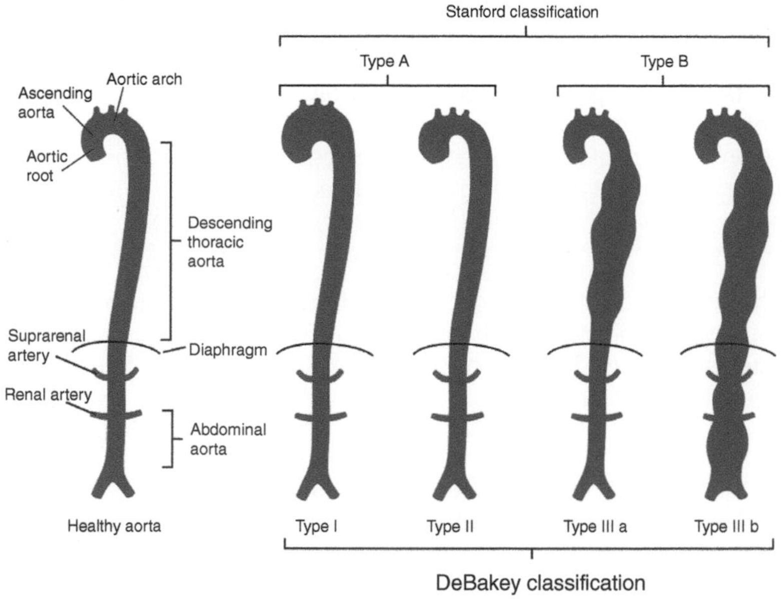

Figure 9.5 Types of dissection per Stanford and DeBakey
Source: Olga Bolbot/Shutterstock

Type A aortic dissection is a surgical emergency and prompt diagnosis is vital. Survival falls with every hour. Management requires input from a multidisciplinary team of cardiothoracic/vascular surgeons, obstetricians, obstetric and cardiac anaesthetists. The primary goal of initial immediate treatment is to reduce the stress on the aorta and provide analgesia. Depending on gestation at presentation, the fetus may be delivered urgently by caesarean section while proceeding to immediate aortic surgery. Aortic surgery should proceed with a non-viable fetus still in utero in the maternal interest, acknowledging a 20–30% fetal mortality associated with cardiopulmonary bypass.

Stanford type B dissection is usually treated conservatively with intravenous antihypertensive medication and the involvement of vascular surgeons for monitoring and assessment.

Diagnostic imaging modalities for diagnosis include *ECG gated computed tomography (CT) aortogram* when the patient is haemodynamically stable (Figure 9.6), or urgent transthoracic echocardiography when the patient is unstable. Commonly taught clinical signs may not be reliable – for example, CXR does not always demonstrate a widened mediastinum, and lack of blood pressure discrepancy in the arms is not a reliable means of excluding aortic dissection.

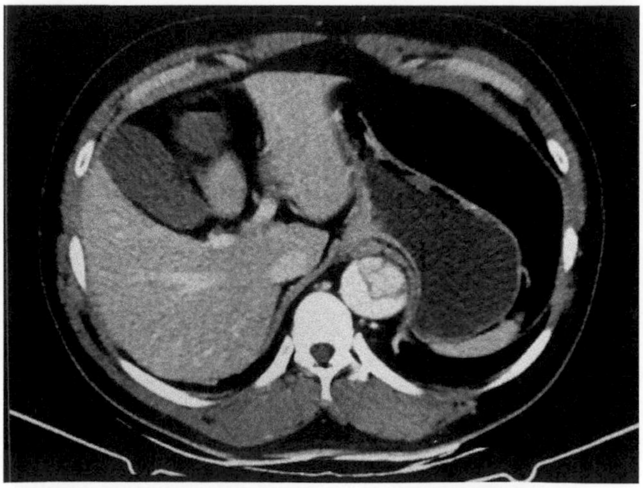

Figure 9.6 Axial CT angiogram of aortic dissection
Source: pp_watchar/Shutterstock

Initial management aortic dissection:

1. Have a systematic ABCDE approach.
2. Relieve aortocaval compression if >20 weeks' gestation and supine by 15° of left lateral tilt or MUD.
3. Initial investigations include ECG, CXR, ECG gated CT aortogram and echocardiogram.
4. There should be early escalation to senior clinicians who should be involved in the assessment and decision making, including obstetrician and anaesthetist, radiologist, cardiologist and cardiothoracic surgeon.

Shortness of breath

As noted previously with chest pain, there are several differential diagnoses to consider for patients presenting with dyspnoea. Furthermore, this symptom is commonly multifactorial, and physiological breathlessness is a common pregnancy symptom. Recognition of red flags including **recurrent re-presentation** with shortness of breath is important (Box 9.2). Remember, not only excluding a condition but diagnosing an alternative condition is essential.

Box 9.2 Red flags in a pregnant patient presenting with breathlessness

- Sudden onset breathlessness
- Orthopnoea
- Breathlessness with chest pain or syncope
- Respiratory rate >20 breaths per minute
- Oxygen saturation <94% or falls to <94% on exertion
- Breathlessness with associated tachycardia

Source: RCP (Royal College of Physicians). *Acute Care Toolkit 15: Managing Acute Medical Problems in Pregnancy*. London: RCP, 2019. © 2019 Royal College of Physicians

In common with all acute presentations, consideration of the medical and obstetric background is important along with the history and clinical findings. Acute respiratory conditions presenting with breathlessness include pulmonary embolism, pneumonia, pneumothorax and exacerbation of asthma. Pulmonary hypertension is a relatively uncommon cause of breathlessness but is important not to miss in pregnancy. Anaemia is usually readily diagnosed from the blood count but acute blood loss may not be immediately evident, and can initially appear well tolerated in younger patients before sudden compromise. Breathlessness may also be a feature of systemic conditions such as sepsis, anaphylaxis or diabetic ketoacidosis.

From a cardiac point of view, dyspnoea can be the presenting symptom of a variety of conditions including left ventricular failure, myocardial ischaemia, valve disease and arrhythmia. Breathlessness may be caused by pulmonary congestion/ oedema or reduced cardiac output, or a combination of both. The cause is usually apparent based on clinical assessment, ECG and echocardiography. The latter is particularly helpful so early investigation and input from a senior cardiologist is required.

Pulmonary oedema

Symptoms may range from mild breathlessness with early pulmonary congestion to acute respiratory distress with florid pulmonary oedema. Orthopnoea and paroxysmal nocturnal dyspnoea are compelling symptoms and the clinical finding of new inspiratory crepitation should raise suspicion, particularly if there are corresponding changes on CXR (Figure 9.7). Signs are usually but not always bilateral. Wheeze or unexplained cough may be present and should not be assumed to be due to asthma, particularly if there is no history of airway disease. Importantly, other commonly associated features of heart failure such as elevation of the jugular venous pressure and peripheral oedema may be absent.

The pathophysiology of pulmonary oedema can be more complex in pregnancy and the presence of significant hypertension, with or without pre-eclampsia, is an important variable. High blood pressure can cause an acute elevation in the left atrial pressure leading to pulmonary congestion with resulting anxiety, worsening hypertension and respiratory distress being rapidly self-perpetuating. This usually responds quickly to intravenous diuretic and blood pressure control.

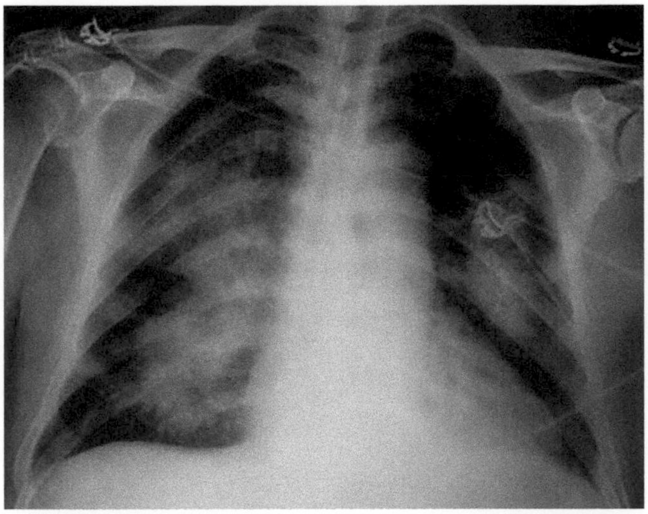

Figure 9.7 Bat wing or butterfly sign in pulmonary oedema
Source: Han J, et al. Bat wing or butterfly sign: pulmonary oedema. *J Med Imag Radiat Oncol* 2018; 62(S1): 18. With permission of John Wiley & Sons. https://doi.org/10.1111/1754-9485.06_12785

In the absence of hypertension, pulmonary oedema is more likely to reflect underlying left ventricular systolic dysfunction, and early echocardiography is particularly important. This finding may reflect a new or acute cause (such as peripartum cardiomyopathy) or decompensation due to a pre-existing condition such as dilated cardiomyopathy, significant heart valve disease or tachyarrhythmia. In some cases, rapid changes in left ventricular size or function can cause acute mitral regurgitation, further exacerbating pulmonary congestion (Figure 9.8).

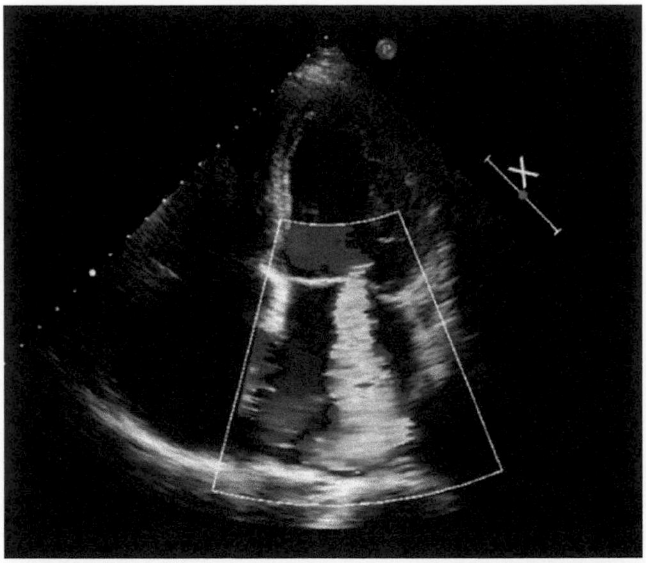

Figure 9.8 Four chamber zoomed image of mitral regurgitation with colour Doppler showing a central jet of mitral regurgitation
Source: Silbiger JJ. Mechanistic insights into atrial functional mitral regurgitation: far more complicated than just left atrial remodeling. *Echocardiography* 2019; 36(1): 164–9. With permission of John Wiley & Sons. https://doi.org/10.1111/echo.14249

Other risk factors or contributing factors for the development of acute pulmonary oedema in pregnancy are:

- Pre-existing conditions – known heart disease, obesity, advanced maternal age, endocrine disorders
- Pregnancy-specific conditions – pre-eclampsia, amniotic fluid embolism, pulmonary embolism, sepsis
- Fetal factors – multiple gestation
- Pharmacological agents – beta-adrenergic tocolytics, corticosteroids, magnesium sulphate, recreational drugs, e.g. cocaine
- Iatrogenic factors – excessive fluid resuscitation

Initial management of pulmonary oedema:

1. Have a systematic ABCDE approach.
2. A patient with pulmonary oedema will be best managed sitting up if conscious and blood pressure is adequate. If supine due to reduced conscious level or hypotension, reduce aortocaval compression if >20 weeks' gestation by left lateral tilt or MUD
3. Give high-flow oxygen if oxygen saturation is <94% on air with early anaesthetic input. Continuous positive airway pressure can be effective in the treatment of pulmonary oedema.
4. ***Give frusemide 40–80 mg IV.***
5. Initial investigations include arterial blood gas, ECG, CXR, and echocardiogram.
6. Senior clinicians should be directly involved with prompt escalation to a multidisciplinary team.
7. Agents that vasodilate can be used to reduce left ventricular afterload – e.g. GTN Infusion (50 mg/50 ml, starting at 1–2 ml/h with close monitoring of blood pressure as it can cause hypotension).
8. Transfer to an appropriate location for ongoing multidisciplinary management and investigation of the underlying cause. Consideration should be given to the timing and place of delivery once maternal stability has been achieved.

For patients with cardiogenic shock or heart failure refractory to initial treatment, escalation for mechanical circulatory support should be considered. This might involve the insertion of an intra-aortic balloon pump, or transfer to a centre with facility for ventricular assist device (VAD), extracorporeal membrane oxygenation (ECMO) or even urgent cardiac transplantation.

Palpitations

Palpitation can simply be defined as an awareness of one's heartbeat. It is a common symptom in pregnancy and usually benign, reflecting an increased heart rate and cardiac output. An important distinction is the presence of arrhythmia versus awareness of the heartbeat in normal sinus rhythm. Palpitation is commonly due to ectopy, giving a sensation of 'skipped beats'. Ectopic beats may be ventricular or supraventricular in origin, and can easily be diagnosed with ECG monitoring. However, it is important to exclude other causes by remembering the red flags (Box 9.3), and to take seriously re-presentation with recurrent palpitations.

Box 9.3 Red flags in a pregnant patient presenting with palpitations

- Palpitations in a woman with a family history of sudden cardiac death
- Palpitations in a woman who has structural heart disease or previous cardiac surgery
- Palpitations with syncope
- Palpitations with chest pain
- Persistent, severe tachycardia

Source: RCP (Royal College of Physicians). *Acute Care Toolkit 15: Managing Acute Medical Problems in Pregnancy*. London: RCP, 2019. © 2019 Royal College of Physicians

Again, the history is particularly useful in the assessment of patients presenting with palpitation. This should include the frequency and duration of symptoms and a detailed description of what the patient feels. Features more suggestive of tachyarrhythmia include a sudden onset/offset of palpitation, a sense of very rapid heart racing and associated dizziness, breathlessness or chest discomfort. Syncope is a red flag, and the wider history should also take account of relevant family background of arrhythmia or sudden cardiac death. Persisting significant sinus tachycardia is not a normal physiological change in pregnancy and an underlying cause such as hypovolaemia, anaemia, sepsis, pulmonary embolism or hyperthyroidism should be considered.

Clinical examination is often normal. Routine assessment comprises blood tests including blood count, electrolytes and thyroid function tests. Close attention should be paid to the 12 lead ECG to assess the rhythm, and also pointers to possible arrhythmic tendency – e.g. PR interval, QRS duration and QTc interval (Figure 9.9).

Depending on the nature and frequency of symptoms, cardiac monitoring may helpful. In patients presenting with cardiac arrhythmia at the time of assessment, prompt further investigation and management is required with senior input and involvement of a cardiologist. For patients in sinus rhythm with red flag symptoms, specialist review should be sought, as a period of inpatient cardiac monitoring may be helpful in establishing an early diagnosis.

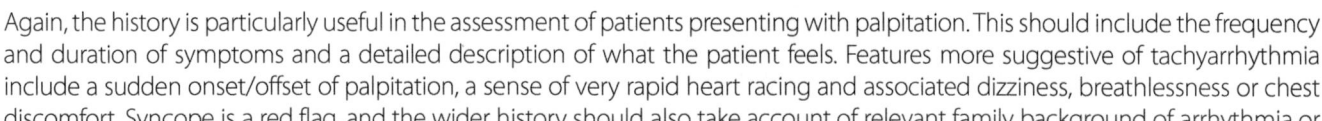

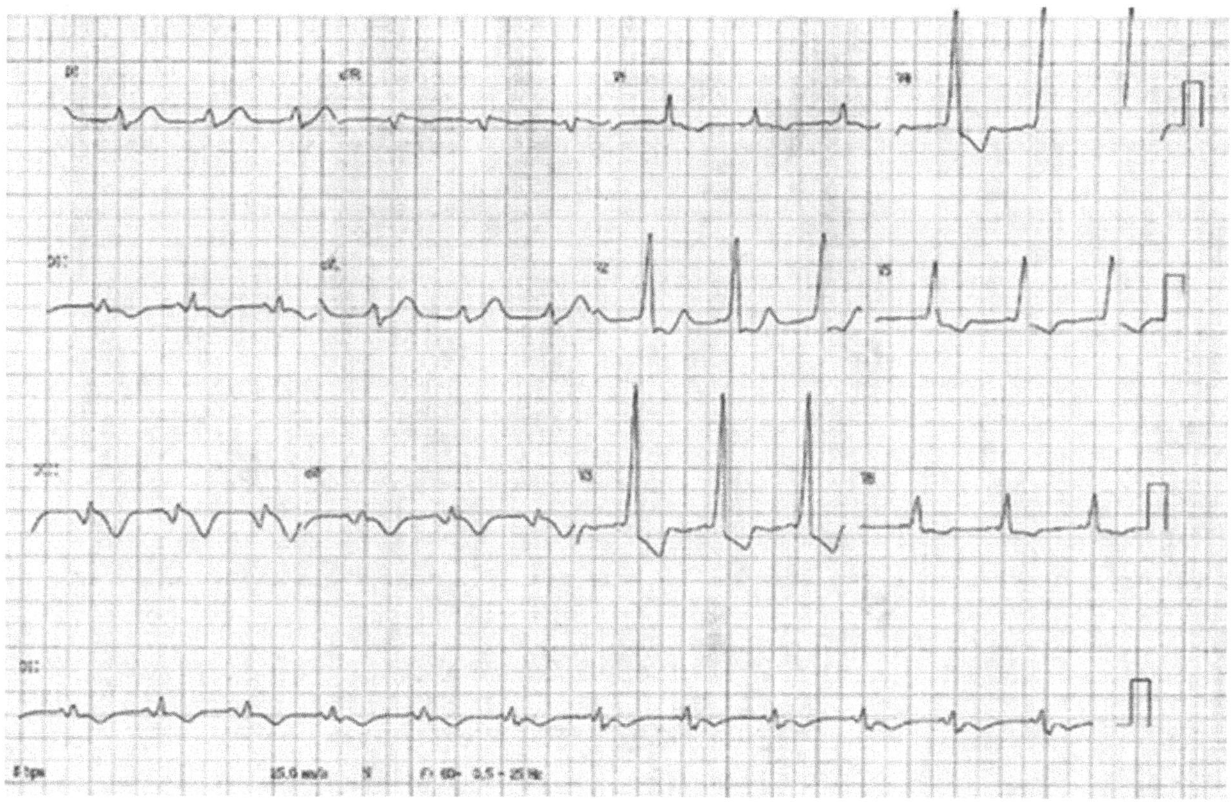

Figure 9.9 Short PR interval with a wide QRS complex and slurred onset of the QRS waveform compatible with delta wave of Wolff–Parkinson–White syndrome

Source: Lessa de Castro R, Jr, et al. Concealed Wolff–Parkinson–White syndrome revealed by acute coronary syndrome. *Ann Noninvasive Electrocardiol* 2020; 25(5): e12735. With permission of John Wiley & Sons. https://doi.org/10.1111/anec.12735

For patients with more benign symptoms, Holter monitoring can be used to assess heart rate trends, quantify ectopy and, importantly, correlate rhythm with symptoms, which can clarify the diagnosis and provide reassurance. If symptoms are infrequent, a patient-activated arrhythmia monitor may be used. In cases of syncope where there is a suspicion of a cardiac cause, an implantable loop recorder can be invaluable in demonstrating the presence or absence of associated arrhythmia.

Tachyarrhythmias such as atrial fibrillation or atrial flutter are relatively uncommon and often reflect an underlying cardiac condition, including pre-existing valvular or congenital heart disease. Ventricular arrhythmias are fortunately rare – they usually indicate serious underlying cardiac pathology requiring urgent escalation and specialty input. **For any patient showing signs of compromise due to tachyarrhythmia, urgent DC cardioversion should be considered**, and early escalation to senior obstetric and anaesthetic colleagues is vital. Relevant adverse clinical signs include shock, syncope, myocardial ischaemia and heart failure.

Supraventricular tachycardia (SVT) due to atrioventricular nodal re-entry or atrioventricular re-entry is relatively common in pregnancy. This is often well tolerated but very fast heart rates may cause hypotension, and prolonged episodes can lead to decompensation due to tachycardia-related cardiomyopathy with impaired left ventricular function.

Initial management of SVT:

1. Have a systematic ABCDE approach.
2. Relieve aortocaval compression if >20 weeks' gestation and supine by left lateral tilt or MUD.
3. Initially assess haemodynamic state.
4. Undergo a trial of vagal manoeuvres under continuous ECG monitoring.
5. If ineffective, give intravenous **adenosine 6–12 mg** under continuous ECG monitoring.
6. If compromised plan for synchronised DC cardioversion.

7. A senior clinician should be directly involved in prompt escalation and clinical decision making to involve a multidisciplinary team.
8. The aim is to stabilise the mother **– do not commence cardiotocography monitoring**. The aim is not to deliver the fetus at this time but to stabilise and revert the mother to sinus rhythm.
9. Transfer to an appropriate location for cardiac monitoring and further management.

9.4 Summary

- Cardiovascular disease remains an important cause of morbidity and mortality in pregnancy. This can be due to pre-existing cardiac problems or acute/new presentation of cardiac disease
- Common presentations include chest pain, breathlessness and palpitation. Symptoms may overlap and red flag features should not be overlooked
- Differential diagnoses should not just be excluded but active diagnosis should be pursued
- Pregnant patients presenting with acute cardiac symptoms should be stabilised and appropriately monitored, with relevant investigation prioritised and early discussion with senior specialists including obstetrician, anaesthetist and cardiologist

9.5 Further reading

ESC (European Society of Cardiology). *Cardiovascular Diseases during Pregnancy (Management of) Guidelines*. Brussels: ESC, 2018.

Knight M, Bunch K, Tuffnell D, et al (eds) on behalf of MBRRACE-UK. *Saving Lives, Improving Mothers' Care – Lessons Learned to Inform Maternity Care from the UK and Ireland Confidential Enquiries into Maternal Deaths and Morbidity 2015–17*. Oxford: National Perinatal Epidemiology Unit, University of Oxford, 2019.

RCoA (Royal College of Anaesthetists), et al. *Care of the Critically Ill Woman in Childbirth; Enhanced Maternity Care*. London: RCoA, 2018. https://www.rcoa.ac.uk/sites/default/files/documents/2020-06/EMC-Guidelines2018.pdf (last accessed January 2022).

RCP (Royal College of Physicians). *Acute Care Toolkit 15: Managing Acute Medical Problems in Pregnancy*. London: ACP, 2019.

PART 3
Resuscitation

CHAPTER 10

Airway management and ventilation

Learning outcomes

After reading this chapter, you will be able to:

- Describe the importance of airway patency, maintenance and protection
- Identify the circumstances in which airway compromise can occur
- Assess and manage the airway and ventilation

10.1 Introduction

An obstructed airway or inadequate ventilation results in tissue hypoxia within minutes and this can lead to organ failure and death. Some organs are more sensitive to hypoxia than others. For example, cerebral hypoxia, even for a short period of time, will cause agitation then a decreased level of consciousness and, eventually, irreversible brain damage. Management of the airway is of first concern because obstruction to the airway can quickly result in hypoxia with brain damage or death. The next presenting threat to life results from inadequate ventilation, so attention to this is given next priority.

Supplementary oxygen must be administered to all seriously injured and ill pregnant patients through a tight-fitting facemask attached to a reservoir bag at a flow of 12–15 l/min. The primary goal in providing supplementary oxygen is to maximise the delivery of oxygen to the vital organs, including the placenta.

Carbon dioxide is produced by cellular metabolism and carried in the blood to the lungs to be exhaled. If there is airway obstruction or inadequate ventilation, carbon dioxide builds up in the blood (hypercarbia). This causes drowsiness, acidosis and a rise in intracranial pressure secondary to vasodilatation.

10.2 Airway assessment

Importance of patency, maintenance and protection of the airway

The airway must be open, maintained and protected if there is risk of regurgitation and aspiration as in the heavily pregnant patient. An awake, fully conscious woman will protect her own airway. Otherwise, in an unconscious woman, the gold standard for providing a patent and protected airway is by placing a cuffed tube in the trachea, usually by endotracheal intubation. If there is a breathing problem, ventilatory support may also be necessary once you have established a patent airway.

A before B before C before D

Managing Medical and Obstetric Emergencies and Trauma: A Practical Approach, Fourth Edition. Edited by Rosamunde Burns and Kara Dent.

Circumstances in which an airway problem is likely to occur

Suspect an airway problem with the following:

- The patient with a decreased level of consciousness (because there is reduced muscle tone and the tongue is likely to slip back into the pharynx)
- Anaphylaxis
- Hypoxia
- Hypotension
- Eclampsia
- Poisoning
- Alcohol
- Intracranial pathology or injury
- Maxillofacial injuries:
  - Midface fractures can move backwards and block the airway
  - Mandibular fractures can allow the tongue to fall backwards
  - Bleeding and secretions caused by these injuries can block or soil the airway
- Open injuries to the neck
- Direct trauma to the larynx and supporting structures
- Bleeding inside the neck compressing the hypopharynx or trachea
- Burns to the face and neck; swelling of the upper and lower airway due to direct burns, or inhaling hot smoke, gases or steam, will cause airway obstruction

Airway problems may have the following features:

- They be immediate (block the airway quickly)
- They be delayed (come on after a time delay – minutes or hours)
- They may deteriorate with time – this is often insidious because of its slow progression and is easily overlooked (as with burns to the upper airway); consider the potential for deterioration during transfer and, if a risk, secure a definitive airway before transfer

An airway that has been cleared may obstruct again:

- If the support for keeping the airway patent is removed (e.g. chin lift)
- If the patient's level of consciousness decreases
- If there is further bleeding into the airway
- If there is increasing swelling in or around the airway

Assessment of the airway

Talk to the patient. Failure to respond implies an obstructed airway or a breathing problem, with inability to exhale enough air to phonate, or an altered level of consciousness with the potential for airway compromise. A positive, appropriate reply in a normal voice indicates that the airway is patent, breathing is normal and brain perfusion adequate.

Look to see if the patient is agitated, drowsy or cyanosed. The absence of cyanosis does not mean the patient is adequately oxygenated. Look for use of accessory muscles of respiration. A patient who refuses to lie down quietly may be trying to sit up in an attempt to keep her airway open or her breathing adequate. The abusive patient may be hypoxic and should not be presumed to be merely aggressive or intoxicated.

Listen for abnormal sounds. Snoring, gurgling and gargling sounds are associated with partial obstruction of the pharynx. Hoarseness implies laryngeal injury. An absence of sound does not mean the airway is patent; if the airway is totally obstructed there may be total silence. Feel for air movement on expiration and check if the trachea is in the midline.

Assessment of ventilation

Establishing a patent airway is the first step, but only the first step. A patent airway allows oxygen to pass to the lungs, but this will only happen with adequate ventilation. Ventilation may be compromised by airway obstruction, altered ventilatory mechanics or by central nervous system depression. If breathing is not improved by clearing the airway, attempt to ventilate by facemask. If ventilation is possible, then the airway is patent but there is a problem with spontaneous ventilation. If ventilation is not possible, this would suggest that the airway continues to be obstructed. If there is a problem with spontaneous ventilation look for a cause within the chest or an intracranial or spinal injury as a cause and assist ventilation.

Inspect	Look for chest movement, use of accessory muscles of respiration and obvious injuries
Palpate	Palpate for chest movement and palpate the back of the patient's chest for injuries Palpate the trachea, checking it is in the midline
Percuss	Percussion note should be resonant and equal bilaterally
Auscultate	Air entry should be equal bilaterally

10.3 Airway management

- Clear the obstructed airway
- Maintain the intact airway
- Recognise and protect the airway at risk

The airway is at risk from aspiration in any patient with reduced level of consciousness, but in the pregnant patient regurgitation is more likely so the potential for aspiration is increased.

Suspected cervical spine injury

Techniques for clearing, maintaining and protecting the airway need to be modified in the trauma patient in whom cervical spine injury is suspected or present. Cervical spine motion restriction should be instituted wherever there is suspicion of injury, either by manual inline immobilisation or by head blocks, backboard and straps.

Clearing the obstructed airway

In the patient with suspected cervical spine injury, manual inline immobilisation of the cervical spine and airway clearance manoeuvres are carried out together. In a patient with an altered level of consciousness, the tongue falls backwards and obstructs the pharynx. This can be readily corrected by the jaw thrust manoeuvre, and blood and debris cleared by suction.

Head tilt/chin lift (no cervical spine injury suspected)

Tilt the head posteriorly with the intention of straightening and slightly extending the neck. At the same time, place the fingers of one hand under the chin and gently lift it upwards to bring the chin anteriorly (Figure 10.1). This will open the upper airway in 70–80% of patients.

Do not hyperextend the neck if a cervical spine injury is suspected. Use a jaw thrust rather than a head tilt.

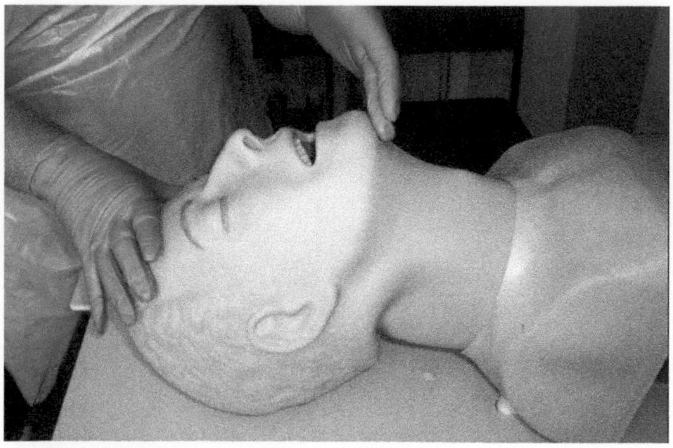

Figure 10.1 Head tilt/chin lift

Jaw thrust

Grasp the angles of the mandible, one hand on each side, and move the mandible forward (Figure 10.2). The jaw thrust is used for the injured patient because it does not destabilise a possible cervical spine fracture and risk converting a fracture without spinal cord injury to one with spinal cord injury. This manoeuvre will open 95% of obstructed upper airways.

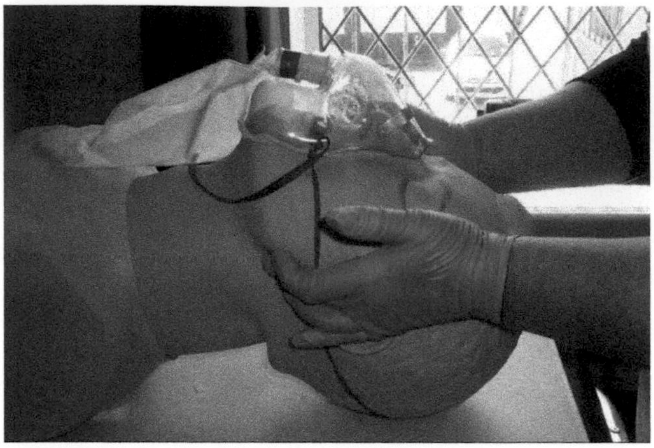

Figure 10.2 Jaw thrust

Suction

Remove blood and secretions from the oropharynx with a rigid suction device (e.g. a Yankauer sucker). A patient with facial or head injuries may have a cribriform plate fracture – in these circumstances suction catheters should not be inserted through the nose, as they could enter the skull and injure the brain.

How to check if the airway is clear

If attempts to clear the airway do not result in the restoration of spontaneous breathing, this may be because the airway is still not patent or because the airway is patent but there is no breathing. The only way to distinguish these two situations is to put either a pocket mask or facemask over the face and give breaths (either mouth to pocket mask or with self-inflating bag and mask). If the chest rises, this is not an airway problem but a breathing problem. If the chest cannot be made to rise, this is an airway problem.

Clearing the airway may result in improvement in level of consciousness, which then might allow the patient to maintain her own airway.

Maintaining the airway

If the patient cannot maintain her own airway, continue with the jaw thrust or chin lift or try using an oropharyngeal airway.

Oropharyngeal airway

The oropharyngeal airway (Guedel type) is inserted into the mouth over the tongue. It stops the tongue falling back and provides a clear passage for airflow. The preferred method is to insert the airway concavity upwards, until the tip reaches the soft palate and then rotate it 180°, slipping it into place over the tongue (Figure 10.3). Make sure that the oropharyngeal airway does not push the tongue backwards as this will block, rather than open, the patient's airway. A patient with a gag reflex may not tolerate the oral airway.

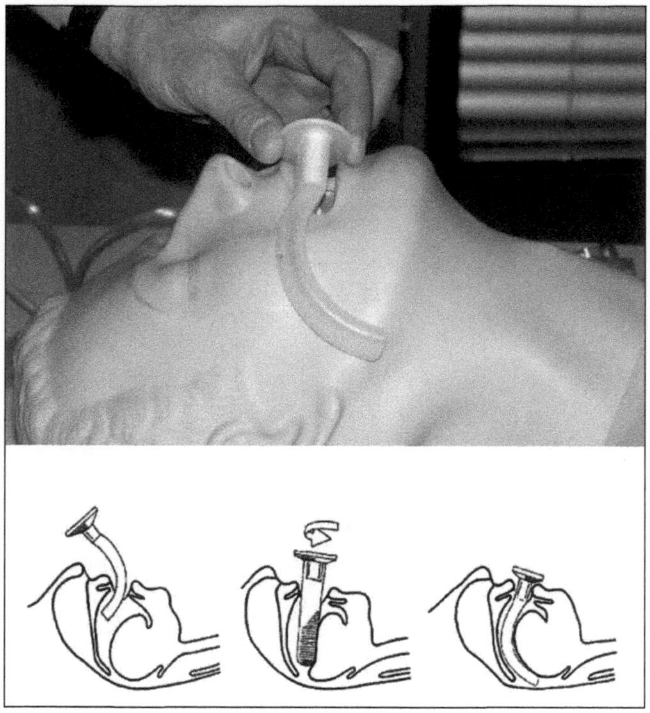

Figure 10.3 Oropharyngeal airway

Nasopharyngeal airway

A nasopharyngeal airway is better tolerated than the oropharyngeal airway by the more responsive patient. Their use is contraindicated if there is a suspected fractured base of the skull. Be aware of the potential for insertion to cause bleeding from the fragile nasal mucosa, which may soil the lungs of a patient with obtunded laryngeal or pharyngeal reflexes (the unconscious or hypotensive patient). This is especially so in pregnancy. Their use is limited to intensive care units where they might be placed by physiotherapists or anaesthetists to facilitate suctioning of pharyngeal secretions. They should only be used if there is an airway problem, an oropharyngeal airway is not being tolerated and an anaesthetist is unavailable. *Be very reluctant to use a nasal airway.* They do not have a large part to play in contemporary UK anaesthetic practice because of their potential to cause bleeding, which is exacerbated in pregnancy.

Lubricate the airway and insert it gently through either nostril, straight backwards – not upwards – so that its tip enters the hypopharynx. A safety pin should be applied across the proximal end before insertion to prevent the tube disappearing into the nasal passages. Gentle insertion, good lubrication and using an airway that passes easily into the nose will decrease the incidence of bleeding.

The oropharyngeal and nasopharyngeal devices maintain the airway but do not protect it from aspiration.

10.4 Advanced airway techniques

A definitive airway is a gold standard for opening, maintaining and protecting the airway. It means that there is a cuffed tube in the trachea attached to oxygen and secured in place. Advanced airway techniques provide a definitive airway.

Advanced airway techniques may be required in the following circumstances:

- In cases of apnoea
- When the above techniques fail
- To maintain an airway over the longer term
- To protect an airway
- To allow accurate control of oxygenation and ventilation
- When there is the potential for airway obstruction
- To control carbon dioxide levels in the unconscious patient, as a way of minimising the rise in intracranial pressure

Advanced airway techniques include:

- Endotracheal intubation
- Surgical cricothyroidotomy
- Surgical tracheostomy

The circumstances and urgency determine the type of advanced airway technique to be used. Note: the pregnant woman is at increased risk of gastric regurgitation because she has a mechanical obstruction to gastric emptying, i.e. the pregnant uterus. She also has reduced tone in the lower oesophageal sphincter as a result of hormonal effects on the smooth muscle. Trauma patients are at increased risk of regurgitation because of reduced gastric emptying. Consequently, the pregnant woman (with or without trauma) without adequate pharyngeal and laryngeal reflexes (unconscious or hypotensive) is at increased risk of pulmonary aspiration. The chemical pneumonitis suffered when a pregnant woman aspirates is more severe than in a non-pregnant woman as the gastric aspirate is more acidic in pregnancy. Consider an early definitive airway, particularly in the context of a reduced conscious level.

Endotracheal intubation

In a patient with airway or respiratory compromise, the primary aim is to oxygenate the patient and this can initially be successfully achieved by positioning, the use of oropharyngeal airways and the use of a facemask and self-inflating bag.

If this cannot be achieved, intubation is needed. This should only be carried out without drugs where there is an urgent need for intubation, i.e. in the case of complete airway obstruction or a respiratory arrest, where the airway cannot be otherwise maintained.

It should be emphasised that heavily pregnant women are difficult to intubate and to ventilate with a bag and mask because of weight gain during pregnancy and the potential for large breasts falling back into the working space. Consequently, for a non-anaesthetist, the use of a supraglottic airway device such as a laryngeal mask airway (LMA) may be the preferred option. It is usually easier to maintain an airway or ventilate by bag–valve–mask if the woman is in a 30° head up position, rather than lying completely supine. This allows the weight of the breasts and abdomen to fall away from the chest, increasing functional residual lung capacity. It will also make intubation easier.

Oral endotracheal intubation is most commonly used. This uses a laryngoscope to visualise the vocal cords. A cuffed endotracheal tube is placed through the vocal cords into the trachea.

Tracheal intubation without using drugs is not possible unless the patient is very deeply unconscious or has sustained a cardiac arrest. If the patient is unconscious, intracranial pathology may be implied and intubation without anaesthetic and muscle relaxation drugs will cause increases in blood pressure and intracranial pressure, which may exacerbate the intracranial condition. Intubation is therefore always a threat to patient well-being unless drugs are used.

Drugs should only be used to intubate by those with adequate anaesthetic training.

Where anaesthetic skills and drugs are available, endotracheal intubation is the preferred method of securing a definitive airway. This technique comprises rapid sequence induction of anaesthesia ('crash induction'):

- Preoxygenation
- Application of cricoid pressure
- Rapid unconsciousness using drugs
- Gentle bagging, maximum 20 cmH_2O pressure
- Rapid placement of endotracheal tube in trachea
- Inflation of cuff before removal of cricoid pressure
- Maintenance of cervical spine immobilisation when indicated

Meticulous care must be taken to keep the cervical spine immobilised if injury to the cervical spine is suspected.

Intermittent oxygenation during difficult intubation

An inability to intubate will not kill. An inability to oxygenate will. If you can oxygenate by bag and mask, this will keep the patient alive.

Avoid prolonged efforts to intubate without intermittently oxygenating and ventilating. Practise taking a deep breath when starting an attempt at intubation. If you have to take a further breath before successfully intubating the patient, abort the attempt and reoxygenate using the bag and mask technique. The joint guidelines from the Obstetric Anaesthetists' Association (OAA) and Difficult Airway Society (DAS) in 2015 suggest a maximum of two attempts, with a third only being attempted by an experienced colleague.

The 2006–2008 *Saving Mothers' Lives* report on maternal deaths in the UK once again identified failure to oxygenate in a patient with a difficult airway as a cause of maternal death (Cantwell et al., 2011).

Correct placement of the endotracheal tube

To check correct placement of the endotracheal tube apply the following steps:

- See the endotracheal tube pass between the vocal cords
- Listen on both sides in the mid-axillary line for equal breath sounds
- Listen over the stomach for gurgling sounds during assisted ventilation for evidence of oesophageal intubation
- Monitor end-tidal carbon dioxide levels; the use of capnography in emergency intubation is recommended to confirm correct tube placement. Primary methods such as auscultation are important, but not reliable, particularly in a noisy environment. In the absence of cardiac output there will still be exhaled carbon dioxide to detect, and an attenuated capnograph trace will be seen. A capnograph will ensure continuing correct placement throughout the arrest and transfer, and presence of increased exhaled carbon dioxide is an indicator of restoration of cardiac output should it occur
- If in doubt about the position of the endotracheal tube, take it out and oxygenate the patient by another method – bag and mask or surgical airway

Failed intubation in the obstetric patient

Failed intubation is more common in the obstetric population. There are a number of agreed algorithms to deal with this situation (the mMOET course refers to the OAA/DAS 2015 guidelines).

Despite the recommendation from the OAA/DAS guidelines, if considering conversion to total intravenous anaesthesia (TIVA) after a failed intubation where there is subsequent concern about uterine tone, we would advise extreme caution.

- Converting to TIVA is adding a complex task in a situation where the anaesthetist is already likely to be stressed and may increase the risk of errors
- Uterine tone can be managed with a number of other pharmacological methods without the need to change from volatile anaesthetic agents. It is worth remembering that judicious use of opioids can also reduce inhalational requirements
- It is a technique associated with a high risk of patient awareness and therefore, if TIVA is used, we would recommend depth of anaesthesia monitoring to minimise the risk of awareness

Other methods for maintaining the airway

These methods are not definitive as the airways are still unprotected.

Supraglottic airway devices

Laryngeal mask airways (and other supraglottic airway devices (SADs)) may be used to establish a patent airway and to maintain it, thereby allowing adequate ventilation to occur. They are relatively easy to insert in non-expert hands compared with tracheal intubation, which is important in the light of evidence from studies of intubation involving non-experts resulting in an unacceptably high level of accidental oesophageal intubation. They may also be inserted with little, if any, interruption to cardiac compressions compared with intubation.

SADs do not protect the airway; consequently, there remains the potential risk of aspiration of gastric contents, which is a particular concern in pregnant women. They could be used by non-anaesthetists in an emergency where the airway can not be maintained or ventilation reliably achieved by bag–mask ventilation in combination with an oropharyngeal (Guedel) airway. Any method of manual ventilation, whether by bag–valve–mask or SAD, can cause the stomach to become inflated, further predisposing to regurgitation. Newer second-generation SADs have a gastric port which allows access to the gastric contents and may offer better airway protection than the older first-generation devices, but they are still not protected airways.

Surgical airway

A surgical airway should not be undertaken lightly, and is used when:

- Trauma to the face and neck makes endotracheal intubation impossible
- The anaesthetist cannot intubate or ventilate, e.g. caesarean section

Surgical cricothyroidotomy places a tube into the trachea via the cricothyroid membrane (Figure 10.4). A small tracheostomy tube (5–7 mm) is suitable. During the procedure, appropriate cervical spine protection must be maintained when indicated. There are also commercially available surgical cricothyroidotomy sets. A cricothyroidotomy can be replaced by a formal tracheostomy (if needed) at a later time.

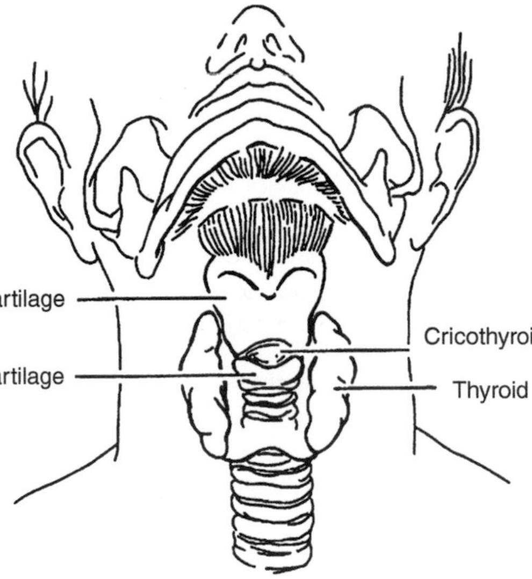

Figure 10.4 Anatomical landmarks for surgical cricothyroidotomy

Needle cricothyroidotomy has a high failure rate and is no longer recommended in UK guidelines for the emergency management of an inability to secure an airway. Instead surgical cricothyroidotomy is the technique of choice and is discussed further in Appendix 10.1.

A formal emergency *surgical tracheostomy* takes longer and is more difficult than a surgical cricothyroidotomy.

10.5 Management of ventilation

Once the airway is patent and maintained, there may be a separate requirement to assist breathing (ventilation). Spontaneous ventilation (self-ventilation) means the same as breathing. Assisted (artificial) ventilation means the patient is receiving help with breathing. The aim is to improve gaseous exchange in the lungs and to breathe for the patient if spontaneous ventilation has stopped or is inadequate.

The indication for assisted ventilation is when ventilation is inadequate as in:

- Chest injury
- Respiratory depression due to drugs (such as opiates)
- Head injury that might be causing respiratory depression and requires end-tidal carbon dioxide levels to be closely controlled to prevent cerebral vasodilatation and a consequent rise in intracranial pressure

Assisted ventilation can be achieved by the following techniques:

- Mouth to mouth (or nose) – unlikely in hospital
- Mouth to pocket mask
- Self-inflating bag to pocket mask or facemask
- Self-inflating bag to endotracheal tube, LMA or tracheostomy tube
- Automatic ventilation via endotracheal tube or tracheostomy tube

As soon as monitoring in the form of pulse oximetry is available and can be reliably interpreted, oxygen delivery should be adjusted to maintain a target oxygen saturation of 94–98%. There is known to be evidence of harm in providing prolonged periods of hyperoxia. Further monitoring can be provided by the use of blood gas analysis.

Extubation

Attention to detail is also needed before extubation of any patient, even 'just' after elective surgery under general anaesthesia. The woman should be fully awake and able to protect her own airway before extubation.

Theoretically, in cases where a mother is known to have a full stomach before emergency anaesthesia, gastric contents can be reduced by gentle use of a soft, wide-bore orogastric tube. However, this is rarely performed in practice as it is difficult to ensure stomach emptying. It is usual to await full awakening and utilise the left lateral or sitting position for extubation to aid the management of vomiting should it occur.

Anaesthetists should be aware of the dangers of extubation, and have a plan for rapid reintubation should problems occur.

10.6 Summary

- Talk, look, listen, feel
- The primary aim is to provide adequate oxygenation
- Try simple manoeuvres, i.e. chin lift, jaw thrust, suction
- Try simple adjuncts, namely the oropharyngeal airway
- Tracheal intubation with a cuffed tube is the gold standard because this achieves a protected airway and maintains patency. SADs may have a role in oxygenation and ventilation but do not provide a protected airway
- Be aware of cervical spine injury during airway management

10.7 Further reading

OAA/DAS (Obstetric Anaesthetists' Association/Difficult Airway Society). *Guidelines for the Management of Difficult and Failed Intubation in Obstetrics – 2015*. https://das.uk.com/guidelines/obstetric_airway_guidelines_2015 (last accessed January 2022).

Appendix 10.1 Practical procedures

Oropharyngeal airway insertion

Equipment

- A range of sizes of oropharyngeal (Guedel) airways
- Tongue depressor (optional)

Procedure

The correct size of airway is selected by comparing it with the distance from the angle of the mandible to the centre of the incisors. The airway is inserted as follows:

1. Open the patient's mouth and check for debris. Debris may be inadvertently pushed into the larynx as the airway is inserted.
2. Insert the airway into the mouth either:
   - 'Upside down' (concave uppermost) as far as the junction between the hard and soft palates and rotate through 180°
   - Or use a tongue depressor to aid insertion of the airway the 'right way up' under direct vision.
3. Insert so that the flange lies in front of the upper and lower incisors or gums in the edentulous patient (Figure 10A.1).
4. Check the patency of the airway and ventilation by 'looking, listening, and feeling'.

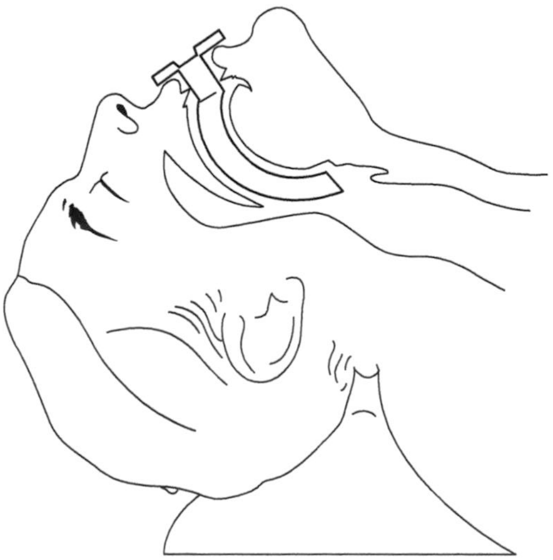

Figure 10A.1 Oropharyngeal airway in situ

Pocket mask use

Equipment

- Pocket mask
- Airway training manikin

Procedure

1. With the patient supine, apply the mask to the patient's face, using the thumbs and index fingers of both hands
2. Use the remaining fingers to exert pressure behind the angles of the jaw (as for the jaw thrust), at the same time pressing the mask on to the face to make a tight seal (Figure 10A.2).
3. Blow through the inspiratory valve for 1–2 seconds, at the same time looking to ensure that the chest rises and then falls.
4. If oxygen is available, add via the oxygen inlet at 12–15 l/min.

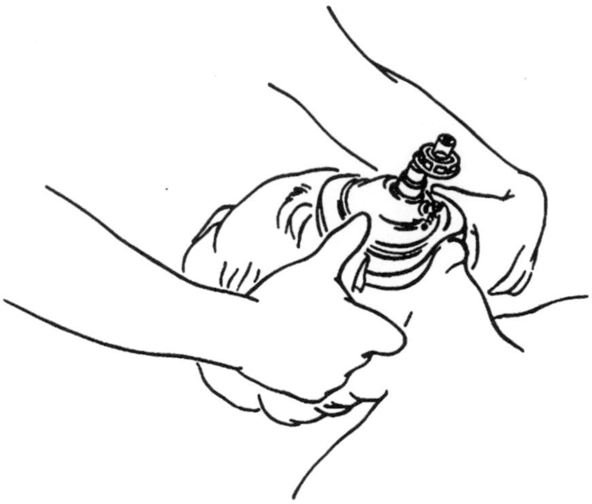

Figure 10A.2 Pocket mask in situ using a jaw thrust technique

Laryngeal mask insertion

Equipment

- LMA
- Lubricant
- Syringe to inflate cuff
- Adhesive tape to secure LMA
- Suction
- Ventilating device

Procedure

Whenever possible, ventilate the patient with 100% oxygen using a bag–valve–mask device before inserting the LMA. During this time, check that all the equipment is present and working, particularly the integrity of the cuff.

1. Deflate the cuff and lightly lubricate the back and sides of the mask.
2. Tilt the patient's head (if safe to do so), open the mouth fully and insert the tip of the mask along the hard palate with the open side facing, but not touching, the tongue (Figure 10A.3a).
3. Advance the LMA, along the posterior pharyngeal wall, with your index finger initially providing support for the tube (Figure 10A.3b). Eventually, resistance is felt as the tip of the LMA lies at the upper end of the oesophagus (Figure 10A.3c). It is extremely helpful if an assistant performs a jaw thrust manoeuvre as the LMA is inserted in order to make more space for the LMA in the posterior pharynx.
4. Fully inflate the cuff using the air-filled syringe attached to the valve at the end of the pilot tube using the volume of air shown in Table 10A.1 (Figure 10A.3d).
5. Secure the LMA with adhesive tape and check its position during ventilation as for a tracheal tube.
6. If insertion is not accomplished in less than 30 seconds, re-establish ventilation using a bag–valve–mask.

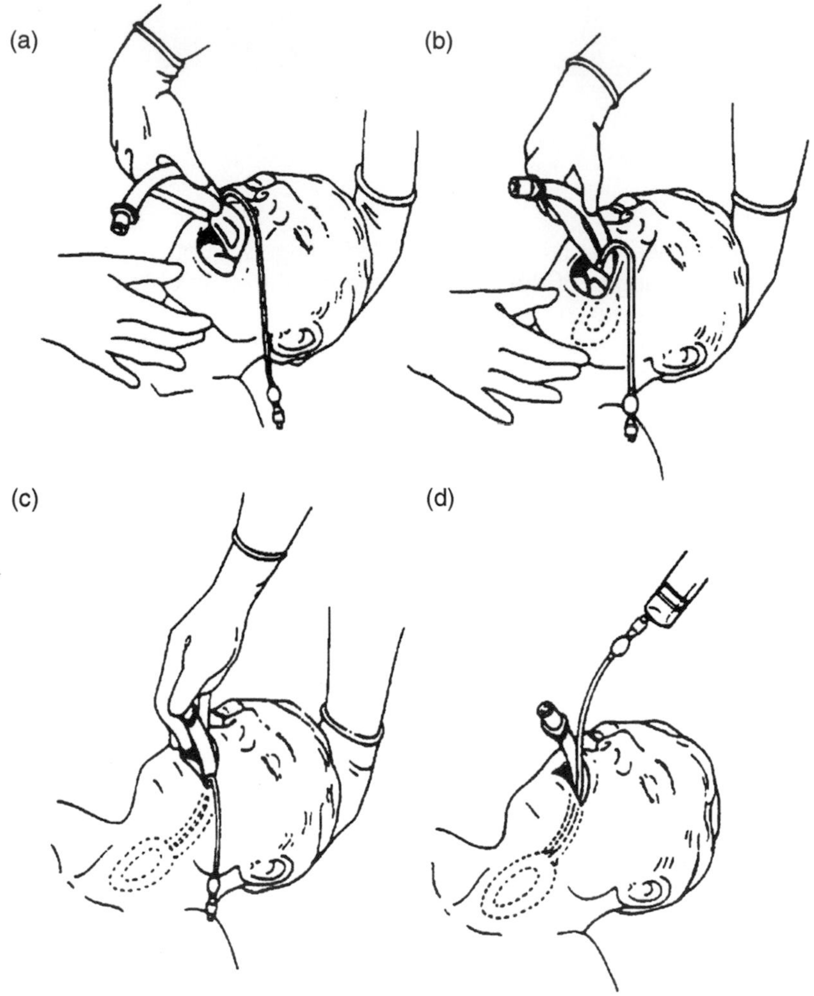

Figure 10A.3 Inserting a laryngeal mask airway

Table 10A.1 LMA sizes and inflation volumes

LMA size	Maximum inflation volume (ml)
3	20
4	30
5	40
6	50

Complications

Incorrect placement is usually due to the tip of the cuff folding over during insertion. The LMA should be withdrawn and reinserted.

Inability to ventilate the patient can be because the epiglottis has been displaced over the larynx. Withdraw the LMA and reinsert it, ensuring that it closely follows the hard palate. This may be facilitated by the operator or an assistant lifting the jaw upwards. Occasionally, rotation of the LMA may prevent its insertion. Check that the line along the tube is aligned with the patient's nasal septum; if not, reinsert.

Coughing or laryngeal spasm is usually due to attempts to insert the LMA into a patient whose laryngeal reflexes are still present.

Surgical airway

It is important to realise that this technique, whilst it provides a secure airway, is not a long-term measure. The following technique is reproduced in Box 10A.1 from the OAA/DAS 2015 guidelines.

Box 10A.1 Scalpel cricothyroidotomy

Equipment
- Scalpel (number 10 blade)
- Bougie
- Tube (cuffed 6.0 mm ID)

Laryngeal handshake to identify cricothyroid membrane

Palpable cricothyroid membrane
- Transverse stab incision through cricothyroid membrane
- Turn blade through 90° (sharp edge caudally)
- Slide coude tip of bougie along blade into trachea
- Railroad lubricated 6.0 mm cuffed tracheal tube into trachea
- Ventilate, inflate cuff and confirm position with capnography
- Secure tube

Impalpable cricothyroid membrane
- Make an 8–10 cm vertical skin incision, caudad to cephalad
- Use blunt dissection with fingers of both hands to separate tissues
- Identify and stabilise the larynx
- Proceed with technique for palpable cricothyroid mambrane as above

Figure 10A.4 shows the laryngeal handshake to identify the cricothyroid membrane. The index finger and thumb grasp the top of the larynx (the greater cornu of the hyoid bone) and roll it from side to side (Figure 10A.4a). The bony and cartilaginous cage of the larynx is a cone, which connects to the trachea. The fingers and thumb slide down over the thyroid laminae (Figure 10A.4b). The middle finger and thumb rest on the cricoid cartilage, with the index finger palpating the cricothyroid membrane (Figure 10A.4c).

(a) (b) (c)

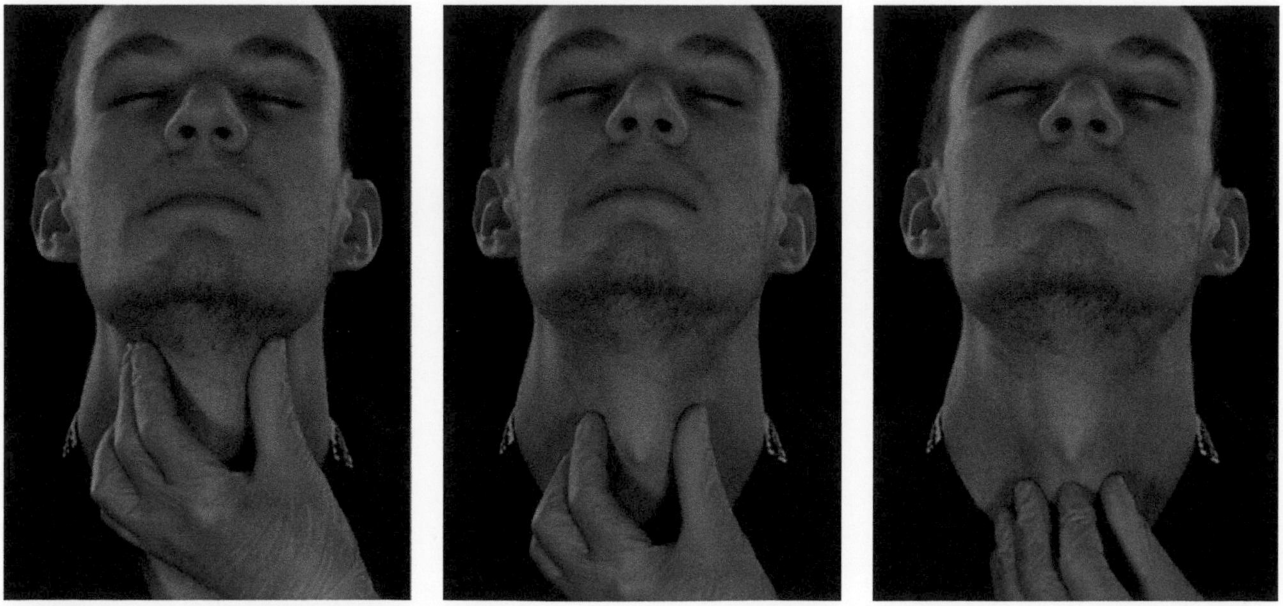

Figure 10A.4 Laryngeal handshake
Source: From Frerk C, Mitchell VS, McNarry AF, et al. Difficult Airway Society 2015 guidelines for management of unanticipated difficult intubation in adults. *Br J Anaesth* 2015; 115(6): 827–48. Courtesy of DAS

Figure 10A.5 shows an example of a surgical cricothyroidotomy kit in use in the UK.

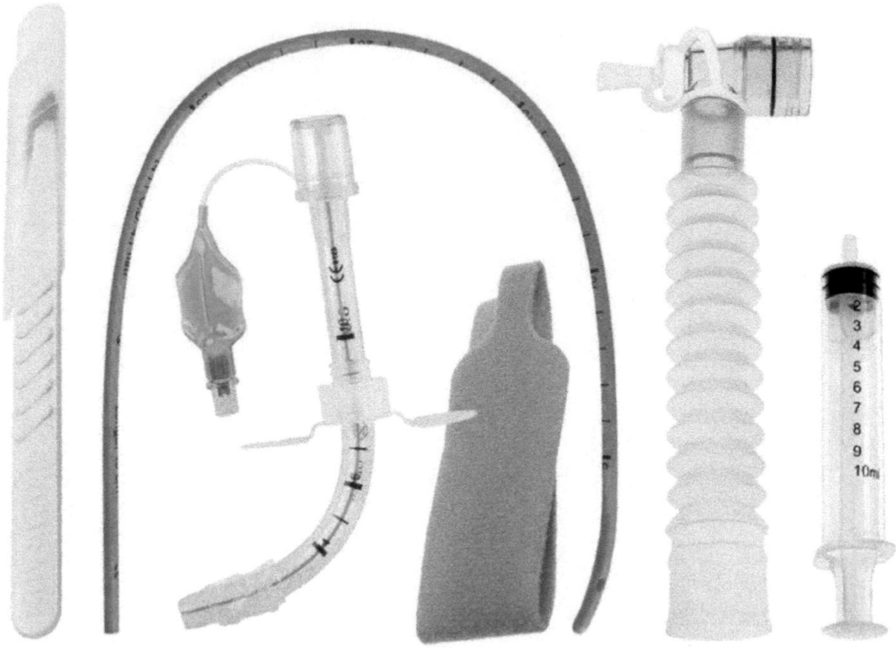

Figure 10A.5 Surgical cricothyroidotomy kit
Source: Figure courtesy of VBM

Complications

Complications of this technique can include:

- Asphyxia
- Pulmonary barotrauma
- Bleeding
- Oesophageal perforation
- Subcutaneous and mediastinal emphysema
- Aspiration

Adult advanced life support (modified for pregnancy)

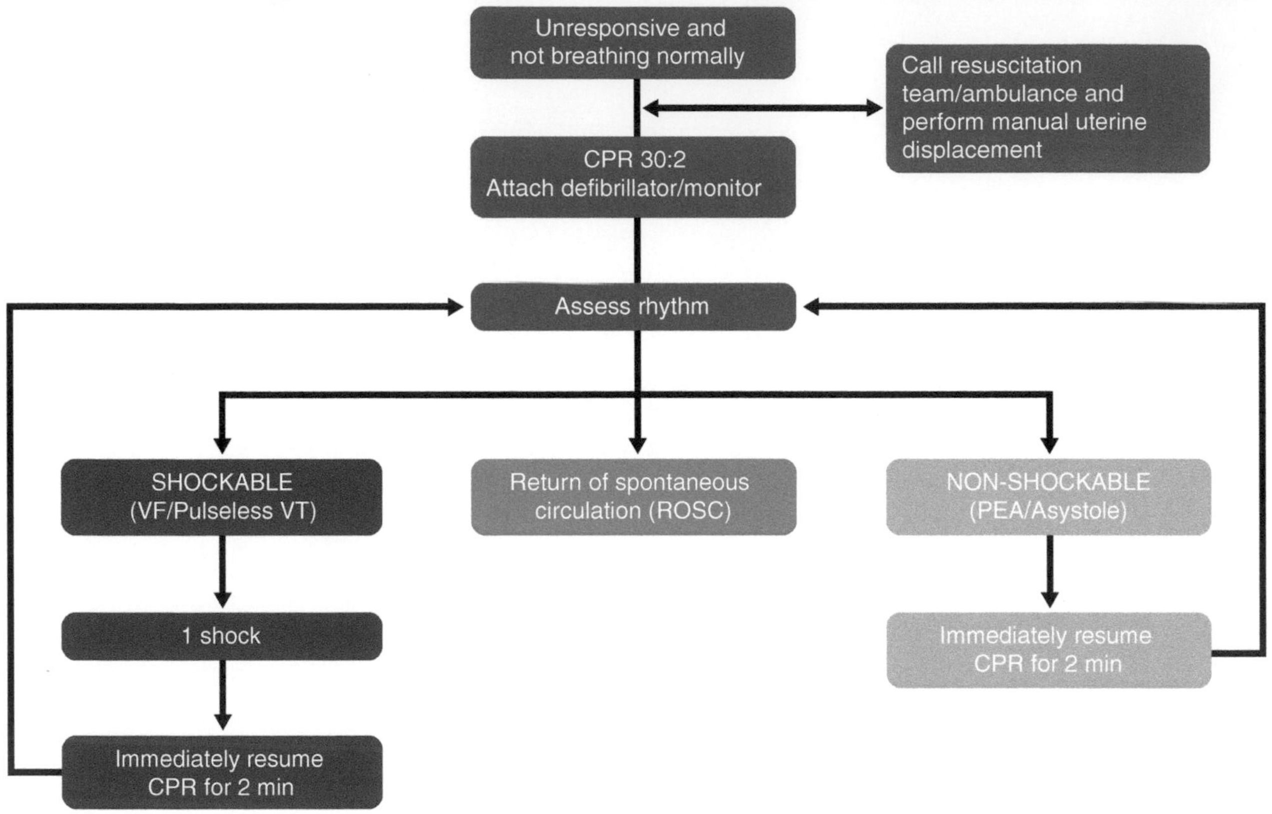

Unresponsive and not breathing normally
Call resuscitation team/ambulance and perform manual uterine displacement
CPR 30:2
Attach defibrillator/monitor
Assess rhythm
SHOCKABLE
(VF/Pulseless VT)
Return of spontaneous circulation (ROSC)
NON-SHOCKABLE
(PEA/Asystole)
1 shock
Immediately resume CPR for 2 min
Immediately resume CPR for 2 min

Give high-quality chest compressions: manually displace the uterus

- Give oxygen
- Use waveform capnography
- Continuous compressions if advanced airway
- Minimise interruptions to compressions
- Intravenous or intraosseous access
- Give adrenaline every 3-5 min
- Give amiodarone after 3 shocks
- Identify and treat reversible causes
- Empty the uterus within 5 minutes of cardiac arrest

Identify and treat reversible causes

- **H**ypoxia
- **H**ypovolaemia*
- **H**ypo-/hyperkalaemia/ metabolic
- **H**ypo/hyperthermia
- **T**hrombosis – coronary*, pulmonary, amniotic
- **T**ension pneumothorax
- **T**amponade – cardiac
- **T**oxins – local anaesthetic, magnesium
- Eclampsia*

Consider ultrasound imaging to identify reversible causes

*more likely in pregnancy

Consider

- Coronary angiography/ percutaneous coronary intervention
- Mechanical chest compressions to facilitate transfer/ treatment
- Extracorporeal CPR

After ROSC

- Use an ABCDE approach
- Aim for SpO_2 of 94-98% normal $PaCO_2$
- 12-lead ECG
- Identify and treat cause
- Targeted temperature management

Algorithm 11.1 Adult advanced life support (modified for pregnancy)
Source: Resuscitation Council (UK)

CHAPTER 11
Cardiopulmonary resuscitation in the pregnant patient

Learning outcomes

After reading this chapter, you will be able to:

- Describe how to perform basic and advanced life support
- Define the importance of early defibrillation where appropriate
- Identify the adaptations of CPR in the pregnant woman
- Describe the role of perimortem caesarean section in maternal resuscitation

11.1 Introduction

In the UK, a cardiac arrest is estimated to occur in every 36 000 maternities. Both thromboembolism and amniotic fluid embolism are important causes of maternal death, which may present with sudden collapse. It is important that healthcare teams know the appropriate actions to take in such an event, to improve outcome for both the mother and fetus.

Basic life support

Basic life support describes the procedures that a trained *lay person* could be expected to provide. These include:

- Recognising an absence of breathing or other signs of life
- Knowing to ask for an automated external defibrillator (AED) when summoning help
- A lone bystander can call for help using a mobile phone (999) in the hands-free mode so they can continue with cardiopulmonary resuscitation (CPR) while summoning help
- Performing chest compressions and mouth-to-mouth or pocket mask breathing
- (If the rescuer is not happy to perform mouth-to-mouth breathing they can continue with only chest compressions)
- Minimising interruptions to chest compression while using the AED

Managing Medical and Obstetric Emergencies and Trauma: A Practical Approach, Fourth Edition. Edited by Rosamunde Burns and Kara Dent.

Adult basic life support in community settings

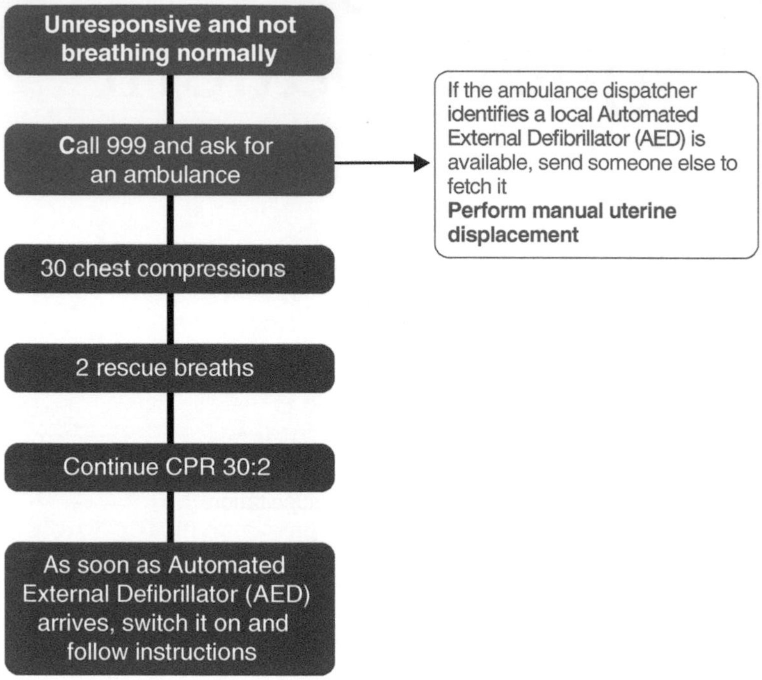

Algorithm 11.2 Adult basic life support in community settings

Advanced life support

Advanced life support describes the procedures that a trained *healthcare professional* could be expected to provide. This includes all of the above, and in addition:

- Use of airway adjuncts to provide more effective ventilation
- Insertion of intravenous cannulae to give drugs
- Use of semiautomated or manual defibrillators

It should not be necessary to perform mouth-to-mouth ventilation in a hospital as airway adjuncts should be close to hand.

In a hospital setting, the distinction between basic and advanced life support is arbitrary. The clinical team should be able to provide CPR, the fundamental components of which are:

- Rapid recognition of cardiopulmonary collapse
- Summoning help using a standard procedure/number
- Starting CPR, with manual uterine displacement (MUD) over 20 weeks' gestation, using appropriate adjuncts
- Early defibrillation, when required, if possible within 3 minutes
- Perimortem caesarean section (PMCS) in the absence of rapid return of spontaneous circulation (ROSC) in pregnant women with a uterus palpable at or above the umbilicus

Recent guidelines place greater emphasis on high-quality cardiac compressions (*'push hard and fast'*) with minimal interruptions.

11.2 Management of CPR

The rescuer must ensure a safe environment. Try to rouse the woman by gently shaking and shouting. If there is no response, call for help, indicating, if required, that the patient is pregnant and that a scalpel may be needed for delivery and then return to the woman. If there is no response but there are still '*signs of life*', then urgent medical attention should be requested and further assessment and appropriate treatment given. Signs of life include:

- Normal breathing (not agonal gasps)
- Movement
- Coughing/gagging

In the event of little or no signs of life, the following instructions are listed in order of importance to guide single- or two-attendant arrests. If there are multiple helpers, one should take a leading role, and the following interventions applied simultaneously.

Perform manual uterine displacement

If a uterus is palpable at or above the level of the umbilicus (i.e. 20 weeks' gestation or more), uterine aortocaval compression will markedly reduce the effect of cardiac compressions. If two attendants are available, one must be assigned to MUD throughout resuscitation. Only if a third attendant is available should an individual be nominated to ventilate the patient.

A left lateral tilt can be adopted in a single-attendant arrest situation, but cardiac compressions will be less effective than if the thorax remained on a flat surface as in MUD.

Open the airway

Open the mouth and briefly check for debris or foreign bodies. Use suction or forceps under direct vision to remove any obstruction, taking care not to cause trauma.

To open the airway, place your hand on the patient's forehead and gently tilt the head back. At the same time, with your fingertips under the point of the patient's chin, lift the chin to open the airway. This manoeuvre will straighten the head and neck from a slumped or flexed position, and may slightly extend the head relative to the neck. It allows more space behind the tongue in the posterior pharynx for air movement. In a conscious person, the pharyngeal muscle tone naturally maintains this space for breathing, but this will be absent in the unconscious person. An oral airway may be used to provide the same space behind the tongue, with less requirement for vigorous head extension.

A jaw thrust may be required to open the airway. Do this by placing fingers *behind* both of the angles of the jaw and pushing the jaw anteriorly to displace the tongue from the pharynx. If an injury to the neck is suspected, use manual inline stabilisation, avoid head tilt and use a jaw thrust to open the airway.

Assess breathing (and signs of life: circulation)

Assess breathing for *no more than 10 seconds* by simultaneously looking for chest movements, listening for breath sounds and feeling for the movement of air. An absence of breathing in the presence of a clear airway is now considered a marker of absence of circulation, along with absence of gagging or movement. Experienced staff may check the carotid pulse for no more than 10 seconds at the same time as assessing breathing, but it is important to be aware of how difficult it is for even experienced clinicians to confirm the absence of a pulse and not to waste time before starting chest compressions. 'Unnecessary' chest compressions are almost never harmful. Gasping or agonal breathing may occur during cardiac arrest and should *not* be taken as a sign of life – it is a sign of dying and CPR should commence immediately.

> If there is no circulation (or you are at all unsure) give 30 chest compressions followed by two ventilations

Start CPR

1. Chest compressions should be applied to the lower half of the sternum. Place the heel of one hand there, with the other hand on top of the first. Interlock the fingers of both hands and lift the fingers to ensure that pressure is not applied over the patient's ribs. Keep in the midline at all times. Do not apply any pressure over the top of the abdomen or lower tip of the sternum.
2. Position yourself above the chest and with your arms straight, press down on the sternum to depress 5–6 cm at a rate of 100–120 beats/min in a ratio of 30:2 compressions to ventilations. Change the person doing chest compressions about every 2 minutes to maintain efficiency, but avoid any delays in the changeover.
3. Ventilation breaths. Keep an open airway and provide ventilation with appropriate adjuncts. This might be a pocket mask, oral airway or self-inflating bag with mask. Oxygen in high flow should be added as soon as possible.
4. Each breath should last about 1 second and should make the chest rise as for a normal breath. Tracheal intubation should only be undertaken by experienced personnel with minimal interruption to chest compressions. The laryngeal mask airway may be useful as an alternative airway adjunct if intubation cannot be achieved swiftly. Once the woman is intubated, ventilation should continue at a rate of 10 breaths/min, but does not need to be synchronised with chest compressions. These should be continued without interruption.
5. Mouth-to-mouth breathing is rarely necessary in the hospital setting – the important thing is to maintain a patent airway during cardiac compressions. If it is undertaken, head tilt and chin lift should be maintained. Close the soft part of the woman's nose with your thumb and index finger. Open her mouth but maintain chin lift. Take a breath and place your lips around the mouth, making sure that you have a good seal. Blow steadily into the mouth for over 1 second, watching for the chest to rise. Maintaining head tilt and chin lift, take your mouth away and watch for the chest to fall as the air comes out. Take another breath and repeat the sequence to give another effective breath. Return to chest compressions quickly.
6. Prepare for a PMCS by ensuring that a knife is available and that one of the attendants is capable of the procedure, or that appropriate help is available imminently.

> If circulation is present but there is no breathing (respiratory arrest), continue rescue breathing at a rate of 10 breaths/min

Recheck the circulation every 10 breaths, taking no more than 10 seconds each time. If the woman starts to breathe on her own but remains unconscious, turn her into the recovery position and apply high-flow oxygen (15 l/min or maximum flow rate available). Check her condition and be ready to turn her back to restart rescue breathing if she stops breathing and/or compressions if necessary.

Capnography can be used in CPR. Although carbon dioxide levels are low, they are not nil and can be used to monitor CPR efficacy. An increase in carbon dioxide will indicate ROSC. There is evidence that post-resuscitation hyperoxaemia is associated with a worse outcome compared with normoxaemia or hypoxaemia and so, once arterial oxygen can be monitored, aim to keep saturation between 94% and 98% by adjusting oxygen flow as needed.

Automated external defibrillation

As soon as possible, apply the defibrillator pads or paddles and pause compressions briefly to assess the rhythm. This is quicker than attaching the electrocardiogram stickers. If a shockable rhythm is identified by the AED, then continue chest compressions while the AED is charging if necessary. Follow the AED voice prompts or use manual defibrillation as appropriate.

The most frequent initial rhythm in the context of sudden collapse in an adult (i.e. not preceded by gradual deterioration or illness) is ventricular fibrillation (VF). The chance of successful defibrillation diminishes over minutes. The AED enables early defibrillation by less trained personnel as it performs rhythm analysis, gives information by voice or visual display and delivers a shock automatically.

Attaching AED pads (or position gel pads for manual defibrillator)

Expose the chest and place one adhesive defibrillator pad on the patient's chest to the right of the sternum below the right clavicle, and one in the left mid-axillary line, taking care to avoid breast tissue. Keep the axillary electrode vertical to maximise efficiency.

If defibrillation is *not* indicated, CPR should be continued for 2 minutes, at which stage the AED will prompt further analysis of rhythm. If a shock is indicated, deliver it (many devices do this automatically) and immediately resume compressions for 2 minutes, after which there will be a further prompt for a rhythm analysis.

11.3 Follow the advanced life support algorithm

When trained support arrives, the rhythm should be identified as shockable or non-shockable and defibrillation instituted if indicated without delay, if not already under way. The airway should be secured and intravenous access obtained.

Shockable rhythms

- Shockable rhythms are treated by a single shock followed by immediate continuation of compressions without stopping for a rhythm or pulse check
- Every 2 minutes, the rhythm should be assessed and, if necessary, a further shock delivered. The pulse is not checked *unless* there is organised electrical activity, i.e. a rhythm that looks as though it might produce an output or signs of life
- The energy used for defibrillation depends on whether a monophasic or biphasic defibrillator is used. Most modern defibrillators are biphasic as this is the most efficient way of delivering energy. The charge needed is therefore lower than on the older monophasic machines
- The initial and subsequent shocks should be 150–200 J from a biphasic machine or 360 J from a monophasic machine
- On the shockable side of the algorithm, adrenaline 1 mg IV is given once chest compressions are started *after the third shock* and then after alternate shocks; i.e. approximately every 4 minutes. Amiodarone 300 mg IV is also given after the third shock

Non-shockable rhythms

- On the non-shockable side of the algorithm (i.e. pulseless electrical activity (PEA) or asystole), adrenaline (epinephrine) 1 mg should be given as soon as intravenous access is available and thereafter every 3–5 minutes while continuing chest compressions and ventilations at 30:2

Reversible causes of cardiac arrest

Reversible causes of cardiac arrest should be considered and treated as necessary. After complications of regional anaesthesia, *hypovolaemia* (from haemorrhage or sepsis) and *thromboembolism* are the most common causes of cardiac arrest/collapse in pregnancy. They are more likely to cause *non-shockable cardiac arrest*. (See Chapters 6, 7, 12, 13 and 28.)

The UK Resuscitation Council advanced life support guidelines (Nolan and Soar, 2021) recognise the increasing role of POCUS (point of care ultrasound) in the peri-arrest scenario to aid diagnosis of maternal collapse. This requires a skilled operator and must not interrupt CPR. Extracorporeal CPR should be considered as a bridge to coronary angiography, percutaneous coronary intervention, pulmonary thrombectomy in massive pulmonary embolism, and rewarming after hypothermic cardiac arrest (Figure 11.1).

Four Hs
- Hypoxia
- Hypovolaemia (haemorrhage or sepsis)
- Hyperkalaemia and other metabolic disorders
- Hypothermia

Four Ts
- Thromboembolism
- Toxicity (drugs, e.g. magnesium overdose or those associated with regional or general anaesthesia)
- Tension pneumothorax
- Cardiac tamponade

Obstetric Cardiac Arrest

Resuscitation Council UK — MBRRACE-UK (Mothers and Babies: Reducing Risk through Audits and Confidential Enquiries across the UK)

Alterations in maternal physiology and exacerbations of pregnancy related pathologies must be considered. Priorities include calling the appropriate team members, relieving aortocaval compression, effective cardiopulmonary resuscitation (CPR), consideration of causes and performing a timely emergency hysterotomy (perimortem caesarean section) when ≥ 20 weeks.

START

1. **Confirm cardiac arrest** and **call for help. Declare 'Obstetric cardiac arrest'**
   - Team for mother and team for neonate if > 20 weeks
2. **Lie flat, apply manual uterine displacement to the left**
   - Or left lateral tilt(from head to toe at an angle of 15–30° on a firm surface)
3. **Commence CPR** and request **cardiac arrest trolley**
   - Standard CPR ratios and hand position apply
   - **Evaluate potential causes (Box A)**
4. **Identify team leader, allocate roles including scribe**
   - Note time
5. **Apply defibrillation pads and check cardiac rhythm** (defibrillation is safe inpregnancy and no changes to standard shock energies are required))
   - if VF / pulseless VT ➔ defibrillation and first adrenaline and amiodarone after 3rd shock
   - If PEA / asystole ➔ resume CPR and give first adrenaline immediately
   - Check rhythm and pulse every 2 minutes
   - Repeat adrenaline every 3-5 minutes
6. **Maintain airway and ventilation**
   - Give 100% oxygen using bag-valve-mask device
   - Insert supraglottic airway with drain port *–or–* tracheal tube if trained to do so (intubation may be difficult, and airway pressures may be higher)
   - Apply waveform capnography monitoring to airway
   - If expired CO_2 is absent, presume oesophageal intubation until absolutely excluded
7. **Circulation**
   - I.V. access above the diaphragm, if fails or impossible use upper limb intraosseous (IO)
   - See **Box B** for reminders about drugs
   - Consider extracorporeal CPR (ECPR) if available
8. **Emergency hysterotomy (perimortem caesarean section)**
   - Perform if ≥ 20 weeks gestation, to improve maternal outcome
   - Perform immediately if maternal fatal injuries or prolonged pre-hospital arrest
   - Perform by 5 minutes if no return of spontaneous circulation
9. **Post resuscitation from haemorrhage - activate Massive Haemorrhage Protocol**
   Consider uterotonic drugs, fibrinogen and tranexamic acid
   Uterine tamponage / sutures, aortic compression, hysterectomy

Version 1.1

Box A: POTENTIAL CAUSES *4H's and 4T's*(specific to obstetrics)	
Hypoxia	Respiratory – Pulmonary embolus(PE), Failed intubation, aspiration Heart failure Anaphylaxis Eclampsia / PET – pulmonary oedema, seizure
Hypovolaemia	Haemorrhage –obstetric(remember concealed), abnormal placentation,uterine rupture, atony, splenic artery/hepatic rupture, aneurysm rupture Cardiac – arrhythmia, myocardial infarction (MI) Distributive – sepsis, high regional block, anaphylaxis
Hypo/hyperkalaemia	Also consider blood sugar, sodium, calcium and magnesium levels
Hypothermia	
Tamponade	Aortic dissection, peripartum cardiomyopathy, trauma
Thrombosis	Amniotic fluid embolus, PE, MI, air embolism
Toxins	Local anaesthetic, magnesium, illicit drugs
Tension pneumothorax	Entonox in pre-existing pneumothorax, trauma

Box B: IV DRUGS FOR USE DURING CARDIAC ARREST	
Fluids	**500 mL IV** crystalloid bolus
Adrenaline	**1mg IV** every 3-5 minutes in non-shockable or after 3rd shock
Amiodarone	**300 mg IV** after 3rd shock
Atropine	**0.5-1 mg IV** up to 3 mg if vagal tone likely cause
Calcium chloride	**10% 10 mL** IV for Mg overdose, low calcium or hyperkalaemia
Magnesium	**2 g IV** for polymorphic VT / hypomagnesaemia, **4 g IV** for eclampsia
Thrombolysis/PCI	For suspected massive pulmonary embolus / MI
Tranexamic acid	**1 g** if haemorrhage
Intralipid	**1.5 mL kg-1 IV** bolus and **15 mL kg-1 hr-1 IV** infusion

Obstetric Anaesthetists' Association — Promoting the highest standards of anaesthetic practice in the care of mother and baby

GUIDELINES 2021

Figure 11.1 Obstetric cardiac arrest
Source: Resuscitation Council (UK)

Doubt about the rhythm

If there is doubt about whether the rhythm is asystole or fine VF, CPR should be maintained and the algorithm for asystole (non-shockable rhythm) followed.

Other drugs

Sodium bicarbonate 50 mmol IV should only be given routinely if the arrest is associated with tricyclic antidepressant overdose or hyperkalaemia. Otherwise, it should not be given, as it exacerbates intracellular acidosis, reduces tissue oxygen availability and has a negative inotropic effect on the myocardium. Arterial blood gases are not reliable in cardiac arrest; venous blood gases provide a better estimation of tissue pH.

Magnesium sulphate 8 mmol (4 ml of 50% solution) may be given for refractory VF. Other indications include hypomagnesaemia, torsade de pointes (a persistent VF) or digoxin toxicity. These are unlikely in pregnancy.

Calcium chloride 10 ml 10% (6.8 mmol Ca^{2+}) IV is indicated if PEA is suspected to be due to hyperkalaemia, hypocalcaemia or overdose of calcium channel blocking drugs. Calcium maybe given as a bolus if the patient has no output, *but not in the same line as sodium bicarbonate* as this will result in precipitation. Magnesium overdose (usually in the context of treatment of pre-eclampsia) is usually reversed with calcium gluconate.

11.4 Physiological changes in pregnancy affecting resuscitation

There are a number of reasons why CPR is more difficult to perform and may be less effective in the pregnant than in the non-pregnant population. The gravid uterus compromises resuscitative efforts from about 20 weeks of gestation, but the effect will become more marked as the mother approaches term.

Vena caval occlusion

At term the vena cava is completely occluded in 90% of healthy *supine* pregnant women and the stroke volume may be only 30% of that of a non-pregnant woman. As soon as the neonate is delivered, the vena caval flow returns towards normal and adequate venous return, and consequently cardiac output, is restored.

During cardiac arrest, the priorities are high-quality CPR and relief of aortocaval compression. The latter should be achieved with MUD (see Figure 6.1), which maintains the supine position and maximum efficiency of compressions, unlike pelvic tilt, which was previously advised. One helper should be assigned to MUD, even if there are only two helpers attending the arrest. Cardiac compressions without MUD are unlikely to achieve adequate perfusion and maternal survival.

Delivery of the fetus during cardiac arrest will immediately relieve aortocaval compression, increase venous return to the heart and reduce oxygen demands on the mother, thereby increasing the chances of successful resuscitation (see next section).

Changes in lung function

Pregnant women become rapidly hypoxic because functional residual capacity is reduced by 20% due to the pressure of the gravid uterus on the diaphragm and the lungs – they have a smaller reservoir of oxygen to withstand apnoea. This is exacerbated by a 20% increase in resting oxygen usage due to the demands of the fetus and uterus. These changes make it difficult to provide adequate oxygen delivery during resuscitation of a pregnant woman who is near term.

Efficacy of ventilation

In the latter half of a pregnancy it is increasingly difficult to provide effective ventilation breaths during CPR, due to the increased weight of the abdominal contents and the breasts. Oesophageal sphincter tone is reduced, so the stomach is more readily inflated and the risk of passive regurgitation of stomach contents and acid aspiration into the lungs is increased. It is imperative that the airway is protected and adequate ventilation established, with a cuffed endotracheal tube, as early as possible, by appropriately trained staff.

11.5 Perimortem caesarean section

At gestations over 20 weeks, unless ROSC occurs immediately, maternal survival is unlikely without PMCS. Emptying the uterus relieves aortocaval compression, reduces maternal oxygen consumption, increases venous return, makes ventilation easier and allows control of non-compressible abdominal haemorrhage, with direct cardiac compressions if required.

Although caesarean section is a very common procedure, it is unusual to perform this procedure entirely for maternal benefit, which may explain the, even momentary, hesitation to proceed. If there is no maternal cardiac output, the aim of PMCS is purely to improve maternal outcome. The outcome for the fetus is a secondary consideration. If sufficient personnel are available, all appropriate efforts should be made to resuscitate the neonate if he or she is of a viable gestation.

When to do it

Preparations for surgical evacuation of the uterus should begin almost at the same time as CPR following cardiac arrest. Pregnant women develop anoxia faster than non-pregnant women and can suffer irreversible brain damage within 4–6 minutes of cardiac arrest. Maternal (and fetal) prognosis are improved by rapid PMCS and, unless ROSC occurs immediately, the uterus should be emptied as soon as the team is ready. In non-survivable arrest, consideration should be given to immediate delivery for fetal benefit. CPR should be continued throughout the PMCS and afterwards, as this increases the chances of a successful neonatal and maternal outcome.

Maternal survival has been described with PMCS at 39 minutes post-arrest.

Where to do it

Unless there is imminent danger to the patient or team, do not move the patient as this will delay delivery. If resuscitation is successful, the woman can be anaesthetised and moved to theatre for surgical repair.

How to do it

Minimal surgical equipment is required and full surgical scrub is unnecessary. The operator should protect themselves with an apron and gloves, but otherwise only a scalpel is required to commence the procedure. Torches or portable lamps will maximise visibility. Once the neonate is delivered, a cord clamp or ligature can secure the cord. A swab can be used to pack the wound while continuing resuscitation but bleeding will be minimal until ROSC occurs. An anaesthetic machine should be obtained so that the anaesthetist can administer a general anaesthetic if ROSC occurs, to allow surgical repair.

Surgery should proceed whilst cardiac compressions and MUD continue. A subumbilical midline incision provides the most rapid entry with maximal exposure to the abdomen, which is particularly important where there has been trauma. If there is blood in the peritoneal cavity on entry this may indicate that there is catastrophic, non-compressible haemorrhage as a cause of the cardiac arrest, such as ruptured splenic artery aneurysm or hepatic or uterine rupture. The team leader should be informed and a general surgeon called.

Obstetricians will be familiar with lower segment caesarean section but this approach is only appropriate at more advanced gestations where the lower segment has formed. If there is any doubt, a vertical incision in the midline of the uterus should be used. Given the circumstances of a patient constantly moving from cardiac compressions, in most circumstances this incision is also likely to be the most practicable. Incise at the fundus anteriorly and continue inferiorly, in the midline, to just above the bladder. The thickness of the uterus depends on the gestation, but can be up to 4 cm deep at the fundus. Once the amniotic sac herniates into the incision or liquor is seen, use digital dissection to minimise operator and fetal injury.

Deliver the baby and clamp the cord with a cord clamp or ligature, cutting the cord on the mother's side of the clamps or tie. Pass the baby to the neonatal team for resuscitation or nominate a team member to dry the baby and keep it warm until help arrives. Manual uterine displacement can cease.

Leave the placenta in situ. If swabs are now available, pack the uterine incision. In cases of catastrophic haemorrhage, aortic compression may assist the resuscitation by limiting the circulatory volume, encouraging cerebral perfusion. The arrest team leader should give instructions to best deploy those available to determine and treat the reversible causes of arrest.

If ROSC occurs, bleeding will commence and uterine tone may return, resulting in placental separation. If not, a uterotonic drug can be given to aid this process, allow placental delivery and reduce blood loss. Swabs can achieve adequate haemostasis until the patient is stable enough to move to an operating theatre environment for surgical repair under general anaesthetic. Careful inspection of the abdomen should be carried out to detect iatrogenic organ damage or any pathology that might have caused the arrest. Broad-spectrum antibiotics should be administered.

An intensivist should be consulted to ensure effective transfer to intensive care.

It is important to note that the coagulopathy may not develop if there is a rapid deterioration and the woman dies. It will be present, or develop, if the woman survives the initial collapse. It is extremely unlikely that bleeding will be the first presentation.

12.4 Symptoms and signs

The initial UK Registry paper describes several initial patterns of presentation:

- Maternal hypotension, shortness of breath, and fetal bradycardia, then delivery (14%)
- Maternal loss of consciousness or seizure, then delivery (35%)
- Maternal collapse after delivery of baby at CS (14%)
- Fetal distress and then maternal collapse (23%)
- Loss of consciousness or seizures immediately following delivery (14%)

In each case it was followed by coagulation difficulties, and usually also profuse haemorrhage.

The UKOSS data describe the presentations and features of AFE as shown in Table 12.1.

Table 12.1 Presentation and features of amniotic fluid embolism (AFE)

Feature	Women exhibiting feature as the main feature* (*n* = 60)	Women exhibiting first symptom or sign of AFE (*n* = 60)
Maternal haemorrhage	39 (65%)	1 (2%)
Hypotension	38 (63%)	5 (8%)
Shortness of breath	37 (62%)	12 (20%)
Coagulopathy	37 (62%)	0 (0%)
Premonitory symptoms (e.g. restlessness, agitation, numbness, tingling)	28 (47%)	18 (30%)
Acute fetal compromise	26 (43%)	12 (20%)
Cardiac arrest	24 (40%)	5 (8%)
Cardiac rhythm problems)	16 (27%)	3 (5%)
Seizures	12 (20%)	4 (7%)

Percentages are of complete data and some women had multiple features.
* Some women presented with more than one feature.

Suspecting an AFE

Amniotic fluid embolism should be part of the differential diagnosis of women who present with any of the above during labour or after delivery. In the MBRRACE-UK maternal mortality report (2013–2015) AFE was again reviewed alongside major obstetric haemorrhage (Knight et al., 2017). Two deaths followed rapid labour related to management of late intrauterine death involving relatively high doses of misoprostol and a specific recommendation was made:

> Misoprostol should always be used with extreme caution for women with late intrauterine fetal death, especially in the presence of a uterine scar. In these women, particularly those with a scar, dinoprostone may be more appropriate.

12.5 Diagnosis of AFE

The diagnosis is a clinical one. Absolute confirmation is only possible following death, with fetal squames in the maternal pulmonary circulation. However, other clinical features still need to be present to confirm the diagnosis. This is because fetal squames have been found in central venous blood in other conditions and even in the non-pregnant woman. In the living, fetal squames, or lanugo, on central venous samples cannot be taken as indicative of the diagnosis without a compatible clinical presentation.

The differential diagnosis involves considering an exhaustive list of the causes of maternal collapse in the peripartum period:

- Postpartum haemorrhage (uterine atony)
- Placental abruption
- Uterine rupture
- Eclampsia
- Septic shock
- Thrombotic embolus
- Air embolus
- Acute myocardial infarction
- Peripartum cardiomyopathy
- Local anaesthetic toxicity
- Anaphylaxis
- Transfusion reactions
- Aspiration of gastric contents

Only after exclusion of all the other causes can a diagnosis be confirmed clinically.

A clotting screen is often very abnormal, even before haemorrhage becomes apparent, and will exclude a large number of other diagnoses. When haemorrhage is already present, abnormal clotting could be secondary to the haemorrhage (but normally considerable blood loss with fluid or blood replacement needs to have occurred in the case of haemodilutional coagulopathy).

An electrocardiogram is helpful, to look for signs of myocardial damage. In AFE, bizarre cardiac rhythms can often be present thus making interpretation difficult. Arterial blood gases and a pulse oximeter may aid management but will not differentiate causes. A ventilation–perfusion scan of the lungs may demonstrate defects with either pulmonary embolism or AFE.

12.6 Management of AFE

The management of AFE is supportive rather than specific. Multidisciplinary treatment with early involvement of senior, experienced staff is essential. Obstetricians, anaesthetists, intensivists and haematologists are mandatory to give the best prospect of survival.

As collapse is the predominant presentation, the initial management is basic resuscitation to maintain vital organ perfusion.

Airway/breathing

- High-flow oxygen with early intubation and mechanical ventilation

Circulation

- Cardiac arrhythmias or cardiac arrest may occur
- Inotropic support is likely to be needed
- Following cardiac arrest, cardiopulmonary resuscitation and rapid delivery, within 5 minutes, aids resuscitation
- Coagulopathy and haemorrhage are likely, requiring blood and blood products
- Uterotonics to minimise/treat uterine atony
- Cardiac output measurement may guide therapy

The MBRRACE-UK report (2013–2015) recommended several other actions related to general management of collapse relevant to both AFE and haemorrhage:

- Fluid resuscitation and blood transfusion should not be delayed because of false reassurance from a single haemoglobin result
- Haemorrhage (which might be concealed) should be considered when classic signs of hypovolaemia are present (tachycardia and/or agitation and the late sign of hypotension) even in the absence of revealed bleeding
- When there has been a major obstetric haemorrhage and the bleeding is ongoing, or there are clinical concerns, then a major obstetric haemorrhage call should be activated
- Early recourse to hysterectomy is recommended where bleeding continues after an unsuccessful intrauterine balloon. In extremis and/or while waiting for assistance there are measures which can help. These include aortic compression and stepwise uterine artery ligation

Ensure that fluid overload does not occur, as this can lead to worsening pulmonary oedema and subsequent acute respiratory distress syndrome. This is particularly important when the coagulopathy and haemorrhage develops, in what has been described as the 'secondary' phase of the condition, when there are high filling pressures reflecting a failing left ventricle.

Vasopressors, such as phenylephrine, ephedrine or noradrenaline, are likely to be needed to restore aortic perfusion pressure.

In this secondary phase of coagulopathy and haemorrhage, prompt transfusion of fluids will be necessary to replace blood loss. This occurs at a variable point after initial presentation. The early consideration of clotting factor replacement with fresh frozen plasma, cryoprecipitate and platelets is important if there are signs of coagulopathy (such as haematuria or bleeding from the gums) even before massive blood loss is apparent. It is appropriate to commence this before receiving the laboratory confirmation of coagulopathy. In all cases, a direct discussion with a haematologist can help to optimise treatment. Cryoprecipitate may be of intrinsic value, beyond its clotting factor components, as it contains fibronectin, which aids the reticuloendothelial system in the filtration of antigenic and toxic particulate matter. The haemorrhage that occurs is usually as a result of uterine atony, which may be exacerbated by hypoxia and the coagulopathy. Hence, cryoprecipitate, by removing fibrin degradation products, may assist in the treatment of the uterine atony. Aggressive treatment of uterine atony with medical products (oxytocics, ergometrine, prostaglandin, tranexamic acid) and adjunctive techniques (packing, tamponade, Rusch balloons) should be used, though early recourse to hysterectomy may be life saving.

The presentation of AFE can sometimes be acute fetal collapse, which is followed, a little time after, by maternal deterioration. Checking coagulation studies and monitoring pulse oximetry in women in whom there has been sudden fetal deterioration, or whose fetus is unexpectedly severely acidotic, may identify abnormalities, providing the opportunity for earlier diagnosis and treatment.

The literature contains a number of case reports suggesting other specific treatments that include:

- Extracorporeal membrane oxygenation (ECMO)
- Prostacyclin
- Nitric oxide
- Plasma exchange
- Haemofiltration
- Cardiopulmonary bypass
- Ligation of the infundibulopelvic ligament and uterine arteries
- Factor VIIa (after discussion with a haematologist)

As the condition is anaphylactoid in nature, it has also been suggested that high-dose hydrocortisone 500 mg 6 hourly might be appropriate, but no studies have examined this. The treatments, which aim to filter or 'cleanse' the circulating blood volume, may be effective in more rapidly reversing coagulation abnormalities and are similar to the use of cryoprecipitate described earlier.

Risk of recurrence

Further pregnancies have been reported in women with a successful outcome after AFE, all with good fetal and maternal outcome.

Neonatal outcome

In the US Registry cases, 22 of 28 fetuses (79%) alive and in utero at the time of collapse survived, but only 11 (50% of survivors) were neurologically intact. In the initial UK series of the 13 women who died:

- Seven neonates survived: four of these were acidotic, and one had hypoxic ischaemic encephalopathy (HIE) and went on to develop cerebral palsy; the outcome of the other three acidotic babies seemed initially uneventful. Three of the babies did well after immediate delivery
- Six neonates died: one died in utero before presentation, one was a fresh stillbirth and the others died in the early neonatal period

Of the 18 surviving women with a fetus alive and in utero at the time of the maternal collapse:

- Twelve neonates survived: four had HIE, with one developing cerebral palsy and two others with low cord pH. The other eight were normal
- Four neonates died

In the later UK series, 10% of babies died.

12.7 Summary

- Amniotic fluid embolism is rare and often devastating for both the woman and her fetus
- Outcomes are improving and prompt resuscitation, assessment and support may lead to a better chance of a good outcome
- Involvement of a haematologist can help to optimise blood product replacement
- Specific therapies have not been evaluated

12.8 Further reading

Fitzpatrick KE, Tuffnell D, Kurinczuk M, Knight M. Incidence, risk factors, management and outcomes of amniotic-fluid embolism: a population-based cohort and nested case–control study. *BJOG* 2016; 123(1): 100–9.

Khan KS, Moore PAS, Wilson MJ, et al. Cell salvage and donor blood transfusion during cesarean section: a pragmatic, multicentre randomised controlled trial (SALVO). *PLoS Med* 2017; 14(12): e1002471.

Knight M, Bunch K, Tuffnell D, et al. (eds), on behalf of MBRRACE-UK. *Saving Lives, Improving Mothers' Care – Lessons Learned to Inform Maternity Care from the UK and Ireland Confidential Enquiries into Maternal Deaths and Morbidity 2016–18*. Oxford: National Perinatal Epidemiology Unit, University of Oxford, 2020.

UKOSS (UK Obstetric Surveillance System). *Amniotic Fluid Embolism*. https://www.npeu.ox.ac.uk/ukoss/current-surveillance/amf (last accessed January 2022).

Chapter 13: Pulmonary thromboembolism

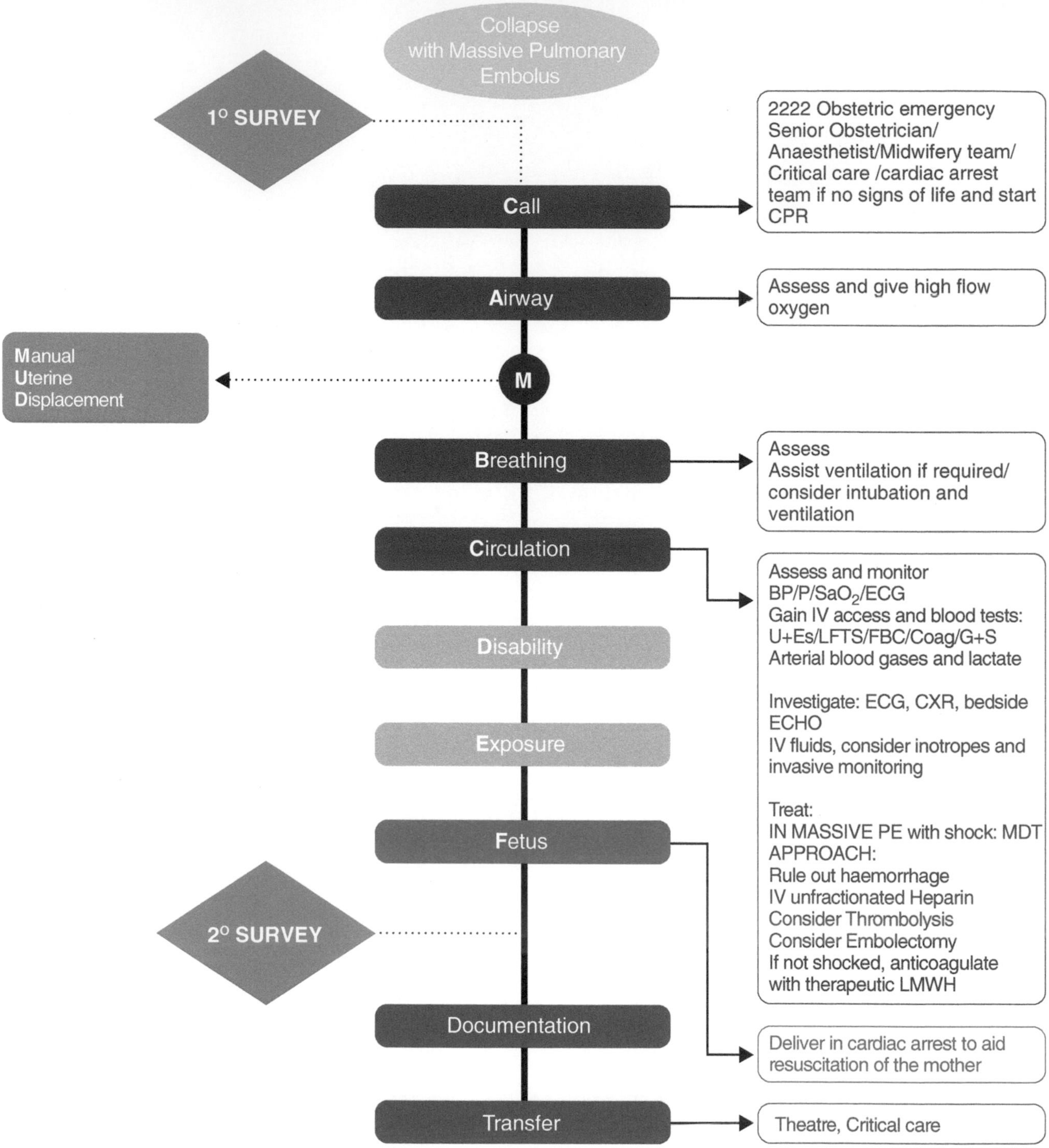
Collapse with Massive Pulmonary Embolus
1° SURVEY
Call
2222 Obstetric emergency
Senior Obstetrician/
Anaesthetist/Midwifery team/
Critical care /cardiac arrest
team if no signs of life and start
CPR
Airway
Assess and give high flow
oxygen
M
Manual
Uterine
Displacement
Breathing
Assess
Assist ventilation if required/
consider intubation and
ventilation
Circulation
Assess and monitor
BP/P/SaO2/ECG
Gain IV access and blood tests:
U+Es/LFTS/FBC/Coag/G+S
Arterial blood gases and lactate
Investigate: ECG, CXR, bedside
ECHO
IV fluids, consider inotropes and
invasive monitoring
Treat:
IN MASSIVE PE with shock: MDT
APPROACH:
Rule out haemorrhage
IV unfractionated Heparin
Consider Thrombolysis
Consider Embolectomy
If not shocked, anticoagulate
with therapeutic LMWH
Disability
Exposure
Fetus
Deliver in cardiac arrest to aid
resuscitation of the mother
2° SURVEY
Documentation
Transfer
Theatre, Critical care

Algorithm 13.1 Pulmonary thromboembolism

CHAPTER 13

Venous thromboembolism

Learning outcomes

After reading this chapter, you will be able to:

- Recognise the risk factors for thromboembolism and understand the need for appropriate risk assessment and thromboprophylaxis
- Recognise the features of pulmonary embolism and have an early suspicion of the diagnosis
- Describe the treatment of suspected pulmonary embolism, including submassive, life-threatening pulmonary embolism

13.1 Introduction

Venous thromboembolism (VTE) remains one of the leading causes of direct maternal mortality and morbidity worldwide. The risk of VTE is significantly increased in pregnancy overall, due to a variety of important changes in the coagulation system and factors that contribute to an individual's risk. The risk of VTE during the antenatal periods is 4–5-fold higher in pregnant women than in age-matched non-pregnant women. However the absolute risk remains low, at 1 in 1000 pregnancies. The puerperium is the time of highest risk, with estimates of relative risk of 20-fold, but can occur during any week of gestation. Timely risk stratification to enable appropriate thromboprophylaxis to be initiated throughout pregnancy is important to reduce the risk of VTE (Table 13.1).

Table 13.1 Risk factors for venous thromboembolism (VTE)

Obstetric risks	Maternal risks	Fetal risks
Premature delivery	Advanced maternal age	Multiple pregnancies
Postpartum haemorrhage	BMI >30 kg/m^2	Stillbirth
Operative delivery	History of VTE	
Pre-eclampsia	Thrombophilia (acquired and congenital)	
	Dehydration (e.g. hyperemesis)	
	Immobility	
	Active pre-existing medical conditions	
	Cancer	
	Travel	

Managing Medical and Obstetric Emergencies and Trauma: A Practical Approach, Fourth Edition. Edited by Rosamunde Burns and Kara Dent.

The risk factors may alter throughout pregnancy and the postpartum period. The importance of reassessment on every admission should be emphasised. The criteria for commencing thromboprophylaxis is steered by national guidelines such as those from the RCOG.

13.2 Pathophysiology of thromboembolism

Virchow's triad of venous stasis, hypercoagulability and vessel wall damage explain the higher risk of thrombus formation in pregnancy. Thrombus occurs more commonly in the left leg because the right common iliac artery compresses the left common iliac vein and this compression is accentuated by the enlarging uterus. Ileofemoral venous thrombosis occurs more commonly in pregnancy than in non-pregnant women.

Pulmonary embolism occurs because of the obstruction of the pulmonary arteries and release of vasoactive substances from platelets elevating pulmonary vascular resistance. The resulting increase in alveolar dead space and redistribution of blood flow impairs gas exchange. Right ventricular afterload increases, resulting in right ventricular dilatation, dysfunction and ischaemia. Stimulation of irritant receptors causes alveolar hyperventilation. Reflex bronchoconstriction increases airway resistance and pulmonary oedema decreases pulmonary compliance.

13.3 Clinical presentation of pulmonary embolism

Pulmonary embolism can present as a life-threatening event, or as a more subtle, varying combination of several symptoms. These symptoms include breathlessness and pleuritic chest pain, but dyspnoea may be absent and there may be haemoptysis or a pyrexia. Clinical diagnosis of pulmonary embolism can, therefore, be challenging and commonly delayed. The significance of symptoms may not be appreciated and there may be few signs on examination (Table 13.2).

Table 13.2 Incidence of clinical findings in pulmonary embolism

Findings	**Occurrence in patients with proven pulmonary embolism**
Tachypnoea	89%
Dyspnoea	81%
Pleuritic pain	72%
Apprehension	59%
Cough	54%
Tachycardia	43%
Haemoptysis	34%
Temperature >37°C	34%

Differential diagnoses include cardiac causes, pneumonia and pneumothorax. If there is suspicion of pulmonary embolism, then treatment should be started immediately and continued until it has been excluded and a different diagnosis confirmed. The importance of not only excluding a VTE but making a diagnosis should be emphasised.

A submassive pulmonary embolism may present (i) with hypotension, severe dyspnoea, cyanosis and circulatory collapse; (ii) with central chest pain as a result of right ventricular myocardial ischemia; or (iii) as sudden collapse, cardiac arrest or death. In this emergency situation, there may be right-sided heart failure, with increased jugular pressure, liver distension and subtle cardiac signs.

13.4 Management of thromboembolism

In the stable patient where VTE is suspected, a therapeutic dose of low molecular weight heparin (LMWH) should be commenced immediately. The multidisciplinary team should decide on the most appropriate investigations and treatment, involving the patient in discussions where possible. Compared with computed tomography pulmonary angiography (CTPA), ventilation/perfusion (V/Q) scanning may carry a slightly increased risk of childhood cancer but is associated with a lower risk of maternal breast cancer, although the absolute risk is small.

The patient must be closely monitored as she may deteriorate and require resuscitation. Remember the risk factors for thromboembolism and maintain a high index of suspicion at all times with women presenting with chest pain, dyspnea, tachycardia or collapse. The approach in this circumstance is 'SAFE approach, call for help' (senior obstetrician, anaesthetists, on-call medical team, resuscitation team if collapsed). Make sure the woman is well tilted and timely perimortem caesarean section (PMCS) is possible if there is no response to cardiopulmonary resuscitation (CPR) with an arrest. If pulmonary embolism is confirmed or in extreme circumstances, consider early thrombolysis once haemorrhage is excluded. Apply an ABCDE approach. If unresponsive and uncertain about respiration and heart rate, follow the cardiac arrest protocol.

Initial management consists of the following:

1. Ensure a safe environment, approach the patient, shake and shout if necessary.
2. Call for help and ensure escalation to senior multidisciplinary team to include a consultant obstetrician, senior anaesthetist, physician and radiologist. If the patient is unresponsive, call the crash team and start CPR.
3. Employ the ABCDE approach.
4. Reduce aortocaval compression if >20 weeks' gestation by manual uterine displacement (or left lateral position in the conscious patient). A PMCS should be performed if immediate return of spontaneous circulation is not achieved with CPR.
5. Give high-flow oxygen if hypoxic.
6. Perform an electrocardiogram (ECG).
7. Perform a chest x-ray (CXR).
8. Secure vascular access and send blood for full blood count, coagulation screen, urea and electrolytes (U&Es) and liver function tests plus group and save. Check arterial blood gases.
9. An urgent portable echocardiogram or CTPA within an hour of presentation should be arranged. Sources of concealed haemorrhage should be excluded, such as intra-abdominal bleeding, or aortic dissection. Point of care ultrasound should be considered. If massive pulmonary embolism is confirmed, or in extreme cases prior to confirmation, intravenous unfractionated heparin is the preferred initial treatment and immediate thrombolysis should be considered. Percutaneous catheter-based embolectomy or surgical embolectomy may also be considered by the multidisciplinary team. Care must be individualised. Thrombolysis may be life saving for the mother and should be given as it would in the non-pregnant patient. Surgical bleeding after thrombolysis may be catastrophic so the consequent delay in delivery may, on occasion, sacrifice the fetus.
   Aim *not* to deliver at this time but to treat the pulmonary embolism.
10. Transfer to an appropriate location for further management, such as a high dependency unit (HDU) or intensive treatment unit (ITU). Monitor BP, pulse oximetry, ECG and hourly urine output.

Once resuscitated, move to a HDU or ITU for investigation, monitoring and definitive treatment. This may include thrombolytic therapy, pulmonary embolectomy, sedation and ventilation with invasive monitoring, as well as anticoagulation.

13.5 Investigations for patients with a possible pulmonary embolism

Chest radiograph

A CXR can exclude pneumonia, pneumothorax or lobar collapse and abnormal features associated with pulmonary embolism, such as atelectasis, effusions, focal opacities, regional oligaemia and pulmonary oedema. Radiation exposure of the fetus from a CXR is negligible. The CXR is normal in 50% of women with subsequently proven pulmonary embolism. A normal x-ray should prompt a bilateral leg Doppler ultrasound as confirmation of a deep vein thrombosis (DVT) will support the diagnosis of pulmonary embolism.

Doppler ultrasound

If a leg Doppler scan confirms the presence of DVT, no further imaging is required to demonstrate pulmonary embolism. As the treatment is the same for both embolus and thrombus, other investigations can be avoided, thereby limiting the radiation dose to the fetus.

Other investigations

- Baseline blood tests include a full blood count, coagulation screen, U&Es and liver function tests
- A thrombophyllia screen will not influence the management but renal and hepatic function may influence coagulation

Further imaging

The V/Q lung scan and CTPA are evolving technologies and local availability varies. Imaging should be discussed with a senior radiologist. A perfusion scan must be carried out in normal working hours but, in a stable patient, therapeutic LMWH can be continued until the test is available. CTPA is more readily available and can identify a wider range of pathology than V/Q scanning.

D-dimer testing

D-dimer testing has no value in the investigation of acute VTE in pregnancy as levels can be raised in a normal pregnancy in the third trimester.

13.6 Treatment of thromboembolism

The LMWH is titrated against the woman's booking weight following national guidance. In a major collapse involving a thromboembolic cause, unfractionated heparin is the recommended initial treatment. If there is haemodynamic compromise, thrombolytic therapy should also be considered once concealed haemorrhage is excluded as the anticoagulant therapy is not enough on its own to reduce the obstruction causing ischaemia.

Maintenance treatment

After the initial acute event, treatment with therapeutic doses of LMWH should be continued throughout the rest of the pregnancy with careful planning for timing of delivery. If possible, delivery should be delayed if appropriate and safe to enable time for the anticoagulant to decrease the burden of clot before delivery. This is more difficult if the pulmonary embolism occurs later in the pregnancy.

Anticoagulant therapy during labour

- Once a woman on LMWH maintenance therapy thinks she is in labour, she should not inject any further LMWH
- In the case of planned delivery, therapeutic maintenance LMWH should be discontinued 24 hours before planned delivery
  Regional anaesthetic techniques should not be undertaken until at least 24 hours after the last dose of therapeutic LMWH

Anticoagulant therapy in the immediate postpartum period

- A thromboprophylactic dose of LMWH should be given 4 hours after a caesarean section, or more than 4 hours after removal of an epidural catheter, if appropriate
- The epidural catheter should not be removed within 12 hours of the most recent injection of LMWH

13.7 Summary

- Venous thromboembolism remains the most common direct cause of maternal death in the UK and a high index of suspicion for possible diagnosis must be considered if a woman presents in pregnancy with red flags
- Risk factors for VTE must be screened for from early pregnancy and throughout the pregnancy, including the postpartum period, to allow for appropriate thrombophylaxis and management. Risk factors can change during the pregnancy journey and must be reassessed on each and every admission
- If VTE is suspected, implement treatment until thromboembolism is excluded as a diagnosis, whilst remembering to investigate other possible causes
- If stroke is suspected in a pregnant woman, early thrombolysis can be life saving once haemorrhage is excluded. Treatment and management is instigated as for a non-pregnant woman

13.8 Further reading

NICE (National Institute for Health and Care Excellence). *Venous Thromboembolic Diseases: Diagnosis, Management and Thrombophilia Testing*. NG158. London: NICE, 2020.

RCOG (Royal College of Obstetrics and Gynaecologists). *Thrombosis and Embolism during Pregnancy and the Puerperium, Reducing the Risk*. Green-top Guideline No. 37a. London: RCOG, 2015.

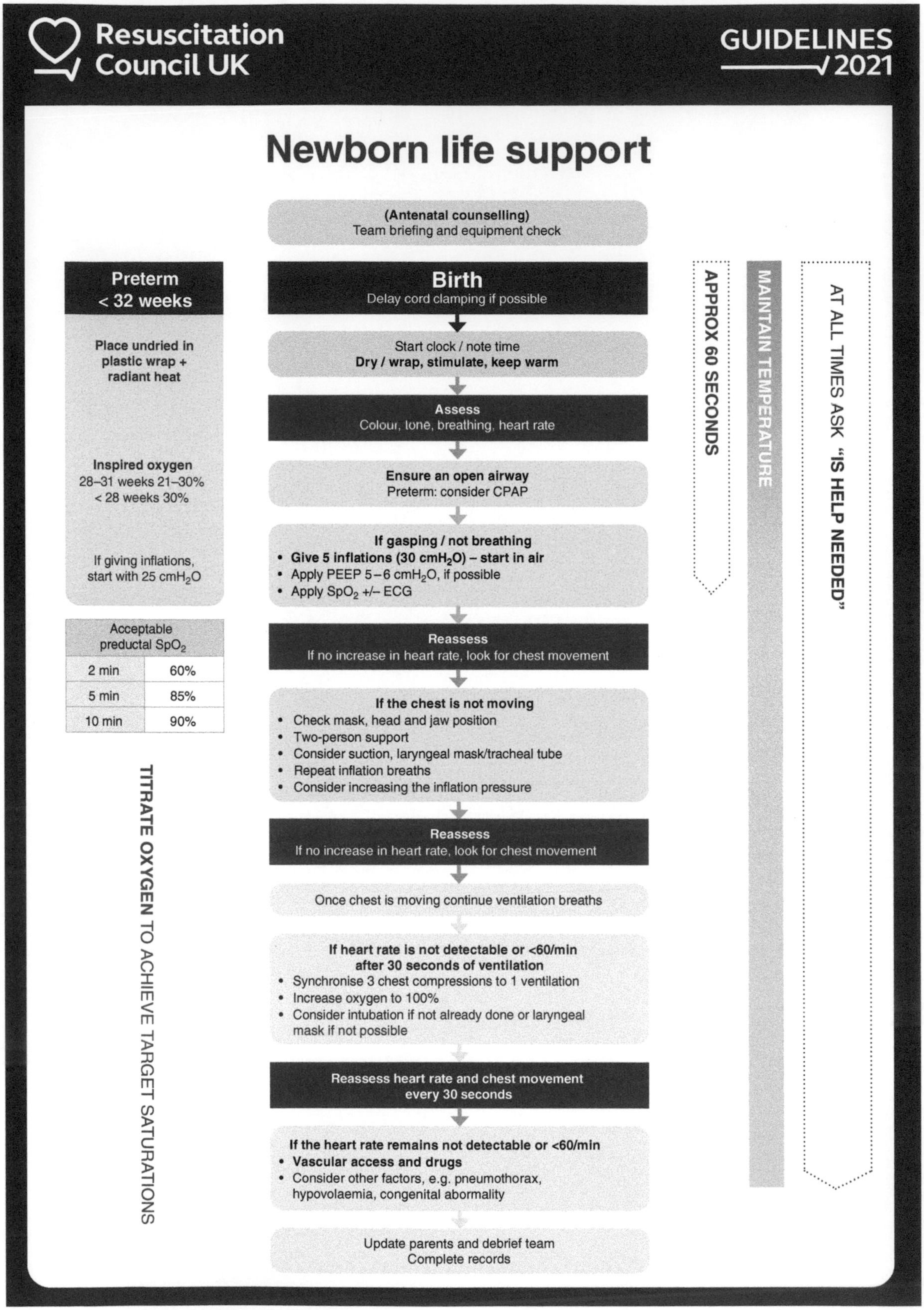

Resuscitation Council UK
GUIDELINES 2021
Newborn life support
(Antenatal counselling)
Team briefing and equipment check
Preterm < 32 weeks
Place undried in plastic wrap + radiant heat
Inspired oxygen
28–31 weeks 21–30%
< 28 weeks 30%
If giving inflations, start with 25 cmH2O
Acceptable preductal SpO2
2 min 60%
5 min 85%
10 min 90%
TITRATE OXYGEN TO ACHIEVE TARGET SATURATIONS
Birth
Delay cord clamping if possible
Start clock / note time
Dry / wrap, stimulate, keep warm
Assess
Colour, tone, breathing, heart rate
Ensure an open airway
Preterm: consider CPAP
If gasping / not breathing
• Give 5 inflations (30 cmH2O) – start in air
• Apply PEEP 5–6 cmH2O, if possible
• Apply SpO2 +/– ECG
Reassess
If no increase in heart rate, look for chest movement
If the chest is not moving
• Check mask, head and jaw position
• Two-person support
• Consider suction, laryngeal mask/tracheal tube
• Repeat inflation breaths
• Consider increasing the inflation pressure
Reassess
If no increase in heart rate, look for chest movement
Once chest is moving continue ventilation breaths
If heart rate is not detectable or <60/min after 30 seconds of ventilation
• Synchronise 3 chest compressions to 1 ventilation
• Increase oxygen to 100%
• Consider intubation if not already done or laryngeal mask if not possible
Reassess heart rate and chest movement every 30 seconds
If the heart rate remains not detectable or <60/min
• Vascular access and drugs
• Consider other factors, e.g. pneumothorax, hypovolaemia, congenital abormality
Update parents and debrief team
Complete records
APPROX 60 SECONDS
MAINTAIN TEMPERATURE
AT ALL TIMES ASK "IS HELP NEEDED"

Algorithm 14.1 Newborn resuscitation algorithm
Source: Reproduced with kind permission from the Resuscitation Council UK

CHAPTER 14

Resuscitation of the neonate at birth

Learning outcomes

After reading this chapter, you will be able to:

- Describe the approach to the resuscitation of the neonate at birth and how this differs from the resuscitation of older children

14.1 Introduction

The resuscitation of neonates at birth is different from the resuscitation of all other age groups as it usually involves a process of assisted transition from intra- to extrauterine life, rather than recovery of a human with serious illness or injury. Knowledge of the physiology of normal transition and how interruption to transition leading to hypoxia affects this is essential in understanding the process outlined in the algorithm for resuscitating newborns (Algorithm 14.1). The majority of neonates will establish normal respiration and circulation without help. A small minority will not, and will require intervention.

As some neonates may be born unexpectedly out of hospital, in a non-maternity setting within a hospital, or are unwell as a result of peripartum circumstances, it is important that clinicians working in 'receiving' specialties have an understanding of the differences between resuscitating older children and a newborn. Ideally, someone trained in newborn resuscitation should be present at all deliveries. It is advisable that all those who attend deliveries regularly should have been on courses such as the Newborn Life Support course organised by the Resuscitation Council UK, European Resuscitation Council courses, or the Neonatal Resuscitation Program organised by the American Academy of Pediatrics.

14.2 Normal physiology

Successful transition at birth involves moving from a fetal state, where the lungs are fluid-filled and respiratory exchange occurs through the placenta, to that of a newly born neonate whose air-filled lungs have successfully taken over that function. Preparation for this in a pregnancy progressing without incident is thought to begin in advance of labour, with detectable cellular changes occurring that may subsequently prime the lung tissues for reabsorption of the intra-alveolar fluid.

After delivery, a healthy full-term neonate usually takes its first breath within 60–90 seconds. Several factors drive this first breath to occur: exposure to the relative cold of the extrauterine environment; the physical stimulus of delivery; and the fact that even an uncomplicated vaginal delivery involves a degree of exposure to hypoxia. In a term neonate, approximately

Managing Medical and Obstetric Emergencies and Trauma: A Practical Approach, Fourth Edition. Edited by Rosamunde Burns and Kara Dent.

100 ml of fluid is cleared from the airways and alveoli, initially into the interstitial pulmonary tissue, and then later into the lymphatic and capillary systems. During vaginal delivery, around 35 ml of fluid from the uppermost airways will be displaced by physical forces experienced by the fetus during passage through the birth canal.

The respiratory pattern in newborn mammals has specifically evolved to facilitate replacement of the fluid in the lungs with air during the first few breaths. Animal studies show that at initiation of breathing, the inspiratory phase is longer than the expiratory phase (expiratory braking): expiration occurs against a partially closed glottis, heard as either crying or sometimes a grunting sound, creating increased pressure in the airways. In a healthy neonate, the first spontaneous breaths may generate a negative inspiratory pressure of between −30 and −90 cmH_2O. This pressure is 10–15 times greater than that needed for later breathing but is necessary to overcome the viscosity of the fluid filling the airways, the surface tension of the fluid-filled lungs, and the elastic recoil and resistance of the chest wall, lungs and airways. These powerful chest movements also aid displacement of fluid from the airways into the interstitial tissue of the lung. As long as the functional residual capacity (FRC) is successfully established, then the fluid displaced into the lung interstitial tissues will be subsequently cleared via the lymphatic system into the circulation.

If this process fails, and the fluid is not cleared from the interstitial tissue or leaks back into the alveolar spaces, then respiratory compromise will be seen with increased respiratory rate and effort of breathing.

Neonatal circulatory adaptation commences at the same time as the pulmonary changes. Lung inflation and alveolar distension releases vasomotor compounds that reduce the pulmonary vascular resistance as well as increasing oxygenation. Evidence shows that as pulmonary vascular resistance falls during establishment of the FRC, pulmonary blood flow increases and consequently venous return to the left atrium increases. This leads to improved left ventricular filling and an increased stroke volume.

If the umbilical cord is clamped prior to the first breath, reduced venous return from the placenta to the right side of the heart results in an immediate decrease in heart size and a bradycardia as the pulmonary vascular resistance drops. There is then a return to its original size and recovery of the heart rate as long as the neonate has successfully started to breath. The increase in size subsequently seen is likely due to an increased volume of blood returning to the left side of the heart from the expanded pulmonary circulation that occurs once the lungs are aerated. The loss of the low resistance placental circulation results in increased systemic resistance and a spike in blood pressure. Immediate cord clamping is associated with a bradycardia that is avoided if cord clamping is delayed, particularly until after the first breath is taken (Figure 14.1).

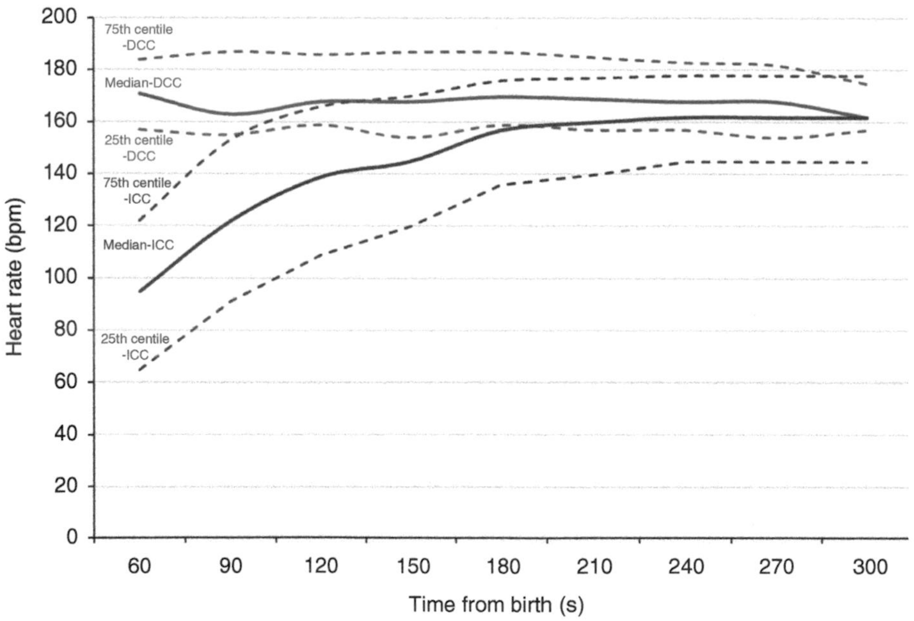

Figure 14.1 Heart rates for babies who received immediate umbilical cord clamping versus those who had their cord clamped after their first breath

DCC, delayed cord clamping; ICC, immediate cord clamping

Source: Northern Neonatal Network

Circulatory adaptation proceeds with closure of the interatrial foramen due to pressure changes as the pulmonary venous return to the left atrium increases and finishes with functional, then permanent, closure of the ductus arteriosus over the following days.

For these reasons, after a neonate is born the drying, thermal care and initial assessment starts with the cord intact. If assessment shows the neonate is well, good thermal care should continue and the cord should remain unclamped for at least 60 seconds (preferably until the first breaths have been taken). If assessment demonstrates compromise warranting immediate resuscitation, then the cord can be clamped and cut to allow the neonate to be taken to the resuscitative platform.

14.3 Pathophysiology

The approach to resuscitating newborn humans evolved from observation of the pathophysiology of induced, acute, fetal hypoxia during pioneering mammal-based research in the early 1960s. The results of these experiments, which followed the physiology of newborn animals during acute, total, prolonged asphyxia and subsequent resuscitation, are summarised in Figure 14.2.

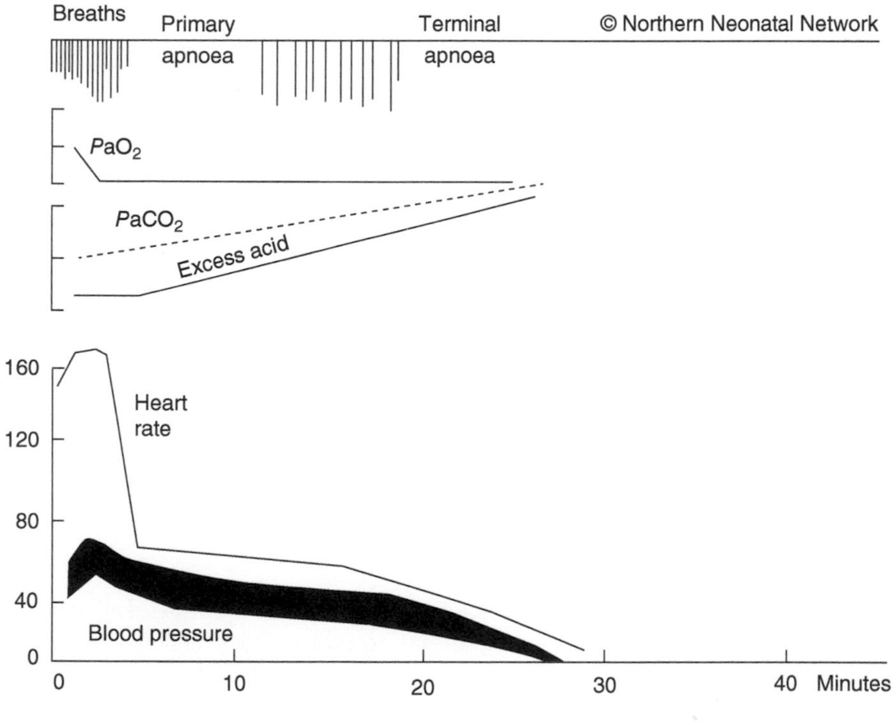

Figure 14.2 Response of a mammalian fetus to total, sustained asphyxia starting at time 0
Source: Northern Neonatal Network

When the placental oxygen supply is interrupted or severely reduced, the fetus will initiate respiratory movements (i.e. attempt to breathe) in response to hypoxia. These breathing efforts fail to provide an alternative oxygen supply as the fetus is still in the womb surrounded by amniotic fluid: consequently the baby will become unconscious. If hypoxia continues, the higher respiratory centre in the brain becomes inactive and unable to continue to drive respiratory movements. The breathing therefore stops, usually within 2–3 minutes. This cessation of breathing is known as **primary apnoea** (Figure 14.3).

At the onset of hypoxia, a marked bradycardia will occur quickly. Intense peripheral vasoconstriction helps to maintain blood pressure with diversion of blood away from non-vital organs. The reduced heart rate allows a longer ventricular filling time, and thus an increased stroke volume, which also helps maintain blood pressure.

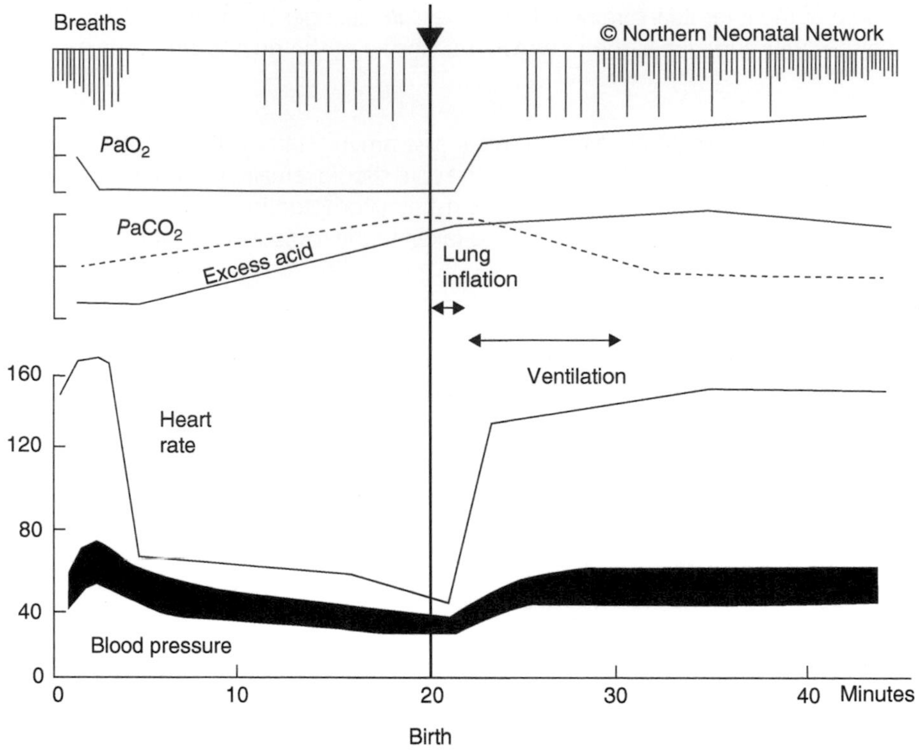

Figure 14.3 Effects of lung inflation and a brief period of ventilation on a neonate born in early terminal apnoea but before failure of the circulation
Source: Northern Neonatal Network

As hypoxia continues, primary apnoea is broken: loss of descending neural inhibition by the higher respiratory centre allows primitive spinal centres to initiate forceful, gasping breaths. These deep, irregular gasps are easily distinguishable from normal breaths as they only occur 6–12 times per minute and involve all accessory muscles in a maximal, 'whole body', inspiratory effort. If this fails to draw air into the lungs and hypoxia continues, even this reflexive activity ceases and **terminal apnoea** begins. Without intervention, no further innate respiratory effort will occur. The time taken for such activity to cease is longer in the newborn than at any other time in life, taking up to 30 minutes.

The circulation is almost always maintained until **after** all respiratory activity ceases. This resilience is a feature of all newborn mammals at term and is largely due to the reserves of glycogen in the heart permitting prolonged, anaerobic generation of energy in the cardiomyocytes. Resuscitation is therefore relatively uncomplicated if undertaken before all respiratory activity has stopped. Once the lungs are aerated, oxygen will be carried to the heart and then to the brain provided the circulation is still functional (Figure 14.3). Recovery will then be rapid. Most neonates who have **not** progressed to terminal apnoea will resuscitate themselves if their airway is open. Once gasping ceases, however, the circulation starts to fail and resuscitation becomes more difficult. Support for the circulation is then required in addition to support for the breathing (Figure 14.4).

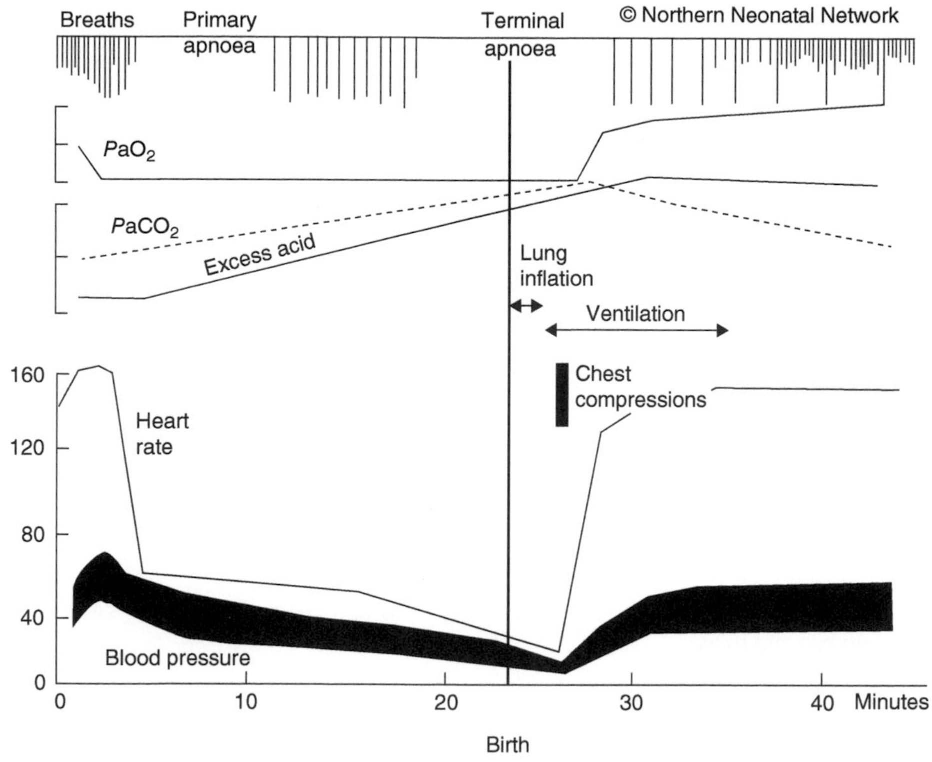

Figure 14.4 Response of a neonate born in terminal apnoea. In this case lung inflation is not sufficient because the circulation is already failing. However, lung inflation delivers air to the lungs and then a brief period of chest compressions delivers oxygenated blood to the heart which then responds
Source: Northern Neonatal Network

14.4 Equipment for newborn resuscitation

For many neonates, especially those born outside the delivery room, the need for resuscitation cannot be predicted. It is therefore useful to plan for such an eventuality. Equipment that may be required to resuscitate a neonate is listed in Box 14.1. Most neonates can be resuscitated if there is access to some key equipment: a firm, flat surface; a means to provide warmth; a way to deliver air or oxygen to the lungs in a controlled fashion to displace fluid present in the airways at delivery if the neonate does not breathe itself (ranging from mouth-to-mouth to equipment-based techniques); and guidance from someone who is familiar with the process of newborn resuscitation (either as part of the resuscitation team or by telephone at the time of need).

Box 14.1 Equipment for newborn resuscitation

- Flat surface
- Radiant heat source and dry towels
- Plastic bag for preterm neonates
- Suitable hats
- Suction with catheters of at least 12 Fr gauge
- Face masks
- Bag–valve–mask or T-piece with pressure-limiting device
- Source of air and/or oxygen
- Laryngeal mask size 1 (such as LMA of iGel)
- Laryngoscopes with straight blades, 0 and 1
- Nasogastric tubes
- Cord clamp
- Scissors
- Tracheal tubes sizes 2.5 to 4.0 mm
- Umbilical catheterisation equipment
- Adhesive tape
- Disposable gloves
- Saturation monitor/stethoscope

14.5 Strategy for assessing and resuscitating a neonate at birth

Resuscitation is likely to be rapidly successful if commenced before the neonate has progressed beyond the point at which their circulation has started to fail. Neonates in primary apnoea can usually resuscitate themselves if they have a clear airway. Unfortunately, it is not possible during the initial assessment to reliably distinguish whether an apnoeic newborn is in primary or terminal apnoea. A structured approach that will work in either situation must therefore be applied to **all** apnoeic neonates. The structured approach is outlined below. In reality the first four steps (up to and including assessment) are completed simultaneously. After this, appropriate intervention can begin following an ABC approach:

1. Call/shout for help.
2. Start the clock or note the time.
3. Dry and wrap the neonate in warmed dry towels. Maintain the neonate's temperature.
4. Assess the situation.
5. Airway.
6. Breathing.
7. Chest compressions.
8. Drugs/vascular access.

Call for help

Ask for help if you expect or encounter any difficulty or if the delivery is outside the labour suite. Where a pre-alert is received in hospital, convene the team for briefing and allocate roles.

Start the clock

Start the clock if available, or note the time of birth.

At birth

There is no need to rush to clamp the cord at delivery. It should be left unclamped while the following steps are completed:

- Dry the neonate quickly and effectively
- Remove the wet towel and wrap the neonate in a fresh, dry, warm towel (for very small or significantly preterm neonates it is better to place the wet neonate in a food-grade plastic bag – and under a radiant heater as soon as possible)
- Put a hat on **all** neonates regardless of gestation
- Assess the neonate during and after drying and decide whether any intervention is needed

If your assessment suggests that the neonate is in need of resuscitation, clamp and cut the cord. Otherwise wait for at least 60 seconds from the complete delivery of the neonate (or if safe, until the neonate has started to breathe) before clamping the cord.

If the neonate is assessed as needing assistance/resuscitation then this becomes the priority. If the equipment and skills are available resuscitation can be started whilst the neonate is still attached to the placenta by a functioning umbilical cord. However, more commonly the cord needs to be clamped and cut in order to deliver assistance/resuscitation.

Keep the neonate warm

The normal temperature range for a newborn neonate is 36.5–37.5°C. For each 1°C decrease in admission temperature below this range in otherwise healthy term newborns, there is an associated increase in baseline mortality of 28%. In environments likely to receive sick neonates or infants, the room temperatures should be kept as close as possible to the recommended minimum for term neonates (23–25°C) and if a preterm neonate is known to be about to deliver the environment should be warmed to at least 26°C if possible. Where delivery or admission of a newborn neonate is imminent **outside** these environments, anticipation and active management of room temperature to achieve this baseline as quickly as possible is required: eliminate any draughts from the room (close windows and doors where possible) and heat the room to above 23°C (term neonates) or 25°C (preterm neonates).

Once delivered, dry the neonate immediately and then wrap in a warm, dry towel. In addition to increased mortality risk, a cold neonate has an increased rate of oxygen consumption and is more likely to become hypoglycaemic and acidotic. If this is not addressed at the beginning of resuscitation it is often forgotten. Most heat loss at delivery is caused by the neonate being wet (evaporation) and in a draught (convection). Neonates also have a large surface area to weight ratio exacerbating heat loss. Ideally an overhead heater or external heat source should be used as well if available, but drying effectively and wrapping the neonate in a warm, dry towel with the head covered by a hat are the most important interventions in avoiding hypothermia. A naked dry neonate can still become hypothermic despite a warm room or use of a radiant heater, especially if there is a draught.

In **all** neonates, the head represents a significant part of the surface area (see Section 14.8 on 'Preterm neonates' later in this chapter) so attention to providing a hat is invaluable in maintaining normothermia.

Out of hospital: neonates of all gestations born outside the normal delivery environment may benefit from placement in a food-grade polyethylene bag or wrap *after* drying and then swaddling. Alternatively, well newborn neonates of more than 30 weeks' gestation who are breathing may be dried, have a hat put on and nursed with skin-to-skin contact (or kangaroo parent care) with a cover over any remaining exposed skin to maintain their temperature whilst they are transferred. Ensure the neonate remains positioned in a way that maintains airway patency.

Assessment of the newborn neonate

During and immediately after drying and wrapping the neonate, make a full assessment.

A/B	Breathing	Regular, gasp, none
C	Heart rate	Fast (>100 beats/min), slow (60–100 beats/min), very slow/absent (<60 beats/min)
D	Tone	Well flexed, reduced tone, floppy

Unlike resuscitation at other ages, **all** three items are assessed in parallel and a rapid ABC assessment helps decide on the need for resuscitation. Once resuscitative measures are started regular reassessment should assess their effect.

This is different to the linear hierarchy of assessment and treatment used at other ages. In the newborn, heart rate and breathing provide the most useful information and are the **only** items that need regular reassessment during resuscitation to assess effectiveness of intervention. At the initial assessment, however, taking note of the neonate's tone can also be informative: a very floppy neonate is likely to be unconscious, suggesting that the neonate may have been subject to hypoxia.

Colour, while no longer formally assessed, is still a potentially useful indicator of status. Normal neonates are born 'blue' and become 'pink' in the first minutes of life. A neonate who is pale and white ('shut down') due to intense peripheral vasoconstriction is more likely to be acidotic: this sort of appearance suggests a significant cardiovascular response to peripartum compromise.

Breathing movements and colour can be determined by observation during drying; tone can be evaluated whilst in the act of drying the neonate. Heart rate is determined by auscultation of the heart using a stethoscope, which can be done during the drying by a second person or immediately afterwards if the responder is on their own.

Breathing

Most well term neonates will take their first breath 60–90 seconds after delivery and establish spontaneous, regular breathing sufficient to maintain the heart rate at ≥100 beats/min within 3 minutes of birth. If there is no breathing (apnoea), gasping or irregular, ineffective breathing that persists after drying, intervention is required.

Heart rate

In the first couple of minutes, auscultating at the cardiac apex is the best method to assess the heart rate. Palpating peripheral pulses is not practical and is not recommended. Palpation of the umbilical pulse can only be relied upon if the palpable rate is ≥100 beats/min. A rate less than this should be checked by auscultation. It may not be possible to feel a cord pulse when there **is** a heart rate that can be detected by auscultation.

In delivery suites, saturation monitors are used by neonatal intensive care unit (NICU) teams when resuscitation is required at term, or when preterm neonates have been delivered. However, applying a saturation monitor should not interrupt the process of resuscitation. It is also good practice to correlate the probe reading (heart rate), once good detection signal strength is achieved, with the auscultated heart rate. An electrocardiogram (ECG), if available, can give a rapid, accurate and continuous heart rate reading during newborn resuscitation, but the use of ECG must not delay the delivery of resuscitative care. In low-resource or non-specialist settings (especially if the only saturation monitor probe available is designed to fit a larger child or adult), the use of a stethoscope is recommended to allow resuscitation to proceed without delay.

The probe for the saturation monitor must be applied to the **right** (not left) hand or wrist in order to accurately reflect the preductal saturations (which are most likely to reflect the oxygenation of blood being distributed to the coronary arteries and cerebral circulation). A correctly applied pulse oximeter can give an accurate reading of heart rate and saturations within 60–90 seconds of application. Oxygen saturation levels in healthy neonates in the first few minutes of life may be considerably lower than at other times (Table 14.1). Attempting to judge oxygenation by assessing colour of the skin or mucous membranes is not reliable, but it is still worth noting the neonate's colour at birth as well as whether, when and how it changes later in the resuscitation. Very pale neonates who remain pale and bradycardic after resuscitation may be hypovolaemic as well as acidotic. Similarly, tone immediately at birth should be assessed, and then changes noted as resuscitation progresses.

Table 14.1 Acceptable preductal saturation levels (SpO_2)

Time from birth	Acceptable preductal SpO_2 levels
2 min	65%
5 min	85%
10 min	90%

An accurate and prompt initial assessment of heart rate is vital because an increase in the heart rate will be the first sign of success during resuscitation.

Outcome of the initial assessment

Initial assessment will categorise the neonate into one of the three following groups:

1. **Vigorous breathing or crying, good tone, heart rate ≥100 beats/min.** These are healthy babies. They should be dried and kept warm, with a hat on, and the umbilical cord clamped after 60 seconds. They can be given to their mothers and nursed skin to skin if this is appropriate, with protection from draughts by covering. The neonate will remain warm through skin-to-skin contact under a cover and may also be put to the breast at this stage.
2. **Irregular or inadequate breathing or apnoea, normal or reduced tone, heart rate <100 beats/min.** If gentle stimulation (drying will be an adequate stimulus in this situation) does not induce effective breathing, consider whether the cord needs to be clamped and cut to allow resuscitation to commence. After drying and wrapping are completed, the airway should be opened. Most of these neonates will improve with inflation of the lungs using a mask and the heart rate should be used to assess the effect of this intervention. Some neonates in this group will then require a period of ventilation by mask until they recover respiratory drive and are able to breathe for themselves.
3. **Breathing inadequately, gasping or apnoeic, globally floppy, heart rate very slow (<60 beats/min) or absent and colour blue or pale (pale often suggests poor perfusion).** Ensure good thermal care and begin intervention as in Algorithm 14.1.

Whether an apnoeic neonate is in primary or terminal apnoea (see Figure 14.2), the initial management is the same although it will be quickly apparent that in this case delayed cord clamping is not appropriate. Cord milking ('stripping') has sometimes been advocated as an alternative to delayed cord clamping in neonates who are in need of immediate assistance. This can be done in neonates of >28 weeks' gestation but is not recommended below this as there is some evidence it is associated with harm (cerebral intraventricular haemorrhage).

Dry and wrap the neonate, assessing as you go and then commence resuscitation. Open the airway and then inflate the lungs using five 2–3-second breaths. A reassessment of heart rate response and chest rise with mask inflation directs further resuscitation. After assessment, resuscitation follows the broad categories of the structured approach seen in Algorithm 14.1:

- Airway
- Breathing
- Circulation
- Drugs, in a few selected cases

Resuscitation of the newborn

Airway

To achieve an open airway, the neonate should be positioned with the head in the neutral position (Figure 14.5) (see also Chapter 19). A newborn's head has a large, often moulded, occiput which tends to cause the neck to flex when they are supine on a flat surface. A 2 cm folded towel placed under the neck and shoulders may help to maintain the airway in a neutral position and a jaw thrust may be needed to bring the tongue forward and open the airway, especially if the neonate is floppy. However, overextension may also collapse the newborn's pharyngeal airway, leading to obstruction. If using a towel under the shoulders, care must be exercised to avoid such overextension of the neck.

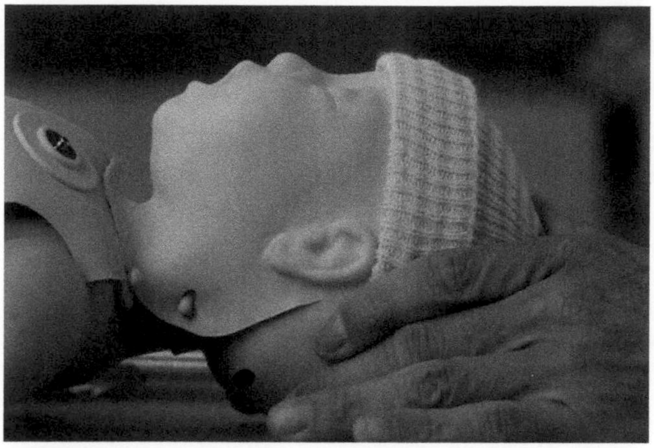

Figure 14.5 Neutral position in neonates

Most secretions found in and around the oropharynx at birth are thin and rarely cause airway obstruction. Priority should be given in **all** neonates to the application of a well-fitting mask and inflating the lungs once airway position and control is established, even in those born through meconium.

If, during resuscitation, there is concern that there might be an airway obstruction (for example if the heart rate is poor and the chest does not move with appropriately applied mask ventilation), then airway opening options including a two-person jaw thrust (Figure 14.6), insertion of a laryngeal mask or suction of the oropharynx under direct vision using a laryngoscope, should be considered. Any obvious material obstructing the airway should be removed by gentle suction with a large-bore suction catheter. Deep pharyngeal suction without direct visualisation should not be performed as it may cause extensive soft tissue injury, vagal nerve-induced bradycardia and laryngospasm. Suction, if it is used, should not exceed −150 mmHg (–20.0 kPa).

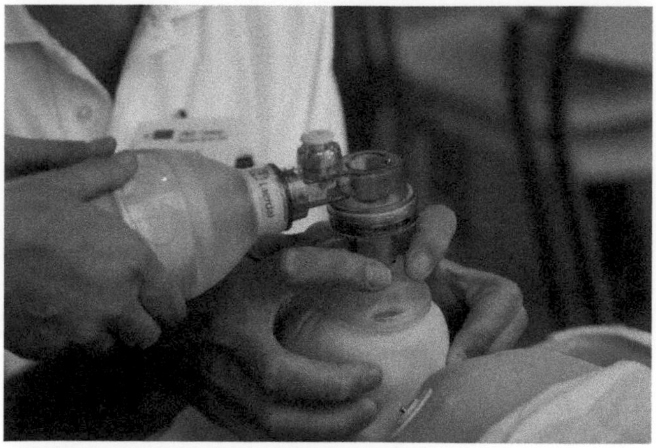

Figure 14.6 Two-person jaw thrust

A two-person jaw thrust or a laryngeal mask are used in preference to oropharyngeal airways as these can occasionally worsen airway obstruction in smaller babies. Oropharyngeal airways can sometimes be useful in the context of a difficult airway.

Meconium aspiration

Meconium-stained liquor (light green tinge) is relatively common and occurs in up to 10% of births. Meconium aspiration is a **rare** event and, when it happens, usually occurs in utero as the fetus approaches term. It requires intrauterine fetal compromise severe enough to have caused both the reflexive passage of meconium and the onset of gasping respiratory movements for meconium to be aspirated.

That meconium has been inhaled *before* delivery means that the previously widely advocated and used combined obstetric–neonatal strategy of suctioning the airways after delivery has not been shown to be of use. No difference in the incidence of meconium aspiration syndrome has been shown in the most obtunded of neonates who were subjected to tracheal intubation followed by suction and those who were not intubated. All that these procedures do is to delay the application of appropriate resuscitative measures to the neonate in need, in a timely fashion. Thus, when faced with a neonate who has been born through meconium-stained liquor, and who needs assistance, lung aeration should be the priority, **not** clearance of meconium.

In the context of a neonate delivered through meconium who needs resuscitation, start with the standard newborn life support (NLS) algorithm. Only suction under direct vision if you fail to get chest movement with inflation breaths delivered for the correct length of time (5 breaths, each 2–3 seconds long) with the head in the correct (neutral) position.

From the perspective of effective resuscitation, the only type of meconium that may cause an immediate issue is that which is thick and viscid and which has the potential to block the airway. If suction under direct vision is required, a suitable wide-bore catheter or Yankauer sucker should be used. Routine tracheal intubation is not recommended for neonates born through meconium, although if very thick meconium blocks the airway then using a meconium aspirator attached to a tracheal tube can be helpful if the team present have the required skills. A small proportion of neonates born through thick meconium will need more advanced intensive care management on a neonatal unit.

Breathing (inflation breaths and ventilation)

The first five breaths in term neonates should be 'inflation' breaths in order to replace the lung fluid in the alveoli with air. These should be 2–3-second sustained breaths ideally delivered using a continuous gas supply, a pressure-limited device (set at a limit of 30 cmH_2O) and an appropriately sized mask. Use a suitable sized facemask that is big enough to cover the nose and mouth of the neonate. If no such system is available then a 500 ml self-inflating bag and a blow-off valve set at 30–40 cmH_2O can be used (Figure 14.7). This is especially useful if compressed air or oxygen is not available. A smaller size of bag (<500 ml) can work but it is harder to sustain the inflation over 2–3 seconds and thus should not be used by choice unless no alternative exists. During these five breaths, it is important to remember that the chest may not be seen to move during the first few breaths as fluid is displaced and replaced by air. After the five breaths, the first reassessment should be done.

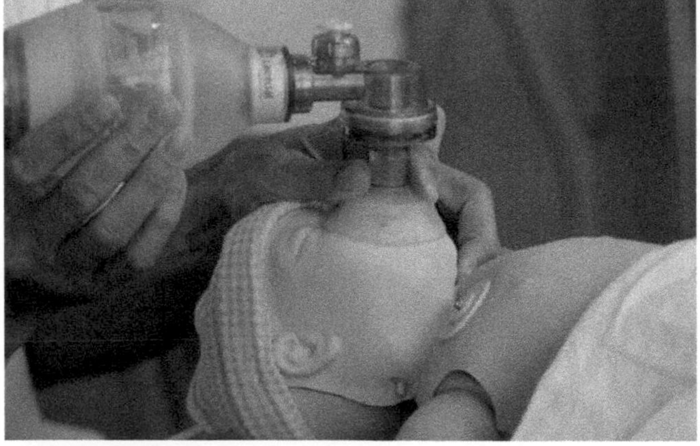

Figure 14.7 Bag–mask ventilation with a one-handed chin lift

Adequate lung inflation is usually indicated by either a rapidly increasing heart rate or a heart rate that is maintained at ≥100 beats/min. It is safe to assume the chest has been inflated successfully if the heart rate responds.

Once the chest is inflated and the heart rate has increased **or** the chest has been seen to move, then ventilation should be continued at a rate of about 30 per minute using shorter breaths (no more than 1 second of inspiratory time). Continue ventilatory support until regular spontaneous breathing is established.

Where possible, start resuscitation of the newborn of > 32 weeks' gestation with air. There is now good evidence for this in term neonates and excessive oxygen should be avoided in premature neonates. For neonates <28 weeks' gestation start in 30% oxygen, and for neonates 28–32 weeks' gestation use 21–30% oxygen. The use of supplemental oxygen should be guided by preductal pulse oximetry (see earlier), with reasonable levels listed in Table 14.1 and on Algorithm 14.1.

If the heart rate has not responded to the five inflation breaths, then check that you have **seen** chest movement. Auscultation by stethoscope of fluid-filled lungs during the administration of inflation or ventilation breaths may erroneously detect 'breath' sounds even **without** effective lung inflation. Go back and check airway opening manoeuvres and repeat the inflation breaths if you have not seen chest movement. If you have seen chest movement and the heart rate has not increased, give 30-second ventilation breaths and reassess the heart rate.

Circulation

If the heart rate remains very slow (<60 beats/min) or absent, despite adequate lung inflation **and** subsequent ventilation for 30 seconds (with demonstrable chest movement), then chest compressions should be started.

Chest compressions in the newborn aim to move oxygenated blood from the lungs to the heart and coronary arteries; they are not intended to sustain cerebral circulation as they do in older children or adults. Once oxygenated blood reaches the coronary arteries it will usually result in a change from anaerobic energy generation to aerobic energy generation and, as a result, the heart rate will increase. This will then provide the required cardiac output to perfuse the vital organs. The blood you move using cardiac compressions **can only be oxygenated if the lungs have air in them**. Newborn cardiac compromise is almost always the result of respiratory failure and can only be effectively treated if effective ventilation is occurring.

The most efficient way of delivering chest compressions in the newborn is to encircle the chest with both hands, so that the fingers lie behind the neonate, supporting the back, and the thumbs are overlapped, overlying the lower third of the sternum (Figure 14.8). Overlapping the thumb tips is more effective than placing the thumb tips side by side, but is more likely to cause operator fatigue. Compress the chest briskly, **by one-third of the anteroposterior diameter** and ensure that **full recoil of the anterior chest wall is allowed** after each compression, before commencing the next compression. The relaxation phase is when the blood returns to the coronary arteries and therefore is essential to effective technique. Evidence clearly supports a synchronised ratio of three compressions for each ventilation breath (3:1 ratio) as the most effective ratio in the newborn, aiming to achieve 120 events (90 compressions and 30 ventilations) per minute.

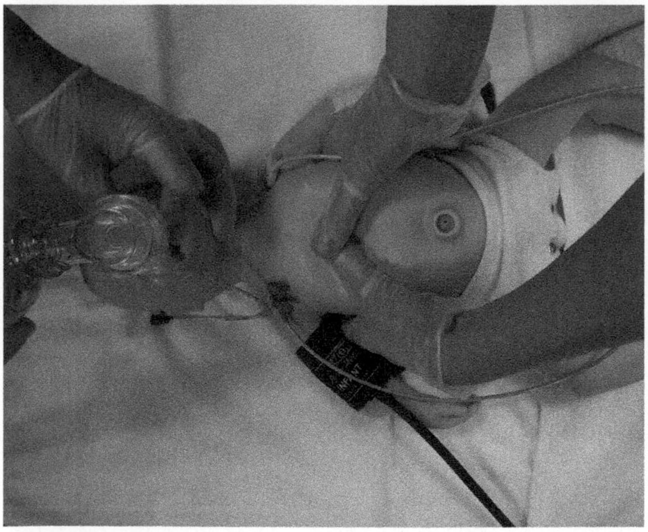

Figure 14.8 Hand-encircling technique for chest compressions

The purpose of chest compression is to move **oxygenated** blood or drugs to the coronary arteries in order to initiate cardiac recovery. Thus there is no point in starting chest compression before effective lung inflation has been established. Similarly, compressions are ineffective unless interposed by ventilation breaths of good quality. Therefore, the emphasis must be upon **good-quality breaths**, followed by effective compressions at a ratio of 1 breath to 3 compressions. Simultaneous delivery of compressions and breaths (otherwise known as chest compression with asynchronous ventilation, as used in older patients with a secure airway) should not be done even when the neonate is intubated, as compressions will reduce the effectiveness of any breath if the two coincide. It is usually only necessary to continue chest compressions for about 20–30 seconds before the heart responds with an increase in heart rate; thus reassessment of the heart rate at regular 30-second intervals is recommended. If chest compressions are required in resuscitation, ensure that 100% oxygen is also being delivered to the neonate by whatever ventilatory system is being used during the period of cardiopulmonary resuscitation. This can then be weaned using pulse oximetry as a guide once return of spontaneous circulation is established.

Once the heart rate is above 60 beats/min and rising, chest compressions may be discontinued. Ventilation breaths will need to be continued, by whichever method has been used successfully thus far, until effective spontaneous breathing commences. In the absence of breathing starting spontaneously, formal mechanical ventilation may need to be instituted.

Drugs

If adequate lung inflation and ventilation with effective cardiac compressions does not lead to the heart rate improving above 60 beats/min, drugs should be considered. The most common reason for failure of the heart rate to respond is failure to achieve or maintain lung inflation, and there is **no point** in giving drugs unless the airway is open and the lungs have been inflated. Airway, breathing (i.e. the observed chest movement) and chest compressions must be reassessed as adequate and effective before proceeding to drug therapy. Drugs are best administered via a centrally placed umbilical venous line or, if this is not possible, an intraosseous needle is an alternative in term neonates. The outcome is likely to be poor if drugs are *needed* for successful resuscitation.

Adrenaline

The alpha-adrenergic effect of adrenaline increases coronary artery perfusion during resuscitation, enhancing oxygen delivery to the heart. In the presence of profound, unresponsive, bradycardia or circulatory standstill, 20 micrograms/kg (0.2 ml/kg of 1:10 000) adrenaline may be given intravenously. This **must** be followed by a flush of 0.9% sodium chloride (3–5 ml) to ensure it reaches the circulation. Further doses of adrenaline at 20 micrograms/kg (0.2 ml/kg 1:10 000), followed by a flush of 0.9% sodium chloride, can be given every 3–5 minutes if there is no response to the intial bolus and resuscitation is ongoing. If intravenous or intraosseous access cannot be established, intratracheal adrenaline can be tried, although a dose of 100 micrograms/kg will be needed. This higher dose **must not** be given intravenously. If intratracheal adrenaline is given and resuscitation is ongoing, then umbilical venous catheter/intraosseous access should be sought.

Glucose

Hypoglycaemia is associated with adverse neurological outcomes and worsened cerebral damage in neonatal animal models of asphyxia and resuscitation. Once the neonatal heart has consumed endogenous glycogen supplies, it also requires an exogenous energy source to continue functioning. Therefore, during prolonged resuscitation it is appropriate to consider giving a slow bolus of 2.5 ml/kg of 10% glucose intravenously. Once a bolus has been given, provision of a secure intravenous glucose infusion is needed to prevent rebound hypoglycaemia. A glucose bolus given during neonatal resuscitation is unlikely to cause harmful hyperglycaemia but may avoid damaging hypoglycaemia. Normoglycaemia is optimal and post-resuscitation glucose levels should be closely monitored. Many strip glucometers are not reliable in neonates and, wherever possible, should not be used for blood glucose estimation unless using the local laboratory arrangements incurs an excessive delay.

Bicarbonate

Any neonate in terminal apnoea will have a significant metabolic component to the acidosis present. Acidosis depresses cardiac function. Sodium bicarbonate 1–2 mmol/kg (2–4 ml/kg of 4.2% solution) may be used to raise the pH and enhance the effects of oxygen and adrenaline in prolonged resuscitation, after adequate ventilation and circulation (with chest compressions) has been established. Bicarbonate use remains controversial and it should only be used in the absence of discernible cardiac output despite all resuscitative efforts, or in profound and unresponsive bradycardia. Its use is not recommended during short periods of cardiopulmonary resuscitation.

Fluids

Very occasionally, hypovolaemia may be present because of known or suspected blood loss (antepartum haemorrhage, placenta/vasa praevia or bleeding from a separated but unclamped umbilical cord). Hypovolaemia secondary to loss of vascular tone following asphyxia is less common. Where a neonate remains pale and shocked in appearance, or where there is a persistent bradycardia despite drug administration, intravascular volume expansion may be appropriate. Balanced crystalloids at 10 ml/kg (or 0.9% sodium chloride) can be used safely. If blood loss is likely, especially where acute and severe, uncrossmatched, cytomegaolovirus-negative, O rhesus D (RhD)-negative blood should be given in preference. Albumin (and other plasma substitutes) cannot be recommended. However, most newborn or neonatal resuscitations do not require the administration of fluid unless there has been known blood loss or septicaemic shock.

As most newborns requiring resuscitation are not hypovolaemic, especially those born preterm, extreme caution should be exercised in order to avoid inappropriately excessive amounts of fluid boluses. Excessive intravascular volume expansion may cause worsened cardiac function in a heart subject to prolonged hypoxia, and is associated with increased rates of (cerebral) intraventricular haemorrhage and pulmonary haemorrhage in preterm neonates.

Naloxone

This is not a drug of resuscitation to be given acutely. Occasionally, a neonate who has been effectively resuscitated, is pink, with a heart rate of ≥100 beats/min, may not breathe spontaneously because of the possible effects of maternal opioid medications. If respiratory depressant effects are suspected in the neonate, then naloxone intramuscularly (200 micrograms in a full-term newborn) could be considered. Smaller doses of 10 micrograms/kg will also reverse opioid sedation but the effect will only last a short time (20 minutes compared with a few hours after intramuscular administration). Intravenous naloxone has a half-life shorter than the opiates it is meant to reverse, and there is no evidence to recommend intratracheal administration.

Bicarbonate, glucose, fluids and naloxone should **never** be given via intratracheally.

Response to resuscitation

The first indication of successful progress in resuscitation will be an increase in heart rate. Recovery of respiratory drive may be delayed. Babies in terminal apnoea will tend to gasp first as they recover before starting normal respirations (see Figure 14.3). Those who were in primary apnoea are likely to start with normal breaths, which may commence at any stage of resuscitation. Depending on circulatory status, skin colour may recover quickly or slowly, but universally the tone (a proxy for consciousness) of the neonate is the last key metric to improve once heart function, circulation and spontaneous, effective breathing are restored.

Discontinuation of resuscitation

The outcome for a neonate with no detectable heart rate for more than 10 minutes after birth outside a planned setting is likely to be poor but innovation in neonatal intensive care means that where there is rapid access to good neonatal intensive care this is no longer universally true. Additionally it commonly takes longer than 10 minutes to complete all the steps in the NLS algorithm.

Place of birth, likely intrauterine aetiology of the presentation and duration of events before delivery, and immediate access to treatment such as therapeutic hypothermia and good quality neonatal intensive care, should be factored into the decision-making process when considering stopping resuscitation. Most recent studies show that if conditions exist to ensure immediate high-quality resuscitation and optimised post-resuscitation with active therapeutic hypothermia then resuscitation can reasonably continue beyond 10 minutes without a detectable heart rate. However, particular attention to correcting reversible causes of arrest should be made beyond this point if not already done, and if the time without recovery of a heart rate approaches 20 minutes proactive consideration of stopping resuscitation should be made.

Resuscitation beyond 20 minutes with no detectable heart rate is most likely to end in death for the neonate or severe disability in the very few survivors regardless of the subsequent provision of NICU care.

Stopping resuscitation is a decision that should be made by the most senior clinicians present, ideally with input from those experienced in resuscitation of the newborn. This may mean consulting with neonatal teams, in other centres, by telephone or video-conferencing.

Where a very slow heart rate has persisted (at less than 60 beats/min without improvement) during 20 minutes of continuous resuscitation, the decision to stop is much less clear. No evidence is available to recommend a universal approach beyond evaluation of the situation on a case-by-case basis by the resuscitating team and (ideally) senior clinicians. In these circumstances, availability and access to ongoing intensive care has a greater bearing on what decision may be appropriate.

A decision to stop resuscitation measures or stop before 20 minutes, or not starting resuscitation at all, may be appropriate in situations of extreme prematurity (<22–23 weeks), a birth weight of <400 g or in the presence of lethal abnormalities such as anencephaly or confirmed trisomy 13 or 18. Resuscitation is nearly always indicated in conditions with a high survival rate and acceptable morbidity. Such decisions should be taken by a senior member of the team, ideally a consultant, in partnership with the parents and other team members.

14.6 Laryngeal masks

The laryngeal mask (LM) may be considered as an alternative to a facemask for positive pressure ventilation among newborns weighing more than 2000 g or delivered ≥34 weeks' gestation. The use of a LM should be considered during resuscitation of the newborn if facemask ventilation is unsuccessful with a two-person technique or where there is a single rescuer. There is limited evidence evaluating its use for newborns weighing <2000 g or delivered at <34 weeks' gestation, and none for babies who are receiving compressions.

Commonly used types of neonatal appropriate LMs include the laryngeal mask airway (which utilises an inflatable cuff to create a seal) and the iGel (which uses a soft thermoplastic that moulds itself to the shape of the neonate's larynx once in place by virtue of the neonate's body heat, to create a seal).

The insertion of a LM should be undertaken only by those individuals who have been trained to use it. However, to achieve proficient use requires only a short training period. Due to constraints on training time and experience, it is more likely that someone can be trained to use a LM than will have opportunity to achieve proficiency in tracheal intubation. Evidence suggests that LMs are not superior to facemasks in trained hands and in most UK settings it will be appropriate to use facemasks as the first line. If there is a need for transfer between settings and respiratory support is ongoing, a LM may be useful to provide a secure airway. In the neonate, it is recommended that a laryngoscope or tongue depressor is used to help move the tongue out of the way before insertion of the LM, as this creates a wider space for the LM to pass through. It also allows examination for any potential oropharyngeal obstruction by particulate matter to be identified and resolved by use of suction before the LM is inserted.

14.7 Tracheal intubation

Most neonates can be resuscitated using a facemask or LM system. Swedish data suggest that if mask ventilation is applied effectively, only 1 in 500 neonates actually **need** intubation. Tracheal intubation only remains the gold standard in airway management but only if the tracheal tube can be correctly placed, without significantly interrupting ongoing ventilation and without causing trauma to the oropharynx and trachea. It is especially useful in prolonged resuscitations, in managing extremely preterm neonates and when a tracheal blockage is suspected. It should be considered if mask ventilation has failed, although the most common reason for this is poor positioning of the head with consequent failure to open the airway. It is, however, a common source of task fixation and can result in a significant interruption of resuscitation. It therefore needs experienced operators carefully marshaled to prevent unwarranted delay in moving along the resuscitative algorithm **especially** if mask ventilation is effective prior to the intubation attempt (see 'Discontinuation of resuscitation' earlier in chapter).

The technique of intubation is the same as for older infants. An appropriately grown, normal, full-term newborn usually needs a 3.5 mm (internal diameter) tracheal tube, but 2.5, 3.0 and 4 mm tubes should also be available.

Tracheal tube placement must be assessed visually during intubation and in most cases will be confirmed by a rapid response in heart rate on ventilating via the endotracheal tube. An exhaled CO_2 detection system (either colorimetric or quantitative) is a rapid, and now widely available, adjunct to confirmation of correct tracheal tube placement. The detection of exhaled CO_2 should be used to confirm tracheal tube placement but it should not be used in isolation. Listening to air entry in both axillae and seeing symmetrical chest movement may help avoid intubation of the right main bronchus, which can give a 'false positive' capnographic test. A number of other false positive reactions can occur with direct contamination of colorimetric detectors by drugs used in the newborn setting. False negatives can occur in low cardiac output states where CO_2 may not be detected despite accurate tracheal tube placement.

14.8 Preterm neonates

Unexpected deliveries outside delivery suites are more likely to be preterm. Whilst moderately preterm neonates (33–36 weeks' gestation) can be managed in the same way as term neonates, many neonates born between 32 and 33 weeks' gestation, and **all** neonates born before 32 weeks' gestation, need to be carefully supported during their transition to extrauterine life. This is described as stabilisation, rather than resuscitation, and aims to prevent problems, rather than providing resuscitation from a hypoxic event.

Premature neonates are more likely to get cold (because of a higher surface area to mass ratio), and are more likely to become hypoglycaemic (fewer glycogen stores). Wrapping the head and body (but not face) of all babies of <32 weeks' gestation in polyethylene wrap or a bag, where there is access to a radiant heater, should be done to aid maintenance of normothermia. The use of a radiant heater overhead theoretically warms the wet neonate through the plastic, creating a warmed, humidified atmosphere to maintain thermal control (Box 14.2). In neonates of <32 weeks' gestation, other interventions may also be needed to maintain temperature, such as use of a thermal mattress and warmed, humidified respiratory gases when ventilated. Where external heat sources are used, continuous temperature monitoring is necessary to prevent hyperthermia. After 30 weeks' gestation, an alternative is to dry and wrap the neonate in a dry, warm towel in a similar fashion to those born at term.

Box 14.2 Guidelines for the use of plastic bags for preterm neonates (<32 weeks' gestation) at birth

1. Preterm neonates born before 32 completed weeks of gestation may be placed in plastic bags or wrap for temperature stability during resuscitation. They should remain in the bag until they are on the NICU and the humidity within their incubator is at the desired level. It is a way of preventing evaporative heat loss and cannot replace incubators, etc. Neither should it replace all efforts to maintain a high ambient temperature around neonates born outside delivery suites.
2. At birth the neonate should not be dried, but should be slipped straight into the prepared plastic bag or wrapping. There is no need to wrap in a towel so long as this is done immediately after birth. This gives immediate humidity. The plastic bag only prevents evaporative heat loss – once in the bag the neonate should be placed under a radiant heater.
3. Suitable plastic bags are food-grade bags designed for microwaving and roasting.
4. The bag should cover the neonate from the shoulders to the feet. Gaps around the neck should be avoided as this allows warm humidified air out and colder air in. The head will stick out of the bag and should be dried as usual and a hat should be placed over the head to further reduce heat loss. Resuscitation/stabilisation should commence as per NLS guidelines.
5. A plastic bag or wrap will not interfere with standard resuscitation measures. If the umbilicus is required for vascular access then a small hole can be made in the bag to facilitate this.
6. The bag should not be removed unless deemed necessary by the registrar or consultant.
7. After transfer to a neonatal unit and stabilising ventilation, if required, the neonate's temperature should be recorded. The bag is only removed when the incubator humidity is satisfactory, the neonate's temperature is normal and further care is provided as per nursing protocols.

The plastic bag is a potentially useful technique for keeping larger neonates warm when born unexpectedly outside the delivery suite or in the community. However, it should be augmented by also wrapping with warm towels and ensuring a warm environment.

The more premature a neonate, the less likely they are to establish adequate spontaneous respirations without assistance. Preterm neonates of less than 32 weeks' gestation are likely to be deficient in surfactant especially after unexpected or precipitant delivery. Surfactant, secreted by alveolar type II pneumocytes, reduces alveolar surface tension and prevents alveolar collapse on expiration. Small amounts of surfactant can be demonstrated from about 20 weeks' gestation, but a surge in production only occurs after 30–34 weeks. Surfactant is released at birth due to aeration and distension of the alveoli. Production is reduced by hypothermia (<35°C), hypoxia and acidosis (pH <7.25). Surfactant deficiency can occur at any gestational age but is especially likely in neonates born before 30 weeks' gestation. Many units will have a policy to address this issue based on the gestation at birth. Nasal continuous positive airway pressure (CPAP) is now widely used to stabilise preterm neonates with respiratory distress and may avoid the need to intubate and ventilate many of these neonates. If, however, intubation and ventilation is necessary, then exogenous surfactant should be given as soon as possible.

The lungs of preterm neonates are more fragile than those of term neonates and thus are much more susceptible to damage from overdistension. Therefore, it is appropriate to start with a lower inflation pressure of 25 cmH_2O (2.5 kPa) but do not be afraid to increase this to 30 cmH_2O (2.9 kPa) if there is no heart rate response. Using a positive end-expiratory pressure (PEEP) helps prevent collapse of the airways during expiration and is normally given using a pressure of 5 cmH_2O (~0.5 kPa). In most situations it will not be possible to measure the tidal volume of each breath given and while seeing some chest movement helps confirm aeration of the lungs, very obvious chest wall movement in premature neonates of less than 28 weeks' gestation may indicate excessive and potentially damaging tidal volumes. This should be avoided and inspiratory pressures should be decreased if chest movement is excessive, the heart rate is ≥100 beats/min and there are adequate oxygen saturations.

Premature neonates are more susceptible to the toxic effects of hyperoxia. Using a pulse oximeter to monitor both heart rate and oxygen saturation from birth makes stabilisation much easier. Exposing preterm neonates at birth to high concentrations of oxygen can have significant long-term adverse effects. The current guidance is that for stabilisation or resuscitation of a preterm nenoate at <28 weeks' gestation, start with 30% oxygen, between 28 and 32 weeks start with with 21–30% oxygen and beyond 32 weeks start in 21% oxygen (air). Inspired oxygen should be titrated to oxygen saturations and acceptable preductal saturations measured on the right arm or wrist are shown in Table 14.2.

Table 14.2 Acceptable preductal saturation monitoring (SpO_2) in premature neonates above which supplemental oxygen is not needed

Time from birth	Acceptable (25th centile) preductal SpO_2 levels
2 min	65%
5 min	85%
10 min	90%

In preterm babies (<28 weeks' gestation) there is association with poorer clinical outcomes if the measured oxygen saturations are <80% at 5 minutes of age. Inspired oxygen concentration should be increased if saturations of 85% have not been met by 5 minutes. If chest compressions are given inspired oxygen should be increased to 100%

CPAP via mask versus intubation

As mentioned, tracheal intubation to 'secure' the airway is rarely needed in term neonates. In addition, it carries with it the inherent risks of: delaying ongoing resuscitation due to task fixation; causing traumatic injury to oropharyngeal and tracheal tissue; and at worst irreversibly destabilising an otherwise well neonate.

In preterm neonates, effective initial respiratory support of spontaneously breathing neonates with respiratory distress can be given using CPAP. Therefore, CPAP should be considered a first line intervention for ongoing support in this population especially where personnel are not skilled in, or only infrequently practice, tracheal intubation. Where a mask plus T-piece system is being used for initial resuscitation, and a PEEP valve is available on the T-piece, CPAP may be given effectively by mask. Other dedicated CPAP devices utilising small nasal masks or prongs are available.

14.9 Actions in the event of poor initial response to resuscitation

1. Check head position, airway and breathing:
   - Repeat five inflation breaths, does the heart rate improve or the chest rise?
   - Do you need a second pair of hands for airway control, or an airway adjunct (e.g. LM)?
2. Check for a technical fault:
   - Is mask ventilation effective? Is there a significant leak around the mask? Observe chest movement
   - Is a longer inflation time or higher inflation pressure required?

   If the neonate is intubated:
   - Is the tracheal tube in the trachea? Auscultate both axillae, listen at the mouth for a large leak and observe chest movement. Use an exhaled CO_2 detector to ensure tracheal tube position
   - Is the tracheal tube in the right main bronchus? Auscultate both axillae and observe chest movement
   - Is the tracheal tube blocked? Use an exhaled CO_2 detector to confirm tracheal position and patency of the tracheal tube. Remove it and retry mask support if there is any concern that the tracheal tube is the problem
   - If starting in air then increase the oxygen concentration. This is the least likely to be a cause of poor responsiveness, although if monitoring saturations it could be a cause for slow increase in observed saturations

3. Does the neonate have a pneumothorax? This occurs spontaneously in up to 1% of newborns, but pneumothoraces needing action in the delivery unit are exceptionally rare. Auscultate the chest for asymmetry of breath sounds. A cold light source can be used to transilluminate the chest – the pneumothorax may show as a hyperilluminating area. If a tension pneumothorax is thought to be present clinically, a 21 gauge butterfly needle should be used to perform needle thoracocentesis via the second intercostal space in the mid-clavicular line. Alternatively, a 22 gauge cannula connected to a three-way tap may be used. Remember that this risks causing a pneumothorax during this procedure (see Chapter 17) but can equally be life saving.
4. Does the neonate remain cyanosed despite a regular breathing pattern, no increased work of breathing and with a good heart rate? There may be a congenital heart malformation, which may be duct dependent, or a persistent pulmonary hypertension.
5. If, after resuscitation, the neonate is pink and has a good heart rate but is not breathing effectively, and there is a history of maternal opiate administration, they may be suffering the effects of maternal opiates. Options include managing the airway and breathing until this effect wears off or rarely naloxone 200 micrograms may be given intramuscularly, which should outlast the opiate effect. Naloxone is not considered a resuscitation drug.
6. Is there severe anaemia or hypovolaemia? In cases of large blood loss, 10–20 ml/kg O RhD-negative blood should be given.

14.10 Birth outside the delivery room

Whenever a neonate is born unexpectedly, the greatest difficulty often lies in keeping them warm. Drying and wrapping, turning up the heating and closing windows and doors are all important in maintaining temperature. Special care must be taken to clamp and cut the cord to prevent blood loss.

Hospitals with an emergency medicine department should have guidelines for resuscitation at birth, summoning help and post-resuscitation transfer of neonates born in, or admitted to, the department.

Neonates born unexpectedly outside hospital are more likely to be preterm and at risk of rapidly becoming hypothermic. However, the principles of resuscitation are identical to the hospital setting. Transport to the place of definitive care will need to be discussed according to local guidelines.

14.11 Communication with the parents

It is important that the team caring for the newborn informs the parents of progress whenever possible. This is likely to be most difficult in unexpected deliveries so prior planning to cover the eventuality may be helpful. Decisions at the end of life must involve the parents whenever possible. All communication should be documented immediately after the event, ideally after a team debriefing. As it is likely to be a stressful and relatively rare occurrence to have unplanned deliveries out of hospital or in the emergency department, teams should ensure that they have mechanisms in place to facilitate timely and effective debriefing of all teams involved.

14.12 Summary

The approach to newborn resuscitation is different from that used for children and adults and is summarised in Algorithm 14.1 at the start of the chapter.

PART 4
Trauma

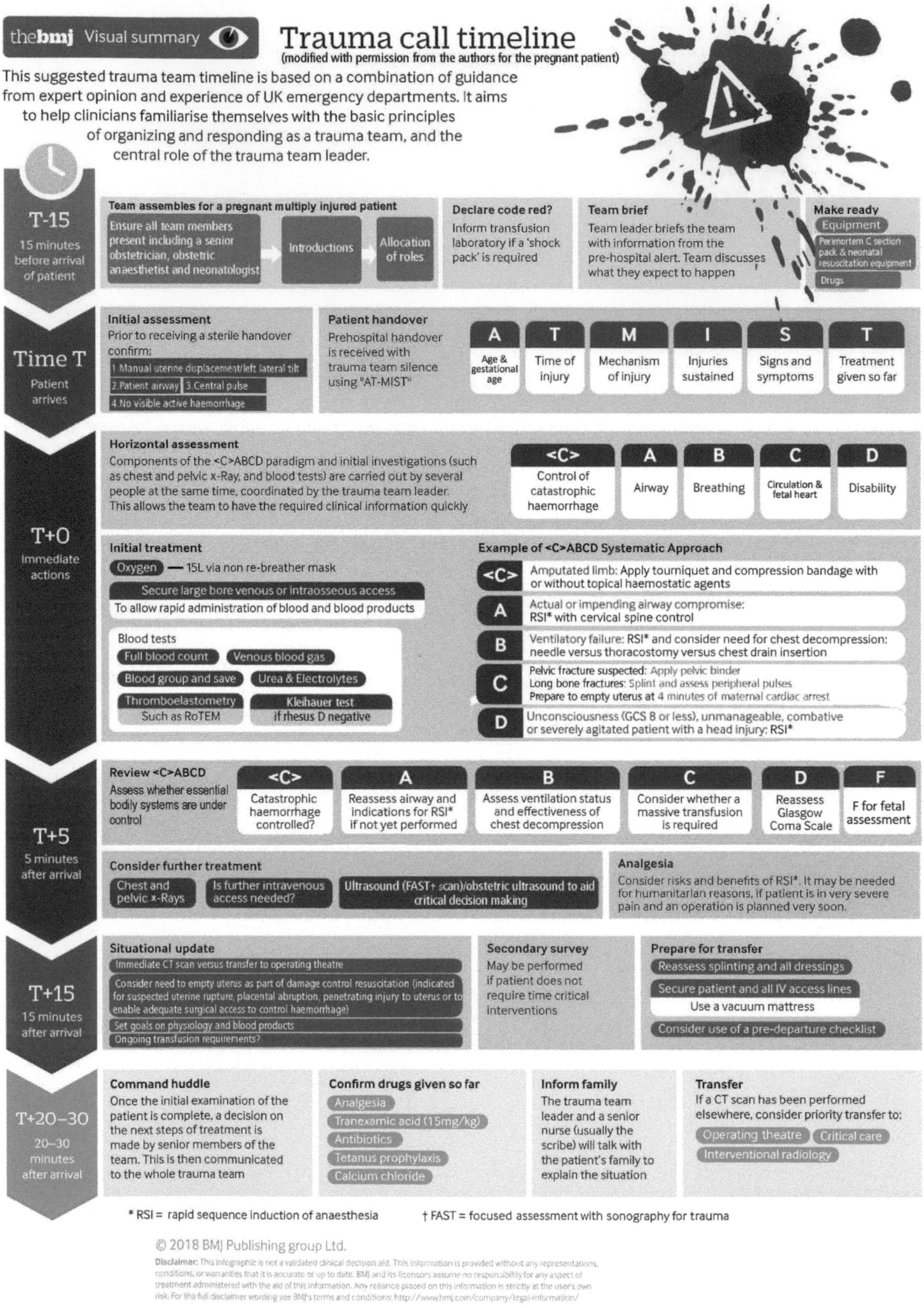

thebmj Visual summary
Trauma call timeline
(modified with permission from the authors for the pregnant patient)
This suggested trauma team timeline is based on a combination of guidance from expert opinion and experience of UK emergency departments. It aims to help clinicians familiarise themselves with the basic principles of organizing and responding as a trauma team, and the central role of the trauma team leader.
T-15
15 minutes before arrival of patient
Team assembles for a pregnant multiply injured patient
Ensure all team members present including a senior obstetrician, obstetric anaesthetist and neonatologist
Introductions
Allocation of roles
Declare code red?
Inform transfusion laboratory if a 'shock pack' is required
Team brief
Team leader briefs the team with information from the pre-hospital alert. Team discusses what they expect to happen
Make ready
Equipment
Perimortem C section pack & neonatal resuscitation equipment
Drugs
Time T
Patient arrives
Initial assessment
Prior to receiving a sterile handover confirm:
1.Manual uterine displacement/left lateral tilt
2.Patient airway
3.Central pulse
4.No visible active haemorrhage
Patient handover
Prehospital handover is received with trauma team silence using "AT-MIST"
A Age & gestational age
T Time of injury
M Mechanism of injury
I Injuries sustained
S Signs and symptoms
T Treatment given so far
T+0
Immediate actions
Horizontal assessment
Components of the <C>ABCD paradigm and initial investigations (such as chest and pelvic x-Ray, and blood tests) are carried out by several people at the same time, coordinated by the trauma team leader. This allows the team to have the required clinical information quickly
<C> Control of catastrophic haemorrhage
A Airway
B Breathing
C Circulation & fetal heart
D Disability
Initial treatment
Oxygen — 15L via non re-breather mask
Secure large bore venous or intraosseous access
To allow rapid administration of blood and blood products
Blood tests
Full blood count
Venous blood gas
Blood group and save
Urea & Electrolytes
Thromboelastometry
Such as RoTEM
Kleihauer test
if rhesus D negative
Example of <C>ABCD Systematic Approach
<C> Amputated limb: Apply tourniquet and compression bandage with or without topical haemostatic agents
A Actual or impending airway compromise: RSI* with cervical spine control
B Ventilatory failure: RSI* and consider need for chest decompression: needle versus thoracostomy versus chest drain insertion
C Pelvic fracture suspected: Apply pelvic binder
Long bone fractures: Splint and assess peripheral pulses
Prepare to empty uterus at 4 minutes of maternal cardiac arrest
D Unconsciousness (GCS 8 or less), unmanageable, combative or severely agitated patient with a head injury: RSI*
T+5
5 minutes after arrival
Review <C>ABCD
Assess whether essential bodily systems are under control
<C> Catastrophic haemorrhage controlled?
A Reassess airway and indications for RSI* if not yet performed
B Assess ventilation status and effectiveness of chest decompression
C Consider whether a massive transfusion is required
D Reassess Glasgow Coma Scale
F F for fetal assessment
Consider further treatment
Chest and pelvic x-Rays
Is further intravenous access needed?
Ultrasound (FAST† scan)/obstetric ultrasound to aid critical decision making
Analgesia
Consider risks and benefits of RSI*. It may be needed for humanitarian reasons, if patient is in very severe pain and an operation is planned very soon.
T+15
15 minutes after arrival
Situational update
Immediate CT scan versus transfer to operating theatre
Consider need to empty uterus as part of damage control resuscitation (indicated for suspected uterine rupture, placental abruption, penetrating injury to uterus or to enable adequate surgical access to control haemorrhage)
Set goals on physiology and blood products
Ongoing transfusion requirements?
Secondary survey
May be performed if patient does not require time critical interventions
Prepare for transfer
Reassess splinting and all dressings
Secure patient and all IV access lines
Use a vacuum mattress
Consider use of a pre-departure checklist
T+20–30
20–30 minutes after arrival
Command huddle
Once the initial examination of the patient is complete, a decision on the next steps of treatment is made by senior members of the team. This is then communicated to the whole trauma team
Confirm drugs given so far
Analgesia
Tranexamic acid (15mg/kg)
Antibiotics
Tetanus prophylaxis
Calcium chloride
Inform family
The trauma team leader and a senior nurse (usually the scribe) will talk with the patient's family to explain the situation
Transfer
If a CT scan has been performed elsewhere, consider priority transfer to:
Operating theatre
Critical care
Interventional radiology
* RSI = rapid sequence induction of anaesthesia
† FAST = focused assessment with sonography for trauma
© 2018 BMJ Publishing group Ltd.
Disclaimer: This infographic is not a validated clinical decision aid. This information is provided without any representations, conditions, or warranties that it is accurate or up to date. BMJ and its licensors assume no responsibility for any aspect of treatment administered with the aid of this information. Any reliance placed on this information is strictly at the user's own risk. For the full disclaimer wording see BMJ's terms and conditions: http://www.bmj.com/company/legal-information/

Algorithm 15.1 Modified trauma call timeline

Source: Mercer SJ, Kingston EV, Jones CPL. The trauma call. BMJ 2018; 361: k2272. © 2018 BMJ Publishing Group

CHAPTER 15
Introduction to trauma

Learning outcomes

After reading this chapter, you will be able to:

- Describe the necessary pregnancy modifications to modern trauma management for the multiply injured pregnant woman

15.1 Introduction

Trauma is an example of a multisystem, life-threatening illness and is the commonest cause of death in young people under 40 years of age. Like all life-threatening emergencies, the management of major trauma requires a systematic approach. The obstetric team is likely to be called to any case of trauma in the pregnant woman. A knowledge of the principles behind modern trauma care will enable the obstetric team to integrate with the trauma team to provide the best care for a pregnant trauma patient.

15.2 Aetiology and epidemiology

Major trauma in pregnancy is rare. Only 1 in 1000 pregnant women will be victims of major trauma (injury severity score >15). The causes of trauma in pregnancy and the early postpartum period are attempted suicide, road traffic collisions, domestic violence, falls and burns. Blunt causes of traumatic injury predominate but penetrating abdominal trauma is associated with much higher fetal and maternal mortality.

In a UK retrospective analysis of a national trauma registry, only 1% of the females of child-bearing age presenting with major trauma were pregnant. However, maternal mortality rates were seen to be higher (5.1%) when compared with the non-pregnant trauma patient (4.1%). Pregnant women were more likely to be seriously injured in road traffic collisions and interpersonal violence than non-pregnant patients. Pregnant trauma victims in this study were more likely to have sustained major thoracic trauma than non-pregnant patients. Fetal survival was 56% from this series. However, it is acknowledged that screening for pregnancy in women of child-bearing age is not routine on admission to the emergency department (ED) and that the incidence of trauma, particularly in early pregnancy, may be underestimated.

15.3 Obstetric complications of trauma

Placental abruption occurs in up to 50% of cases of major trauma in pregnancy and in 5% of cases of minor injuries. Traumatic uterine rupture is much less likely, occurring in less than 1% of major injuries, but it is associated with likely fetal loss and a 10% maternal mortality rate. The seat belt advice for pregnant women remains: 'Above and below the bump, not over it'. Minor trauma cannot be assumed to be benign for the fetus as in addition to the risk of abruption it is associated with increased rates of preterm delivery and low birth weight.

Managing Medical and Obstetric Emergencies and Trauma: A Practical Approach, Fourth Edition. Edited by Rosamunde Burns and Kara Dent.

15.4 Organisation of trauma care

The NCEPOD report in 2007 *Trauma: Who Cares?* found substandard care in 60% of trauma patients studied and recommended the establishment of 24/7 regional trauma networks. Improvements in survival had been brought about in the USA and Australia from the reorganisation of trauma care. The development of regionalised trauma care in England in 2012 with ambulance bypass of local hospitals to newly designated major trauma centres has resulted in significant improvements in outcomes for patients after severe injury (19% increase in the odds of survival for trauma patients who reach hospital alive).

15.5 Trauma call timeline for a pregnant trauma patient

Obstetricians, obstetric anaesthetists and midwives understand the anatomical and physiological changes of pregnancy and are able to bring that knowledge to the trauma team to enable the safe adaptation of standard trauma care for the pregnant woman. At the pre-arrival briefing in the resuscitation room, the obstetric team and neonatologist should introduce themselves to the trauma team leader and scribe. A perimortem caesarean section (PMCS) pack should be available together with the equipment for neonatal resuscitation.

The obstetrician should remind the trauma team leader of:

- The need to relieve aortocaval compression with manual uterine displacement (MUD) to prevent compounding hypotension associated with hypovolaemia. The 30 second ATMIST handover (Algorithm 15.1) should be preceded by relief of aortocaval compression
- Pregnant women have an expanded circulating volume in pregnancy of 100 ml/kg at term compared with 70 ml/kg outwith pregnancy. This means that the pregnant woman may appear cardiovascularly stable despite significant blood loss and will **show signs of shock late**. If shocked, a pregnant trauma patient will be potentially closer to hypovolaemic cardiac arrest than a non-pregnant patient because of this greater ability to compensate following haemorrhage
- The setting of priorities is such that the life of the mother takes precedence over the life of the fetus. The obstetric team know the mother takes priority and resuscitating her is the best hope for the fetus
- However, fetal monitoring can help to identify the extent of maternal hypovolaemia (as the uteroplacental circulation shuts down to preserve maternal circulation). Signs of fetal distress may also aid in the diagnosis of the potential concealed haemorrhage associated with uterine abruption or rupture
- The obstetric team may have a role at **C** as part of 'damage control resuscitation' to potentially empty the uterus to help manage non-compressible haemorrhage. The only equipment needed in the perimortem caesarean section pack is a scalpel and clamp/ligature for the cord. If circulation is restored, the woman can then be taken to theatre

The sequence of care on arrival of the patient should be as per the modified trauma call timeline. This trauma call timeline is led by time T intervals, showing the actions that need to happen from 15 minutes before the arrival of the patient to the 30 minute post-arrival point (Algorithm 15.1). It allows the team to work concurrently making patient management more efficient and gaining information on life-threatening conditions quickly. It uses <C>ABCD throughout where <C> comes first to control catastrophic haemorrhage as a priority.

Streamlined assessment

Major obstetric haemorrhage accounts for over a quarter of all trauma deaths, so the trauma team must be focused on the early *identification* of bleeding and rapid *effective haemostasis* by *targeting* life-saving interventions. Effective use of diagnostic modalities will lead to faster and more accurate diagnosis of the source of bleeding:

- Immediate total body computed tomography (CT) for the bleeding patient if haemodynamically stable and responding to resuscitation
- If haemodynamically *unstable and not responding to fluid resuscitation*, do chest and pelvis x-rays and focused assessment with sonography for trauma (FAST)

15.6 Damage control resusucitation

This is summarised in the aide memoire **TRAUMATIC** (Figure 15.1).

Major Trauma?
Major Haemorrhage? Then...

T	**Tranexamic acid**	• Initial 1 g bolus:
		  • Often already given pre-hospital
		  • Otherwise, administer only if within 3 hours of injury or ongoing hyperfibrinolysis
		  • Do not delay, every minute counts
		• Subsequent 1 g infusion over 8 hours

R	**Resuscitation**	• Activate Major Haemorrhage Protocol
		• Initial transfusion ratio 1:1:1 and consider:
		  • Rapid infuser and cell salvage
		  • Time-limited hypotensive resuscitation
		  • Pelvic binder / splint fractures / tourniquet
		• Limit crystalloid use

A	**Avoid hypothermia**	• Target temperature > 36°C
		  • Increase ambient theatre temperature
		  • Remove wet clothing and sheets
		  • Warm all blood products & irrigation fluids
		  • Warm the patient using forced-air warming device / blanket /mattress

U	**Unstable? Damage control surgery**	• If unstable, coagulopathic, hypothermic or acidotic, perform damage control surgery of: • Haemorrhage control, decompression, decontamination and splintage • Time surgery aiming to finish < 90 min and conduct surgical pauses at least every 30 min
M	**Metabolic**	• Perform regular blood gas analysis • Base excess and lactate guide resuscitation • Adequate resuscitation corrects acidosis • If lactate > 5 mmol/l or rising, consider stopping surgery, splint and transfer to ICU • Haemoglobin results are misleading
A	**Avoid vasoconstrictors**	• Use of vasoconstrictors doubles mortality • However, use may be required in cases of spinal cord or traumatic brain injury • Anaesthetic induction - suggest ketamine • Maintenance - when BP allows, titrate high dose fentanyl and consider midazolam
T	**Test clotting**	• Check clotting regularly to target transfusion: • Laboratory or point of care (TEG / ROTEM) • Aim platelets $>100\times10^9$/l • Aim INR & aPTTR ≤ 1.5 • Aim fibrinogen > 2 g/l

I	**Imaging**	• Consider:
		  • CT:
		  Most severely injured / haemodynamically unstable patients gain most from CT
		  • Interventional radiology

C	**Calcium**	• Maintain ionised calcium >1.0 mmol/l • Administer 10 ml of 10% calcium chloride over 10 minutes, repeating as required • Monitor potassium and treat hyperkalaemia with calcium and insulin / glucose

Figure 15.1 TRAUMATIC mnemonic

Source: May L, Kelly A, Wyse M. University Hospitals Coventry and Warwickshire NHS Trust. © University Hospitals Coventry and Warwickshire NHS Trust

Modern trauma management targets ***early haemorrhage control and preservation of coagulation***.

It is now widely believed that ***large volumes of crystalloid/colloid*** are associated with worse outcomes in major trauma, and that blood loss is best replaced with warmed red cells, plasma and platelets.

The volume resuscitation strategies of the past using crystalloid and colloid have focused on restoring perfusion and eliminating oxygen debt, but this has been shown to be harmful. Attempts to volume resuscitate not only fail to reach these targets in multiply injured patients, but also cause haemodilution, coagulopathy, hypothermia, tissue oedema, abdominal compartment syndrome, organ dysfunction and death.

In major trauma centres, the prehospital team may call a 'code red' major obstetric haemorrhage protocol in the haemorrhagic shock situation, enabling a 'shock pack' of O-negative red cells and fresh frozen plasma to be available on arrival of the patient in the ED. Once the patient's blood group has been determined, the blood transfusion laboratory will issue type-specific blood products. ***If blood is not immediately available*** then 250 ml boluses of warmed crystalloid, up to a maximum of 1000 ml, are recommended while awaiting urgent blood products in the trauma haemorrhagic shock situation. On arrival of blood, transfusion is commenced guided by clinical signs, blood gas analysis (lactate, base excess) and near patient testing of coagulation such as rotational thromboelastometry (ROTEM®) or thromboelastography (TEG®).

The strategy of 'permissive hypotension' described in modern trauma guidelines for actively bleeding multiply injured *non-pregnant* trauma patients implies accepting an adequate (to maintain central circulation) blood pressure ***for as short a time as possible*** during active bleeding until haemostasis is achieved. During this period of lower mean arterial pressure during active bleeding, blood and blood products should be transfused to an acceptable mean arterial pressure. Crystalloid fluid resuscitation should be limited to preserve coagulation.

This is *controversial for the obstetric team*, who know that pregnant women show signs of shock **late** and that placental blood supply depends on mean arterial pressure. A pragmatic approach for pregnancy may therefore be:

- **If haemorrhagic shock is the presentation of the multiply injured pregnant woman** then maternal life saving through aggressive blood transfusion and 'turning off the tap' as soon as possible is appropriate
- With our knowledge of pregnancy physiology, we know that for a pregnant woman to be shocked she will have **lost more of her circulating volume** than a non-pregnant patient and therefore the need to 'turn off the tap' and aggressively replace blood with blood and blood products is **even more urgent**
- The trauma team should move rapidly to control the source of the bleeding as the shocked, multiply injured, pregnant woman will be closer to hypovolaemic arrest in this situation than a non-pregnant patient

In all other circumstances (for example a pregnant woman with an isolated femoral fracture) **maintenance of placental perfusion by ensuring a normal maternal blood pressure is the appropriate management**. The fetus is vulnerable in any situation where there is potential for maternal haemodynamic instability and should be appropriately monitored. Placental vasoconstriction can occur following trauma in the presence of normal/near normal maternal observations. Therefore fetal monitoring can provide important information about the adequacy of maternal resuscitation.

'Turning off the tap' at C

Non-fluid responsive haemorrhagic shock is managed by early recourse to 'damage control surgery' as part of damage control resuscitation in modern trauma management. Damage control surgery is time-limited surgery to stop bleeding and prevent contamination, with definitive care deferred to a later time. Emptying the uterus may form part of the damage control surgery at **C**, if the patient remains haemodynamically unstable and is not responding to volume resuscitation. The indications for emptying the uterus in multiple trauma remain the same:

- Cardiac arrest
- Placental abruption
- Uterine rupture
- Penetrating injury
- To enable surgical access for haemorrhage control within the abdomen/control bleeding from an unstable pelvis

The cardiac arrest situation aside, the order of surgical priorities to stop bleeding will require the obstetric team to be part of the surgical team planning the damage control surgery.

15.7 Interventional radiology

The 2016 National Institute for Health and Care Excellence (NICE) trauma guidelines recommend the following:

> Use interventional radiology techniques in patients with active arterial pelvic haemorrhage, unless immediate open surgery is needed to control bleeding from other injuries. Consider interventional radiology techniques in patients with solid organ (spleen, liver or kidney) arterial haemorrhage. Consider a joint interventional radiology and surgery strategy for arterial haemorrhage that extends to surgically inaccessible regions. Use an endovascular stent graft in patients with blunt thoracic aortic injury.

The multidisciplinary team will need to ensure relief of aortocaval compression if there is a continuing pregnancy at the time these techniques are proposed. Consideration would have to be given to any potential compromise of the uterine blood supply by the interventional radiology technique itself and timing of delivery. The technique should be modified if possible to minimise radiation exposure to a developing fetus.

15.8 Summary

- Major trauma is life threatening and a systematic approach to its management can save lives
- The obstetrician, obstetric anaesthetist and midwife are a valued part of the trauma team. They bring their expertise of pregnancy physiology which has important implications for the modification of trauma care to ensure the best outcome for mother and fetus in this high-risk situation

15.9 Further reading

ACS (American College of Surgeons). *Advanced Trauma Life Support® Student Course Manual*, 10th edn. Chicago: ACS, 2018.

Battaloglu E, McDonnell D, Chu J, Lecky F, Porter K. Epidemiology and outcomes of pregnancy and obstetric complications in trauma in the United Kingdom. *Injury* 2016; 47: 184–7.

Battaloglu E, Porter K. Management of pregnancy and obstetric complications in prehospital trauma care: faculty of prehospital care consensus guidelines. *Emerg Med J* 2017; 34(5): 318–25.

Cameron PA, Gabbe BJ, Cooper DJ, Walker T, Judson R, McNeil J. A statewide system of trauma care in Victoria: effect on patient survival. *Med J Aust* 2008; 189(10): 546–50.

Celso B, Tepas J, Langland-Orban B, et al. A systematic review and meta-analysis comparing outcome of severely injured patients treated in trauma centers following the establishment of trauma systems. *J Trauma Acute Care Surg* 2006; 60(2): 371–8.

Findlay G, Martin IC, Carter S et al. on behalf NCEPOD (National Confidential Enquiry into Patient Outcome and Death). *Trauma: Who Cares?* London: NCEPOD, 2007. www.ncepod.org.uk/2007report2/Downloads/SIP_report.pdf (last accessed January 2022).

Knight M, Bunch K, Tuffnell D et al. (eds) on behalf of MBRRACE-UK. *Saving Lives, Improving Mothers' Care – Lessons Learned to Inform Maternity Care from the UK and Ireland Confidential Enquiries into Maternal Deaths and Morbidity 2015–17*. Oxford: National Perinatal Epidemiology Unit, University of Oxford, 2019.

Mercer SJ, Kingston EV, Jones CPL. The trauma call. *BMJ* 2018; 361: k2272.

Moran CG, Lecky F, Bouamra O, et al, Changing the system – major trauma patients and their outcomes in the NHS (England) 2008–2017. *EClinicalMedicine* 2018; 2: 13–21. https://doi.org/10.1016/j.eclinm.2018.07.001 (last accessed January 2022).

Nevin DG, Brohi K. Permissive hypotension for active haemorrhage in trauma. *Anaesthesia* 2017; 72: 1443–8.

NICE (National Institute for Health and Care Excellence). *Head Injury: Assessment and Early Management*. CG176. London: NICE, 2014 (updated September 2019).

NICE (National Institute for Health and Care Excellence). *Major Trauma: Assessment and Initial Management*. NG39. London: NICE, 2016.

Wiles MD. Blood pressure in trauma resuscitation: 'pop the clot' vs. 'drain the brain'? *Anaesthesia* 2017; 72: 1448–55.

CHAPTER 16
Domestic abuse

Learning outcomes

After reading this chapter, you will be able to:
- Appreciate the incidence of domestic abuse in UK
- Understand the implications for the woman and her baby, during pregnancy and postnatally
- Plan to identify victims of abuse
- Plan to familiarise yourself with support services
- Familiarise yourself with local support services

16.1 Introduction

Domestic abuse (also known as intimate partner abuse) is a major public health concern that threatens the lives, health and emotional well-being of women and their families.

Domestic violence and abuse is defined, by the UK Home Office as:

> Any incident or pattern of incidents of controlling, coercive or threatening behaviour, violence or abuse between those aged 16 or over who are or have been, intimate partners or family members regardless of gender or sexuality. The abuse can encompass, but is not limited to: psychological, physical, sexual, financial, emotional.

In heterosexual relationships, women are more likely to be victims than are men. Domestic abuse affects all social classes and all ethnic groups, occurs worldwide and affects all age groups. The broader definition allows for forced marriage, honour killings and female genital mutilation to be recognised as being part of the issue.

Scale of the problem

The lifetime prevalence of domestic abuse is estimated at between 15% and 71% globally.

- The Office for National Statistics (ONS) domestic abuse prevalence and trends showed an estimated 1.6 million women (8.4% of those aged 16–59 years) experienced domestic abuse in England and Wales in the year ending March 2019
- It is estimated that 30% of domestic abuse starts in pregnancy
- Of women who are murdered, 40% are killed by a current or ex partner

Managing Medical and Obstetric Emergencies and Trauma: A Practical Approach, Fourth Edition. Edited by Rosamunde Burns and Kara Dent.

The 2018 report of MBRRACE-UK (*Saving Lives, Improving Mothers' Care*) reported that 8% of the women who died in the triennium 2014–2016 were documented to have been subject to domestic abuse. In 64% of those who died, there was no documentation of enquiry about domestic abuse having been made by carers during the pregnancy. MBRRACE states that the key message from the National Institute for Health and Care Excellence (NICE) antenatal care guidelines must be reiterated as follows:

> Healthcare professionals need to be alert to the symptoms and signs of domestic abuse, and women should be given the opportunity to disclose domestic abuse in an environment in which they feel secure.

What keeps women in abusive relationships?

To outsiders it seems almost bizarre that anyone would stay within an abusive relationship, but nonetheless they do. The reasons for staying are often multiple:

- *Fear*: She is afraid that, if she leaves, she or other family members will experience more abuse or possibly be killed
- *Financial*: Control of her resources by her abuser
- *Family*: Pressures to stay with the abuser
- *Father*: Wanting a father figure for her children
- *Faith*: That she places in a religious doctrine
- *Forgiveness*: The abuser is often contrite
- *Fatigue*: From living under high and constant stress and erosion of self-esteem

16.2 Domestic abuse and pregnancy

The incidence of domestic abuse in pregnancy ranges from 2% in Australia to 13.5% in Uganda and is therefore more common than many other conditions routinely screened for in the antenatal period. The prevalence of intimate partner violence during pregnancy ranged from approximately 2.0% in Australia, Cambodia, Denmark and the Philippines to 13.5% in Uganda among ever-pregnant, ever-partnered women; half of the surveys estimated prevalence to be between 3.9% and 8.7%. Prevalence appeared to be higher in African and Latin American countries relative to the European and Asian countries surveyed.

Domestic abuse often begins or escalates during pregnancy; in some cases, it commences in the puerperium. The risk of moderate to severe abuse appears to be greatest in the postpartum period. Women suffering physical abuse are at increased risk of miscarriage, premature labour, placental abruption, low birth weight infants, fetal injury and intrauterine fetal death. Women who are subject to abuse are 15 times more likely than average to misuse alcohol, nine times more likely to misuse drugs, three times more likely to be clinically depressed and five times more likely to attempt suicide. These factors all have implications for both the mother and fetus.

Classically, injuries towards the pregnant abdomen, genitals and breasts are seen in pregnancy. However, the injuries can be multiple, affecting any part of the woman's body.

Recognising domestic violence in pregnancy

Women who are being abused often book late and may be poor attenders. Their partners may withhold the money required to travel to the hospital. Alternatively, women may attend repeatedly with trivial symptoms and appear reluctant to be discharged home. If the partner accompanies the woman, he may be constantly present, not allowing for private discussion. The woman may seem reluctant to speak in front of, or contradict, her partner.

Any signs of abuse on the woman's body will tend to be minimised. As with child abuse, the stated mechanism of injury often does not fit with the clinical findings. There may be untended injuries of different ages, or the late presentation of injuries. A history of behavioural problems or abuse in the woman's existing children may be suggestive of domestic violence. Often these patients will give a history of mental health problems.

Diagnosing domestic abuse

As domestic abuse often begins or escalates during pregnancy, it is essential that we, as obstetricians and midwives, routinely ask women whether they are subject to mistreatment. Abusive pregnancies are high risk, and domestic abuse is much more prevalent than other complications of pregnancy, such as pre-eclampsia or gestational diabetes mellitus. Standard questions should therefore be included, in the same way as we would ask about medical disorders, smoking or alcohol use. Systematic multiple assessment protocols lead to increased detection and reporting of abuse during pregnancy. The mnemonic **RADAR** was developed, by the Massachusetts Medical Society in 1992, as a tool to guide enquiry about domestic abuse.

R Routinely enquire
A Ask direct questions
D Document your findings
A Assess safety
R Review options and choices

Health professionals should be given appropriate training and education to improve awareness. Questions should be asked in a non-judgemental, respectful, supportive manner. Obstetricians and midwives should be aware of what help is available if a woman requests help. Questions, such as the following, may allow the woman to disclose the fact that she is subject to violence:

'I have noticed you have several bruises. Did someone hit you? You seemed frightened by your partner. Has he ever hurt you?'

'You mention that your partner loses his temper with the children. Does he ever do so with you?'

'How does your partner act when drinking or on drugs?'

Referral for help

It is essential that local guidelines are developed for referral to appropriate agencies. Many such organisations exist, both locally and nationally, including the Women's Aid, Welsh Women's Aid and SafeLives. These three organisations collect and hold data on the provision of domestic abuse services in England and Wales.

Other strategies, such as questionnaires or information about emergency helplines in the female toilets or printed on the patient-held notes, may help those women whose partners are constantly present. Community midwives visiting women at home may have the privacy to discuss such sensitive matters. The provision of professional interpretation services is essential; it is not adequate or acceptable to rely on family members to act as interpreters, as this does not allow free dialogue to occur.

Documentation in the medical notes is important, even if the woman does not wish to pursue prosecution at the current time. Women often seek prosecution many years later, and evidence of the pattern of domestic abuse may help to secure a conviction. Care must be taken to avoid documenting sensitive information in hand-held notes, which will certainly be scrutinised by controlling partners.

Medicolegal aspects

Following the Domestic Violence Crime and Victims Act 2004, a case against an alleged perpetrator can now proceed, if there is sufficient evidence, even if the victim withdraws their statement. Healthcare workers may be approached for a statement.

Safeguarding of children

Children who live with women who are abused are at significant risk of violence and neglect, and it is crucial to consider the well-being of these children in the overall plan.

Police officers called to deal with domestic abuse are required to investigate the welfare of children who have witnessed abuse and/or are resident at the relevant address. A notification to the Police Child Abuse Investigation Unit may then ensue.

If a woman discloses domestic abuse to a healthcare professional, then steps must be taken to safeguard her existing children. Many units now have safeguarding midwives who are au fait with procedures for referral to social services.

Communication and teamwork

Domestic abuse is an area where multiagency working is essential. No one agency can address all domestic abuse factors. Working collaboratively will ensure appropriate help and support is given. Unit guidelines should incorporate referral pathways for multiagency working.

Audit standard

All women should be seen on their own at least once during the antenatal period to enable the disclosure of such information.

16.3 Summary

- Domestic abuse is a major health and social problem in pregnancy
- Domestic abuse represents a serious threat to the physical and emotional health of women and their children
- All health professionals have an obligation to identify cases of domestic abuse and provide support and help to the victims

16.4 Useful contacts

Scotland: https://sdafmh.org.uk
Scotland: https://www.mygov.scot/domestic-abuse/support-for-female-victims/
Scotland: https://www.scotland.police.uk/keep-safe/domestic-abuse/what-can-i-do-if-this-is-happening-to-me/
UK: https://www.gov.uk/report-domestic-abuse

Rape Crisis
PO Box 69, London, WC1X 9NJ
Tel: 020 7837 1600 (24-hour helpline)
Email: info@rapecrisis.co.uk
Website: www.rapecrisis.org.uk

Refuge
4th Floor, International House, 1 St Katharine's Way, London E1W 1UN
Tel: 0808 2000 247 (24-hour national helpline)
Website: www.refuge.org.uk

Samaritans
Tel: 08457 90 90 90
Email: jo@samaritans.org
Website: www.samaritans.org

Victim Support
Cranmer House, 39 Brixton Road, London, SW9 6DZ
Tel: 020 7735 9166 (enquiries)/Victim Support Line 0845 30 30 900
Email: contact@victimsupport.org.uk
Website: www.victimsupport.org.uk

Women's Aid
PO Box 391, Bristol BS99 7WS
Tel: 0117 944 4411 (office)/0808 2000 247 (helpline)
Email: helpline@womensaid.org.uk
Website: www.womensaid.org.uk
(All websites last accessed January 2022)

16.5 Further reading

Bewley S, Welch J. *ABC of Domestic and Sexual Violence*. BMJ Books, 2014.

Department of Health and Social Care. *Responding to Domestic Abuse: a Resource for Health Professionals Responding to Domestic Abuse. A Handbook for Health Professionals*. London: Department of Health and Social Care, 2017.

Knight M, Bunch K, Tuffnell D, et al. (eds) on behalf of MBRRACE-UK. *Saving Lives, Improving Mothers' Care – Lessons Learned to Inform Maternity Care from the UK and Ireland Confidential Enquiries into Maternal Deaths and Morbidity 2014–16*. Oxford: National Perinatal Epidemiology Unit, University of Oxford, 2018.

CHAPTER 17
Thoracic emergencies

Learning outcomes

After reading this chapter, you will be able to:
- Identify life-threatening injuries in the chest
- Identify potentially life-threatening injuries in the chest
- Be aware of the skills required to manage these life-threatening injuries

17.1 Introduction

This chapter focuses on thoracic emergencies, mainly caused by trauma but occasionally arising spontaneously, as in the case of spontaneous pneumothorax or aortic dissection.

Chest injuries are common in patients with major trauma and they are responsible for around one-quarter of deaths due to trauma. Pregnant trauma patients are more likely than non-pregnant to sustain major thoracic trauma. Many of these deaths can be prevented by the prompt recognition of life-threatening conditions in the primary survey and the early initiation of basic treatments. Few patients will require surgery. Most can be treated by needle decompression or finger thoracostomy followed by tube thoracostomy (chest drain insertion). Prompt and effective resuscitation of the mother, including the avoidance of aortocaval compression, is the most effective way of optimising fetal perfusion.

Types of injury to the chest

Chest injuries are usually classified as penetrating, blunt or both. When there are external signs of thoracic injury, intra-abdominal organs, including the gravid uterus, may also have been damaged, particularly in the later stages of pregnancy. The reverse is also true, in that obvious abdominal trauma may extend into the chest.

17.2 Initial assessment and management of thoracic emergencies

An accurate history of the incident is vital. For example, the driver of a car in collision with a tree would be at risk of a traumatic brain injury, spinal trauma, traumatic aortic rupture, lung and myocardial contusion and abdominal trauma, in addition to many other bony and soft-tissue injuries.

The principles of management are as follows.

Managing Medical and Obstetric Emergencies and Trauma: A Practical Approach, Fourth Edition. Edited by Rosamunde Burns and Kara Dent.

Primary survey and resuscitation

- Life-threatening injuries discovered during the primary survey should be dealt with immediately as they are found
- Catastrophic bleeding – stop this
- Airway maintenance with cervical spine control and displacement of the uterus
- Breathing including delivery of high-flow oxygen through a non-rebreathing reservoir mask
- Circulation with haemorrhage control
- Disability/neurological status
- Exposure and environmental control
- Consider immediate chest x-ray and/or extended focused assessment with sonography for trauma (eFAST; ultrasound for qualified staff members) during the primary survey to assess chest trauma in adults with severe respiratory compromise

Assessment of fetal well-being and viability

- This can be achieved using a Doppler or by ultrasound to locate fetal heart, whichever is available

Secondary survey

- A careful head-to-toe examination should identify any other injuries sustained
- Definitive care is started by the trauma team with early involvement of a multidisciplinary team (including emergency medicine, general surgery, orthopaedic surgery, thoracic surgery, obstetrics, neonates, anaesthetics, critical care and interventional radiology) to maximise successful treatment

17.3 Life-threatening chest injuries

Use the mnemonic for life-threatening injuries in the chest – **ATOM TC**.

A	Airway obstruction
T	Tension pneumothorax
O	Open pneumothorax
M	Massive haemothorax
T	Tracheobronchial injury
C	Cardiac tamponade

Airway obstruction

See Chapter 10.

Tension pneumothorax

Tension pneumothorax should be considered in any trauma patient with severe respiratory distress and also, in some cases, shock. There are usually decreased breath sounds, decreased chest expansion and hyper-resonance on the affected side. The classic signs of tracheal deviation away from the affected side and distended neck veins may be very late or absent.

If there is any doubt, needle decompression or open (finger) thoracostomy to decompress the air, and subsequent chest drain insertion, should be performed without delay. This should be performed before imaging of the chest if the patient is unstable (haemodynamic instability or severe respiratory compromise).

The Advanced Trauma Life Support (ATLS) group recommend either needle decompression or open thoracostomy. In the UK, the National Institute for Health and Care Excellence (NICE) recommend open thoracostomy for trauma patients in hospital because it is more effective, however needle decompression still has a role particularly when the patient is unstable, where needle decompression will probably be faster. Needle decompression is preferably done anterior to the mid-axillary line (third or fourth intercostal space in pregnancy, compared with the fifth intercostal space when not pregnant); the second intercostal space in the mid-clavicular line is an acceptable alternative.

Open pneumothorax (sucking chest wound)

A large open chest wall defect will suck air through it with each inspiration and cause a progressive decline in pulmonary function.

The principle of management is to cover the defect in such a way as to prevent air being sucked in, but allow accumulated air to escape. A sterile dressing large enough to cover the wound and taped securely on *three sides only* will achieve this. Monitor closely for the development of a tension pneumothorax whilst preparing for a tube thoracostomy (chest drain insertion). A tube thoracostomy should then be placed *remote* to the site of chest wall injury.

Massive haemothorax

Massive haemothoraces are usually caused by damage to a systemic or pulmonary vessel. Clinical signs include evidence of hypovolaemia, decreased breath sounds, decreased chest expansion and dullness to percussion on the affected side.

The drainage of a large collection, without wide-bore intravenous access for fluid replacement, can lead to circulatory collapse, so intravenous access must be secured *prior* to chest drainage and restoring blood volume. Most haemothoraces are managed conservatively, but if after the placement of an intercostal drain the initial loss is massive (that is greater than 1500 ml, or continuing losses exceed 200 ml/h), operative intervention may be needed. The major obstetric haemorrhage protocol should be activated.

Tracheobronchial injury

Injuries to the larynx, trachea or bronchi need urgent attention from a senior anaesthetist and thoracic surgeon. Laryngeal and tracheal injuries are rare and present with airway obstruction, subcutaneous emphysema and hoarseness of the voice. In addition, they suggest the presence of other injuries to thoracic or abdominal structures. Bronchial injuries are often fatal. They may present as a pneumothorax with a persisting air leak despite tube thoracostomy (chest drain). Surviving patients usually require surgical repair.

Cardiac tamponade

Cardiac tamponade (compression of the heart by accumulation of fluid in the pericardial sac) may occur following blunt or penetrating trauma to the chest. It may be difficult to detect. It may also be seen in association with spontaneous dissection of the aorta, a well-recognised feature of women with Marfan's syndrome.

Signs include tachycardia, hypotension, distended neck veins and muffled heart sounds. It should be suspected in a hypotensive patient with a penetrating injury to the chest over the cardiac outline (examine the front, back and side of the chest wall). Ultrasound (echocardiography or as part of a FAST scan) can quickly confirm the diagnosis. The definitive management is urgent surgical exploration, but needle pericardiocentesis can be performed, under ultrasound and electrocardiogram (ECG) control, if the patient is deteriorating.

Radiological investigations in chest trauma

A chest radiograph taken during the primary survey should be reviewed. This should be examined for lung expansion, presence of fluid or air in the pleural cavity, mediastinal diameter, any shift of midline structures, bony injury and evidence of contusion. Ultrasound (FAST) may be undertaken by qualified staff. In most cases of multiple trauma, a full body computed tomography (CT) scan will be considered.

17.4 Potentially life-threatening chest injuries

These may not be obvious during the primary survey. They can be categorised into two 'contusions' and four 'disruptions':

- Pulmonary contusion
- Myocardial contusion
- Diaphragmatic disruption
- Oesophageal disruption
- Traumatic aortic disruption
- Chest wall disruption (flail chest)

Pulmonary contusion

Pulmonary contusion is usually as a result of blunt trauma to the chest and presents as hypoxia that may progress to respiratory failure. The key to successful management is to maintain a high index of suspicion. Pregnancy increases oxygen consumption and any problems with oxygen delivery which may be seen with thoracic trauma will make pregnant mothers become hypoxic faster. Any signs of respiratory impairment such as tachypnoea, increased work of breathing including the use of accessory muscles, low oxygen saturations, cyanosis or raised CO_2 on arterial blood gas should prompt early referral to critical care. Patients may require intubation and ventilation for refractory hypoxia. Young pregnant patients should have excellent oxygenation when breathing high-flow oxygen. If they have not, then significant contusion must be suspected.

Myocardial contusion

Myocardial contusion should be considered whenever there is a history of blunt chest injury. Patients may have abnormal electrical activity including extrasystoles through to significant arrhythmias or unexplained hypotension. These patients must have continuous ECG monitoring.

Diaphragmatic disruption

Diaphragmatic disruption is usually associated with blunt abdominal injury and is usually found on the left side. Compression causes a radial tear in the diaphragm, allowing abdominal contents to herniate into the chest. Abdominal structures may have been damaged by the injury itself, by the placement of an intercostal drain or may become ischaemic while in the chest cavity. Oxygenation and ventilation can be severely impaired.

The diagnosis should be suspected with blunt trauma to the chest or abdomen and is confirmed by chest radiograph, e.g. bowel loops on the chest or the presence of a gastric tube above the diaphragm. The diaphragm is usually repaired surgically without delay.

Oesophageal disruption

This is usually the result of a penetrating injury, although it can be caused by blunt trauma to the upper abdomen. Rupture of the oesophagus can also occur after prolonged vomiting (Boerhaave's syndrome). The diagnosis is suggested by:

- History with: pain out of proportion to other injuries; left-sided pneumothorax; particulate matter coming out of the chest drain
- Mediastinal air and surgical emphysema

Surgical repair is the treatment of choice if the diagnosis is made early; mediastinitis can be fatal.

Traumatic aortic disruption

The mechanism of injury here is usually a decelerating injury, such as a road traffic collision or fall from a height. Those that survive to hospital have a tear in the area of the aortic arch as it joins the descending aorta and a contained haematoma. The diagnosis is made using a high index of suspicion from the history and the chest radiograph appearance of a widened mediastinum. This leads to further investigation and will probably be identified during the trauma CT, on angiography or with transoesophageal echocardiography. The treatment is through interventional radiology or direct surgical repair.

Chest wall disruption (flail chest)

When a segment of the chest wall loses continuity with the rest of the thoracic cage from multiple rib fractures, that segment moves paradoxically with respiration and the segment is called a flail segment. Hypoxia is caused by pulmonary contusions due to trauma in the underlying lung, which can be severe. The bony injury can be extremely painful and this impairs oxygenation further. The principles of management include humidified oxygen, careful fluid management and effective analgesia often with local anaesthetic techniques (including intercostal nerve blocks or a thoracic epidural). A period of mechanical ventilation may be required in severe cases.

17.5 Summary

- Chest trauma in pregnancy combines injury to major thoracic structures with the challenge of the gravid uterus which impairs venous return and compromises respiration
- Most injuries can be identified by careful assessment and managed with simple but life-sustaining treatments, including the avoidance of aortocaval compression
- Knowledge of the pathophysiology of these injuries allows the obstetrician to take part in the decision-making process and prioritise maternal and fetal treatment appropriately

17.6 Further reading

ACS (American College of Surgeons) Committee on Trauma. Thoracic trauma. In: ACS Committee on Trauma. *Advanced Trauma Life Support® Student Course Manual*, 10th edn. Chicago: ACS, 2018: pp. 62–81.

Battaloglu E, McDonnell D, Chu J, Lecky F, Porter K. Epidemiology and outcomes of pregnancy and obstetric complications in trauma in the United Kingdom. *Injury* 2016; 47(1): 184–7.

Battaloglu E, Porter K. Management of pregnancy and obstetric complications in prehospital trauma care: faculty of prehospital care consensus guidelines. *Emerg Med J* 2017; 34(5): 318–25.

Havelock T, Teoh R, Laws D, Gleeson F, on behalf of the British Thoracic Society Pleural Disease Guideline Group. Pleural procedures and thoracic ultrasound: British Thoracic Society Pleural Disease Guideline 2010. *Thorax* 2010; 65 (Suppl 2): ii61–76.

NICE (National Institute for Health and Care Excellence). *Major Trauma: Assessment and Initial Management*. NG39. London: NICE, 2016.

Appendix 17.1 Practical procedures

Needle decompression

Equipment

- Antiseptic
- Intravenous cannula (14 gauge)
- 10 ml Luer-Lok™ syringe

Procedure (modified from the principles of ATLS)

1. Administer high-flow oxygen.
2. In a patient with thin subcutaneous tissue, identify the second intercostal space in the mid-clavicular line on the side of the tension pneumothorax.
3. In a patient with thick subcutaneous tissue (more likely in most pregnant patients), use the *third* or *fourth* intercostal space, anterior to the mid-axillary line on the side of the tension pneumothorax. (This would normally be the fifth intercostal space, however in late pregnancy the diaphragm may be raised so the *third* or *fourth* intercostal space should be used.)
4. Swab the chest wall with antiseptic.
5. Insert the cannula into the chest wall horizontally, just over the rib and into the intercostal space, with a 10 ml Luer-Lok syringe, aspirating continuously until air enters the syringe and there is a sudden loss of resistance.
6. Remove the Luer-Lok syringe from the cannula and listen for the escape of air.
7. Remove the needle, leaving the plastic cannula in place.
8. Fix the cannula in place with tape, avoiding kinks in the cannula; proceed to chest drain insertion as soon as possible.

Complications

These can include:

- Failure to reach the pleura (may require longer needle/cannula, or proceed with finger thoracostomy)
- If successful and the cannula kinks or becomes occluded, a tension pneumothorax may redevelop requiring a further decompression
- Lung laceration
- Allergy to antiseptic
- If needle thoracocentesis is attempted, and the patient does not have a tension pneumothorax, the chance of causing a pneumothorax is 10–20%; patients must have a chest radiograph and will require chest drainage if mechanically ventilated

Finger and tube thoracostomy (chest drain insertion)

Equipment (Figure 17A.1)

- Antiseptic
- Sterile drapes
- Local anaesthetic
- 10 ml syringe with orange, blue and green needles
- Sterile gloves
- Scalpel
- Scissors
- Artery forceps
- Two large clamps
- Chest drain tube (without trocar)
- Underwater seal and connector
- Suture
- Dressing

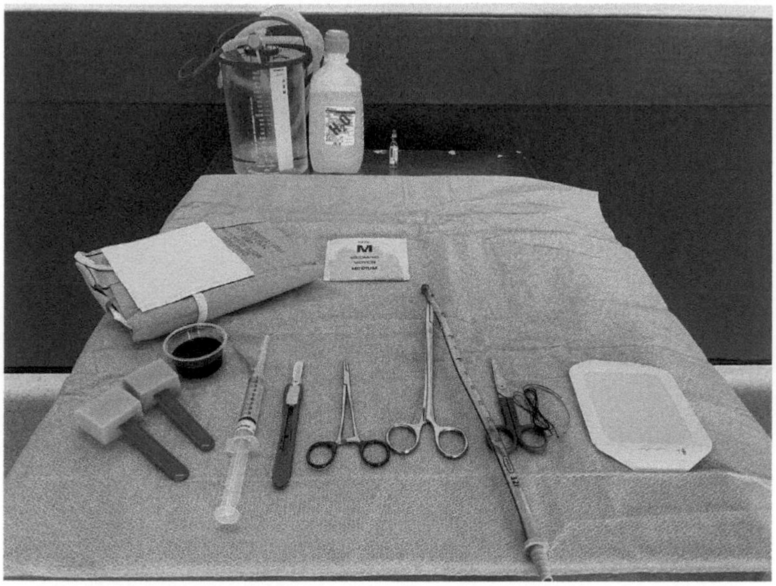

Figure 17A.1 Chest drain kit

Procedure (modified from the principles of ATLS)

1. Position the patient with their ipsilateral arm extended overhead and flexed at the elbow (as long as there is no arm injury).
2. Apply antiseptic to the site of the intended tube thoracostomy and widen this field further with antiseptic, including the nipple.
3. Put on sterile gloves and apply a sterile drape over the site for thoracostomy.
4. Identify relevant landmarks. This is usually the fifth intercostal space anterior to the mid-axillary line, beneath and behind the breast tail, on the side with the pneumothorax. However, in late pregnancy the diaphragm may be raised so the *third* or *fourth* intercostal space should be used. Bedside ultrasound may be helpful.
5. Inject local anaesthetic to the skin, subcutaneous tissue, rib periosteum and parietal pleura.
6. With the scalpel, make a 2–3 cm horizontal skin incision along the inferior line of the intercostal space (to avoid the neurovascular bundle), pushing the breast tail up so that it is out of the way.
7. Bluntly dissect through the subcutaneous tissues just above the rib using blunt forceps.
8. Puncture the parietal pleura with the tip of the forceps; advance them over the rib and spread to widen the opening in the pleura.
9. Air/fluid will be released.
10. Perform a finger sweep to clear any adhesions or clots. This is a finger thoracostomy.
11. Advance the thoracostomy tube with the aid of forceps into the pleural space (i.e. without the trocar).
12. Ensure that the tube is in the pleural space by listening for air movement and by looking for fogging of the tube during expiration.
13. Connect the chest drain tube to an underwater seal below the level of the patient and ensure the water level is swinging.
14. Suture the drain in place.
15. Secure with a sterile dressing and tape.
16. Reassess the patient.
17. Obtain a chest radiograph.
18. Consider administering appropriate antibiotics following chest drain insertion associated with trauma.

Complications

These can include:

- Failure to perform the procedure successfully
- Damage to the intercostal nerve, artery or vein
- Infection
- Lung laceration
- Tube kinking, dislodging or blocking
- Subcutaneous emphysema
- Persistent pneumothorax (due to incorrect tube insertion, leaking around chest drain, leaking underwater seal or bronchopleural fistula)
- Failure of lung to expand (if bronchus is blocked)
- Allergy to antiseptic or local anaesthetic

CHAPTER 18

Abdominal trauma in pregnancy

Learning outcomes

After reading this chapter, you will be able to:

- Assess the patient who has sustained abdominal trauma, and recognise the possibility of injury
- Recognise the need for timely resuscitation and treatment, including surgical intervention
- Describe the changes in anatomy and physiology that occur in pregnancy, and how such changes may alter the response to trauma
- Appreciate the diagnostic procedures available for the investigation of abdominal trauma, and the indications for their use

18.1 Introduction

Abdominal injuries are a significant cause of preventable deaths associated with major trauma in the pregnant and non-pregnant woman alike, and may be due to accidental or non-accidental causes. Prompt and accurate assessment of the presence of intra-abdominal injury, and its likely site, can be challenging; the existence of a gravid uterus makes the task even more complex.

Obstetricians should become involved early in the management of victims of trauma when pregnancy is obvious or suspected. They need to be familiar with the patterns of abdominal injury in the pregnant and non-pregnant patient, and their degree of priority. They need to be aware, also, of the effects of pregnancy on the response to blood loss, affecting both mother and fetus. The mother, especially in later pregnancy, tends to tolerate blood loss well; the fetus tolerates maternal blood loss very badly, and reflects maternal hypovolaemia by demonstrating fetal distress on monitoring.

A specific challenge posed by pregnancy in assessment of the abdomen is that organ displacement occurs as the uterus enlarges. The bowel is pushed upwards, and this anatomical distortion can cause diagnostic uncertainties.

The 2019 MBRRACE-UK report records that between 2015 and 2017 of the 17 women who died from accidents, 11 women died from road traffic collisions. The report emphasised the need for trauma teams to remember to relieve aortocaval compression in the multiply injured pregnant patient and to perform timely perimortem caesarean section (PMCS) to aid maternal resuscitation.

Managing Medical and Obstetric Emergencies and Trauma: A Practical Approach, Fourth Edition. Edited by Rosamunde Burns and Kara Dent.

Injuries may be blunt or penetrating. The vast majority in the UK are of blunt origin, mainly associated with road traffic collisions. Deceleration injuries predispose to blunt trauma, with the resulting risk of damage to viscera, including the uterus and its contents. It is important to identify those patients who require immediate or emergency intervention, either obstetric or surgical. A high index of suspicion is required, and early consultation with other specialties is crucial. Up to 50% of young patients with significant intra-abdominal haemorrhage will have minimal or no signs on initial assessment. Unrecognised or underestimated abdominal injury is still a cause of preventable death.

18.2 Trauma to the uterus

In the first trimester, the uterus is protected from injury by its relatively thick wall, as well as by the bony pelvis. As pregnancy progresses, it is the uterus that provides some protection to the abdominal contents, thereby becoming increasingly vulnerable.

The obstetrician should remind the trauma team leader that uterine rupture, amniotic fluid embolus and placental abruption are possible differential diagnoses in the multiply injured pregnant woman.

Abruption

As pregnancy progresses, the uterine wall becomes thinner. The uterus is elastic but the placenta is not, leading to the risk of trauma-induced abruption as the placenta shears off the uterine wall. Abruption occurs in up to 50% of major trauma in pregnancy and in 5% of minor injuries. What may seem fairly trivial trauma to the uterus may cause significant placental abruption, leading to fetal death, and also possibly leading to disseminated intravascular coagulation in the mother.

Uterine rupture

The possibility of uterine rupture should always be considered. This may be caused in a road traffic collision by blunt trauma from striking the dashboard or steering wheel, or by pressure from an injudiciously placed car seat or seat belt. The recommendation for the use of seat belts in pregnancy is 'Above and below the bump – not over it'. Three-point seat belts should be worn throughout pregnancy, with the lap strap placed as low as possible beneath the 'bump', lying across the thighs, with the diagonal shoulder strap above the bump, lying between the breasts (Figure 18.1). The seat belt should be adjusted to fit as snugly as comfortably possible and, if necessary, the seat should be adjusted to enable the seat belt to be worn properly. Lap belts alone are unsuitable in pregnancy.

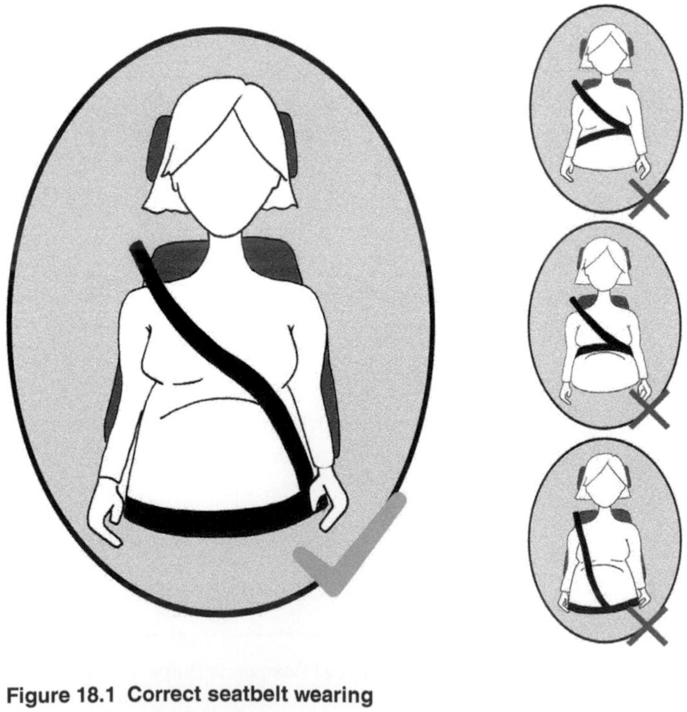

Figure 18.1 Correct seatbelt wearing

Traumatic uterine rupture is much less likely than traumatic abruption, occurring in <1% of major injuries, but is associated with probable fetal loss and a 10% maternal mortality rate. Signs of uterine rupture include abdominal tenderness with guarding and rigidity, associated with signs of hypovolaemia. The fetal lie may be transverse or oblique, with easily palpable fetal parts and inaudible fetal heart sounds. Management of suspected uterine rupture is urgent operative exploration, with a view to delivery of the fetus and repair or removal of the uterus, according to the findings.

Penetrating injury

Penetrating injury, causing uterine rupture and fetal trauma, may be sustained by knife wounds, gunshot wounds or high-velocity fragments due to a blast. Other abdominal viscera, including bladder, bowel, liver and spleen, are likely to be involved in such circumstances.

Amniotic fluid embolus

Amniotic fluid embolus may occur as a result of uterine trauma. This is particularly important to recognise in view of its high associated mortality from respiratory compromise as well as from disseminated intravascular coagulation (see Chapter 12).

Trauma-related haemorrhage

The pregnant woman has an increased tolerance to the effects of blood loss, due to the increase in plasma volume during pregnancy (50% increase by the third trimester).

The opposite is true for the fetus. Significant abdominal trauma in pregnancy is associated with a high likelihood of fetal death, either early or delayed. As the fetoplacental unit is an end organ, it is subject to reduced blood flow as part of the maternal response to hypovolaemia, via the release of catecholamines. Thus, whilst maternal tolerance to blood loss is increased, the fetus is highly sensitive to comparatively small reductions in maternal circulating blood volume.

As a consequence, fetal distress may be evident long before the mother shows any of the classic signs of significant blood loss.

> The trauma team must be focused on the early identification of bleeding and rapid effective haemostasis by targeting life-saving interventions. Effective use of diagnostic modalities will lead to faster and more accurate diagnosis of the source of bleeding.

18.3 Primary survey and resuscitation

The **ATMIST** handover tool in trauma is in widespread use in the UK between the pre-hospital and hospital teams, and from the contained information the risk of abdominal injury can be assessed.

A	Age and gestational age
T	Time of incident
M	Mechanism of injury
I	Injuries seen or suspected
S	Signs, and if improving or deteriorating
T	Treatment pre-hospital

The mechanism of restraint, if any, should be noted as well as the details of the pregnancy. Women may carry their own obstetric notes.

Using the mnemonic **AMPLE** further targeting of the history can be obtained in the emergency situation.

A	Allergies
M	Medication
P	Previous medical history
L	Last meal (and date of last period)
E	Events and environments related to the injury

Airway with cervical spine control

Life-threatening compromise to airway and breathing must be dealt with immediately. Cervical spine control is crucial where there is a possibility of spinal injury.

Breathing, manual uterine displacement

High-flow facial oxygen should be administered promptly. It is essential to avoid aortocaval compression, which occurs due to pressure from the gravid uterus in the supine position, with resulting functional hypovolaemia. The mMOET course emphasises approaching the woman with hands extended, ready to stabilise the cervical spine, while at the same time saying 'Hello, Ms MUD'. This acronym acts as an aide memoire for manual uterine displacement, which is preferable to lateral tilt when spinal injury is suspected.

Circulation

Abdominal injuries may cause a C problem. Blood should be taken for a full blood count, group and crossmatch, venous blood gas and urea and electrolytes. Thromboelastometry and Kleihauer testing should be undertaken. Volume resuscitation should be commenced as described in Chapter 15. A Kleihauer test should be carried out, even if the woman is Rhesus positive, to give an indication of the extent of any fetomaternal transfusion as a consequence of any abruption. If a woman is known to be Rhesus negative, anti-D should be administered within 72 hours, unless the injury is remote from the uterus (e.g. isolated distal extremity injury).

It may be clear from a brief examination during the primary survey – including focused assessment with sonography for trauma (FAST) scan and obstetric ultrasound for fetal heart rate – that continuing haemorrhage is from an abdominal source. Further investigation may therefore be judged inappropriate because of the need to 'turn off the tap'. Resuscitation should continue on the way to theatre for laparotomy.

More commonly, there may be suspicion rather than certainty of intra-abdominal bleeding. Further investigation for a multiply injured pregnant woman who is responding to volume resuscitation and is haemodynamically stable would be trauma computed tomography (CT) performed within 30 minutes of patient arrival in the emergency department.

A fuller examination of the abdomen and pelvis, including vaginal and rectal examinations, should be performed as soon as is practicable, as part of the secondary survey. For further discussion of pelvic fracture, see Chapter 21.

The presence of uterine contractions should be noted, as should the presence of amniotic fluid in the vagina, cervical effacement and dilatation, and the relationship of the fetal presenting part to the ischial spines. A urinary catheter should be put in place.

Bleeding into the uterine muscle or into the uterine cavity is an irritant, and contractions may be the first sign of a developing abruption. Distension, tenderness, guarding and rigidity suggest injury, although a seemingly normal examination does not exclude a potentially serious injury.

Diagnosis

FAST scans

This is a brief ultrasound examination of the left and right upper quadrant, the pelvis and the pericardium by an experienced operator, and is typically available in the resuscitation room as part of the primary survey. The FAST scan will demonstrate if there is intra-abdominal free fluid suggesting intra-abdominal bleeding and enable visualisation of a fetal heart pulsation but is an unreliable guide to the *nature* of the abdominal injury.

A negative examination should be viewed with caution after major trauma, and an emergency abdominal CT should be sought by the trauma team in the stable patient to more clearly understand the nature of the injuries. FAST scans may be more difficult to interpret in the presence of obesity, subcutaneous air and abdominal scarring.

Computed tomography

Computed tomography scanning provides a highly sensitive and specific examination in suspected abdominal trauma, and is superior to FAST scanning in detecting retroperitoneal injuries. Radiation risks have been considerably reduced in recent years. CT scans should be undertaken only in haemodynamically stable patients, where there is, as yet, no clear indication for emergency laparotomy.

Indications for caesarean section in multiple trauma

See the trauma call timeline (Algorithm 15.1) in Chapter 15.

The indication for emptying the uterus as part of the primary survey at C is maternal cardiac arrest. The indications for emptying the uterus as part of 'damage control resuscitation' in the primary survey are uterine rupture, placental abruption, penetrating injury to the uterus or to enable surgical access to control haemorrhage. In the patient with a pregnancy of a viable gestation, abdominal delivery followed by a trauma laparotomy is likely to be the safer option for mother and baby (using a midline skin incision).

It must be emphasised that the best way of achieving a good fetal outcome is by thorough evaluation and resuscitation of the mother, thereby ensuring good placental perfusion and oxygenation.

Solid and hollow visceral injury

Injuries to the liver and spleen are less common in late pregnancy, due to the protection afforded by the gravid uterus, but, nevertheless, they do still occur and will be identified at trauma CT. When such injuries are present, there should be a low threshold for laparotomy and caesarean section.

Experienced staff may occasionally elect to treat selected patients conservatively if the cardiovascular system is stable. This is particularly the case where the fetus is not of a viable gestation.

Injuries to the genitourinary tract, gastrointestinal tract, the pancreas and the diaphragm may be difficult to detect. Specialised radiological investigations may be required, including urethrography, cystography, intravenous pyelography and gastrointestinal contrast studies.

18.4 Secondary survey

A resuscitative laparotomy may be required as part of the primary survey, but if not then a complete examination of the abdomen must be carried out as part of the secondary survey, regardless of whether serious injury is suspected.

Pregnant patients with even apparently *minor* abdominal injuries should be *carefully observed* as placental abruption and fetal loss may occur. It is therefore necessary that a robust plan for ongoing maternal and fetal monitoring in an appropriate location should be made. Clear routes of *communication* and *escalation* should be agreed by a senior multidisciplinary team to facilitate timely delivery if indicated.

Pelvic trauma

See Chapter 21.

18.5 Summary

- Abdominal trauma in pregnancy is most commonly due to road traffic collisions in the UK, but may also be due to domestic violence
- The structured approach should be followed, bearing in mind that resuscitative laparotomy may be required as part of the primary survey
- It must always be remembered that pregnant women tend to compensate well for blood loss. A drop in blood pressure is a late and ominous sign
- Few clinicians in the UK are experienced in dealing with major trauma in pregnancy
- The obstetrician will be involved early, and is an essential core member of the trauma team to ensure optimum outcomes for mother and fetus

18.6 Further reading

ACS (American College of Surgeons) Committee on Trauma. *Advanced Trauma Life Support® Student Course Manual*, 10th edn. Chicago: ACS, 2018.

Hayden B, Plaat F, Cox C. Managing trauma in the pregnant woman. *Br J Hosp Med* 2013; 74(6): 327–30.

Knight M, Bunch K, Tuffnell D et al (eds) *on behalf of MBRRACE-UK. Saving Lives, Improving Mothers' Care – Lessons Learned to Inform Maternity Care from the UK and Ireland Confidential Enquiries into Maternal Deaths and Morbidity 2015–17*. Oxford: National Perinatal Epidemiology Unit, University of Oxford, 2019.

Tran A, Yates J, Lau A, Lampron J, Matar M. Permissive hypotension versus conventional resuscitation strategies in adult trauma patients with hemorrhagic shock: a systematic review and meta-analysis of randomized controlled trials. *J Trauma Acute Care Surg* 2018; 84(5): 802–8.

CHAPTER 19
The unconscious patient

Learning outcomes

After reading this chapter, you will be able to:
- Describe the principles of treatment of the unconscious patient
- Describe the concept of secondary brain injury and how to prevent it
- Identify types of intracranial lesion amenable to urgent surgical intervention (extradural and subdural haematoma)

19.1 Introduction

The immediate management of the unconscious pregnant patient from any cause (Box 19.1) should be a basic skill of every obstetrician and midwife. The obstetric team should be aware of the potential causes of a decreased level of consciousness and treat the underlying cause, with appropriate specialist assistance where necessary.

Box 19.1 Causes of a decreased level of consciousness in the pregnant patient

A/B Failure of airway or breathing: hypoxia/hypercarbia
C Failure of circulation: shock or cardiac arrest
D Failure of central nervous system:
- Eclampsia or epilepsy
- Intracranial haemorrhage, trauma, thrombosis, tumour or infection
- Drugs including opiates and local anaesthetic, alcohol or poisoning
- Hypoglycaemia

19.2 Principles of treatment of the unconscious patient

Although these principles were developed in the context of trauma cases and traumatic brain injury, the same principles apply to any medical situation that threatens the supply of oxygen to the injured or uninjured brain.

Managing Medical and Obstetric Emergencies and Trauma: A Practical Approach, Fourth Edition. Edited by Rosamunde Burns and Kara Dent.

Primary and secondary brain injury

Primary brain injury is the neurological damage produced by the initial event, such as a brain haemorrhage. Secondary (further) brain injury is the neurological damage caused by lack of oxygen delivery to the brain. This may be caused by:

- **A/B** – failure of ventilation, caused by airway obstruction or inadequate breathing, resulting in poor oxygenation. In addition, both airway obstruction and inadequate breathing may lead to a rise in arterial carbon dioxide levels. This has direct consequences on intracranial pressure (ICP)
- **C** – failure of circulation due to shock including hypotension
- **D** – intracerebral damage may cause an excessive rise in ICP, leading to reduced cerebral perfusion pressure (CPP)

Cerebral perfusion

Cerebral perfusion refers to the supply of oxygenated blood to the brain. The blood supply to the brain is more complex than other organs, because the brain is enclosed inside a rigid box. The main components inside the box are:

- Brain substance or space-occupying lesions
- Cerebrospinal fluid
- Cerebral blood vessels and the blood contained within these vessels
- Extracellular fluid

The volume of this box is fixed, so one component can only increase in volume at the expense of another, or at the expense of an increase in ICP.

CPP is the mean arterial pressure (MAP) of blood in the brain minus the resistance to flow from the mean ICP:

CPP = MAP – ICP

- An adequate blood pressure (MAP) must be maintained to maintain CPP
- A reduction in MAP or rise in ICP will affect CPP and potentially contribute to further neuronal damage
- Any rise in volume of intracranial contents may need to be controlled if the normal mechanism of cerebral autoregulation of ICP has failed
- Brain tissue can increase in volume as a result of tumour growth or there may be increased volume caused by blood clot; both conditions may require surgery
- Cerebrospinal fluid pressure can increase if there is an obstruction to free drainage of the fluid, e.g. by blood clots leading to hydrocephalus, and can be drained by temporary or permanent surgical shunts
- Cerebral blood volume can increase if the arterial carbon dioxide levels are allowed to rise resulting in cerebral vasodilatation; carbon dioxide levels can be reduced by maintaining a clear airway and controlling ventilation to restore a low normal level of $PaCO_2$ (hyperventilation is no longer recommended)
- Extracellular fluid levels can increase as a result of response to injury, such as around tumours or following cell damage caused by a major head injury; this is difficult to treat but careful fluid management avoiding excess intravenous fluids will be part of the care
- Raised ICP may also be due to obstruction of venous drainage from the head from pressure on the neck veins, head-down position or excess intrathoracic pressure

Normal MAP = 70–90 mmHg

Normal ICP = 10 mmHg

If CPP is less than 50 mmHg, cerebral hypoxia may follow

The following discussion of priorities in management to prevent secondary brain injury uses the trauma patient as an example and covers:

1. Primary survey and resuscitation.
2. Assessment of fetal well-being and viability.
3. Secondary survey.

It follows that preventing a rise in ICP or a fall in MAP, and so cerebral perfusion, is vital for the overall management and prevention of brain injury.

19.3 Primary survey and resuscitation

Airway

Clear the airway. A patient with a reduced level of consciousness is more likely to have a compromised airway as the tongue falls back into the posterior pharynx. Further, she is at risk of aspiration as she has obtunded laryngeal reflexes

Breathing

Adequate ventilation ensures that the brain receives blood containing enough oxygen, thereby preventing further brain injury. Adequate ventilation prevents the accumulation of carbon dioxide. Ventilation may be impaired by a reduced level of consciousness. Raised intrathoracic pressure (as happens in tension pneumothorax) will compromise venous drainage from the head and raise ICP.

Circulation

An adequate MAP is required to maintain CPP. Use fluids and vasopressors appropriately. In a trauma situation, hypotension resulting from other injuries must be swiftly recognised and managed to prevent secondary brain injury. It is equally important to remember that excessive fluids are rarely needed in an isolated head injury and may contribute to worsening cerebral oedema associated with the injury.

In trauma, never assume that an isolated head injury is the cause of hypotension. Scalp lacerations may bleed profusely and possibly sufficiently to cause shock but this is uncommon. Always presume that hypotension is due to injury outside the brain, not brain injury, and look for a source of blood loss elsewhere or other cause of hypotension such as tension pneumothorax, cardiac tamponade or spinal lesion.

Cushing's response (progressive hypertension, bradycardia and slowing of respiratory rate) is an acute response to rapidly rising ICP and is a premorbid sign. This needs urgent attention, which may include establishing controlled ventilation, use of mannitol and/or urgent surgery with the aim of reducing the ICP.

Disability

A decrease in level of consciousness is a marker of brain injury. Generally, the more deeply unconscious a patient becomes and the longer this persists, the more serious is the injury.

ACVPU is a method of rapid assessment of conscious level in the primary survey. Is the patient:

- **A**lert?
- Suffering from new-onset **C**onfusion, disorientation and/or agitation?
- Responsive to **V**oice?
- Only responding to **P**ain?
- **U**nresponsive?

In 2017 the Royal College of Physicians launched the second version of the national track and trigger observation chart for *non-pregnant* adults: NEWS2. This added **C** to the existing **AVPU** to enable the important signs of new-onset confusion, disorientation and/or agitation to be noted and not missed. These signs score 3 on the NEWS2 system.

Pupillary responses may help to identify the degree of intracranial compromise and the possibility of a unilateral space-occupying lesion, typically an expanding extradural haematoma.

Additional measures include:

- Avoid the head-down position, with the head held up 30° if possible
- Avoid ties around the neck, e.g. for an endotracheal tube
- Consider if a neck collar is required in the presence of block immobilisation and check that it is not compressing the neck veins
- Rapid access to surgery may be required to evacuate a blood clot if present to help manage and reduce ICP

19.4 Assessment of fetal well-being and viability

When the mother is adequately resuscitated, the further well-being of the fetus must be considered. Timing of delivery should be considered in the patient about to undergo neurosurgical treatment, or a prolonged period of intensive care, or who is unlikely to recover consciousness. Delivery of the term fetus may be appropriate if a prolonged period of intensive care is anticipated. Physiological complications that develop in the long-term intensive care patient (coagulopathy, sepsis, etc.) may complicate a continuing pregnancy.

19.5 Secondary survey

The head and neurological examination assesses:

- Pupillary function
- Lateralising signs, e.g. limb weakness
- Level of consciousness; ACVPU is quick to perform. The Glasgow Coma Scale (GCS) is a more formal assessment
- Evidence of a base of skull fracture such as 'panda eyes' (periorbital bruising), Battle's sign (bruising on the mastoid) or otorrhoea/rhinorrhoea
- Evidence of a depressed fracture found on palpation or computed tomography (CT) scan

The mini-neurological examination (ACVPU, pupils, and assessing limbs for power, tone reflexes and sensation) serves to determine the severity of the brain injury and the likelihood of a surgically treatable lesion. When applied repeatedly, it can be used to determine objectively any neurological deterioration. It is supplemented by CT scanning.

Pupillary function

Evaluate the pupils for their equality and response to bright light. A difference in diameter of the pupils of more than 1 mm is abnormal but a local injury to the eye may be responsible for this. Normal reaction to a bright light is brisk constriction of the pupil; a more sluggish response may indicate brain injury. Pressure on the third cranial nerve (oculomotor) will result in a dilated pupil on the same side ('ipsilateral') as the injury.

Lateralising signs, such as limb weakness

Observe spontaneous or to command limb movements, limb tone and reflexes for equality. If movement is negligible then assess the response to supraorbital nerve pressure. Any delay in onset of movement or lateralisation of movement following a painful stimulus is significant. Obvious limb weakness localised to one side suggests an intracranial injury causing brain compression on the opposite side. Damage to the motor or sensory cortex (or tracts leading from them) will result in a motor or sensory deficit on the opposite side to the injury.

Level of consciousness

The GCS provides a quantitative assessment of the level of consciousness. It is the sum of scores awarded (Table 19.1) for three types of response.

Eye opening (E)

The scoring of eye opening is not possible if the eyes are so swollen as to be closed shut. This fact should be documented.

Table 19.1 GCS scoring

Response	Score
Eye opening response	
Spontaneous (open with normal blinking)	4
Eye opening to speech	3
Eye opening only to painful stimulus	2
No eye opening despite painful stimulus	1
Verbal response	
Orientated, spontaneous speech	5
Confused conversation but answers questions	4
Inappropriate words, i.e. recognisable words without sense	3
Incomprehensible sounds	2
No verbal response	1
Motor response	
Obeys commands	6
Localises purposive response to painful stimulus	5
Withdraws from painful stimulus	4
Abnormal flexion to painful stimulus (decorticate response)	3
Abnormal extension to painful stimulus (decerebrate response)	2
No response to painful stimulus	1

Verbal response (V)

The scoring of verbal response is not possible if the patient cannot speak because of endotracheal intubation. This fact should be documented.

Motor response (M)

The best response obtained at the time of assessment for either of the upper extremities is recorded even though worse responses may be present in other extremities.

Reassessment

Serial reassessment of the GCS score and limb movement can be used to detect any deterioration. A decrease is a cause for concern and requires immediate treatment. The severity of head injuries is classified as:

Score 8 or less = severe

Score 9 to 12 = moderate

Score 13 to 15 = minor

Changes in vital signs

Changes in the GCS score may be accompanied by changes in physiological vital signs indicating deterioration. Rising ICP due to brain swelling or expanding haematomas inside the head can cause pressure on the respiratory and cardiovascular centres in the brain stem. This produces respiratory or cardiovascular abnormalities such as changes in heart rate (slows down) and blood pressure (rises), change in breathing pattern and rate (slows down) – the Cushing response or triad.

19.6 Types of head injury

The severity of head injury is classified based on the GCS score (Table 19.1).

There are two types of brain injury: primary injury at the time of trauma, which may be diffuse or focal and about which nothing preventive can be done, and **secondary brain injury, through lack of oxygen delivery and tissue perfusion, which can be mitigated by applying resuscitation measures**.

Diffuse primary brain injury

Blunt injury to the brain may cause diffuse brain injury, particularly when rapid head motion (acceleration or deceleration) leads to widespread damage within the brain substance. Such injuries form a spectrum, extending from mild concussion to severe injury known as diffuse axonal injury.

Concussion is a brain injury often accompanied by a brief loss of consciousness, and in its mildest form may cause only temporary confusion or amnesia. With mild forms of concussion, most patients will be only slightly confused and may be able to describe how the injury occurred. They are likely to complain of headache, dizziness or nausea. The mini-neurological examination will not show lateralising signs.

With more severe injury there may be a longer period of unconsciousness, longer amnesia (for time both before and after the injury) and there may be focal signs. The type (pre or post) and duration of amnesia needs to be recorded.

Diffuse axonal injury is present in nearly all of those who sustain loss of consciousness in a motor vehicle collision and is associated with coma following traumatic brain injury. The treatment of such injury involves controlled ventilation in an intensive care unit and prolonged neurorehabilitation.

Focal primary brain injury

Contusions are caused by blunt injury producing acceleration and deceleration forces on the brain tissue, resulting in tearing of the small blood vessels inside the brain. Contusions can occur immediately beneath the area of impact, when they are known as coup injuries, or at a point distant and opposite from the area of impact in the direction of the applied force, when they are known as contre-coup injuries. If the contusion occurs near the sensory or motor areas of the brain, these patients will potentially present with a neurological deficit. Precise diagnosis requires appropriate imaging (CT scanning).

Haematoma within the cranial vault may arise either from torn meningeal vessels or from vessels within the brain substance. They are defined anatomically; such a classification is useful as it has implications in terms of remedial surgery, urgency and prognosis.

Intracranial and extracerebral bleeding

Extradural haemorrhage

Extradural haemorrhage is caused by a tear in a dural artery, most commonly the middle meningeal artery. This can be torn by a linear fracture crossing the temporal or parietal bone and injuring the artery lying in a groove on the deep aspect of the bone.

Isolated extradural haemorrhage is unusual, accounting for only 0.5% of all head injuries and less than 1.0% of injuries causing coma. The importance of early recognition of this injury lies in the fact that, when treated appropriately and within the first hours, the prognosis is good. If unrecognised, the rapidly expanding haematoma causes the ICP to rise, reducing cerebral perfusion and leading to cerebral hypoxia, coma and death.

The pathognomic symptoms and signs of extradural haemorrhage are:

- Loss of consciousness followed by a lucid interval (which may not be a complete return to full consciousness)
- Dilated pupil on the side of injury
- Weakness of the arm and leg on the contralateral side to the injury

Subdural haemorrhage

Acute subdural haematomas due to trauma are the most lethal of all head injuries and have a high mortality rate if not treated by surgical decompression. In addition to the compression caused by the subdural blood clot, there is often major injury to the underlying brain tissue. The haematoma can arise from tears in the bridging veins between the cortex and the dura or from laceration of the brain substance and the cortical arteries.

The typical symptoms and signs of subdural haemorrhage are:

- Varying levels of consciousness, depending on the underlying brain damage and rate of haematoma formation
- Dilated pupil on the side of the injury
- Weakness of the arm and leg on the contralateral side to the injury

Initial treatment:

- Aims to prevent secondary brain injury
- Involves urgent evacuation of the haematoma where surgically amenable

Subarachnoid haemorrhage

Where haemorrhaging has occurred into the subarachnoid space, the irritant effect of the bloody cerebrospinal fluid causes headache, photophobia and neck stiffness. On its own, this is not critical, but prognosis is poor if it is associated with a more severe head injury.

Intracerebral penetration

Through-and-through injuries, side-to-side injuries and injuries in the brain stem all have a poor outcome.

All foreign bodies found protruding from the skull should be left in place. They should only be removed at a neurosurgical unit. Care must be taken during transfer to ensure that there is no further penetration. Open brain injury in a conscious patient carries a good prognosis if surgery is not delayed.

Scalp haemorrhage should be stopped, entrance and exit wounds covered with sterile dressings, and the patient transferred to a neurosurgical unit.

Other injuries

Scalp wounds

The scalp is arranged in layers. It is highly vascular and a laceration will often result in profuse haemorrhage. The bleeding point should be located and the haemorrhage arrested. This may include the use of haemostatic surgical clips or ligatures, particularly where the laceration is deep. Direct pressure may not be sufficient. The wound should be inspected carefully for signs of skull fracture and irrigated to remove debris and dirt.

Gentle palpation of the scalp wound, wearing a sterile glove, may enable the clinician to diagnose the presence of a skull fracture. If an open or depressed fracture is detected, close the wound with sutures, apply a dressing, consider antibiotics and transfer the patient to a neurosurgical unit. Do not remove any bone fragments.

Skull fractures

Although skull fractures are quite common, many major brain injuries will occur without the skull being fractured, and many skull fractures are not associated with severe brain injury. The current primary investigation of choice for the detection of acute, clinically important brain injuries is CT imaging of the head. Skull radiography is rarely undertaken.

Linear skull fractures

These are particularly important when the fracture crosses the line of intracranial vessels, indicating an increased risk of intracranial haemorrhage.

Depressed skull fractures

All depressed skull fractures should be referred for neurosurgical assessment. They may be associated with underlying brain injury and may require operative elevation to reduce the risk of infection in more serious cases.

Open skull fractures

By definition, there is direct communication between the outside of the head and the brain tissue, because the dura covering the surface of the brain is torn. This can be diagnosed if brain tissue is visible on examination of the scalp wound or if cerebrospinal fluid is seen to be leaking from the wound. These fractures all require operative intervention and the risk of infection is high. Discuss the use of prophylactic antibiotics with the neurosurgical team.

Basal skull fractures

The base of the skull does not run horizontally backwards but diagonally. Basal skull fractures will produce signs along this diagonal line. They can be diagnosed clinically in the presence of cerebrospinal fluid leaking from the ear (otorrhoea) or the nose (rhinorrhoea). When cerebrospinal fluid is mixed with blood it may be difficult to detect. Bruising in the mastoid region (Battle's sign) also indicates basal skull fracture, but the bruising can take 36 hours to develop. Blood seen behind the tympanic membrane (haemotympanum) may also indicate a basal skull fracture. Fractures through the cribriform plate are frequently associated with bilateral periorbital haematomas. Subconjunctival haematoma may occur from orbital fractures and there is no posterior limit to the haematoma. All these signs may take several hours to develop and may not be present in a patient seen immediately after injury. Basal skull fractures are seen on a CT scan of the head. Discuss with the neurosurgical team.

19.7 Summary

- Remember the ABCDE routine
- Prevent secondary injury by preventing hypoxia, hypercarbia and hypovolaemia
- Establish a working diagnosis
- Serially repeat the mini-neurological examination
- Consider the best management of the fetus

19.8 Further reading

NICE (National Institute for Health and Social Care Excellence). *Head Injury: Assessment and Early Management*. CG176. London: NICE, 2014 (updated September 2019).

RCP (Royal College of Physicians). *National Early Warning Score (NEWS) 2: Standardising the Assessment of Acute-Illness Severity in the NHS. Updated Report of a Working Party*. London: RCP, 2017.

CHAPTER 20
Spine and spinal cord injuries

Learning outcomes

After reading this chapter, you will be able to:
- Recognise circumstances in which spinal trauma is likely to occur
- Understand the importance of motion restriction and techniques for spinal immobilisation

20.1 Introduction

In the context of this chapter, spinal injuries refer to injuries to the bony spinal column, the spinal cord or both. There can be an injury to the bony spine without injury to the spinal cord, but there is significant risk of cord injury in these circumstances.

Failure to immobilise a patient with a spinal injury can cause or exacerbate neurological damage. Failure to immobilise a patient with an injury to the bony spine (without cord injury at that stage) can cause avoidable injury to the spinal cord. Evaluation of the spine and exclusion of spinal injuries can be safely deferred so long as the patient's spine is protected. Spinal injuries occur most commonly in road traffic collisions (50%), falls from a height more than 3 m (43%) and sport (7%).

A spinal injury should always be suspected in the following circumstances:

- In vehicle collisions, even at low speed
- When pedestrians have been hit by a vehicle
- In falls from a height (however it is possible to injure the spine in a fall from a standing position, e.g. a fall due to a convulsion)
- In sports field injuries, e.g. rugby
- In a person with multiple injuries *including from acts of violence*
- In a person with an injury above the clavicle (including the unconscious patient – 15% of unconscious patients have some form of neck injury)
- In the conscious patient complaining of neck pain and sensory and/or motor symptoms
- In drowning victims

Persons who are awake, sober, neurologically normal and have no neck pain are extremely unlikely to have a cervical spine fracture. However, a specialist opinion from the emergency department physician, neurosurgeon or orthopaedic surgeon should always be sought if an injury is suspected or detected.

The cervical spine is more vulnerable to injury than the thoracic or lumbar spine.

Approximately 10% of patients with a cervical spine fracture have a second associated non-contiguous fracture of the vertebral column. Hence, if a cervical spine fracture is diagnosed, other spinal fractures should be suspected.

Managing Medical and Obstetric Emergencies and Trauma: A Practical Approach, Fourth Edition. Edited by Rosamunde Burns and Kara Dent.

20.2 Immobilisation and motion restriction techniques

If injury to the spine is suspected, the whole spine should be immobilised until examination and radiological investigations have excluded spinal injury.

In recent years the concept of spinal immobilisation has been challenged because of the lack of evidence of benefit and reports of adverse events caused by certain techniques. Since true immobilisation is impossible, the term motion restriction is preferred. Established international guidelines aim to determine which patients benefit from motion restriction techniques (Figure 20.1), for example, the Canadian C-spine rule.

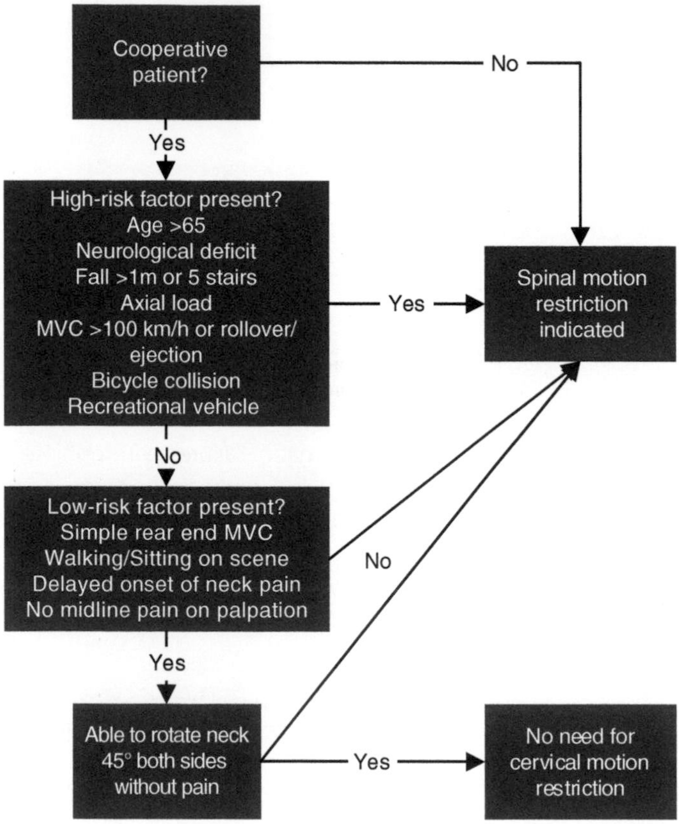

Figure 20.1 High- and low-risk factor decision process for cervical spine motion restriction from the Canadian C-spine rule
MVC, motor vehicle collision

Motion restriction should be carried out by maintaining the spine in the neutral position.

Cervical spine

The strict use of rigid cervical collars is not recommended. Care in the management of the cervical spine is achieved by:

- Manual inline immobilisation of the head
- Application of blocks on a backboard ((which may be a headboard or vacuum mattress) and straps), possibly with a collar, in a comfortable position using other soft devices if needed (Figure 20.2)

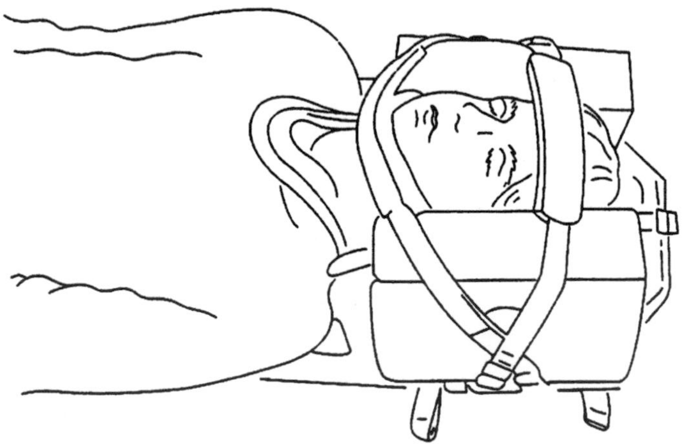

Figure 20.2 Immobilisation of the cervical spine using blocks, tape and headboard (collar shown as may still be used in some circumstances)

Thoracic and lumbar spine

Movement of the thoracic and lumbar spine should be restricted by a vacuum mattress for trauma which may be placed on a scoop stretcher for transportation. Previously, the use of a long spine board led to inadequate movement restriction and pressure complications from the tissue board interface, with the possibility of worsening any injury and the risk of pressure sores. Early assessment by the trauma team is undertaken to allow removal from the device.

To avoid supine hypotension in the heavily pregnant trauma patient, aortocaval compression must be relieved. Either deploy a team member to perform manual uterine displacement or, alternatively, the whole patient can be tilted to the left on a scoop stretcher, on a long board or vacuum mattress by using a wedge under the stretcher.

20.3 Evaluation of a patient with a suspected spinal injury

Spinal injuries may cause problems that are identified in the primary survey, affecting airway, breathing or circulation, or the injury may itself be identified during the secondary survey.

Spinal assessment

A log-roll must be performed to inspect the back of the patient when deemed appropriate by the trauma team leader. This is a coordinated, skilled manoeuvre by trained personnel because it has the potential to cause harm. At least five persons are required to perform this: one to maintain manual inline stabilisation of the patient's head and neck, one for the torso, with one for the hips and one the legs. There needs to be a fifth person to undertake any inspection or procedure. The leader of the movement should be the person maintaining head and cervical spine movement restriction. The fifth person looks for bruising, deformity and localised swelling of the vertebral column. They should palpate for localised tenderness or gaps between the spinous processes. At this point it may be appropriate to carry out a per rectum examination if clinically indicated.

Neurological assessment

Of the many tracts in the spinal cord, the three that can be assessed clinically are:

- Corticospinal tract: controls muscle power on the same side of the body and is tested by voluntary movement and involuntary response to painful stimuli
- Spinothalamic tract: transmits pain and temperature sensation from the opposite side of the body and is tested generally by pinprick
- Posterior columns: carry position sense from the same side

Each can be injured on one or both sides.

If there is no demonstrable sensory or motor function below a certain level bilaterally, this is referred to as a complete spinal injury. If there is remaining motor or sensory function with some loss this is an incomplete injury (and has a better prognosis).

Sparing of sensation in the perianal region may be the only sign of residual function. Sacral sparing is demonstrated by the presence of sensation perianally and/or voluntary contraction of the anal sphincter.

An injury does not qualify as incomplete on the basis of preserved sacral reflexes, e.g. bulbocavernous or anal wink.

The neurological level is the most caudal myotome or dermatome segment with normal sensory and motor function on both sides. For completeness, the main dermatomes are given in Figure 20.3.

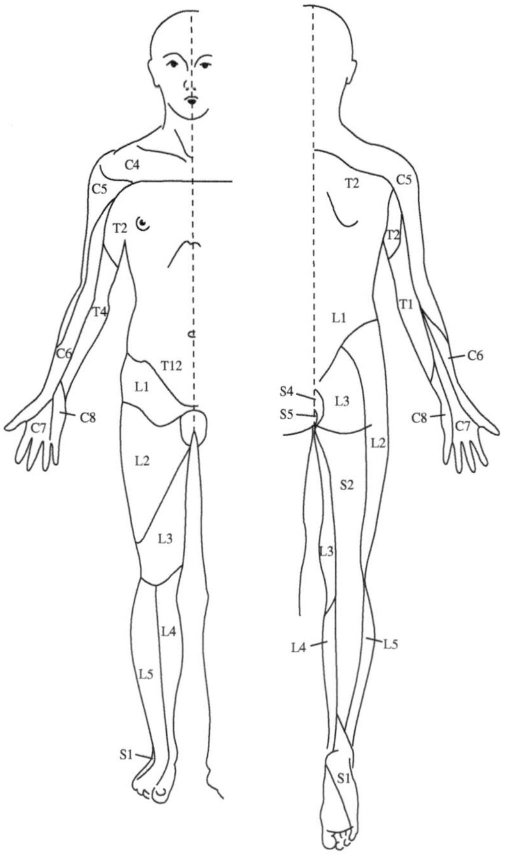

Dermatome	Area
Sensory	
C5	Area over deltoid
C6	Thumb
C7	Middle finger
C8	Little finger
T4	Nipple
T8	Xiphisternum
T10	Umbilicus
T12	Symphysis
L4	Medial aspect shin
L5	Web of first and second toes
S1	Lateral border of foot
S4/5	Perianal
Motor	
C5	Deltoid (shoulder abduction)
C6	Wrist extension
C7	Elbow extension
C8	Flexion of middle finger
T1	Abduction of small finger
L2	Hip flexion
L3	Knee extension
L4	Dorsiflexion
L5	Extension of big toe
S1	Plantar flexion

Figure 20.3 Myotomes/dermatomes used for sensory and motor testing

Each nerve root innervates more than one muscle and most muscles have innervation from more than one nerve root. Certain movements, however, are identified as representing a single nerve root.

A broad distinction can be made between lesions above and lesions below T1 (as determined by sensory and motor testing). Lesions above T1 can result in quadriplegia and lesions below T1 in paraplegia. There is often a discrepancy between neurological injury level and level of bony injury because spinal nerves travel up or down the canal from the point of entry through the bone to join the spinal cord. The level quoted is the neurological level.

20.4 Principles of treatment in spinal injuries

The principles of treatment are primary survey and resuscitation, assessment of fetal well-being and viability, and then secondary survey and protection from further injury.

A spinal injury may be identified in either the primary survey or the secondary survey.

- Deal with life-threatening conditions according to ABC but avoid any movement of the spinal column
- Establish adequate motion restriction and maintain it until you are certain there is no spinal injury
- Make an early referral to a neurosurgeon or orthopaedic surgeon if a spinal injury is detected
- Be aware of associations of spinal injury with effects on other systems and injuries

Primary survey

Airway

Trauma that has caused damage to the spine is likely to be sufficient to cause injury above the clavicle. This may take the form of an injury to the airway or a head injury, which puts the patient at risk of airway problems.

Breathing

If the injury is above the fourth cervical vertebra, there is potential diaphragmatic compromise. With injuries between the fourth cervical and the 12th thoracic vertebrae there will be intercostal embarrassment and, depending on the level, there may be only diaphragmatic breathing.

Complicating factors are: rib fractures; flail chest; pulmonary contusion; haemopneumothorax; and aspiration pneumonitis. Vigorously address these problems by providing ventilatory support, chest drainage and, if the patient can feel pain, analgesia.

Circulation

Spinal injury may cause a circulation problem. Neurogenic shock results from impairment of the descending sympathetic pathways. Below the level of the lesion, there is loss of sympathetic tone to the vessels and therefore vasodilatation, which causes a marked fall in blood pressure. In this situation, blood pressure is not restored by fluid alone and may require the judicious use of vasopressors. Central venous pressure monitoring may be indicated, particularly in the heavily pregnant woman.

Injury above the T4 level causes loss of sympathetic innervation to the heart and therefore bradycardia. With an injury above the T4 level, the combination of vasodilatation below the level of the lesion and the bradycardia caused by impaired sympathetic outflow to the cardiac accelerators can cause profound hypotension.

Atropine may be needed to counteract bradycardia. If ineffective, an isoprenaline infusion may be required. Specialist advice and support will be needed.

Abdominal injuries

Abdominal injuries may only present as a **C** problem. Inability to feel pain due to spinal injury may mask serious intra-abdominal injury that will present only as shock. The only symptom pointing to an intra-abdominal problem may be referred shoulder-tip pain. Ileus is usual in a paralysed patient, so an oro- or nasogastric tube should be passed to empty the stomach.

Locomotor injuries

Musculoskeletal injuries may present with life-threatening hypovolaemia but can be less readily localised in a patient with spinal cord injury, because of the inability to feel pain.

Skin

In a high cord lesion, temperature control function is lost and the patient may become hypothermic or hyperthermic. Spinally injured patients are at severe risk of ischaemic skin loss if not nursed to avoid pressure sores.

Secondary survey

Any injury may be masked by the absence of pain. A vigilant approach to detection is needed. Correct management of upper limb injuries may have a profound effect on the eventual mobility of a quadriplegic.

Bladder

Patients with spinal cord injury and urinary retention need continuous catheter drainage. Urinary output is a good monitor of response to resuscitation.

20.5 Summary

- Appropriate immobilisation of the injured patient during primary resuscitation is a vital part of care until further investigation can be carried out
- Spinal injuries may be a cause of ABC problems, which should be treated first
- Hypotension due to spinal shock may require vasopressors rather than excess fluids

20.6 Further reading

NICE (National Institute for Health and Care Excellence). *Head Injury: Assessment and Early Management*. CG176. London: NICE, 2014 (updated September 2019).

NICE (National Institute for Health and Care Excellence). *Trauma*. QS166. London: NICE, 2018.

CHAPTER 21

Musculoskeletal trauma

Learning outcomes

After reading this chapter, you will be able to:

- Describe the principles of management of a patient with musculoskeletal trauma
- Be aware of how to identify and treat life-threatening injuries
- Be aware of how to identify and treat limb-threatening injuries

21.1 Introduction

The primary survey and resuscitation, secondary survey and definitive care are outlined in this chapter. Within the primary survey, life-threatening injuries are identified and treated. Musculoskeletal injuries can threaten life as a cause of catastrophic haemorrhage and exsanguinating injuries mandate immediate attention. The need to address exsanguinating injuries resulted in the <c>ABC paradigm where during <c> a tourniquet or direct pressure is applied to massive bleeding before commencing the standard airway, breathing, circulation assessment and management sequence.

Immobilisation is an important adjunct to the primary survey in musculoskeletal trauma and has the following beneficial effects:

- Prevents further blood loss
- Protects circulation
- Prevents further soft tissue damage
- Helps to control pain
- Reduces the risk of fat embolism

Beyond the initial resuscitation phase, renal failure can result from traumatic rhabdomyolysis caused by crush injuries. Fat embolism is an uncommon, but lethal, complication of long-bone fractures and presents with hypoxia and respiratory distress.

It is important to realise that the patient may have multiple injuries. Knowledge of the mechanism of the injury can help to predict the pattern of injuries: a fall from a height can result in cervical spine and other vertebral fractures and/or fractures of the long bones. Some fractures are not easy to detect, such as around the shoulder or knee, and are found only after repeated examination.

Managing Medical and Obstetric Emergencies and Trauma: A Practical Approach, Fourth Edition. Edited by Rosamunde Burns and Kara Dent.

21.2 Primary survey

Life-threatening injuries include:

- Major pelvic disruption with haemorrhage
- Major arterial haemorrhage
- Long-bone fractures
- Crush injuries

Major pelvic disruption with haemorrhage

There is limited literature concerning the management of serious pelvic injuries in the later stages of pregnancy. However, uncontrolled haemorrhage from pelvic fractures continues to be a cause of potentially avoidable death after major trauma in the non-pregnant population, and the management principles should be common to both groups. In a multiply injured patient there should be a high index of suspicion for pelvic injury and the pelvis should be immobilised with a pelvic binder at the pre-hospital scene.

Pelvic fractures in pregnant women may cause fracture to the fetal head, especially if the head is engaged. The precise mechanism of injury may provide an indication of the type of pelvic injury sustained. A trauma computed tomography (CT) scan would typically be undertaken and demonstrate the nature and extent of the pelvic injury. A plain pelvic x-ray can be used if the CT scan is not quickly available.

Under no circumstances should there be an attempt to demonstrate the 'open book fracture' by 'springing' the pelvis. Massive retroperitoneal bleeding from pelvic fracture may be more likely in pregnancy because of engorgement of the pelvic vessels. Major pelvic disruption tears the pelvic venous plexus.

The input of an orthopaedic surgeon as part of the trauma team is required urgently as stabilisation of the pelvis by external fixation may be part of resuscitation, in order to 'turn off the tap'.

Major arterial haemorrhage

Venous and arterial haemorrhage should be treated initially with manual attempts to return the pelvis to its anatomical position. This manoeuvre and the application of an external fixator to maintain anatomical reduction may be difficult in the later stages of pregnancy. Often, delivery by caesarean section will be required to achieve control of pelvic haemorrhage. It may be necessary to empty the uterus by caesarean section, even if the fetus is dead, in order to gain pelvic access and to control haemorrhage. Interventional radiological techniques in the angiography suite may be required to embolise the veins and arteries. A high index of suspicion of the pelvis as a potential source of life-threatening bleeding should be maintained.

Long-bone fractures

Assess for bleeding and suspect arterial damage if there are changes in colour, temperature or pulse volume in the extremity concerned. Treatment of visible external bleeding comprises limb immobilisation or traction, compression, fluid resuscitation and orthopaedic input.

Haemorrhage from limb injuries is often compressible. Compression is carried out by:

- Pressing on an obvious source of bleeding or applying a tourniquet (important to note the time of application)
- Immobilising to reduce bleeding, e.g. splinting or definitive surgery/external fixator

With open limb wounds, blood loss may be evident or suspected when a limb is swollen and deformed. Equally, blood loss may only be detected by recognising the signs of hypovolaemia; a closed fracture of the femoral shaft may easily result in the loss of 2 litres of blood into the surrounding tissues. Loss into long bones is one of the five areas for major occult blood loss (chest, abdomen, pelvis, retroperitoneum and long-bone fractures). This requires resuscitation, immobilisation and orthopaedic input.

Crush injuries

Crush injuries cause damage to muscle cells (rhabdomyolysis) and a subsequent release of muscle cell contents. Damage to the sarcolemmal membrane causes fluid sequestration within the muscle cell, and the muscle cells release the toxic substances myoglobin, potassium, phosphate and urate into the circulation. This causes shock, hyperkalaemia (which may precipitate cardiac arrest), hypocalcaemia, metabolic acidosis, compartment syndrome and acute renal failure. The acute renal failure is due to the combination of hypovolaemia, metabolic acidosis and the nephrotoxins myoglobin, urate and phosphate. Beyond the initial resuscitation, invasive monitoring of blood pressure and central venous pressure should be established with ongoing input from critical care to optimise the complex fluid and electrolyte management required to limit acute kidney injury.

21.3 Secondary survey

Limb-threatening injuries are identified in the secondary survey and must be treated promptly. The system of examination of the limbs is look, feel and circulatory assessment. Radiographs of skeletal injuries form part of the secondary survey.

Types of limb-threatening injuries

These include:

- Open fractures and joint injuries
- Vascular injuries and traumatic amputations
- Compartment syndrome
- Nerve injuries secondary to fracture dislocation

Open fractures and joint injuries

With an open fracture, control haemorrhage by direct pressure, firm compression, bandaging and elevation of the limb. Gross contamination, such as with earth and bits of clothing, should be removed and the wound copiously irrigated before applying a dry, sterile dressing. Severe soft tissue wounds are immobilised to relieve pain and to control haemorrhage. Wounds should be described in the notes to avoid repeated disturbance of the dressing before definitive treatment. A photograph or a drawing is helpful. Repeated wound inspection increases the risk of infection. The fracture is then treated as appropriate.

Dislocations are extremely painful when attempts are made to move the joint and this helps early recognition. Such early recognition can allow prompt reduction, especially if there is altered blood supply to the limb, for example in posterior dislocation of the knee occluding the popliteal artery.

All dislocations are reduced at the earliest opportunity. They are often relatively easy to reduce soon after injury. Distal circulation is checked and the joint immobilised after reduction.

Vascular injuries and traumatic amputations

A major vascular injury may be suspected by:

- Obvious arterial or venous haemorrhage from the wound
- An expanding haematoma
- Absent distal pulses
- Delayed capillary refill
- Differing skin colour and temperature compared with the contralateral limb
- Increasing pain at the site of the injury
- Decreased or absent sensation

Repeated assessment of the circulation is necessary.

Fractures or fracture-dislocations around the knee or elbow are commonly associated with injury to the femoral and brachial artery, respectively.

Compartment syndrome

Compartment syndrome occurs when the interstitial pressure in a fascial compartment exceeds the capillary pressure as a result of haemorrhage or oedema within the involved compartment. Initially, venous *outflow* stops and, as the pressure increases, the arterial supply then also stops.

The presence of a distal pulse does not exclude a compartment syndrome.

Ischaemia of the nerves and muscles occurs with rapid and irreversible damage. The distal pulses may be present throughout. The compartments most commonly affected are the anterior tibial compartment and the flexor compartment of the forearm, *especially in young people.*

Causes include crush injuries, prolonged limb compression, open or closed fractures, ischaemia of the limb and tight plasters or dressings.

In an obstetric rather than trauma context, there are reports of iatrogenic compartment syndrome associated with the Lloyd Davies position and the lithotomy position. This is possibly caused by venous obstruction from kinking of the veins at the groin, or external pressure from stirrups or compression cuffs with arterial hypoperfusion to a leg being above the level of the heart. Other factors might include an increase in compartment pressure owing to the weight of limb in stirrups or passive plantar flexion of the foot.

The main presenting symptom is severe pain in an injured limb that is adequately immobilised out of proportion to the injury seen. The pain is aggravated by passive stretching of the muscles in the involved compartment. Active movements are absent. The compartment may be swollen and tense with reduced distal sensation, although this is not always obvious clinically.

If left untreated or with delayed intervention, this injury will lead to permanent disability and even loss of the limb. Prompt recognition and emergency surgical decompression are needed. If the limb is in plaster, or has circumferential dressings, split them completely down to the skin and open them widely. If symptoms do not improve within 15 minutes, any dressings overlying open wounds should be removed and the underlying muscle examined (see also Chapter 22 on burns and escharotomy).

Nerve injuries secondary to fracture dislocation

Some injuries are often associated with neurological damage; for example, a dislocated hip and sciatic nerve injury or a dislocated elbow and median nerve injury. Altered sensation or motor power, or both, suggests nerve involvement. Orthopaedic surgeons should be involved urgently.

Definitive care continues in the hands of the orthopaedic surgeons.

21.4 Summary

- Manage life-threatening injuries first; they usually present as a circulation problem
- Suspect, detect and treat limb-threatening injuries

21.5 Further reading

Chavez LO, Leon M, Einav S, Varon J. Beyond muscle destruction: a systematic review of rhabdomyolysis for clinical practice. *Crit Care* 2016; 20: 135.

Chapter 22: Burns

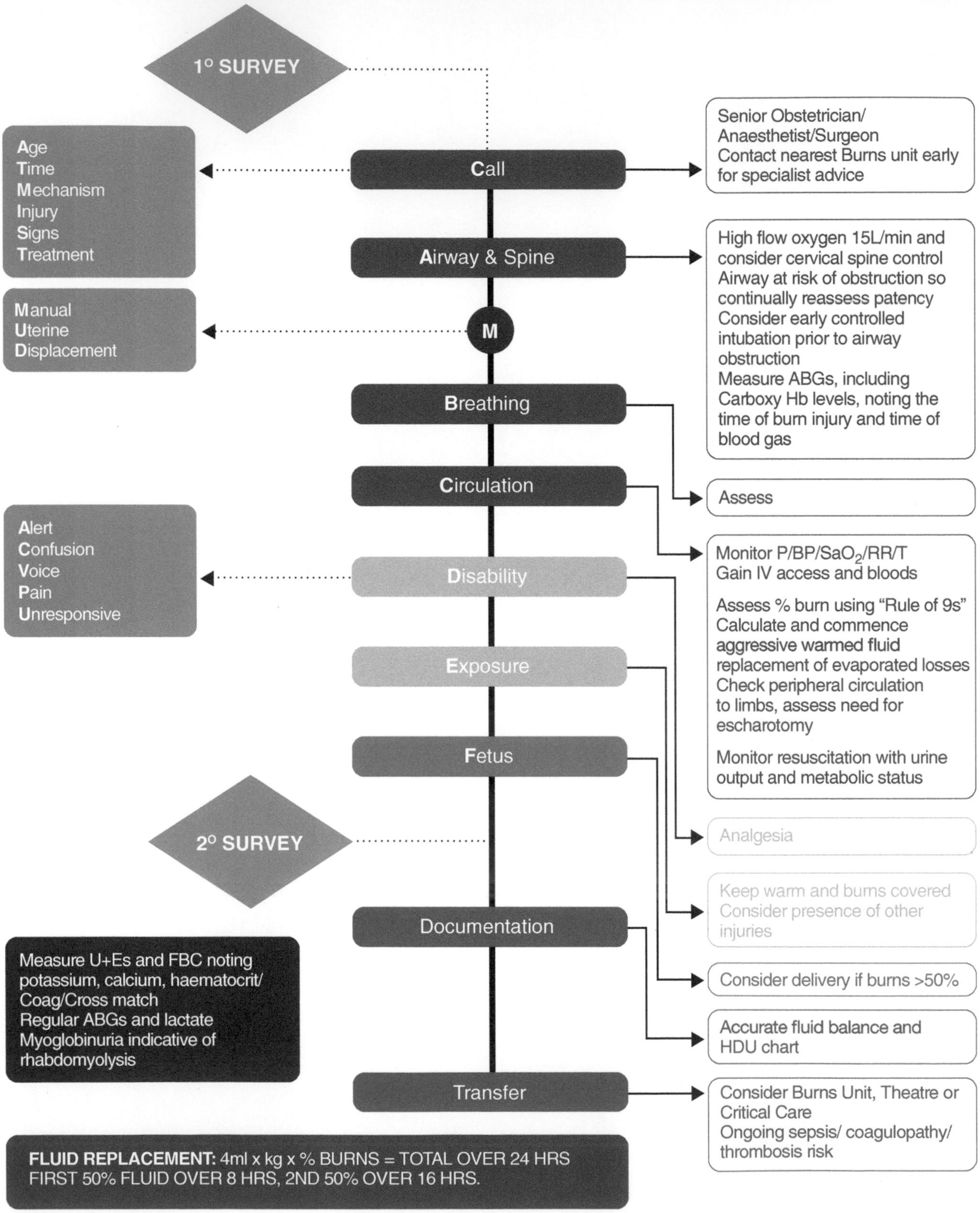

1° SURVEY
Call
Age
Time
Mechanism
Injury
Signs
Treatment
Senior Obstetrician/
Anaesthetist/Surgeon
Contact nearest Burns unit early for specialist advice
Airway & Spine
High flow oxygen 15L/min and consider cervical spine control
Airway at risk of obstruction so continually reassess patency
Consider early controlled intubation prior to airway obstruction
Measure ABGs, including Carboxy Hb levels, noting the time of burn injury and time of blood gas
M
Manual
Uterine
Displacement
Breathing
Assess
Circulation
Monitor P/BP/SaO2/RR/T
Gain IV access and bloods
Assess % burn using "Rule of 9s"
Calculate and commence aggressive warmed fluid replacement of evaporated losses
Check peripheral circulation to limbs, assess need for escharotomy
Monitor resuscitation with urine output and metabolic status
Disability
Alert
Confusion
Voice
Pain
Unresponsive
Analgesia
Exposure
Keep warm and burns covered
Consider presence of other injuries
Fetus
Consider delivery if burns >50%
2° SURVEY
Documentation
Accurate fluid balance and HDU chart
Measure U+Es and FBC noting potassium, calcium, haematocrit/
Coag/Cross match
Regular ABGs and lactate
Myoglobinuria indicative of rhabdomyolysis
Transfer
Consider Burns Unit, Theatre or Critical Care
Ongoing sepsis/ coagulopathy/ thrombosis risk
FLUID REPLACEMENT: 4ml x kg x % BURNS = TOTAL OVER 24 HRS
FIRST 50% FLUID OVER 8 HRS, 2ND 50% OVER 16 HRS.

Algorithm 22.1 Burns

CHAPTER 22
Burns

Learning outcomes

After reading this chapter, you will be able to:

- Describe the impact of a thermal injury on airway, breathing and circulation
- Describe the immediate management of airway, breathing and circulation problems in a patient with burns
- Assess the severity of burns
- Discuss the management of the fetus in the pregnant patient with burns

22.1 Introduction

Most burns are caused by thermal injury but chemical, electrical and radiation burns may also occur. The severity of the injury is characterised by the area and depth of the burn and the effect of smoke inhalation and inhalational burns on the airway.

Burns may cause immediately life-threatening problems that need to be simultaneously identified and treated in the primary survey.

The literature about burns in pregnancy is limited (historical, case reports and small series primarily from the developing world) and care is based on standard non-pregnant burns protocols. In the UK, care is centralised into facilities, units and regional centres for burns. Pregnancy should be considered to be a special feature and may warrant early/prompt consultation with a regional centre.

The British Burns Association have recently published standards of care:

- Fluids within 1 hour
- Wound cleaned and dressed within 6 hours
- Consultant review
- Dietary, physiotherapy, occupational therapy, and psychological input available in regional centres

Severity of the burn

The severity of the burn depends on the:

- Total body surface area burned – measured with the 'rule of nines' (Figure 22.1 and Table 22.1)
- Depth of the burn

The increased abdominal girth of pregnancy or morbid obesity increases the area of the burn – if there is difficulty assessing, the patient's palm represents 1% of body surface area.

Managing Medical and Obstetric Emergencies and Trauma: A Practical Approach, Fourth Edition. Edited by Rosamunde Burns and Kara Dent.

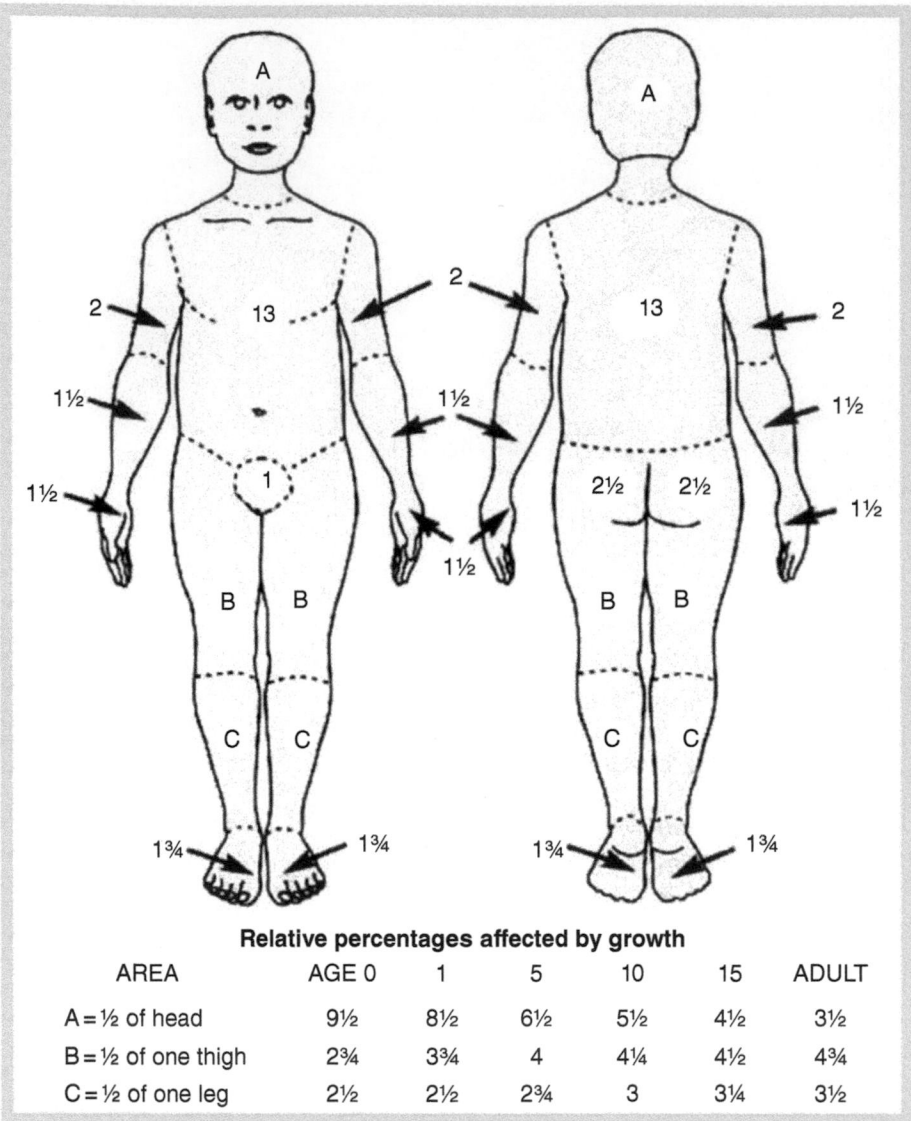

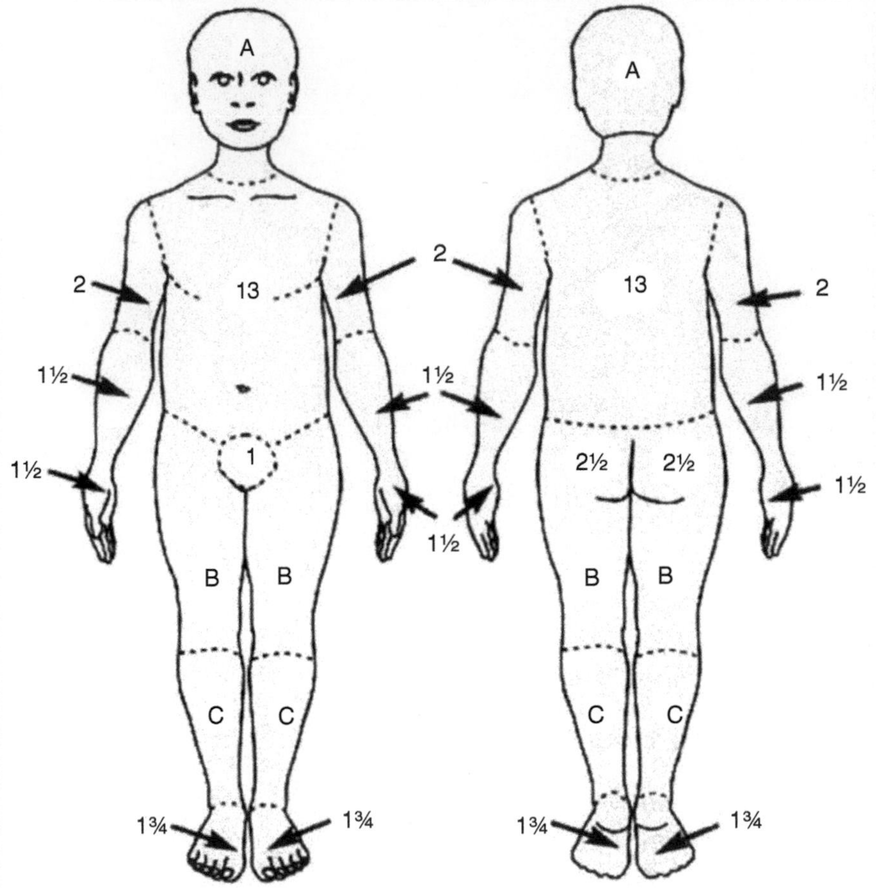

Relative percentages affected by growth

AREA	AGE 0	1	5	10	15	ADULT
A = ½ of head	9½	8½	6½	5½	4½	3½
B = ½ of one thigh	2¾	3¾	4	4¼	4½	4¾
C = ½ of one leg	2½	2½	2¾	3	3¼	3½

Figure 22.1 Percentage burn by body area
Source: COBIS, NHS National Services Scotland

Assessment of burn depth

In the past (and still in some countries) the depth of a burn was classified by degrees - first, second, third or fourth degree. A new classification system has been introduced in the UK to help decide the need for surgery, to guide treatment and predict outcomes:

- **Simple erythema**: reversible redness of the skin, typical of mild sunburn
- **Superficial partial thickness:** involves only the upper layers of the skin, is pink coloured and painful. It usually heals within 2 weeks with minimal or no scarring
- **Deep partial thickness**: involves superficial and deeper layers of skin, has a creamy white base and is less painful. Without surgery it will usually be associated with delayed healing and risk of significant scarring
- **Full thickness**: involves all layers of skin and sometimes underlying tissues. The surface is initially grey-white and leathery, which if left to dry a transparent brown eschar will form. This is painless and without surgery will lead to scarring and contractures

Table 22.1 The 'rule of nines'

Body surface area	Area burned
Head and neck	9%
Each upper limb	9%
Front of trunk*	18%
Back of trunk	18%
Each lower limb	18%
Perineum	1%

* The gravid abdomen would represent a larger proportion of the total body surface area. The area of the patient's palm represents about 1% of the body surface area.

22.2 Pathophysiology of burns

Airway and respiratory effects

Airway injury from burns can be immediate or delayed, so the airway must be continually assessed and early intubation should be considered, particularly if the patient is to be transferred. Although maximum oedema is likely to occur at 24 hours post injury, changes in airway patency can be rapid and disastrous. Clinical changes of impending airway obstruction, i.e. stridor (airway noise on inspiration), increased work of breathing with falling SaO_2 and decreasing conscious level, must be acted on.

Obstruction of the lower airways may be caused by deposition of soot particles.

Injury to the lung parenchyma may be caused directly by hot gas or steam and may result in critically impaired gas exchange. However, impairment of respiratory function can occur in the burns patient in the absence of obvious respiratory injury. The mechanism for this is unclear, but can involve ventilation/perfusion mismatch, secondary infection or adult respiratory distress syndrome (ARDS) and may occur up to 2 weeks after the initial injury.

Carbon monoxide inhalation

Inhalation of carbon monoxide is common, especially if the burn has been sustained in an enclosed area with low levels of oxygen or, without any burn injury, due to inhalation of exhaust fumes or from faulty household heaters.

Oxygen delivery relies on haemoglobin binding to oxygen, however carbon monoxide has a greater affinity for haemoglobin than oxygen and so displaces oxygen from the binding sites on the haemoglobin molecule, resulting in reduced oxygen delivery to the tissues. Pulse oximetry will be misleading because carboxyhaemoglobin is interpreted as oxygenated haemoglobin.

Diagnosis is made by measuring carboxyhaemoglobin in the venous or arterial blood – a level of greater than 10% indicates significant inhalation of carbon monoxide. However, there are usually no physical symptoms at less than 20%, hence the danger of this condition and the risk of failing to make the diagnosis.

The 'cherry red' discoloration of carbon monoxide poisoning is usually a terminal sign, and should not be relied upon for diagnostic purposes. Carbon monoxide levels of 60% are likely to result in death.

Treatment is high-flow oxygen. Hyperbaric oxygen therapy should be considered for the more severe cases.

There can be serious effects on the fetus if the mother has carbon monoxide poisoning. Carbon monoxide crosses the placental barrier and binds with even higher affinity to fetal haemoglobin, leading to fetal tissue hypoxia. This may result in fetal death, injury, miscarriage or preterm labour even if the mother's injury appears mild.

Circulatory effects

Localised tissue damage causes oedema and fluid leak into the tissues. In addition, circulating inflammatory mediators cause an increase in systemic capillary permeability. This leads to generalised extravasation of fluid from the intravascular compartment into the tissues, producing massive peripheral and pulmonary oedema. These inflammatory mediators can have a direct effect on cardiac function, which, when combined with relative hypovolaemia and vasodilatation, result in a marked reduction in tissue perfusion. A summary of these effects can also be simply defined as 'shock', which in the case of a severe burn may be classified as hypovolaemic, cardiogenic or distributive shock.

Immediate first aid

The burning process must be stopped: extinguish the flames by lying the affected patient on the ground in the left lateral position and wrapping them in a blanket or equivalent. Gently remove burned clothing and any jewellery unless stuck to the burnt skin. Small burns can be cooled with clean, cold water. Burns should be covered to avoid hypothermia – non-sterile, domestic cling film is useful as a first aid dressing as it allows visualisation of the wound, but protects it from contamination and fluid loss whilst reducing pain.

22.3 Primary survey and resuscitation

Remember tilt or manual uterine displacement.

Airway and breathing

Airway and breathing injuries should be suspected if:

- The burn was sustained in an enclosed space
- There is hoarseness, loss of voice, stridor or wheeze
- There is evidence of burns around the lips, mouth and nose
- There is singeing to the nasal hair or eyebrows
- There is soot around the mouth or nose, or the patient is coughing up carbonaceous sputum
- There is respiratory distress and alteration in level of consciousness
- There is carbon monoxide poisoning

If there is a suspicion of an airway and breathing problem, or in the presence of carbon monoxide poisoning, urgent assessment by an experienced anaesthetist is required, as early intubation and ventilation may be indicated. Airway burns rarely occur in the absence of facial burns.

Anaesthetic considerations include:

- Suxamethonium can be used safely for the first 72 hours but after that there is a risk of hyperkalaemia and should be avoided
- Use an uncut endotracheal tube as significant facial swelling is to be expected
- Normal lung protective strategies should be used in ventilation

Management of suspected carbon monoxide inhalation

High-flow oxygen should be administered to all patients.

Cyanide may also be absorbed by inhalation as a product of combustion of certain materials, and impairs respiration at the cellular level with equivalent reduction in cellular oxygenation. However, routine testing is not recommended unless there is a profound metabolic acidosis with no other explanation.

Circulation

Significant circulatory losses are anticipated.

Secure intravenous access, through non-burned skin, where possible. It will be difficult to secure intravenous lines in burned areas and may increase the risk of infection, but on occasions this may be the only option. In extreme difficulty, intraossseous cannulae or central lines may be required.

Different formula exist to guide fluid resuscitation based on the time elapsed from the burn, the weight of the patient and the extent of the burn. The most common one in use is the Parkland formula:

4 ml × actual body weight (kg) × % burn = total volume of fluid of resuscitative fluid required in 24 hours from time of burn

Fluids:

- Warmed Ringer's lactate/Hartmann's solution
- First half – given over first 8 hours
- Second half – given over next 16 hours
- Additional fluid will be required for maintenance and additional losses

Monitor circulatory status by heart rate, urine output, blood pressure and haematocrit. Fluid replacement should result in a urine output of 0.5–1.0 ml/kg/h based on ideal body weight.

The combination of smoke inhalation and a burn increases fluid requirements compared with a burn alone. Critical care should be involved in ongoing care.

Pain relief

As soon as time allows, give pain relief. Covering the burn, where practicable, with a transparent film will help to relieve pain while maintaining wound visibility. Opiates will be necessary in most cases, which should be titrated intravenously to achieve satisfactory pain relief, do not give intramuscularly or subcutaneously.

22.4 Secondary survey

A burned patient may have other injuries being masked by the pain of the burn. A full top-to-toe secondary survey is necessary to identify injuries that were not apparent in the primary survey.

Assess fetus

Obstetric management must be individualised by the multidisciplinary team (obstetricians, obstetric anaesthetists, critical care physicians and burns specialists). Fetal outcome depends on fetal age and the degree of maternal harm (sepsis, hypoxia, hypovolaemia).

Within hours, the mother may become hypermetabolic which leads to hyperthermia, increased oxygen consumption, tachypnoea, tachycardia and an increase in serum catecholamine levels. Maternal acidosis is predictive with regard to progression of the metabolic insult. Nigerian studies have demonstrated that mortality from significant burns in pregnancy is three times that of equivalent burns in non-pregnant woman.

If the burn area is 50% or more and in the second or third trimester, urgent delivery should be carried out with multidisciplinary involvement after the initial resuscitation. Fetal survival is not improved by waiting, and the additional metabolic requirements may compromise the mother. If the total body surface area injuried is significant, spontaneous onset of labour commonly occurs within a few days.

Earlier in pregnancy there appears to be no evidence that pregnancy affects maternal survival. However, with increasing burn injury there will be an increased risk of miscarriage, preterm labour or fetal death, especially in the first week post burn.

If the burn is less than 30% body surface area, the prognosis is good for both mother and fetus, dependent on gestational age and avoidance of sepsis.

Electrical burns

There are limited data on the management of electrical burns in pregnancy with the amniotic fluid and uterus being good conductors of electricity. There are reports of long-term oligohydramnios and intrauterine growth restriction. However, it is generally felt that there is an 'all or nothing' effect on the fetus: either death results or the prognosis is comparatively good.

22.5 Definitive care

Escharotomy – Burned tissue may constrict the blood supply to the limbs. Check peripheral circulation by capillary refill and estimating perfusion. Call for general/plastic surgical assistance for assessment and treatment. The procedure of cutting through burned tissue to restore blood supply (and prevent rhabdomyolysis) is called escharotomy.

Sepsis – Prevention of sepsis by appropriate dressings, early excision and grafting is important. Sepsis is the major cause of death due to burns in pregnancy.

Thrombosis – There should be a high index of suspicion for venous thrombosis and use of thromboprophlaxis.

Coagulation – There may be disturbance of coagulation either by dilutional effects where there is large fluid loss or by development of disseminated intravascular coagulopathy.

22.6 Summary

- Management of the burned pregnant woman involves multiple specialities
- Assess the severity and depth of surface burns, and treat
- Assess the actual or potential effect of the burn on the ABCs and treat appropriately
- Arrange the timely delivery of the fetus when appropriate
- Conduct a secondary survey and definitive care

22.7 Further reading

British Burn Association. *National Standards for Provision and Outcomes in Adult and Paediatric Burn Care.* https://www.britishburnassociation.org/standards/ (last accessed January 2022).

Care of Burns in Scotland. www.cobis.scot.nhs.uk (last accessed January 2022).

PART 5

Other obstetric medical and surgical emergencies

Chapter 23: Abdominal emergencies

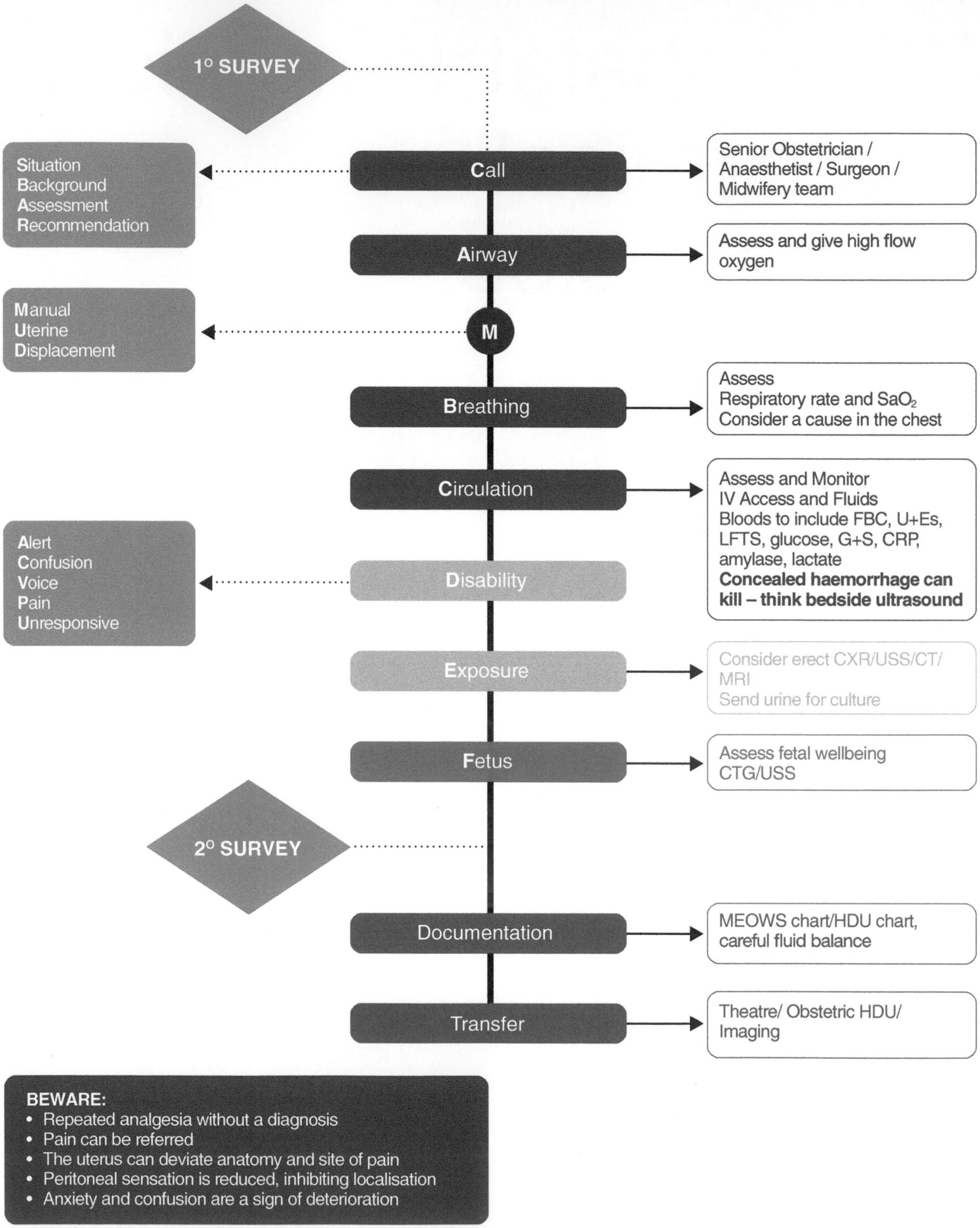

1° SURVEY
Call
Situation
Background
Assessment
Recommendation
Senior Obstetrician / Anaesthetist / Surgeon / Midwifery team
Airway
Assess and give high flow oxygen
M
Manual
Uterine
Displacement
Breathing
Assess
Respiratory rate and SaO2
Consider a cause in the chest
Circulation
Assess and Monitor
IV Access and Fluids
Bloods to include FBC, U+Es, LFTS, glucose, G+S, CRP, amylase, lactate
Concealed haemorrhage can kill – think bedside ultrasound
Disability
Alert
Confusion
Voice
Pain
Unresponsive
Exposure
Consider erect CXR/USS/CT/MRI
Send urine for culture
Fetus
Assess fetal wellbeing
CTG/USS
2° SURVEY
Documentation
MEOWS chart/HDU chart, careful fluid balance
Transfer
Theatre/ Obstetric HDU/ Imaging
BEWARE:
• Repeated analgesia without a diagnosis
• Pain can be referred
• The uterus can deviate anatomy and site of pain
• Peritoneal sensation is reduced, inhibiting localisation
• Anxiety and confusion are a sign of deterioration

Algorithm 23.1 Abdominal emergencies

CHAPTER 23
Abdominal emergencies

Learning outcomes

After reading this chapter, you will be able to:

- Describe how to assess the pregnant woman with abdominal pain
- Describe how to suspect and promptly diagnose potentially life-threatening conditions
- Consider the changes in anatomy and physiology that occur in pregnancy and understand how these may affect the response to, and presentation of, acute abdominal conditions
- Outline the investigation and treatment of abdominal pain in pregnancy

23.1 Introduction

The incidence of an acute abdomen within pregnancy is common at 1 in 500–635 pregnancies. Frequently, minor ailments such as lower urinary tract infections are found to be the cause, but significant serious pathology does occur and can present in subtle ways. This can result in serious diagnoses being missed or delayed, which can, in turn, result in death of the mother and/or fetus. In the UK, all maternal deaths in pregnancy are reported, through MBRARACE-UK, and the last report in 2020 showed that there were 11 women who died from gastrointestinal disorders, more than in previous years. Five of these were from pancreatitis or complications, four from bowel perforations or ulcers, one from a volvulus and the other from hyperemesis.

Many of the women who died received substandard care, which often included a delay in diagnosis. Recurrent problems highlighted throughout the confidential reports include:

- Failure to entertain the possibility of a non-obstetric diagnosis
- Readmission, or multiple admissions, with no consultant input
- Repeated doses of opiate analgesia, without consultant review or an adequate cause for pain being established
- High-risk women being looked after in a disjointed way by junior clinicians, with lack of communication between services
- Anxiety and confusion too readily being attributed to a psychiatric cause rather than to the underlying (undiagnosed) organic disease

Women who have received bariatric surgery previously are now being seen more often in obstetric practice and need to be considered high risk. Evidence shows that there is a risk of 'stomal ulceration' (ulceration at the anastomosis of the small bowel and stomach), which can be worsened and even perforate if non-steroidal anti-inflammatory drugs (NSAIDs) are used. One patient in the MBRRACE-UK report had received NSAIDs in the postnatal period for pain relief and this was thought to add to her resulting gastric perforation and collapse. She died of subsequent organ failure. The report recommends that these women should be looked after by a multidisciplinary team with expertise in pregnancy. NSAIDs should be relatively contraindicated.

Managing Medical and Obstetric Emergencies and Trauma: A Practical Approach, Fourth Edition. Edited by Rosamunde Burns and Kara Dent.

23.2 Pathophysiology of abdominal pain in pregnancy

Abdominal pain, especially of acute onset, in the pregnant woman, is a medical emergency that requires urgent assessment. As pregnancy advances, the assessment of the abdomen becomes more challenging:

- Areas of maximum pain or tenderness may shift due to organ displacement
- The uterus inhibits abdominal palpation
- The peritoneum is less sensitive.

The other problem produced by the gravid uterus is that of hampering the omentum from its role as 'policeman' of the intra-abdominal contents, with the consequence of an inability to contain local inflammation. In turn, this results in more rapid progression of conditions such as appendicitis or perforation.

Intra-abdominal bleeding can also confuse the clinician, as the mother, especially in later pregnancy, tolerates blood loss well. The reader is referred to Chapters 6 and 28, and reminded that the signs of bleeding, including tachycardia, narrowing of the pulse pressure, oliguria and confusion, all occur after significantly more blood is lost in the pregnant than the non-pregnant woman, and that hypotension is an *extremely* late sign. What does help with assessment in pregnancy is that the fetus tolerates maternal blood loss very badly and is a good 'monitor' of maternal hypovolaemia, demonstrating heart rate abnormalities on monitoring. Early fetal heart rate monitoring is therefore extremely useful in women presenting with abdominal pain from the late second trimester onwards.

23.3 Clinical approach to diagnosis: history, examination and investigations

History

A detailed history around the *nature of the pain* is a vital step in beginning the diagnostic process, and is especially important in pregnancy, where abdominal examination can be so inhibited by the gravid uterus. The following should be found from general and then direct enquiry.

Pain onset: acute versus gradual

- ***Acute onset*** with *persistent severe pain* suggests rupturing or tearing including ruptured ectopic, ruptured uterus, ruptured aneurysm (splenic, renal, epigastric or aortic), rupture of an abscess or perforation of an ulcer. Acute abruption also presents with severe acute abdominal pain and should be the presumptive diagnosis until ruled out. Acute onset with *colicky pain* suggests either intestinal or ureteric obstruction. Hernial orifices should be checked (sometimes difficult in a heavily pregnant and/or obese woman). If colicky pain becomes constant then the possibility of underlying ischaemia must be considered (e.g. bowel or ovary)
- ***Gradual onset*** increasing over a comparatively short time is more characteristic of 'inflammation' such as might occur with acute appendicitis, acute degeneration of a fibroid, acute cholecystitis, acute pancreatitis and acute diverticulitis

Other important characteristics

- ***Quality*** and severity (colicky pain suggests an obstruction or something twisting, while continuous pain is more likely to suggest inflammation/infection)
- ***Location*** (think uterine, intraperitoneal, retroperitoneal and referred)
- ***Radiation*** (remembering diaphragm to shoulder, renal to groin and ovary down inner thigh)
- ***Exacerbating or relieving factors*** (movement, coughing, voiding, position)
- ***Associated symptoms*** (anorexia, nausea, vomiting, constipation, dysuria, haematuria, frequency)

Location of the pain and its likely cause

Uterine pain: abruption, degeneration of fibroids, chorioamnionitis or uterine contractions

The location of this is usually straightforward and confirmed by tenderness on palpation of the uterus, but fibroids can lie posteriorly and be inaccessible to palpation, and a posteriorly located placenta can abrupt without producing local tenderness. Remember to check:

- The placental location (by ultrasound scan) relative to any uterine pain or tenderness
- The fetal heart rate pattern (by cardiotocography)

Intraperitoneal (abdominal) pain

Visceral peritoneal, compared with parietal peritoneal, irritation stimulates the afferent nerve fibres running within the sympathetic part of the autonomic system back to the sympathetic chain and spinal cord. This, therefore, produces a vague 'referred pain', usually in the central region, corresponding to the cutaneous nerves that arise from the corresponding level of the spinal cord. For example, in appendicitis this produces pain in the region of T10, which is around the umbilicus.

Once the parietal peritoneum becomes involved, segmental somatic innervation comes into play and produces sensation in the location of the problem, hence vague pains 'move' to localise as the disease process progresses. Inflammation and infection tend to produce constant pain that evolves as described earlier, but is also usually associated with constitutional upsets of nausea, anorexia, vomiting and fever. In many conditions, initial inflammation leads to subsequent infection, such as in appendicitis and cholecystitis.

Obstruction produces colicky pain that can be severe, and can also be associated with nausea and vomiting if the obstruction is in the small intestine. There may be a change in bowel habit depending if the distal small bowel or colon is involved. Perforation of a viscus usually follows deterioration of the above conditions or more directly from a peptic ulcer, or sigmoid diverticulum. This leads to the severe constant pain of generalised peritonitis, worsened by movement of any sort.

- Examples of inflammation without infection include oesophagitis (heartburn) and (simple) peptic ulceration. These lead to epigastric pain, whereas a flare up of either Crohn's disease or ulcerative colitis leads to more central abdominal pain, which may be colicky and usually associated with diarrhoea. It is worth noting that the administration of steroids, either to promote fetal lung maturation, or as treatment for inflammatory bowel disease, can not only exacerbate peptic ulceration, but also, importantly and dangerously, mask intra-abdominal signs and add to confusion in the diagnostic process
- Examples of inflammation, which lead to infection, include cholecystitis and appendicitis. Both these conditions present with increasing pain that settles into a specific location. The appendix migrates superiorly with advancing gestation, progressing from the right iliac fossa upwards to the right paraumbilical region and can even reach the right hypochondrium
- Examples of obstruction include sigmoid volvulus and pseudo-obstruction, the latter characteristically occurring post caesarean section. Whilst a sigmoid volvulus is usually associated with absolute constipation, pseudo-obstruction may not be so, and small amounts of liquid stool are not uncommon. Colonic neoplasms, although rare, can also occur
- Perforations from peptic ulceration arise de novo and are rarely associated with any prodromal symptoms of an underlying ulcer. Perforations from appendicitis, sigmoid volvulus or pseudo-obstruction occur due to delay in both diagnosis and management
- Rupture or torsion of an ovarian cyst can also produce a colicky pain, which can progress to a constant pain with constitutional upset once ischaemia develops. Whilst this pain is in the iliac fossa region in early pregnancy, as with appendicitis, it can occur relatively higher in later pregnancy

Inflammation and swelling of an organ (liver)

Hepatic pain from inflammation or infection can be severe and even result in spontaneous rupture secondary to gross swelling. The pain is often epigastric rather than right subcostal and this, together with local tenderness in the pre-eclamptic patient, should alert to the possibility of the HELLP (haemolysis, elevated liver enzymes, low platelet count) syndrome.

Vascular accident

- Spontaneous rupture of an artery can occur. Most commonly this is a splenic artery aneurysm that produces sudden onset of severe pain rapidly progressing to collapse. This can be mistaken for an acute abruption and the diagnosis only realised after blood is discovered free in the abdominal cavity at caesarean section. In its less dramatic form it can present with left upper quadrant pain; this is a very unusual location for pain in pregnancy and should always be taken seriously
- Deep vein thrombosis of the pelvic vessels can produce a vague, generalised abdominal pain
- A bleeding peptic ulcer is not associated with abdominal pain unless there is a concomitant anterior perforation. It usually presents with haematemesis and/or melaena along with hypovolaemia. A history of indigestion may give a clue as to the cause. If the bleed is catastrophic, collapse and death may occur before melaena is ever passed

Retroperitoneal

- Loin pain is usually due to pyelonephritis and, because of the dextro-rotation of the uterus, this is invariably on the right side. (Serious consideration should be given to the accuracy of this 'diagnosis' if pain is left-sided.) The pain tends to be constant and is usually associated with a fever although the urine may be clear. Loin tenderness can also occur with cholecystitis, but anterior tenderness in this condition helps to distinguish it from renal pain
- Colicky pain commencing in the loin, but migrating towards the groin, may be produced by renal/ureteric colic and the passage of a stone. Haematuria may also be present
- Pancreatitis causes constant, severe, epigastric pain that radiates through to the back. It is sometimes relieved by leaning forward. It can often present as a much more vague abdominal pain and sometimes in an atypical upper abdominal location

Referred and neurological pain

- Pathology in the chest can present with abdominal discomfort or pain. Examples include myocardial ischaemia, pneumonia, pulmonary embolus and aortic dissection
- Cholecystitis is commonly referred to the area of the lower ribs posteriorly or between the shoulder blades; hyperaesthesia may be present over the lower ribs to the right (Boas's sign)
- Irritation under the diaphragm (usually from sepsis or blood) will produce pain in the shoulder region. This is more common on the left than the right, due to the presence of the liver on the right-hand side
- Herpes zoster can produce abdominal pain before the vesicular eruption occurs

Examination

Obstetricians tend to forget to perform a general examination and instead go straight to the abdomen. This must be avoided, and a systematic, thorough general examination is needed, including assessment of:

- Pulse rate, pulse character and vascular perfusion
- Colour, temperature, hydration and fetor oris
- Lymphadenopathy and jugular venous pressure
- Chest, including respiratory rate
- Legs

An abdominal examination will then include:

- Looking – does the patient move or lie still? Is there shallow breathing?
- Are there any scars? (Remembering that laparoscopic procedures will leave no characteristic scars as clues)
- Palpation for tenderness with guarding or rebound
- Auscultation for the presence and character of the bowel sounds

Abdominal examination is further confounded by obesity, which is an ever-increasing problem in the pregnant population.

The site of the pain can be very useful in distinguishing where it originates from. A focal pain is more likely to be peritoneal pain whereas visceral pain is less localised. If the pain is related to foregut structures, it is normally felt in the upper abdomen. Pain from the midgut structures are felt around the umbilicus, whereas pain from the hindgut structures are more often perceived in the lower abdomen.

Investigations

Cardiotocography

Cardiotocography should be performed early to assess uterine activity and fetal condition.

Blood tests

Blood tests can help make a diagnosis in patients with abdominal pathology, for example a grossly elevated amylase in acute pancreatitis or deranged liver function tests in HELLP. More commonly, however, they can be less useful and even on occasions misleading. An elevated white cell count can be a normal finding in pregnancy due to a neutrophilia (typically white cells rise from about 7×10^9 to 15×10^9/litre). Therefore the danger here is for obstetricians to assume an elevated count is normal, while surgeons might read too much into it. Inflammatory and infective conditions can occur with remarkably normal white cells. Elevated C-reactive protein (CRP) levels are a good indication of an underlying inflammatory condition and these levels do not change in normal pregnancy. D-dimers are unhelpful in diagnosing thrombosis in pregnancy. It is important to remember that if acute pancreatitis has been ongoing for more than a day, the peak of serum amylase may be missed and the raised amylase detected only in the urine.

Ultrasound

This is useful to check the viability of the pregnancy, the location of the placenta and any fibroids, and can also be useful to check for intra-abdominal bleeding. It may, however, fail to identify small amounts of intraperitoneal fluid, or other pathology (particularly retroperitoneal). A negative examination should therefore be viewed with caution, and may need to be repeated. It is not good at diagnosing an early, or evolving, abruption.

Radiographs

Chest radiographs can be helpful for cardiac and chest pathology, and for excluding air under the diaphragm from a visceral perforation. (Remember, the latter may not be beneficial in women who have had a recent caesarean section or other surgery.)

Abdominal plain radiographs are rarely used during pregnancy, but can be used post-delivery in assessing colonic dilatation in pseudo-obstruction.

CT and MRI

It is always useful to discuss the best imaging modality with the radiologist in the first instance. Understandably, there are concerns regarding computed tomography (CT) and ionising radiation. It is known now that exposure of <5 rads has not been associated with fetal defects or loss. (A CT of the abdomen/pelvis carries an exposure of 3.5 rads.) Care should be taken to shield the pregnant patient to reduce unnecessary exposure. The risks and benefits should be carefully discussed with the patient and documented.

One problem with these advanced imaging modalities is that the pregnant woman may not fit into the scanner. Care should be taken during these tests so that the woman is placed tilted in the left lateral position to avoid aortocaval compression during the scan.

23.4 Clinical management of abdominal emergencies

When a junior doctor has taken a history and performed a thorough examination and the diagnosis is not obviously obstetric related, the consultant obstetrician should be called for an opinion. This focuses attention on the problem, helps to identify who is the best specialist to involve and adds weight to the referral – which in most circumstances should be on a consultant to consultant basis. These are high-risk women, and making a diagnosis can not only be extremely difficult, but the cost of failure is high for both mother and fetus, not to mention the hospital. Assessment and referral between junior doctors is fraught with potential errors and should be avoided.

In cases where the diagnosis is not clear, but surgical intervention is required, a midline incision is advisable. The risk of miscarriage (0.7%) and preterm labour (3.2%) with surgical intervention needs to be discussed.

Acute appendicitis

Acute appendicitis is the commonest cause for acute abdominal pain with an incidence of 1 in 800–1500 pregnancies. It is more common in the first two trimesters, but perforation is more common in the third, probably due to the difficulties in establishing an early diagnosis or the peritoneum being stretched. It has long been recognised that there is a higher morbidity for mother and fetus in pregnancy and therefore a relatively high negative operation rate is acceptable. Laparoscopy may be helpful in early pregnancy, and laparoscopic appendicectomy is usually possible. Later in pregnancy, the position of the appendix shifts upwards and laterally and, because of access difficulties due to the enlarged uterus, a muscle-splitting incision should be made over the site of maximum tenderness. This is often in the right upper quadrant. There is, however, increasing published evidence to suggest that the management of an imaging-proven non-perforated acute appendicitis with antibiotics and regular review is perfectly safe.

Acute cholecystitis

In the general population, acute cholecystitis is best managed by early laparoscopic cholecystectomy in patients fit for surgery. In pregnant patients, the severity of symptoms needs to be weighed up against the risk of losing the pregnancy from either surgery or sepsis. Patients who have simple biliary colic without obvious signs of acute inflammation (ultrasonographic features of a thickened gall bladder wall, localised tenderness and free fluid) are better treated non-operatively as the symptoms are usually short-lived and the gall bladder can be removed at some stage after the pregnancy has been completed. Patients who develop significant and recurrent biliary colic during pregnancy should be considered for cholecystectomy, preferably in the second trimester, as this is associated with less risk to the fetus than in the first or third trimesters. In patients with obvious acute cholecystitis, the decision is more difficult, and other factors will need to be considered such as the state of the patient and the stage of the pregnancy.

In general, because of the risk of fetal loss during surgery, non-operative management should be attempted in the first instance. However, persistence of symptoms and/or progression of disease should lead to cholecystectomy. If a common bile duct stone is the cause of obstruction and pain, the British Society of Gastroenterology recommends endoscopic retrograde cholangiopancreatography (ERCP). In the advanced stages of pregnancy, laparoscopic access may be difficult, and open surgery may be required.

Acute pancreatitis

Acute pancreatitis is rare in pregnancy, occurring in approximately three in 10 000 pregnancies. It is most commonly due to cholelithiasis, but the oestrogenic effects of hyperlipidaemia can also be responsible. If severe, it is associated with a maternal and perinatal mortality rate of almost 40%. Whilst symptoms are usually gastrointestinal with pain, nausea and vomiting, 10% of cases are associated with respiratory effects, which can progress to acute respiratory distress syndrome (ARDS).

Acute pancreatitis should be considered in any woman with unexplained abdominal pain, with early clinical suspicion leading to laboratory assessments. Oxygen saturations should also be measured. Amylase levels are used to help make the diagnosis as they are often more than three times the normal range. However, in a chronic condition these can normalise and be in the lower levels and may be misleading. Serum lipase may be more sensitive. As above, do not forget that a urine amylase can be useful to confirm diagnosis once the serum peak has passed. Once a diagnosis is made, prompt multidisciplinary care is needed. When caused by gall stones, early cholecystectomy is recommended, again taking into account the various factors discussed earlier. Otherwise, management is essentially non-operative and supportive in the initial period, and in the severe form may require critical care support. In such circumstances, early delivery will be required.

Colonic pseudo-obstruction

This was first described secondary to retroperitoneal malignancy by William Ogilvie, and is sometimes referred to as Ogilvie's syndrome (incorrectly, unless malignancy is the cause).

This functional (i.e. non-mechanical) colonic obstruction can be a complication of pregnancy and delivery, most commonly caesarean section. Many (especially junior) surgeons will not be familiar with it in young women. The main features are:

- Increasing abdominal distension, which may be dramatic
- Bowel sounds may sound obstructive or absent
- Constipation is rarely absolute

Investigation and treatment includes the following:

- Abdominal radiographs will show generalised, and often relatively non-specific, distension of the colon. There is often, but not invariably, a cut-off seen in the region of the splenic flexure (where the parasympathetic fibres of the vagus nerve distribution meet those ascending from the pelvic nerves). Distension of the small bowel may also be present. As the condition progresses, the caecum will enlarge to a greater extent than the rest of the colon. If greater than 9 cm the risk of perforation is high. Patients may or may not complain of right iliac fossa pain. Tenderness, almost always present in the normal population, may be masked by the enlarged uterus. This is an absolute surgical emergency and immediate colonoscopic decompression is indicated
- A CT scan and colonoscopy can be used to decompress the bowel if simple measures to manage the ileus are not successful

- Opiate analgesia is often used to keep these patients comfortable and this can compound the problem. Avoiding opiates, and administering metoclopramide, can help. Whilst neostigmine use has been reported, it is rarely used nowadays even in the non-obstetric population. It is contraindicated in pregnancy as its stimulant effect on the myometrium can precipitate preterm labour
- If surgery is required due to failure of resolution (despite correction of electrolyte abnormalities, attempted colonoscopic decompression, mobilising the patient and withdrawing opiates), it should be carefully planned by an experienced consultant general surgeon taking into consideration the available imaging and individual patient features (previous abdominal surgery, habitus and so on). The aims of surgery are to assess the viability of and decompress the distended bowel in the safest way possible
- If diagnosis has been delayed and perforation has occurred with faecal peritonitis, an emergency laparotomy is required with full support from the intensive treatment unit and in line with NELA (National Emergency Laparotomy Audit) recommendations for emergency laparotomy, in addition to delivery of the fetus

Sigmoid volvulus

The incidence of volvulus is increased in pregnancy. Pain is left-sided and colicky in nature, whilst examination confirms an obstructive picture. A plain abdominal radiograph is usually diagnostic, and a flexible sigmoidoscopy is therapeutic.

Intestinal obstruction

Intestinal obstruction can be due to small or large bowel pathology. Small bowel obstruction is primarily related to adhesions, which are either congenital or follow previous abdominal surgery. External hernias should always be searched for and, if present, surgery will be required. Always check the femoral canal. Causes of large bowel obstruction are more likely to require intervention. Volvulus and pseudo-obstruction have already been discussed. Neoplasms and diverticular strictures can still occur in more elderly pregnant patients, and adequate investigation of suspected 'pseudo-obstruction' is essential to avoid missing an underlying mechanical cause, which will require either colonoscopic stenting or surgical resection.

The management of small bowel obstruction due to suspected adhesions is initially non-operative, with a high chance of success, in line with NASBO (National Audit of Small Bowel Obstruction), National Institute for Health and Social Care Excellence (NICE) and National Confidential Enquiry into Patient Outcome and Death (NCEPOD) guidelines. The patient is made 'nil by mouth', nasogastric aspiration is commenced and intravenous fluids administered. A CT scan is ideal to confirm the diagnosis in the first 24 hours. If unresolved at 24 hours, the administration of oral gastrograffin is recommended as a therapeutic modality. If the patient does not have a significant resolution within 24 hours then surgery is indicated. Depending on the gestation and fetal assessment, the fetus may need to be delivered at the time of laparotomy. Obviously if there are any signs of possible underlying bowel ischaemia, urgent laparotomy should be undertaken.

23.5 Summary

- Acute abdominal problems in pregnancy are difficult to diagnose and can be associated with a high morbidity and mortality to mother and fetus. Prompt diagnosis and treatment is therefore essential
- A high index of suspicion is required in all patients, together with early obstetric and general surgical consultant input
- When non-obstetric conditions are suspected, obstetricians should call on other specialists for advice, while remembering that few specialists have experience of dealing with pregnancy. The obstetrician must therefore ensure that a specialist of appropriate seniority is involved, and the consultant obstetrician must coordinate any multidisciplinary input
- It must always be remembered how well young, fit, pregnant women compensate for blood loss. Subtle early signs of shock must be sought, rather than waiting for a fall in blood pressure
- Be aware that obesity adds greatly to the diagnostic challenge

23.6 Further reading

Knight M, Bunch K, Tuffnell D, et al. (eds), on behalf of MBRRACE-UK. *Saving Lives, Improving Mothers' Care – Lessons Learned to Inform Maternity Care from the UK and Ireland Confidential Enquiries into Maternal Deaths and Morbidity 2016–18*. Oxford: National Perinatal Epidemiology Unit, University of Oxford, 2020.

Woodhead N, Nkwam O, Caddick V, Morad S, Mylvaganam S. Surgical causes of acute abdominal pain in pregnancy. *Obstet Gynaecol* 2019; 21: 27–35.

CHAPTER 24
Diabetic emergencies

Learning outcomes

After reading this chapter, you will be able to:

- Understand how pregnancy affects diabetes in order to manage it effectively
- Anticipate the health problems of women with pre-existing disease
- Appreciate the critical diagnostic features to recognise diabetic ketoacidosis in order to implement prompt treatment
- Take part in the urgent multidisciplinary care of pregnant and puerperal women with diabetic ketoacidosis

24.1 Introduction

The incidence of diabetes in pregnancy has increased significantly over the last 10–20 years, with a rise mainly being seen in the type 2 diabetics and gestational diabetes cohorts, a consequence of increased maternal age and obesity rates. For the first time, the National Pregnancy In Diabetes Audit (2018) showed that type 2 diabetes is now more prevalent than type 1 diabetes (NICE, 2020). Figures in the UK show that 16 out of 100 pregnant women will go on to develop gestational diabetes (Mohan et al., 2017). The fact that the number of women with a body mass index of 18–25 in pregnancy are in the minority helps explain these rising statistics; ethnicity is also relevant, as are changing population demographics.

Background to diabetic ketoacidosis (DKA)

Diabetic ketoacidosis (DKA) is a medical emergency in obstetrics that has serious consequences for both mother and baby, with fetal mortality reported between 9% and 36% in the published literature; new unpublished UK data show this rate to be 15%. Maternal mortality has improved and been reported as being 4–15%, however more recent UK data show that to be negligible, but morbidity is not insignificant. Long-term effects on the fetus are less understood. Potentially, there is an effect on placental blood flow with the overall maternal volume depletion seen during DKA. Maternal acidosis and electrolyte imbalance combined may cause fetal hypoxia.

In order to be able to treat DKA quickly and effectively, we need to understand why pregnancy makes a woman with diabetes more prone to this condition. The incidence of DKA is between 0.5% in non-pregnancy and nearly 9% in pregnancy. Whilst historically it has been recognised to affect type 1 diabetics in pregnancy, it must be remembered that it can potentially affect type 2 and gestational diabetics, although rarely. That is why the priority with any sick diabetic patient in pregnancy is to **exclude DIABETIC KETOACIDOSIS**.

24.2 Pathophysiology of DKA

Diabetic ketoacidosis occurs because there is a relative or complete absence of insulin at the same time as a relative increase in hormones such as catecholamines, cortisol and glucagon. This imbalance then results in an increase in gluconeogenesis and glycogenolysis, hence the classic triad of ketosis, hyperglycaemia and an acidosis. The ketosis is a result of increased free fatty acids available to the liver, secondary to the lipolysis that has occurred.

Managing Medical and Obstetric Emergencies and Trauma: A Practical Approach, Fourth Edition. Edited by Rosamunde Burns and Kara Dent.

The normal physiology of pregnancy means that the body has a lower buffering capacity than usual. Together with an increase in hormones such as human placental lactogen from the placenta, progesterone and cortisol, the pregnant woman is more resistant or less sensitive to insulin and therefore more prone to DKA. In addition, DKA can develop more rapidly than outside pregnancy. This hormonal effect becomes more pronounced throughout the pregnancy which is why DKA is seen more often in the latter two trimesters.

Risk factors such as socioeconomic deprivation, mental health disorders, poor pregnancy glycaemic control and precipitants such as infection, hyperemesis gravidarum and steroid administration are all relevant when considering risk of DKA. Sepsis and hyperemesis are both conditions that effectively dehydrate a pregnant woman, making them more susceptible to DKA. Known non-compliance with insulin therapy in pregnancy should alert clinicians to the risk of complications such as DKA as these patients can account for nearly a third of cases seen. Gastroperesis is a condition in diabetics to remember where there has been an autonomic neuropathy affecting the vagal nerve. It leads to the stomach working slower and more erratically, affecting the predictability of food absorption and good sugar control.

Changes in practice have seen important changes in the management of diabetics in pregnancy, enabling better control and reducing the risk of DKA. There is now central funding for continuous glucose monitoring (CGM) (using a sensor just under the skin) in most centres for type 1 or 2 diabetics who are pregnant. Type 1 diabetics should be given a ketone meter at the start of pregnancy to enable them to measure blood ketones as well as glucose levels, raising awareness of ketogenesis. Perhaps one of the most interesting developments is the use of insulin pumps. It should be remembered, however, that these pumps only contain short-acting insulin. Therefore, if there is an unrecognised blockage or malfunction in the delivery of this pump, the effects of no insulin will be quickly realised and the potential for DKA and hyperglycaemia increases.

24.3 Presentation of DKA

Diabetic ketoacidosis presents with an unwell pregnant patient who may complain of feeling generally unwell, blurred vision, nausea and vomiting and lethargy. Ketotic breath (classically smells like pear drops) may be noted. Initial observations may detect hypotension with tachycardia and hyperventilation. An altered mental state is a dangerous sign and is predictive of deteriorating DKA and imminent coma.

It is, however, very important to note that euglycemic ketoacidosis is more common in pregnancy than in the non-pregnant population and therefore should be considered.

Investigations are needed to confirm the diagnosis:

- Known diabetic and blood glucose >11.0 mmol/l
- Capillary blood ketone level ≥3 mmol/l or ++ ketones or more on urinalysis
- Venous bicarbonate <15 mmol/l ± venous pH <7.3

These immediate investigations will confirm your clinical suspicions and help you to assess the severity of the condition.

24.4 Treatment of DKA

Diabetic ketoacidosis is therefore a medical emergency that can affect the mother and fetus. The priority is prompt treatment with a multidisciplinary approach that involves the senior obstetric team, obstetric anaesthetists, endocrinologist or on-call physician and midwifery team in a high dependency unit (HDU) level 2 environment.

Hyperglycaemia causes loss of glucose into the urine and a resultant osmotic diuresis, which explains why there is a massive fluid depletion in DKA that then affects the electrolyte balance causing hypokalaemia. This loss can be dramatic, in the region of 6–10 litres or 100 ml/kg body weight.

The treatment of DKA should address four main areas to guide treatment. Observations should include measurement of blood pressure (particularly systolic), urine output and pulse oximetry. The four areas require a simultaneous approach in a timely fashion using the multidisciplinary team, as appropriate to their skills:

- **Aggressive fluid replacement**
- **Insulin infusion**
- **Electrolyte correction**
- **Identification and correction of cause**

Considering each individually:

1. **IV fluid replacement.** Most guidance recommends 0.9% normal saline (isotonic) infusion at a rate of 10–15 ml/kg/h for the first hour – which translates into approximately 1 litre in a 70 kg patient. Depending on the monitoring and observations, the patient will then then require 500 ml/h for the next 4 hours and 250 ml/h over the next 8 hours. When the blood glucose falls below 14 mmol/l, 10% dextrose can run simultaneously at a rate of 125 ml/h.
   The effect of the IV infusion is to restore the volume, thereby improving tissue perfusion and lowering the hyperglycaemic effect. This is best monitored by the response of the blood pressure and ultimately adequate urine output. An adequate urine output is 0.5 ml/kg/h or 30 ml in a patient weighing 60 kg.
2. **Insulin infusion.** DKA is a condition in which there is either no or very little insulin available. By treating with insulin immediately, the high levels of glucose are addressed and thereby the vicious cycle of gluconeogenesis and glycogenolysis is interrupted. This effect will be seen by a correction of the blood glucose levels and decrease in ketone levels. Intravenous treatment is essential to ensure optimal absorption as intramuscular/subcutaneous perfusion will be compromised.
3. **Electrolyte correction.** Insulin has the effect of pushing K^+ (potassium) into the intracellular space and causing hypokalaemia (which can cause significant cardiac effects). Insulin therapy should be administered with careful concurrent monitoring of K^+. If the serum K^+ is <5.5 mmol/l, potassium needs to be added to the intravenous fluids to correct the hypokalaemia. National recommendations are to give not more than 20 mmol of potassium per hour aiming for a K^+ level of between 3.3 and 5.5 mmol/l.
4. **Identification and correction of cause.** Without simultaneously addressing the cause or trigger for DKA, its effects are not going to be adequately reversed. The most common cause will be infection and its source needs to be identified by clinical examination and a screen for sepsis (e.g. urine, chest, chorioamnionitis) and subsequent administration of appropriate antibiotics (broad spectrum as per local protocol in the first instance). The white cell count is commonly elevated and non-specific in pregnancy; hence C-reactive protein (CRP) and neutrophil count are useful adjuncts.

The most important rule in dealing with DKA is to be vigilant for its presence and to treat it promptly. Fetal monitoring during a DKA crisis can be distracting as it may reflect the acidotic status and be abnormal. Monitoring will usually normalise as the DKA is corrected over a period of up to 4–6 hours. What is difficult to predict and not as well known is the potential long-term effect for the fetus, but stabilisation of the mother has to take priority before delivery is considered.

Urinary ketones take longer to disappear, even after the acidosis is corrected and there is an improvement in the maternal and fetal condition.

Management of DKA

Management of DKA follows the mMOET principles of a structured approach, concentrating on the four main areas outlined above.

1. Call for help.
2. ABC – Airway, breathing and circulation assessment. Signs of DKA include tachypnoea, tachycardia, hypotension and reduced hourly urine output.
3. D – Assessment using the ACVPU (**a**lert, new **c**onfusion, responds to **v**oice, responds to **p**ain, **u**nconscious) and Glasgow Coma Scale (GCS) score. Signs of agitation, altered mental state and lethargy may signal a deteriorating status with coma a possible consequence.
4. EF – Abnormal fetal cardiotocography (CTG) tracing may be evident.

Investigations in DKA

Investigations for assessment of DKA and possible causes include:

- Glucose: BM stix and formal blood glucose levels
- Ketones: urinary and serum levels
- Electrolytes: particularly K^+
- Arterial blood gases (ABG): for pH, bicarbonate and lactate levels and ketones
- Urine: urinalysis/mid-stream urine specimen for possible infection
- Full blood count/CRP/blood lactate/blood cultures
- Consider if a chest x-ray or electrocardiogram are needed

Monitoring of blood glucose and ketones should be hourly until stable. Urinary ketones will take some time to clear. Electrolytes and ABG may be required as frequently as 2 hourly if unstable. Patients should be being looked after in an HDU environment with multidisciplinary input from the obstetric team, on-call endocrinologist, physician or obstetric physician, anaesthetists and midwives.

24.5 Hypoglycaemia in pregnancy

Hypoglycaemia is seen commonly in pregnancy complicated by type 1 diabetes because of the need to have tight sugar control. Whilst it is believed to have little effect on the fetus, it can cause significant risks to the mother. Many women with diabetes will have reduced hypoglycaemia awareness in pregnancy. In trying so hard to achieve normoglycaemia, they are three times more at risk of hypoglycaemia, especially in the first trimester. It is important to educate them and their close contacts to look for signs in order to check their blood sugar levels, especially if they are driving. They also need to know how to treat themselves, including how to give glucagon; the diabetes specialist nurse may need to teach their partner this at the start of pregnancy.

Precipitants for hypoglycaemia are giving insulin for a predicted meal which is then missed, too much insulin given inadvertently and alcohol consumption. Risk factors are impaired awareness, strict control and disordered sleep. A classic cause is giving insulin for a predicted meal and then not eating as much as anticipated or underestimating the amount of exercise/energy expended. Quinine and beta-blockers can also cause hypoglycaemia.

Obstetric causes of hypoglycaemia in the non-diabetic population include acute fatty liver of pregnancy, severe sepsis and Sheehan's syndrome. Medical causes such as Addison's disease, end-stage renal/liver disease or an insulinoma should be excluded but are very rare.

Signs and symptoms of hypoglycaemia present with either autonomic (activation of the sympathoadrenal system) or neuroglycopenic (due to cerebral glucose deprivation) features. Warning symptoms are feeling hot and sweaty, hungry or perhaps more drowsy and lethargic. Speech may become blurred or vague, behaviour more irrational; women may complain of headache or nausea and feeling generally unwell. This should prompt checking of the blood glucose and immediate treatment of any abnormality. The new CGM systems and flash glucose monitoring systems alert patients of a low glucose event. The even newer CGM/pump systems should almost abolish the risk of hypoglycaemia in patients with diabetes.

Management of hypoglycaemia

Treating hypoglycaemia in pregnancy depends on whether the woman is conscious and able to swallow. If she can swallow (i.e. the GCS score is not affected) some quick acting carbohydrate is the first line – orange juice is a common choice or three Jelly Babies. If the patient is disorientated, glucogel or dextrogel can be administered between the teeth and gums where it is well absorbed. Glucagon 1 mg IM is the next step if treatment has been ineffective or in a situation where the woman cannot swallow or is losing consciousness.

If the hypoglycaemia is more severe with a woman who is unconscious or having seizures, a structured approach is needed:

1. Call for help.
2. **M**anual **u**terine **d**isplacement.
3. ABC – Check airway, breathing and circulation.
4. DE – DE-Assess disability with the ACVPU and reassess after each form of treatment.
5. Fetus – Performing a CTG during this episode is not helpful as treatment of the mother is the priority.
6. Glucose – This is needed intravenously. Start with 100 ml of 20% glucose over 15 minutes via a pump. Check the capillary blood glucose 10 minutes later and if <4.0 mmol/l, consider using 150–200 ml 10% glucose over the same time period. If this is still ineffective, give 1 mg glucagon IM.

24.6 Summary

- With an increasing prevalence of both pre-existing diabetes and gestational diabetes being seen in the pregnant population, a high index of suspicion of DKA or hypoglycaemic episodes is needed for prompt treatment
- Any diabetic pregnant woman should have her blood sugar monitored and be screened for ketones on admission if attending feeling unwell
- Successful treatment of DKA requires prompt aggressive fluid replacement, insulin infusion and correction of electrolytes whilst identifying and treating the underlying cause

24.7 Further reading

Mohan M, Baagar KAM, Lindow S. Management of diabetic ketoacidosis in pregnancy. *Obstet Gynaecol* 2017; 19: 55–62.

NICE National Institute for Health and Care Excellence. *Diabetes in Pregnancy: Management from Preconception to the Postnatal Period*. NG3. London: NICE, 2020.

Chapter 25: Neurological emergencies

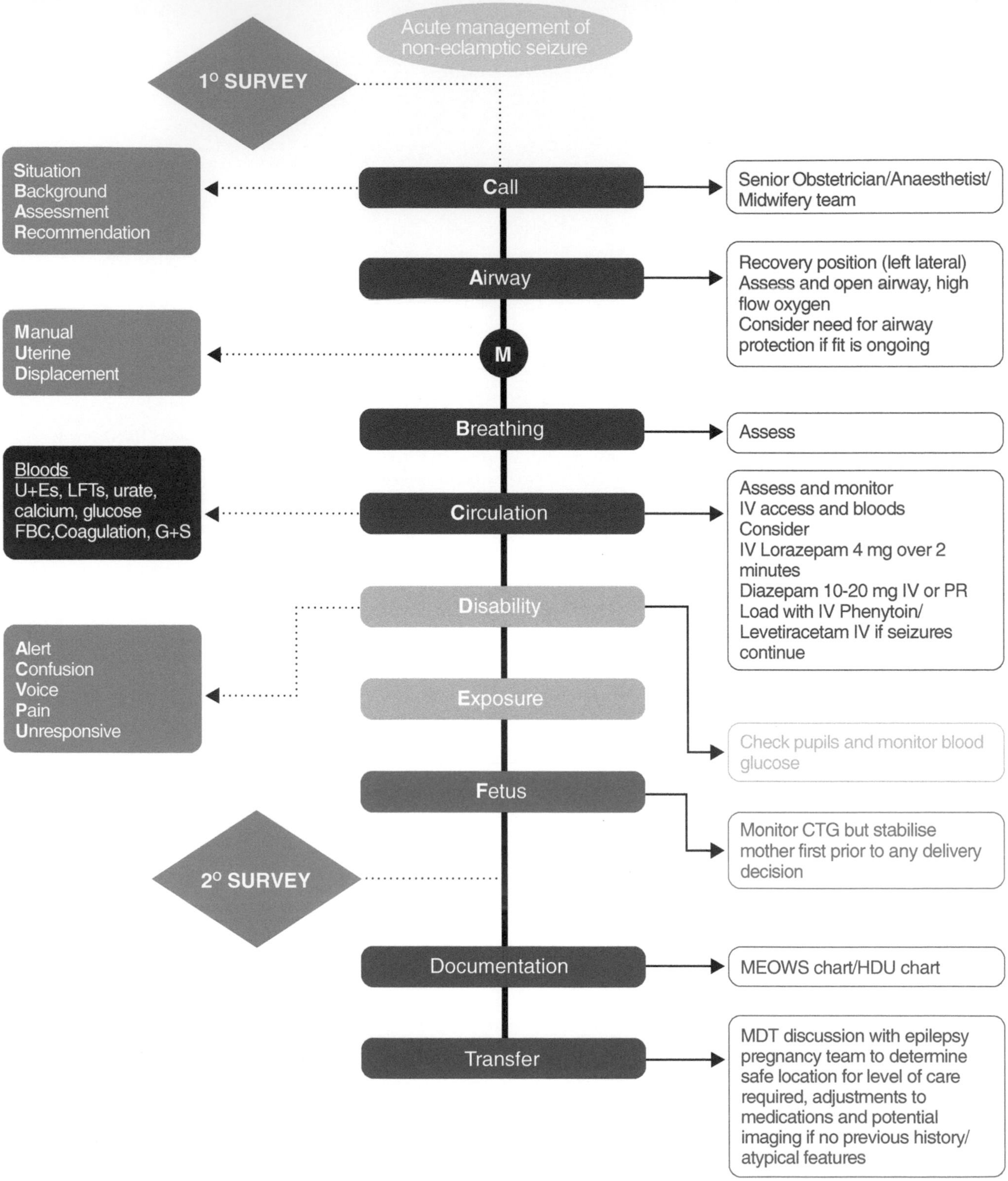

Acute management of non-eclamptic seizure
1° SURVEY
Situation
Background
Assessment
Recommendation
Call
Senior Obstetrician/Anaesthetist/ Midwifery team
Airway
Recovery position (left lateral)
Assess and open airway, high flow oxygen
Consider need for airway protection if fit is ongoing
Manual
Uterine
Displacement
M
Breathing
Assess
Bloods
U+Es, LFTs, urate, calcium, glucose
FBC,Coagulation, G+S
Circulation
Assess and monitor
IV access and bloods
Consider
IV Lorazepam 4 mg over 2 minutes
Diazepam 10-20 mg IV or PR
Load with IV Phenytoin/ Levetiracetam IV if seizures continue
Disability
Alert
Confusion
Voice
Pain
Unresponsive
Exposure
Check pupils and monitor blood glucose
Fetus
Monitor CTG but stabilise mother first prior to any delivery decision
2° SURVEY
Documentation
MEOWS chart/HDU chart
Transfer
MDT discussion with epilepsy pregnancy team to determine safe location for level of care required, adjustments to medications and potential imaging if no previous history/ atypical features

Algorithm 25.1 Neurological emergencies

CHAPTER 25

Neurological emergencies

Learning outcomes

After reading this chapter, you will be able to:

- Appreciate there are many causes of headache in pregnancy
- Understand that the 'red flag' symptoms of headache are key
- Appreciate the important clues in a detailed history and neurological examination
- Describe the causes and management of seizures in pregnancy
- Recognise the importance of investigation, management and referral outwith pregnancy

25.1 Introduction

Neurological diseases in general were the second most common cause of indirect maternal death in the 2021 MBRRACE-UK report after cardiac disease (Knight et al., 2021). These conditions can present at any point in pregnancy, with varying symptoms, and have the potential to cause serious and life-threatening outcomes. In particular, if these symptoms are initially mild and vague, the challenge for the clinician is to use their skill, judgement and experience to decide which patients should be investigated further. Early discussion with a neurologist to simply gain advice or make a referral is important. Pregnancy should not alter investigation and treatment of a patient presenting with headache or potential stroke.

25.2 Headache

Acute headache is a common but important symptom in pregnancy. Headache in pregnancy will usually have a benign cause but can indicate a more serious life-threatening problem. Failure to consider and recognise early potentially serious conditions can lead to significant morbidity and mortality (Revell and Morrish, 2014). The challenge for those caring for pregnant patients is therefore to systematically assess the pregnant patient complaining of headache and act promptly upon significant findings.

Classification of headache

Headache can be classified into primary and secondary (Table 25.1).

Managing Medical and Obstetric Emergencies and Trauma: A Practical Approach, Fourth Edition. Edited by Rosamunde Burns and Kara Dent.

Table 25.1 Possible causes of headache

Causes of primary headache	Causes of secondary headache
Migraine	Pre-eclampsia
Cluster headache	Posterior reversible encephalopathy syndrome (PRES)
Tension headache	Cerebral venous thrombosis (CVT)
	Subarachnoid haemorrhage (SAH)
	Stroke (thrombotic or haemorrhage)
	Reversible cerebral vasoconstriction (RCVS)
	Idiopathic intracranial hypertension
	Postdural puncture headache (PDPH)
	Meningitis/encephalitis
	Anaemia
	Caffeine withdrawal
	Intracranial mass lesions

Source: Adapted from Revell K, Morrish P. Headaches in pregnancy. *Obstet Gynaecol* 2014; 16: 179–84; Nelson-Piercy C. *Handbook of Obstetric Medicine*, 6th edn. Abingdon: CRC Press, 2020

Primary headache is the most likely diagnosis in pregnancy and is more common in the first trimester. Secondary causes of headache are more likely in the third trimester or postpartum period (Revell and Morrish, 2014; RCP, 2019).

These conditions can be difficult to identify, however an initial clinical assessment including a thorough history and neurological examination often helps to identify the correct diagnosis.

Clinical history

A thorough history can distinguish between benign and more serious causes of headache. Onset (e.g. thunderclap headache, think subarachnoid haemorrhage), duration, location, associated symptoms, presence of fever, and relationship to the current and previous pregnancies should be enquired about. The presence of any specific focal neurological symptoms such as limb weakness or cognitive disturbance should be sought. Confusion is an important finding in young women and could be a sign of cerebral thrombosis or other serious diagnoses (Revell and Morrish, 2014). A headache that wakes the patient from sleep is characteristic of a migraine or raised intracranial pressure (ICP).

Any postural nature of a headache is an important distinction. A headache that is worse on sitting up and improved on lying down implies a ***low cerebrospinal fluid pressure*** cause such as a postdural puncture headache. Conversely, a headache that is worse on lying down and improved when sitting up implies a ***high-pressure headache*** caused by, for example, intracranial neoplasm or hydrocephalus. A headache precipitated by physical exercise or a Valsalva manoeuvre should prompt consideration of a subarachnoid haemorrhage or raised ICP.

Any 'red flag' symptoms should also be elicited:

Red flags in the history and examination of a pregnant patient presenting with headaches:

- Sudden-onset headache/thunderclap or worst headache ever
- Headache that takes longer than usual to resolve or persists for more than 48 hours
- Has associated symptoms – fever, neck stiffness, drowsiness, seizures, focal neurology, photophobia, diplopia
- Excessive use of opioids

Source: RCP (Royal College of Physicians). *Acute Care Toolkit 15: Managing Acute Medical Problems in Pregnancy*. London: RCP, 2019. © 2019 Royal College of Physicians

Any patient with a severe or atypical headache or with a 'red flag' symptom should be discussed with a neurologist promptly and urgent imaging considered (RCP, 2019).

Examination

A full neurological examination should be carried out on all women with headache. This involves cranial nerve assessment including pupillary response to light, visual fields, eye movements, speech and swallow. Tone, power, reflexes, sensation and co-ordination should be tested in all four limbs. Examination for neck stiffness is a mandatory part of the examination of a patient with new or atypical headache and is a very simple and quick to do (Knight et al., 2020).

For patients in whom pre-eclampsia is being considered, the routine tests of blood pressure, proteinuria and clonus should be investigated.

Fundoscopy is an important examination to look for papilloedema, a sign of raised ICP (Figure 25.1). MBRRACE-UK recommends that fundoscopy should be mandatory in the assessment of a patient with new or atypical headache (Knight et al., 2020). However, it is clear that not all clinicians may feel comfortable doing this or may lack the required skill, and hence referral to a clinician who can perform fundoscopy is a priority while further investigation of the headache is ongoing.

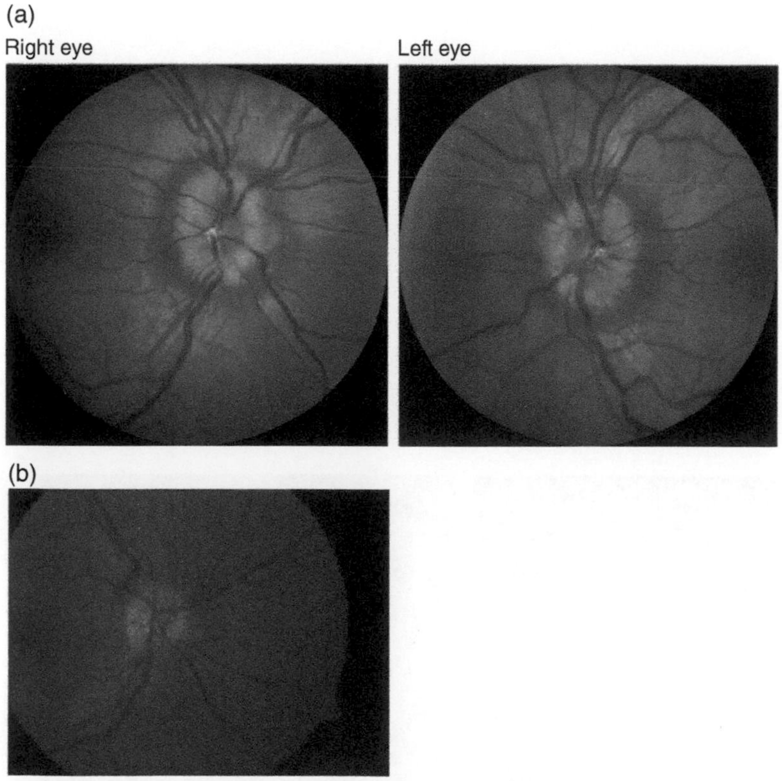

Figure 25.1 (a) Fundoscopy examination showing papilloedema. (b) Normal retina
Source: (a) Friedman DI. *Headache Curr* 2005; 2(1): 1–10. https://doi.org/10.1111/j.1743-5013.2005.20101.x. (b) Machner B, et al. *Eur J Neurol* 2008; 15(7): e68–9. https://doi.org/10.1111/j.1468-1331.2008.02152.x

25.3 Primary headache

Migraine

Migraine is the most common cause of primary headache in women and especially during child-bearing years. Pregnancy can lead to a reduction in frequency and severity of migraine without aura. A patient suffering a migraine will classically describe a moderate to severe, unilateral, pulsating pain which builds up over minutes to hours. A migraine can be associated with nausea and vomiting and sensitivity to light and sound, and can be made worse by routine physical activity. Interestingly, pregnancy can alter the aura associated with migraine and can trigger an aura without a headache, associated with increased oestrogen levels. This can manifest as fully reversible disturbances of vision, motor function and sensation. Hemiplegic migraine can mimic a transient ischaemic attack. Postpartum exacerbation of symptoms is common as oestrogen levels fall (Revell and Morrish, 2014; OAA, 2018).

Management involves avoidance of precipitants, rest and hydration. In an acute attack, paracetamol-based analgesics with metoclopramide is the treatment of choice. Other antiemetics (e.g. cyclizine), dihydrocodeine or short courses of non-steroidal anti-inflammatory drugs (NSAIDs) (in the first and second trimester) may be considered. Sumatriptan and other 5-HT1 agonists are used frequently in non-pregnant patients. There are limited data of their use in pregnancy that are reassuring, and thus they can be used occasionally where they are the only therapy found to gain control of an attack. For frequent attacks, prophylaxis may be considered: low-dose aspirin (75 mg daily) is first line, while beta-blockers (propranolol 10–40 mg tds) can be used in resistant cases. Together these are successful for 80% of patients. Thereafter tricyclic antidepressants (amitriptyline 25–50 mg at night) or calcium channel blocker (verapamil 40–80 mg at night) may be considered in refractory cases (Nelson-Piercy, 2020).

25.4 Secondary headache

Pre-eclampsia

Headache and/or flashing lights can be part of the clinical presentation of pre-eclampsia. It is worth noting that headache is the most common prodromal symptom prior to a seizure (Revell and Morrish, 2014).

Posterior reversible encephalopathy syndrome (PRES) is a clinical condition associated with pre-eclampsia, characterised by headache, vomiting, visual disturbance, seizures and altered mental state. Radiologically, oedema can be seen in the posterior circulation of the brain (Figure 25.2). This is usually a transient disturbance and symptoms and signs usually resolve quickly with treatment (Revell and Morrish, 2014; Nelson-Piercy, 2020).

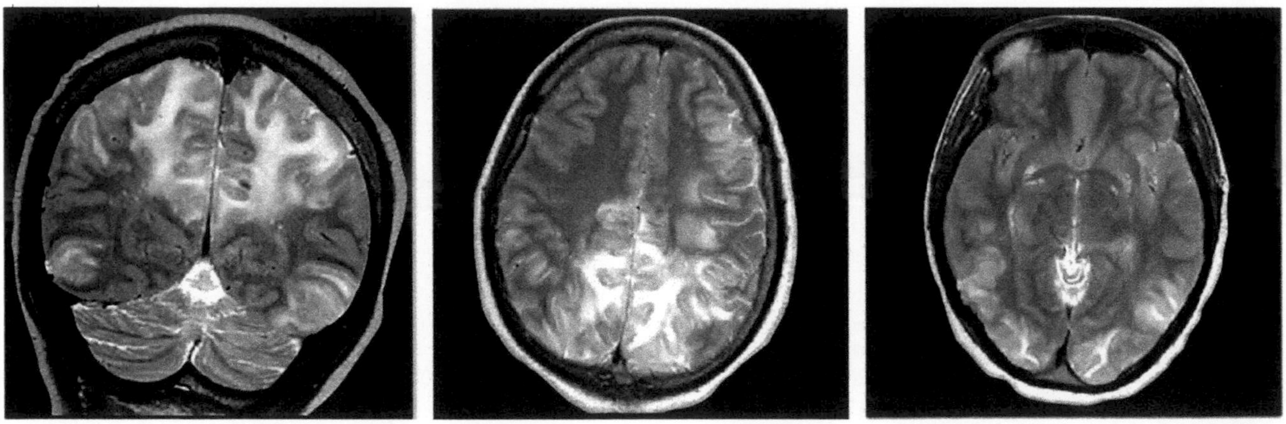

Figure 25.2 MRI images demonstrating posterior reversible encephalopathy syndrome (PRES). These coronal and axial images show increased signal uptake (white) in the parietal and occipital lobes bilaterally which demonstrates cerebral oedema in the typical pattern

Source: Ayanambakkam A, et al. A postpartum perfect storm. *Am J Hematol* 2017; 92(10): 1105–10. https://doi.org/10.1002/ajh.24848

Prompt recognition and management is key. When PRES is caused by pre-eclampsia, the management follows the same treatment protocol with particular attention to blood pressure control, management of seizures and expedited delivery of the fetus (Revell and Morrish, 2014).

Cerebral venous thrombosis

Pregnancy is a recognised risk factor for cerebral venous thrombosis (CVT), thought to be due to prothrombotic changes and dehydration. Caesarean section, anaemia, infection and accidental dural puncture can also increase the risk. Risk is increased in the third trimester and for 4 weeks postpartum. Thrombosis of the sagittal sinus with extension into the cortical veins or primary thrombosis of one of the cortical veins are the most common sites.

Severe headache is usually the first symptom; this can be acute in onset, localised and continuous in nature. Headache can rarely be the only complaint but other clinical findings often include focal neurology, altered Glasgow Coma Scale (GCS) score and seizures. Cranial nerve signs, in particular a sixth nerve palsy resulting in diplopia, can be seen. The onset of symptoms can in some cases be insidious over days or weeks.

Plain computed tomography (CT), which is usually the first radiological investigation in a patient with headache, does not show CVT well and is abnormal in only 30% of cases. Magnetic resonance imaging (MRI) and magnetic resonance venography (MRV) are the investigations of choice (Figure 25.3) (Revell and Morrish, 2014).

When CVT is suspected, prompt referral to neurology is key. Management involves full-dose anticoagulation after haemorrhage is excluded.

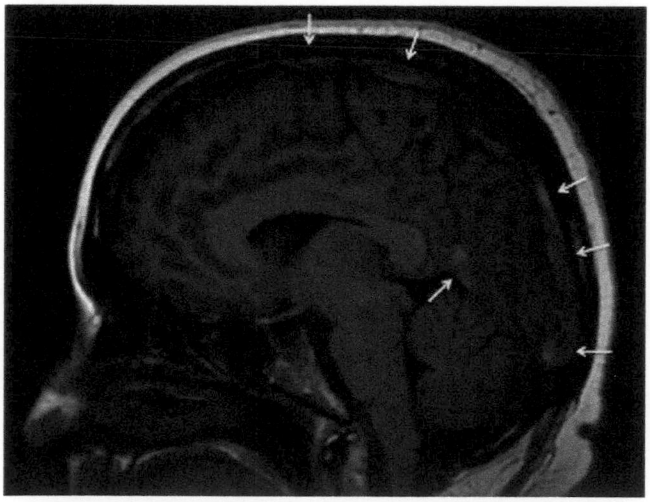

Figure 25.3 Magnetic resonance venography of a filling defect showing extensive filling defects in all the major cerebral veins consistent with extensive cerebral venous sinus thrombosis (yellow arrows)
Source: Ho P, et al. *Intern Med J* 2015; 45(6): 682–3

Subarachnoid haemorrhage

This is most common in the third trimester of pregnancy. Incidence is approximately 20 in 100 000 pregnancies. It characteristically presents with a sudden onset, severe headache known as a 'thunderclap', with the maximum intensity lasting less than 1 minute. Other symptoms include reduced GCS score, photophobia and neurological deficits. If suspected, an urgent CT scan of the head should be performed (Figure 25.4). The sensitivity of this investigation reduces with time (almost 100% sensitive at 24 hours, 50% at 1 week). If CT of the head is negative the patient should have a lumbar puncture to investigate for xanthochromia.

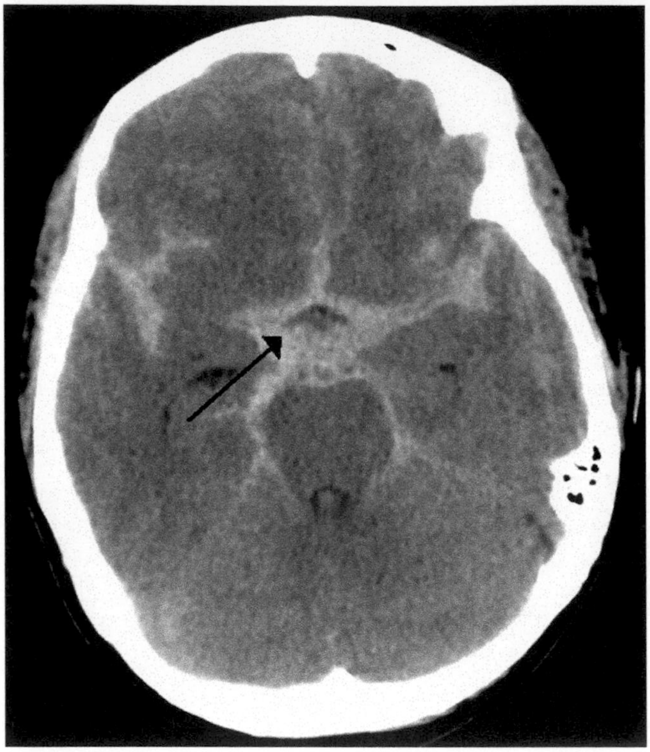

Figure 25.4 Computed tomography scan of the head showing blood in the subarachnoid space
Source: James Heilman, MD / Wikipedia Commons / Public Domain

Neurosurgical or radiological management should be the same as for non-pregnant patients. Nimodipine, used to limit neurological deficits following subarachnoid haemorrhage, should be given in pregnancy and postpartum (Nelson-Piercy, 2020).

Stroke

As with non-pregnant patients, stroke can be caused by arterial thrombosis (ischaemic) or intracerebral haemorrhage. The incidence of 30 per 100 000 is three times higher in pregnancy compared with non-pregnant women of the same age. Patients may present with headache, slurred speech, seizures or neurological deficits. Urgent CT or MRI investigation is recommended. Antenatal stroke is rare, and more likely to occur peripartum or within 6 weeks postpartum.

Ischaemic stroke

Pregnancy is associated with an increased risk of cerebral infarction. Most strokes occur in the distribution of the carotid and middle cerebral arteries and occur in the first week after delivery.

Haemorrhagic stroke

This is almost as common as ischaemic stroke in pregnancy and is often associated with pre-eclampsia/eclampsia and rupture of an arteriovenous malformation. Medical therapy involves careful blood pressure management.

Management

Management of stroke is as for the non-pregnant patient. Being pregnant or in the immediate postpartum state or having had an operative delivery are not absolute contraindications to thrombolysis (intravenous or intra-arterial), clot retrieval or craniectomy and this should not alter investigation or treatment. Optimising oxygenation and haemodynamics is key and thereafter the cause will dictate management. Urgent referral to a stroke unit is recommended (Knight et al., 2020; Nelson-Piercy, 2020).

Reversible cerebral vasoconstriction syndrome

Reversible cerebral vasoconstriction syndrome (RCVS) usually presents in the early postpartum period. It is characterised by recurrent, severe, 'thunderclap' headache together with nausea and vomiting, photophobia and confusion. Cerebral angiography confirms segmental arterial narrowing, which is characteristic and signifies dysregulation of cerebral arterial tone (OAA, 2018).

Conservative treatment is with calcium channel blockers such as nimodipine, corticosteroids and magnesium sulphate. The condition is self-limiting and usually lasts 1–3 months; however, permanent neurological damage and death can occur. RCVS is a differential of subarachnoid haemorrhage and is often diagnosed when the 'thunderclap' headache reoccurs (Revell and Morrish, 2014).

Idiopathic intracranial hypertension

This is a rare condition and mostly occurs in young obese women. It can present for the first time during pregnancy and pre-existing disease can be worsened by becoming pregnant.

The headache is described as generalised and constant, and is intensified by coughing or straining. Visual signs such as diplopia (38%) or visual loss (31%) and papilloedema can occur. Diagnosis requires demonstration of elevated ICP >20 cmH_2O on lumbar puncture.

Management involves encouraging weight loss; a therapeutic lumbar puncture and acetazolamide (after the first trimester) can reduce the ICP and give symptomatic relief. Monitoring of the visual fields and acuity is important as optic nerve infarction can occur (Revell and Morrish, 2014).

Postdural puncture headache

Postdural puncture headache (PDPH) can occur in patients who have had an epidural or spinal anaesthetic during labour or delivery. PDPH usually develops within 24–72 hours of the procedure but can be delayed for 5 days postnatal. The incidence is 1 in every 100 women who have an epidural and 1 in 500 for spinals (OAA, 2018).

The headache is caused by cerebrospinal fluid leaking out from a hole in the dura, made by the epidural or spinal needle, into the epidural space, resulting in low-pressure headache. Classically this is a postural headache where the patient has worsening symptoms on sitting up from a lying position.

Diagnosis is made clinically; radiological investigations are not very useful. A careful history and examination should be carried out to exclude other potential causes of postnatal headache. The woman usually complains of a frontal or occipital headache, postural in nature, which can be of sudden onset. She may also complain of neck pain, diplopia, nausea and vomiting and abnormal hearing as if 'hearing underwater'.

PDPH can in severe cases be complicated by a subdural haematoma that occurs due to the stretching of the bridging veins as the brain sags. It is also a risk factor for CVT.

Patients with PDPH should be reviewed daily by the anaesthesia team and given information on who to contact if symptoms change or worsen when they are discharged from hospital. Follow-up should continue until the headache resolves. The patient's GP and community midwife should be informed of treatments received and what follow-up has been arranged (OAA, 2018).

Management

The patient may gain symptomatic relief by lying in bed for prolonged periods but this is not recommended as it can increase the risk of thromboembolic complications. Patients should be prescribed thromboprophylaxis. Adequate fluid intake should be encouraged and simple analgesia prescribed (paracetamol, NSAIDs and weak opioids if there are no contraindications). Stronger opioids may be required but should only be offered for a maximum of 3 days. There is limited evidence of the benefit of caffeine in the treatment of PDPH.

An epidural blood patch should be considered when symptoms are significant and are affecting the woman's ability to care for her child. This procedure results in permanent relief of symptoms in approximately 30% of patients following epidural and partial relief in 50–80% of cases. This procedure can be repeated in some circumstances (OAA, 2018).

25.5 Differential diagnosis of seizures in pregnancy

Eclampsia

Any woman presenting with a seizure in the second half of her pregnancy that cannot be clearly attributed to epilepsy should be treated as having eclampsia. Immediate treatment is with magnesium sulphate until a definitive diagnosis is made (RCOG, 2016).

Epilepsy

This is the most common neurological disease in pregnancy. Approximately 2500 pregnancies in the UK involve women with epilepsy. During pregnancy, these patients should be seen early by an epilepsy specialist to optimise seizure control, and their diagnosis and treatment plan should be documented and available, particularly out of hours. Patients with nocturnal, poorly controlled seizures or those patients whose seizure treatment is ineffective are high risk for sudden unexpected death in epilepsy (SUDEP). These patients warrant urgent referral to an epilepsy service (Knight et al., 2019, 2020).

Other causes of seizures

Other causes of seizures include the following (RCOG, 2016; Nelson-Piercy, 2020).

Intracranial

- Stroke
- Subarachnoid haemorrhage (SAH)
- Cerebral venous thrombosis (CVT)
- Posterior reversible encephalopathy syndrome (PRES)
- Space occupying lesions
- Reversible cerebral vasoconstriction syndrome (RCVS)
- Infection, e.g. toxoplasmosis
- Thrombotic thrombocytopenic purpura

Cardiac (collapse with jerking movements which could be mistaken for seizure activity)

- Syncope secondary to cardiac arrhythmia
- Aortic stenosis
- Carotid sinus sensitivity
- Vasovagal syncope

Metabolic

- Hypoglycaemia
- Hyponatraemia
- Hypocalcaemia
- Addisonian crisis

Neuropsychiatric

- Non-epileptic attack disorder (pseudo-seizures)

Other

- Drug or alcohol withdrawal

25.6 Acute management of a seizure

- The obstetric emergency team should be alerted immediately
- If >20/40 weeks' gestation, aortocaval compression should be relieved by manual uterine displacement or full left lateral position
- Systematic ABCDE approach
- If eclampsia is considered, give magnesium sulphate 4 g loading dose over 5–15 minutes, then 1 g/hour infusion as per the eclampsia protocol
- If not thought to be eclampsia, give IV lorazepam 4 mg over 2 minutes or diazepam 10–20 mg IV or PR
- Load with IV levetiracetam or IV phenytoin if seizure continues
- If ongoing seizure activity continues despite medical management, the patient may require a general anaesthetic, intubation and ventilation by the anaesthesia team. Stabilise the mother before any surgical input, the aim is not to deliver at this time. Cardiotocographic (CTG) monitoring is not helpful at this point (Nelson-Piercy, 2020)

25.7 Summary

Headache is a very common neurological symptom in pregnancy. It is usually caused by a benign process and can be managed conservatively. However, there are some rarer causes of headache which are very serious and require prompt investigation and treatment to prevent or limit long-term sequelae. These conditions can be difficult to diagnose, however an initial clinical assessment including a detailed history and neurological examination often helps to identify those patients who should be investigated further. Any patient with a severe or atypical headache or who complains of a 'red flag' symptom should be discussed with a neurologist promptly and urgent imaging considered.

A patient who is pregnant or recently pregnant should not be excluded from optimal investigation or management. Specialist neurology advice should be sought.

There are many causes for seizures in pregnancy. Eclampsia should be considered in any patient presenting with a seizure, particularly in the second trimester onwards. Patients with known epilepsy should be closely monitored by an epilepsy specialist during their pregnancy. The immediate management of a seizure aims for seizure control before a surgical decision to deliver the fetus is made.

25.8 Further reading

Knight M, Bunch K, Tuffnell D, et al. (eds), on behalf of MBRRACE-UK. *Saving Lives, Improving Mothers' Care – Lessons Learned to Inform Maternity Care from the UK and Ireland Confidential Enquiries into Maternal Deaths and Morbidity 2015–17*. Oxford: National Perinatal Epidemiology Unit, University of Oxford, 2019.

Knight M, Bunch K, Tuffnell D, et al. (eds), on behalf of MBRRACE-UK. *Saving Lives, Improving Mothers' Care – Lessons Learned to Inform Maternity Care from the UK and Ireland Confidential Enquiries into Maternal Deaths and Morbidity 2016–18*. Oxford: National Perinatal Epidemiology Unit, University of Oxford, 2020.

Knight M, Bunch K, Tuffnell D, et al. (eds), on behalf of MBRRACE-UK. *Saving Lives, Improving Mothers' Care – Lessons Learned to Inform Maternity Care from the UK and Ireland Confidential Enquiries into Maternal Deaths and Morbidity 2017–19*. Oxford: National Perinatal Epidemiology Unit, University of Oxford, 2021.

Nelson-Piercy C. *Handbook of Obstetric Medicine*, 6th edn. Abingdon: CRC Press, 2020.

OAA (Obstetric Anaesthetists' Association). *Treatment of Obstetric Post-Dural Puncture Headache*. London: OAA, 2018.

RCOG (Royal College of Obstetrics and Gynaecologists). *Epilepsy in Pregnancy*. Green-top Guideline No. 68. London: RCOG, 2016.

RCP (Royal College of Physicians). *Acute Care Toolkit 15: Managing Acute Medical Problems in Pregnancy*. London: RCP, 2019.

Revell K, Morrish P. Headaches in pregnancy. *Obstet Gynaecol* 2014; 16: 179–84.

CHAPTER 26

Perinatal psychiatric illness

Learning outcomes

After reading this chapter, you will be able to:

- Outline the prevalence of mental health problems in the pregnant population
- Recognise the importance of identifying the at-risk woman
- Be aware of the need for team working with mental health teams
- Be prepared for the onset of acute mental health problems after delivery
- Understand the effects on the baby of maternal mental health medications and the need to collaborate with other specialties, both in pregnancy and after birth

26.1 Introduction

Mental health problems are common in the community at large. The most common mental health problems are anxiety and depression. Women are at least twice as likely to suffer from these conditions as men and they are particularly prevalent among younger women with children under the age of 5 years. Serious mental illnesses, such as schizophrenia and bipolar disorder (manic depressive illness), are less common, with a prevalence of approximately 1% for each condition and are equally common in women and men.

26.2 Mental health problems in pregnancy

Conception rates in women with mental disorder (with the exception of severe learning disability and anorexia nervosa) are the same as the general population. Antenatal depression and anxiety are therefore common and as common after delivery, affecting 10–20% of all women. In addition, personality disorders, panic disorder, obsessive compulsive disorder, psychoses, substance misuse and eating disorders can all be encountered in pregnant women.

The incidence (new onset) of serious mental illness (schizophrenia, psychoses and bipolar disorder) during pregnancy is markedly reduced compared with other times. However, serious mental illness can occur for the first time during pregnancy and poses particular management problems. A more frequent situation is that of a woman who already has a chronic serious mental illness and becomes pregnant. Approximately two per 1000 births are to women with chronic serious mental illness. Pregnancy is not protective against a relapse of these conditions, particularly if patients stop taking their medication. However, continuing medication can occasionally pose problems for the fetus, management during labour and for the care of the newborn, and a careful risk–benefit analysis must be undertaken before any decision is made whether to continue or not.

Managing Medical and Obstetric Emergencies and Trauma: A Practical Approach, Fourth Edition. Edited by Rosamunde Burns and Kara Dent.

26.3 Mental health problems after delivery

By contrast, there is a dramatic increase in the incidence of serious affective illness following delivery. Women face an increased risk (relative risk of 32) of developing a psychotic illness in the first 3 months following delivery. Postpartum psychosis is often thought to be somewhere on the bipolar spectrum of illnesses. There is also an increased risk (relative risk of 10) of developing a severe unipolar depressive illness whereas there is no increase in risk of developing schizophrenia. Women who have a previous history of bipolar illness, schizoaffective disorder, puerperal psychosis or severe postnatal depression (PND) have at least a 25–50% risk of recurrence of this condition following delivery (if untreated), even if they have been well for many years and are in comfortable social circumstances. The early postnatal period is particularly vulnerable with 50% of puerperal psychoses having presented by day 7, 75% by day 14 and all by 42 days. Women without a personal history but with a family history of bipolar illness (particularly if it is of postpartum onset or who have a first degree relative who has had a puerperal psychosis) also face an elevated albeit smaller risk of developing postpartum psychosis following delivery (~1%) compared with the general population risk of 0.001–0.002%.

These serious postpartum mental illnesses, which become manifest in the early days following delivery, are life threatening. Although the early symptoms can be non-specific (e.g. insomnia, irritability and/or agitation), women can very quickly become acutely disturbed, very frightened and bewildered, and their illness poses a risk to their physical health and safety. They require urgent psychiatric assessment and treatment and should be admitted to a mother and baby unit rather than to a general psychiatry ward.

Severe, but non-psychotic, depressive illness tends to develop more gradually and present later with a bimodal peak at 6 and 12 weeks following delivery. While it benefits from specialist psychiatric care, it can frequently be managed at home with the usual treatments for severe depressive illness, mindful of whether the woman is breastfeeding.

The more common mild to moderate depressive illness, often associated with marked features of anxiety (PND), is in fact no more common following childbirth than in women who have not given birth. These conditions usually occur less acutely and generally not in the early postnatal period, and are best managed in primary care involving more psychological/talking therapies where appropriate. For these conditions, psychosocial treatments are often as effective as antidepressants.

26.4 Confidential Enquiries into Maternal Deaths (CEMD)

The triennial reports of the CEMD over the period from 1997 to 2005 revealed that if late deaths are included, then up to 25% of maternal deaths were caused by psychiatric disorders and 15% by suicide, with suicide identified as the leading cause of maternal death in the UK. The 2006–2008 report only includes late deaths up to 6 months, so direct comparisons cannot be made with previous figures. This report also highlighted the fact that many of the psychiatric deaths that occurred took place shortly after a child protection case conference, or a child being removed into care. A third of the women who committed suicide, and half of the women who were substance misusers, appeared to be avoiding maternity care. Furthermore, substandard care associated with psychiatric deaths is present in approximately 50% of patients.

Women who died from suicide were in the main older, more socially advantaged and better educated than in other causes of maternal death. Suicide is not associated with the same socioeconomic factors as other causes of maternal death. The majority were seriously mentally ill before they died. They had been well during pregnancy and developed either a puerperal psychosis or very severe depressive illness. Over 50% of these women had had a previous episode requiring inpatient psychiatric treatment, even though they had been well for some time before giving birth. This identifiable risk factor had, in most cases, neither been identified at booking, nor had the management of this risk been planned during pregnancy. Both psychiatric and maternity services had failed to take the opportunity to anticipate the risk following delivery. The rapid deterioration of a sudden onset illness appears to have taken all by surprise.

There was little evidence of communication taking place between psychiatric and maternity teams and the lack of planning was reflected in the paucity of information that was passed between involved professionals.

The remainder of the psychiatric deaths, those not due to suicide, were due to women dying from physical illness that could either be directly attributable to their psychiatric disorder (in half the cases, the consequences of alcohol or drug misuse) or because their life-threatening illness was missed or misattributed to psychiatric disorder. Obstetricians and midwives are reminded that serious physical illness can present as, complicate or coexist with psychiatric disorder.

Women who are substance misusers should have integrated specialist care. They should not be managed solely by their GP or midwife. Integrated care should include addiction professionals, child safeguarding and specialist midwifery and obstetric care. Care of the mother should continue once a child has been removed.

The most recent MBRRACE-UK report (2020) confirms that maternal suicide is now the fifth largest cause of death during pregnancy and the first 42 days after delivery, but it is the leading cause of death when considering a year post delivery, similar to previous reports. Looking at the deaths in pregnancy and up to 1 year, one in nine women die by suicide. The 2017 report previously made some strong recommendations:

- Women with a past history of ***any*** psychotic disorder (even when not diagnosed as postpartum psychosis or bipolar disorder) should be referred for an individual assessment and mental health plan, recognising they will be at risk. Ideally this plan should be made by 28–32 weeks into the pregnancy
- There is a responsibility for the mental health team to ensure women who do experience postpartum psychosis on recovery receive a clear explanation of their risks in the future, together with risk-minimising strategies. The need for re-referral in subsequent pregnancies should be shared with relevant professionals in order to try and minimise future risk

Implications for obstetric practice

The long-standing knowledge of the epidemiology and distinctive clinical features of perinatal psychiatric disorder, together with the findings of the confidential enquiries, provide the evidence base for obstetric and midwifery practice and for the psychiatric care of pregnant and postpartum women.

- All women of childbearing age with serious mental illness, and those taking psychotropic medication, should discuss with their general practitioner, psychiatrist or obstetrician their plans for becoming pregnant, the risks to their mental health and the risks to the developing fetus of their medication. Specialist perinatal mental health services offer pre-conceptual counselling and advice
- All women should be asked in a systematic and sensitive way about their previous, as well as current, psychiatric history at booking in early pregnancy. These questions should be structured so that those with a previous or current history of serious mental illness, previous psychiatric care and/or admission can be identified. Those responsible for booking should receive training to enable them to distinguish between serious psychiatric disorders and common mental health problems
- Women with serious mental health problems currently, or those with a past history of a serious psychiatric disorder, should have a written management plan shared between the woman, the general practitioner, obstetrician and psychiatrist, with regard to her peripartum management and the management of her risk in the early weeks following delivery
- Women with serious mental health problems complicating pregnancy and the early postpartum period should have access to a specialist psychiatrist in perinatal mental health, supported by a specialist multidisciplinary team and, if this is not available, to general psychiatric services
- In child protection cases, while the needs of the child must remain paramount, extra support and vigilance is needed for the mother and communication between all agencies involved in her care is essential. Further efforts are required to retain women who are substance misusers in treatment programmes after their child has been removed. Social workers should liaise with, and refer pregnant women in their care to, the local maternity services if necessary

Despite many national recommendations, specialist perinatal mental health teams have yet to be developed in the majority of maternity localities and there are insufficient mother and baby units in the UK to ensure equity of access for all. In addition, both the psychiatric and maternity professions have yet to fully acknowledge and implement the need for screening and proactive management of this high-risk group of women. Therefore, sadly, midwives and obstetricians will still be presented with women in late pregnancy and shortly after delivery with serious psychiatric disorders who have not been previously identified, as well as those who develop illnesses at this time that could not have been anticipated.

26.5 Management of mental health problems

Management of well 'at-risk' women

The well 'at-risk' woman will have been well often for many years, but will have a previous history of either puerperal psychosis or severe PND or a previous episode of bipolar illness. She may not have been in contact with psychiatric services for some time, will not be taking any medication and may be in very comfortable social circumstances and be well educated. Ideally, she should have been detected at the booking clinic and should have been seen by a specialist psychiatrist during pregnancy. The risk of a recurrence of the condition and a management plan should have been drawn up during pregnancy. However, often this has not happened and the risk may be identified only in late pregnancy or on admission to the labour suite.

There are no particular management concerns during labour. If no management plan is in place then the risk of recurrence of the puerperal psychosis or bipolar illness should be explained to the woman and her family. She should be seen by the psychiatrist serving the maternity hospital as soon as possible following delivery, preferably before she is discharged. The maximum risk of a recurrence of the condition is in the first 2 weeks following delivery, with the most frequent onset on day 1 postnatally, so early contact is essential. The minimum requirement will be that the community midwife and GP are alerted and that, together with the psychiatric team, the woman's mental health should be closely monitored over the first 6 weeks following delivery. Ideally, there should be a specialist perinatal mental health team involved, but these are not available to all maternity services.

The psychiatrist may consider using prophylactic medication including a mood stabiliser such as lithium or an antipsychotic (such as olanzapine or quetiapine), if this is acceptable to the woman. There needs to be discussion regarding breastfeeding and the woman made aware that breastfeeding is contraindicated in those taking lithium.

Management of women with chronic severe mental illness

Women with chronic severe mental illness are usually still under the care of psychiatric services. They may be suffering from either chronic schizophrenia and receiving antipsychotic medication, or from bipolar illness and receiving mood stabilisers, antidepressants or antipsychotic medication. Ideally, these women should not present unannounced. There should have been frequent communication and joint management during the pregnancy, consideration given to the choice of medication and its management during pregnancy. There should also be clear, written management plans for both the peripartum period and for her care following delivery.

Women with bipolar illness may be taking lithium carbonate or other mood stabilisers. The haemodynamics of later pregnancy and increased clearance of lithium may well have resulted in increasing oral doses of lithium in order to maintain a therapeutic lithium level (0.4–1.0 mmol/l) during pregnancy. High levels at delivery can be associated with toxicity in the mother and neonate and for this reason lithium should not be administered after labour starts. Close monitoring of her serum lithium levels postnatally, at least twice in the first week following delivery, to guard against increasing levels and the possibility of lithium toxicity (levels higher than 1.5 mmol/l). Following delivery, the dosage of lithium will need to be reinstated at her usual pre-pregnancy dose. The neonatal paediatricians should be made aware. Some women with bipolar disorder will be taking an anticonvulsant mood stabiliser as an alternative to lithium. The most common preparation in use for the management of bipolar illness is sodium valproate. Despite clear guidance from the National Institute for Health and Care Excellence (NICE) and the Coordination Group for Mutual and Decentralised Procedures – human (CMDh) on the management of both epilepsy and bipolar disorder – ***that sodium valproate should not be used in pregnancy and in women of reproductive age***, unless there is no reasonable alternative – this situation still occurs. The government advice is that it must no longer be used unless there is a pregnancy prevention programme in place. If it does arise, the neonatal paediatrician should be alerted. Following delivery, the dose of sodium valproate should be adjusted back to the pre-pregnancy dose and continued, because of the high risk of a relapse of the bipolar disorder following delivery. If the woman wishes to breastfeed, then sodium valproate, or other antiepileptic mood stabiliser, should be given in divided dosage and the neonate monitored for drowsiness and rashes.

A variety of antipsychotic medications may be taken by women with chronic serious mental illness. Some will still be taking the older antipsychotics (such as trifluoperazine and haloperidol). These preparations do not appear to be associated either with an increased risk of major congenital abnormalities or with any particular problems during pregnancy. Most women will be taking atypical antipsychotics (including olanzapine, quetiapine, risperidone and aripiprazole). There are fewer data available on these newer drugs. There is a concern that these medications may potentially be associated with an increased risk of gestational diabetes. In an ideal world, these concerns will have been discussed by the psychiatrist and obstetricians prior to delivery and the pros and cons of the medication considered. The neonatal paediatrician should be made aware of the neonate's exposure to these medications in utero. Following delivery, the pre-pregnancy dose will need to be reinstated because of the risk of relapse postpartum.

Many women take antidepressants during pregnancy. These may be the older tricyclic antidepressants (e.g. imipramine or amitriptyline), but most will be taking selective serotonin reuptake inhibitors (SSRIs) such as sertraline, citalopram and fluoxetine or some newer drugs such as venlafaxine, duloxetine and mirtazepine. There has been some concern that antidepressants may be associated with an increased risk of cardiac abnormalities, e.g. ventricular septal defect (odds ratio of 2 for paroxetine), with first trimester exposure. There is more robust evidence that their use at term is associated with the neonatal adaptation syndrome. Previously, if time allowed and the woman's mental health was stable, tapering the dose of antidepressants prior to delivery was considered. However, recent data have shown that this does not reduce the incidence of neonatal adaptation syndrome. In either case, the neonate should be observed for withdrawal symptoms. Following delivery, the maternal medication should be continued.

26.6 Labour ward crises

True psychiatric emergencies occurring in the labour ward are extremely uncommon. Women with chronic serious mental illness who are under the care of psychiatric teams should probably be accompanied during labour by a familiar mental healthcare professional if they are frightened, unable to fully comprehend what is happening to them or if they are symptomatic. Women who are well, but at risk because of a previous history, should be managed as other women are, but attention paid following delivery to their need for close surveillance in the early postpartum period. If a woman's mental health is predicted to be likely to be unstable around delivery, consider discussing advance directives during pregnancy when her mental state is stable.

Occasionally, acute episodes of distress may occur in women either in early labour or in the minutes and hours following delivery. These acute episodes of distress will usually be understandable (if not proportional) to the contextual meaning of events or procedures in the light of previous experience. Examples would be: previous sexual abuse, previous experience of a traumatic delivery or loss of a baby, misattribution of sensations or procedures, to name but a few. Women will be more vulnerable to the possibility of this occurring if they have previous experience of panic attacks, if they cannot speak English or if they are frightened for a wide variety of reasons.

The overwhelming majority of women in these situations will respond to calm kindness and reassurance. However, some women will be suffering from panic attacks. These will usually be evident because of hyperventilation and are associated with feelings of imminent disaster, a fear of dying or suffocation, losing control or even imminent insanity. Panic attacks are the great imitators. A recurring theme in the CEMD reports describes individual cases where women with cardiac and respiratory disease were mistaken as having panic attacks, but, conversely, panic attacks can be mistaken for pulmonary embolus and other physical emergencies. Swift differential diagnosis is therefore necessary. In many cases, encouragement to control hyperventilation is sufficient, together with an explanation to the woman of what is happening to her. However, on other occasions, after excluding physical disease, it may be necessary to use a short-acting benzodiazepine. Lorazepam 0.5–1.0 mg is best suited to use in labour because of its swift action and short duration.

26.7 Neonatal paediatricians

The neonatal paediatrician needs to be alerted in the following circumstances.

Lithium – Babies born to mothers taking lithium during pregnancy are at increased risk of suffering from cardiac abnormalities. Ebstein's anomaly is rare (approximately two per 1000 exposed pregnancies), but other cardiac abnormalities are more common (up to 10% of all exposed pregnancies). Continuing use throughout pregnancy is associated with an increased risk of: hypothyroidism; heavy weight babies; nephrogenic diabetes insipidus; and floppy baby syndrome following delivery.

Sodium valproate – Babies born to mothers taking sodium valproate are at increased risk of: neural tube defects; fetal valproate syndrome; and cardiac abnormalities following first trimester exposure. Continuing use throughout pregnancy is associated with an increased risk of neurodevelopmental and cognitive problems in later childhood.

Antipsychotic medication – Babies born to mothers receiving antipsychotic medication may experience withdrawal symptoms, jitteriness and convulsions, as well as short-term and reversible extrapyramidal symptoms.

Antidepressants – Babies born to mothers receiving tricyclic antidepressants at full therapeutic dosage may be at risk of withdrawal symptoms, neonatal jitteriness and convulsions, as well as anticholinergic adverse effects.

SSRI medication – Babies born to mothers receiving SSRI medication may experience: withdrawal effects; jitteriness; irritability; feeding difficulties; and problems maintaining blood sugar and temperature.

26.8 Summary

- Most perinatal psychiatric disorders can be predicted and avoided by the identification of potential psychiatric problems in early pregnancy, proactive management and collaborative perinatal management plans between psychiatry and obstetrics
- Occasionally, crises and emergencies arise during labour and more frequently in the early days following delivery. The effective management of these requires the rapid response of a specialist perinatal mental health team
- The possibility of neonatal consequences of maternal psychiatric medication needs to be borne in mind following delivery

26.9 Further reading

Knight M, Bunch K, Tuffnell D, et al. (eds), on behalf of MBRRACE-UK. *Saving Lives, Improving Mothers' Care – Lessons Learned to Inform Maternity Care from the UK and Ireland Confidential Enquiries into Maternal Deaths and Morbidity 2014–16*. Oxford: National Perinatal Epidemiology Unit, University of Oxford, 2018.

Knight M, Bunch K, Tuffnell D, et al. (eds) on behalf of MBRRACE-UK. *Saving Lives, Improving Mothers' Care – Lessons Learned to Inform Maternity Care from the UK and Ireland Confidential Enquiries into Maternal Deaths and Morbidity 2016–18*. Oxford: National Perinatal Epidemiology Unit, University of Oxford, 2020.

Knight M, Nair M, Tuffnell D, Shakespeare J, Kenyon S, Kurinczuk JJ (eds) on behalf of MBRRACE-UK. *Saving Lives, Improving Mothers' Care – Lessons Learned to Inform Maternity Care from the UK and Ireland Confidential Enquiries into Maternal Deaths and Morbidity 2013–15*. Oxford: National Perinatal Epidemiology Unit, University of Oxford, 2017.

Scottish Intercollegiate Guidelines Network (SIGN). *Management of Perinatal Mood Disorders*. SIGN 127. Glasgow: SIGN, 2012. https://www.sign.ac.uk/assets/sign127_update.pdf (last accessed January 2022).

PART 6
Obstetric emergencies

Chapter 27: Pre-eclampsia and eclampsia

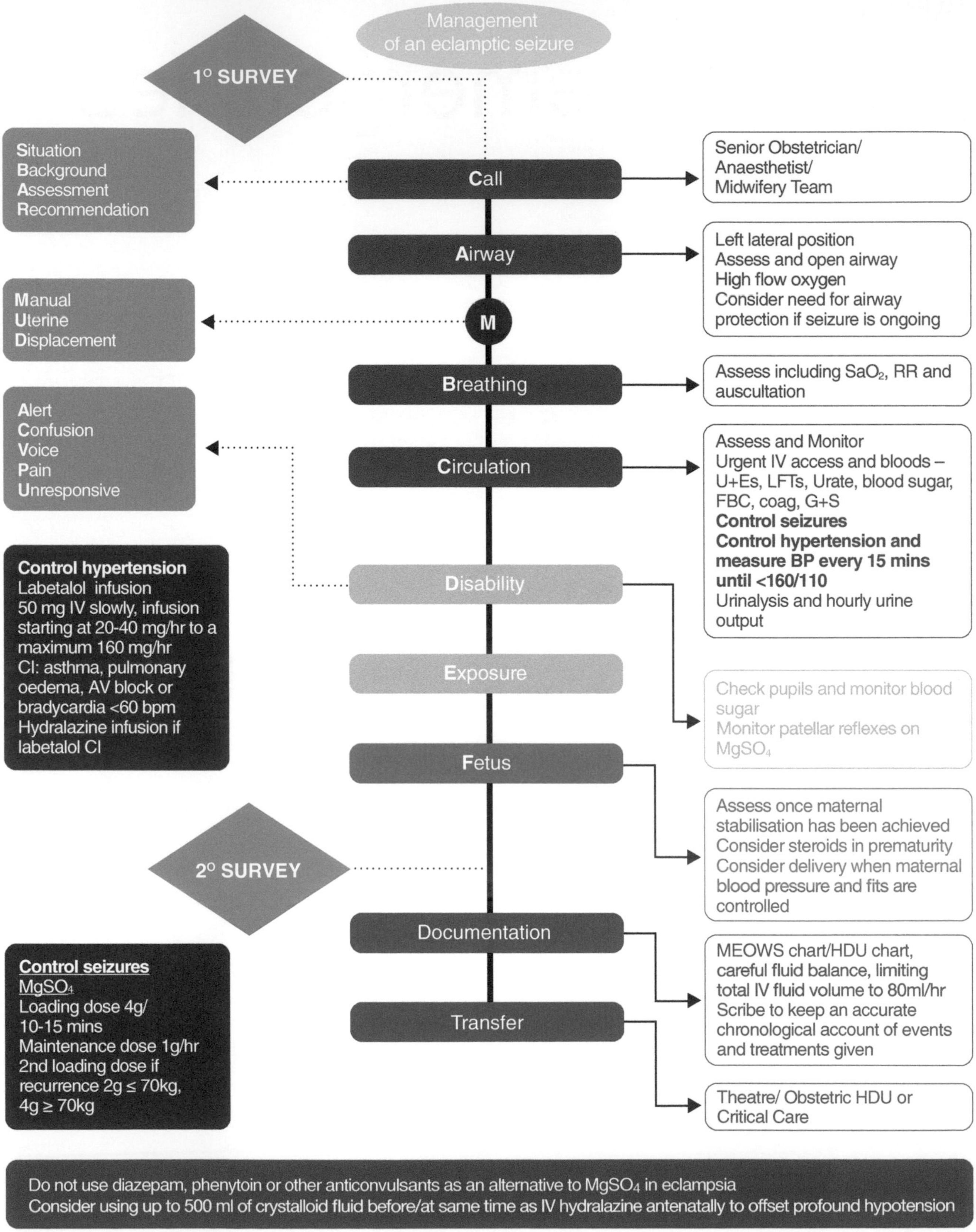
Management of an eclamptic seizure
1° SURVEY
Situation
Background
Assessment
Recommendation
Call
Senior Obstetrician/ Anaesthetist/ Midwifery Team
Airway
Left lateral position
Assess and open airway
High flow oxygen
Consider need for airway protection if seizure is ongoing
Manual
Uterine
Displacement
M
Breathing
Assess including SaO_2, RR and auscultation
Alert
Confusion
Voice
Pain
Unresponsive
Circulation
Assess and Monitor
Urgent IV access and bloods – U+Es, LFTs, Urate, blood sugar, FBC, coag, G+S
Control seizures
Control hypertension and measure BP every 15 mins until <160/110
Urinalysis and hourly urine output
Control hypertension
Labetalol infusion
50 mg IV slowly, infusion starting at 20-40 mg/hr to a maximum 160 mg/hr
CI: asthma, pulmonary oedema, AV block or bradycardia <60 bpm
Hydralazine infusion if labetalol CI
Disability
Exposure
Check pupils and monitor blood sugar
Monitor patellar reflexes on $MgSO_4$
Fetus
Assess once maternal stabilisation has been achieved
Consider steroids in prematurity
Consider delivery when maternal blood pressure and fits are controlled
2° SURVEY
Documentation
MEOWS chart/HDU chart, careful fluid balance, limiting total IV fluid volume to 80ml/hr
Scribe to keep an accurate chronological account of events and treatments given
Transfer
Theatre/ Obstetric HDU or Critical Care
Control seizures
$MgSO_4$
Loading dose 4g/ 10-15 mins
Maintenance dose 1g/hr
2nd loading dose if recurrence 2g ≤ 70kg, 4g ≥ 70kg
Do not use diazepam, phenytoin or other anticonvulsants as an alternative to $MgSO_4$ in eclampsia
Consider using up to 500 ml of crystalloid fluid before/at same time as IV hydralazine antenatally to offset profound hypotension

Algorithm 27.1 Pre-eclampsia and eclampsia

CHAPTER 27
Pre-eclampsia and eclampsia

Learning outcomes

After reading this chapter, you will be able to:

- Recognise the signs and symptoms of severe pre-eclampsia
- Understand the urgency of management of severe hypertension (systolic BP ≥160 mmHg) in pregnancy
- Prevent and treat eclamptic fits effectively
- Understand the ongoing monitoring required when a woman is on magnesium sulphate
- Manage fluid balance in pre-eclampsia/eclampsia

27.1 Introduction

Definitions

Pre-eclampsia is new hypertension presenting after 20 weeks' pregnancy with significant proteinuria. Virtually any organ system may be affected.

Severe pre-eclampsia is defined as:

- Severe hypertension (systolic blood pressure (BP) ≥160 mmHg and/or diastolic BP ≥110 mmHg on two separate readings) with significant proteinuria (urinary protein: creatinine ratio >30 mg/mmol)

Or:

- Mild or moderate hypertension (BP ≥140/90 mmHg) and significant proteinuria with at least one of:
  - Severe headache
  - Problems with vision such as blurring or flashing lights
  - Severe pain just below the ribs or vomiting
  - Papilloedema
  - Signs of clonus (≥3 beats)
  - Liver tenderness
  - HELLP (haemolysis, elevated liver enzymes and low platelets) syndrome
  - Platelet count falls to $<150 \times 10^9$/litre
  - Abnormal liver enzymes (alanine aminotransferase (ALT) or aspartate aminotransferase (AST) rises to >70 IU/l)

Managing Medical and Obstetric Emergencies and Trauma: A Practical Approach, Fourth Edition. Edited by Rosamunde Burns and Kara Dent.

Eclampsia is defined as one or more generalised seizures in association with pre-eclampsia. Pre-eclampsia, gestational hypertension or proteinuria may not be present prior to the first eclamptic seizure. Most seizures are self-limiting, usually lasting less than 90 seconds; 38% of seizures occur antepartum, 44% postpartum and 18% intrapartum.

HELLP syndrome is an important variant of pre-eclampsia. Strictly, a diagnosis of HELLP syndrome needs confirmation of haemolysis, either by measuring lactate dehydrogenase levels or by a blood film to look for fragmented red cells. In addition, ALT levels above 70 IU/l and a fall in platelet count to less than 100×10^9/litre are significant.

Epidemiology

Hypertensive disorders of pregnancy are the second most common cause of maternal death worldwide, responsible for an estimated 40 000 deaths every year. This equates to about five deaths every hour. In the UK, pre-eclampsia affects around 3% of pregnancies and remains a leading cause of maternal, fetal and neonatal morbidity and mortality. Maternal deaths from pre-eclampsia and eclampsia have fallen significantly since the 1980s (1.19 cases per 100 000 maternities in 1985–1987 compared with 0.18 cases per 100 000 maternities in 2016–2018). Improvements such as the introduction of magnesium sulphate and widespread use of management guidelines have had a positive impact on the care of women with hypertensive disorders in pregnancy. The maternal death rate from pre-eclampsia and eclampsia continues to be low, with a further small decrease in 2018.

Maternal deaths from pre-eclampsia and eclampsia are largely avoidable. The major failing in the clinical setting is inadequate treatment of severe hypertension. The 2012–2014 MBRRACE-UK report identified intracranial haemorrhage as the most common cause of maternal death from pre-eclampsia in the UK. Failure to administer effective antihypertensive treatment was implicated in most cases. Systolic hypertension poses the greatest risk and severe hypertension (≥160 mmHg) is extremely dangerous and must be treated as a medical emergency.

27.2 Pre-eclampsia

Pre-eclampsia is a multisystem disorder of pregnancy. The clinical manifestations reflect widespread vascular endothelial dysfunction, resulting in vasoconstriction, end-organ ischaemia and increased vascular permeability. Maternal and fetal complications of pre-eclampsia are detailed in Box 27.1 and predisposing risk factors for pre-eclampsia in Box 27.2.

Box 27.1 Maternal and fetal complications of pre-eclampsia

Maternal complications
- Severe hypertension
- Intracranial haemorrhage (leading cause of maternal death from severe pre-eclampsia in the UK)
- Placental abruption
- Eclampsia
- HELLP syndrome
- Renal failure
- Liver failure (including rupture and infarction)
- Disseminated intravascular coagulation
- Pulmonary oedema
- Acute respiratory distress syndrome

Fetal complication
- Prematurity (leading cause of iatrogenic preterm birth in UK)
- Intrauterine growth restriction
- Oligohydramnios
- Hypoxia from placental insufficiency
- Placental abruption
- Intrauterine death

Box 27.2 Predisposing risk factors for pre-eclampsia

- Hypertensive disease during previous pregnancy
- Chronic kidney disease
- Autoimmune disease (e.g. systemic lupus erythematosus or antiphospholipid syndrome)
- Type 1 or 2 diabetes
- Chronic hypertension
- First pregnancy
- Age ≥40 years
- Pregnancy interval >10 years
- Body mass index ≥35 kg/m^2
- Family history of pre-eclampsia
- Multiple pregnancy

27.3 Management of severe pre-eclampsia

Symptoms and signs

Pre-eclampsia is a multisystem disorder and its clinical presentation reflects this. Women may present with atypical symptoms such as convulsions, abdominal pain or simply general malaise, and should be investigated if there is a suspicion of pre-eclampsia. Awareness of the complications (Box 27.1) that can occur allows anticipation and prompt management.

The following should raise concern:

- Severe hypertension (BP ≥160/110 mmHg)
- Severe frontal headache
- Visual disturbance such as blurring or flashing
- Severe epigastric or right upper quadrant abdominal pain
- Vomiting
- Papilloedema
- Signs of clonus (≥3 beats)
- Liver tenderness
- Rapidly changing biochemical/haematological picture
- Non-dependent (especially facial) or pulmonary oedema

General principles of management

- Work to local guidelines based on current national guidelines. The management of severe pre-eclampsia and eclampsia requires the use of complex treatment plans
- Senior and multidisciplinary involvement. Early involvement of senior medical staff including obstetrician, midwife, anaesthetist and, where appropriate, neonatologist, intensivist and haematologist is essential
- Stabilise. Urgent BP control (especially systolic) is essential
- Seizure prophylaxis
- Regular review of all parameters with an awareness of complications
- Meticulous fluid balance to avoid iatrogenic fluid overload
- Fetal monitoring
- Senior multidisciplinary team plan for delivery if antenatal
- Consider magnesium sulphate and steroids if the fetus is premature

Stabilise

Control of hypertension

Effective and timely antihypertensive treatment is essential and can be life saving. In the 2012–2014 MBRRACE-UK report (as in previous reports), intracranial haemorrhage was the most common cause of death in women with pre-eclampsia and eclampsia. Inadequate treatment of systolic hypertension contributed to the majority of deaths.

Automated methods can systematically underestimate BP, particularly the systolic BP. It has been suggested that a mercury sphygmomanometer with an appropriately sized cuff should be used to initially cross-check the automated BP values. Relying on mean arterial or diastolic BP may provide false reassurance as systolic hypertension poses the greatest risk. As part of the initial assessment the BP should be checked every 15 minutes until the woman is stabilised and then repeated half hourly. If intravenous antihypertensive drugs are administered, the BP may need to be measured every 5 minutes in order to titrate treatment against the response. Consideration should be given to the use of an arterial line particularly if there are additional complications.

The National Institute for Health and Care Excellence (NICE) 2010 guideline for hypertension in pregnancy recommends that maternal BP should be maintained below 135/85 mmHg. More recently, the CHIPS study found that women with tighter control of hypertension (diastolic BP target 85 mmHg) had fewer episodes of severe hypertension than women where the target diastolic BP was 100 mmHg.

Antihypertensive medications should be continued in labour and at caesarean section. Severe hypertension should be controlled before a general anaesthetic due to the hypertensive effects of laryngoscopy, intubation and extubation.

Choice of antihypertensive

The NICE 2010 guideline on hypertension in pregnancy recommends the use of labetalol as first line treatment but recognised that there are other antihypertensive options. Labetalol is less effective in women of Afro-Caribbean origin and should be avoided for women with asthma. Nifedipine may be used as an alternative after considering the side effect profile for mother, fetus and newborn. The guideline does not make any recommendation for hypertension resistant to monotherapy. Many units pragmatically use a combination of nifedipine and labetalol. Nifedipine, labetalol or hydralazine are all suitable agents for the treatment of severe hypertension for women with severe pre-eclampsia.

Labetalol

Labetalol is a combined alpha- and beta-blocker and is less likely to decrease uteroplacental blood flow than pure beta-blockers.

If the woman can tolerate *oral therapy*, an initial 200 mg dose can be given immediately, before venous access is established, to achieve as quick a result as an initial intravenous dose. This reduces delay in treatment whilst putting in a cannula for intravenous options. There should be a reduction in BP within 30 minutes and a second dose administered if the BP is still above the threshold. If the BP is controlled below the threshold a maintenance dose of labetalol 200 tds should be commenced. If systolic BP is ≥160 mmHg and/or diastolic BP ≥110 mmHg after 30 minutes, parenteral options should be considered.

The procedure for *intravenous therapy* is as follows:

- If there is no initial response to oral therapy or if it cannot be tolerated, control should be by IV labetalol bolus followed by a labetalol infusion
- The bolus dose is 50 mg (10 ml labetalol 5 mg/ml) given over 2 minutes. This may be repeated every 5 minutes (maximum four doses) until BP is controlled
- Following this a labetalol infusion should be commenced. An infusion of (neat) labetalol 5 mg/ml should be started at 4 ml/h via a syringe pump. The infusion rate is doubled every 30 minutes until BP is controlled. The maximum infusion rate is 32 ml (160 mg) per hour
- Oral antihypertensives should be commenced once intravenous treatment has been discontinued

It should be remembered that women on beta-blockers may fail to mount a tachycardia. Early signs of haemorrhage may be missed by a falsely reassuring pulse rate.

Nifedipine

Nifedipine is a vasodilator and is recommended as an alternative to oral labetalol in women who are asthmatic and/or Afro-Caribbean. Theoretically, the effect of nifedipine may be exacerbated by magnesium sulphate. Clinically this is rarely a problem. In the Magpie study large numbers of women were treated with no adverse events reported. An initial 10 mg dose of nifedipine (not sublingual) may be repeated after 30 minutes if the BP is still above the threshold. If the BP is controlled a maintenance dose of 10 mg tds should be commenced.

Hydralazine

Intravenous hydralazine may be used if labetalol is contraindicated or is less likely to be effective. Hydralazine is an effective vasodilator. In the antenatal period this can precipitate fetal distress secondary to a reduction in uteroplacental blood flow. A 250–500 ml bolus of crystalloid may be considered before or at the same time as the first dose of hydralazine for women who are not yet delivered. An initial 5 mg (5 ml of hydralazine 1 mg/ml) is given as a slow bolus over 15 minutes. If systolic BP is ≥160 mmHg after 20 minutes a further 5 mg (5 ml of 1 mg/ml) bolus should be given over 15 minutes. An infusion of 2 mg/h can be established for maintenance, with increasing increments of 0.5 mg/h to a maximum of 20 mg/h. The rate should be titrated to response aiming for a systolic BP of 140–150 mmHg. The usual rate is 2–3 mg/h. The rate should be reduced if there are significant adverse effects or if the maternal pulse is >120 beats/min.

A systematic review of hydralazine and labetalol revealed that hydralazine was associated with more maternal hypotension (OR 3.29, 95%CI 1.50–7.13), more caesarean sections (OR 1.30, 95%CI 1.08–1.59), more placental abruptions (OR 4.17, 95%CI 1.19–14.28) and more adverse effects on fetal heart rate (OR 2.04, 95%CI 1.32–3.16). It was suggested that, although the results were not robust, they did not support hydralazine as a first line treatment.

The NICE guidelines on hypertension in pregnancy support the use of all three treatments described.

Prevent seizures

Consider giving intravenous magnesium sulphate to reduce the risk of seizures if the birth is planned within 24 hours in women with severe pre-eclampsia. The risk of eclampsia is low, at around 1% even in women with severe pre-eclampsia. The Magpie trial, designed to establish the clinical efficacy of magnesium sulphate in pre-eclampsia, found that treatment with magnesium sulphate reduced the risk of seizures by 58%. Overall the number needed to treat (NNT) to prevent a seizure was 63 (range of 38–181) in severe pre-eclampsia. In countries with a low mortality rate, the NNT may be over 300. In the UK, the decision to use prophylactic magnesium sulphate should be based on consideration of risk and benefit.

The regimen for magnesium sulphate is the same as for eclampsia: a loading dose of 4 g intravenously over 5 minutes followed by a maintenance infusion of 1 g/h for 24 hours. In cases where it is used for prophylaxis, it may be discontinued before 24 hours if all other features of pre-eclampsia have settled.

Magnesium sulphate protocol

Clinicians need to be aware that there are differing concentrations of magnesium sulphate available, and to avoid confusion over dosing, each unit should have access to one stock only and clear guidance on how to draw it up. The safest approach is for hospitals within the same network to all stock the same preparation. This will reduce the potential risk of dose error, particularly for junior doctors when they move to a new unit. The easiest and least confusing preparation to use is 20% magnesium in 20 and 50 ml ampoules.

Dose of magnesium sulphate

If using 10% magnesium:

- Loading dose: 4 g (40 ml) bolus over 5 minutes (each 10 ml ampoule contains 1 g magnesium sulphate; therefore four ampoules are needed = 40 ml)
- Maintenance dose is then 10 ml/h via a syringe pump

If using 20% magnesium:

- Loading dose: 4 g bolus over 5 minutes (20 ml ampoule contains 4 g magnesium sulphate)
- Maintenance dose is then 5 ml/h via a syringe pump (50 ml ampoule contains 10 g magnesium sulphate)

If using 50% magnesium:

- Loading dose: 4 g bolus over 5 minutes. Draw up 8 ml of 50% magnesium sulphate solution (4 g) followed by 12 ml of 0.9% normal saline into a 20 ml syringe. This will give a total volume of 20 ml
- Maintenance dose is 5 ml/h via a syringe pump. Draw up 20 ml of 50% magnesium sulphate solution (10 g) followed by 30 ml of 0.9% normal saline into a 50 ml syringe

Monitor

Maternal clinical condition can deteriorate rapidly in severe pre-eclampsia. Regular monitoring and assessment is required and observations recorded on a modified early obstetric warning score (MEOWS) chart. The following observations should be performed:

- Blood pressure and pulse every 15 minutes until stabilised, then every 30 minutes. If intravenous antihypertensive drugs are administered, the BP may need to be measured every 5 minutes in order to titrate treatment against response
- Hourly respiratory rate
- Hourly oxygen saturation
- Urine dipstick and protein: creatinine ratio
- Hourly urine output
- Strict fluid balance. Limit input to 1 ml/kg/h unless there are other ongoing fluid losses (e.g. haemorrhage)
- Four-hourly temperature especially for women in labour, postpartum or immediately postoperative
- Neurological examination if there is new onset severe headache or headache with atypical features particularly focal symptoms
- Blood samples every 6–24 hours for renal function, liver function, haematology and magnesium levels if the patient is on magnesium sulphate

Additional observations for woman on magnesium sulphate should include:

- Hourly respiratory rate
- Continuous monitoring of oxygen saturation with hourly charting
- Hourly deep tendon reflexes

Stop magnesium sulphate infusion and check level if:

- Reflexes are absent:
  - If level is less than 4 mmol/l, recommence infusion at 0.5 g/h
- Respiratory rate is less than 10 breaths/min
- Oxygen saturation is less than 90% on air
- Urine output is less than 100 ml in 4 hours

Magnesium is excreted in urine by the kidneys. In women with renal impairment or where there is oliguria, magnesium will not be excreted and magnesium levels are more likely to become toxic. In these circumstances only the loading dose is required. If oliguria develops during treatment, the infusion should be stopped and blood taken to measure the serum magnesium level. Magnesium sulphate has a narrow therapeutic range of 2–4 mmol/l. At toxic levels, magnesium causes muscle weakness, a loss of deep tendon reflexes, respiratory depression, cardiac arrythmia and respiratory and ultimately cardiac arrest (Table 27.1). If toxicity is suspected, immediately stop the magnesium sulphate infusion and take blood for magnesium levels. An overdose of magnesium (whether relative or absolute) should be treated with 10 ml of 10% calcium gluconate, given by a slow intravenous bolus.

Table 27.1 Levels of magnesium sulphate at which adverse effects occur

Symptoms	$MgSO_4$ levels (mmol/l)
Feeling of warmth, flushing, double vision, slurred speech	3.8–5.0
Loss of tendon reflexes	>5.0
Respiratory depression	>6.0
Respiratory arrest	6.3–7.0
Cardiac arrest	>12.0

Assessment of the fetus

Fetal well-being should be assessed by cardiotocography. The fetus is at risk of growth restriction and a Doppler ultrasound assessment for fetal growth, amniotic fluid volume and umbilical artery may be appropriate.

Fluid balance

Close monitoring of fluid input and output is essential. Women with severe pre-eclampsia are at risk of pulmonary oedema and previous confidential enquiries have highlighted the risk of fluid overload. Reassuringly, there have been no maternal deaths as a consequence of inappropriate fluid management since 2003.

The aim of fluid management is to 'run dry'. Fluid intake should be restricted to 1 ml/kg/h (often approximately 80 ml/h). All women with severe pre-eclampsia should have an indwelling urinary catheter and hourly urine output recorded.

In the immediate post-delivery phase, women commonly have a degree of oliguria. Women with severe pre-eclampsia should remain fluid restricted until a natural diuresis occurs, 24–36 hours following delivery.

Persistent oliguria of less than 100 ml over 4 hours requires careful management. Central venous pressure (CVP) monitoring is usually not necessary and may be misleading. This is because pulmonary oedema can occur in the presence of low CVP because of left ventricular dysfunction and increased pulmonary interstitial fluid. A central line may be helpful to aid fluid management when there are added complications such as a postpartum haemorrhage in a woman with severe pre-eclampsia. The aim is to maintain a CVP in the range 0–5 mmHg. Women requiring large volumes of blood and fresh frozen plasma (FFP) are a particular challenge. In cases where fluid balance measurements are likely to be inaccurate, owing to difficulties measuring blood loss, early recourse to central monitoring may be appropriate. CVP line insertion may be difficult or hazardous (for example in the presence of coagulopathy, or if lying head down is impossible due to severe pulmonary oedema) and the consultant anaesthetist and consultant obstetrician should be involved.

If oxygen saturation levels fall this may indicate pulmonary oedema. Symptoms include shortness of breath, inability to lie flat, inability to talk in full sentences with confusion and agitation. The woman should be examined for signs of tachypnoea, crepitations at the lung bases, decreasing oxygen saturations, tachycardia and frothy pink sputum. Appropriate treatment may include sitting the woman upright or giving furosemide and oxygen. A chest x-ray should be performed. If there is no diuresis and oxygen saturation does not improve, urgent referral to intensive care/renal referral should be considered.

Coagulopathy

Disseminated intravascular coagulation is a potential complication of severe pre-eclampsia. If platelet levels are less than 100×10^9/litre, a coagulation screen and fibrinogen should be sent. If results are abnormal, treatment with platelets, FFP and cryoprecipitate may be required and the involvement of senior haematology input is essential.

Planning delivery

Once the maternal condition has been stabilised, a decision should be made regarding timing and mode of birth. The choice of caesarean section or induction of labour should be made on an individual basis. After 34 weeks' gestation, vaginal delivery should be considered. Antihypertensive treatment should be continued throughout labour and postpartum.

Antenatal steroids

If the pregnancy is preterm and can be prolonged safely beyond 24 hours, intramuscular steroids should be given for fetal lung maturation.

Magnesium sulphate

If the pregnancy is less than 30–32 weeks, magnesium sulphate should be given prior to delivery for fetal neuroprotection. Ideally, it should be administered 4 hours prior to delivery and for a maximum of 24 hours using the standard PET regime described earlier.

First stage of labour

Continuous electronic fetal monitoring is recommended as there is an increased risk of fetal hypoxia and abruption.

The use of epidural anaesthesia should be considered to prevent a rise in BP associated with pain in labour, providing there is no coagulopathy. Women with severe pre-eclampsia should not be given a preload with intravenous fluid prior to an epidural or spinal. Consider if below 34 weeks.

During labour, BP should be measured every 15 minutes in women with severe hypertension and hourly if their hypertension is mild or moderate.

Second stage of labour

If the BP is less than 160/110 mmHg and the woman does not have a severe headache, visual disturbance or epigastric pain the duration of second stage should not be limited.

Vaginal birth should be expedited if the BP is ≥160/110 mmHg despite treatment or the woman is symptomatic.

Third stage of labour

The third stage should be managed with oxytocin, either 5 units via slow IV infusion or 10 units intramuscularly, or after caesarean section cabetocin 100 micrograms IV over 1 minute. **Ergometrine or syntometrine should not be given to women with pre-eclampsia or eclampsia because of the risk of precipitating a rapid rise in blood pressure.**

Organisation and transfer

If transfer to a bigger unit is required, maternal safety must not be compromised and the woman must be stabilised prior to transfer. The following are necessary prior to transfer:

- Blood pressure should be stabilised
- All basic investigations should have been done and results clearly recorded in the accompanying notes or telephoned through as soon as available
- Fetal well-being must be assessed to be certain that transfer before delivery is in the fetal interest; steroids should be given if the woman is preterm
- Appropriate personnel are available to transfer the woman; this will normally mean at least the presence of a senior midwife with medical staff as appropriate
- Transfer has been discussed with the appropriate consultant and relevant medical and midwifery staff at the receiving unit

Postnatal care

Women with severe pre-eclampsia require continued critical care after birth. This may last for hours or days depending on the clinical situation. Pre-eclampsia can deteriorate postnatally, and it is worth remembering that most eclamptic seizures occur in the postnatal period. BP may fall initially but usually rises again at around 24 hours' postpartum. Antenatal antihypertensive should be reduced if BP falls below 130/80 mmHg. Postnatal hypertension is often more resistant to treatment and may require a rapid increase in dose and number of antihypertensive medications to achieve control. If symptoms arise this should prompt appropriate monitoring and investigation. Women should be assessed for venous thromboembolic risk, and thromboprophylaxis will be required in almost all cases. Before discharge, a care plan should be written outlining management in the community, including:

- Frequency of BP monitoring
- Thresholds for reducing or stopping antihypertensive medication
- Indications for referral for medical review

27.4 Management of eclampsia

The incidence of eclampsia in the UK has fallen since the introduction of the use of magnesium sulphate. The UK obstetric surveillance study in 2005 reported a rate of eclampsia of 2.7 per 10 000 births compared with 4.9 per 10 000 births in 1992. This has further fallen in 2017 to 0.08/100 000 maternities. There is a high rate of maternal complications associated with eclampsia with 1 in 10 women experiencing a major morbidity after a seizure. Perinatal mortality is 10 times higher than in normal pregnancy.

Eclampsia presents as a generalised tonic-clonic seizure. The mother may become cyanosed and tongue biting and urinary incontinence may occur. Most seizures are self-limiting, usually lasting less than 90 seconds. The recurrence rate of seizure is 5–30%, even with treatment.

Immediate resuscitation

Management should start with basic life support measures. Do not leave the woman alone and protect her from injury. Activate the emergency buzzer to summon help, or call 999 if working in the community. Help should include a senior midwife, the most senior obstetrician and anaesthetist available and additional midwives and maternity support worker. Team working is essential for effective timely management. The consultant obstetrician and consultant anaesthetist should be contacted as soon as possible. Contemporaneous documentation should be delegated to a team member once there are enough people. The time and duration of the seizure, the time of pressing the emergency buzzer and the arrival of staff should be documented. Many units have an ECLAMPSIA BOX containing laminated treatment algorithms for eclampsia and severe hypertension, as well as equipment, blood test packs and treatment for the immediate management of eclampsia. This should be brought into the room as soon as possible.

A Monitor and maintain the airway. Place the woman in the left lateral position and ensure she has an open airway
B Assess breathing and administer high-flow oxygen using a non-rebreathing mask with reservoir bag. Pulse oximetry is useful once the seizure has stopped. Lungs should be auscultated after the convulsion has ended to detect aspiration or pulmonary oedema
C Check pulse and blood pressure. Site a large-bore cannula and take blood for a full blood count, urea and electrolytes, liver function tests, clotting and group and save

Control of seizure

- Give magnesium sulphate to manage eclampsia
- Most eclamptic seizures are self-limiting
- The intravenous route is associated with fewer adverse effects than the intramuscular route
- Dosage: see 'Prevent seizures', earlier in this chapter
- Continue maintenance treatment for 24 hours after the last seizure or 24 hours from delivery, whichever is longest

The results of the Collaborative Eclampsia Trial demonstrated that woman treated with magnesium sulphate had fewer recurrent seizures than women treated with diazepam or phenytoin. Magnesium sulphate appears to act primarily by reducing cerebral vasospasm.

Management of recurrent seizures while on magnesium sulphate

- Seek immediate senior help
- Give a single further dose of 2–4 g over 5 minutes
- Take blood for magnesium level prior to giving the bolus dose

In the Collaborative Eclampsia Trial, a further bolus of 2 or 4 g of magnesium sulphate was administered depending on maternal weight. The larger dose is appropriate for women over 70 kg.

If there are recurrent or prolonged seizures that are unresponsive to magnesium sulphate then alternative agents such as lorazepam IV or diazepam PR may be used. Urgent anaesthetic assistance should be sought as women with prolonged seizures may require other agents such as thiopentone or propofol in conjunction with intubation to protect the airway and maintain oxygenation, with transfer to intensive care.

Other differential diagnoses including hypoglycaemia or hyponatremia, intracranial haemorrhage, epilepsy, a space occupying lesion or cerebral vein thrombosis should be considered and urgent neuroimaging arranged.

Eclampsia box

It has been recommended that each maternity unit should have an emergency box for eclampsia, based on the treatment packs that were available for the Collaborative Eclampsia Trial. This will ensure that appropriate drugs are readily available. The box should be regularly checked to keep drugs in date.

27.5 HELLP syndrome

HELLP is a syndrome comprising haemolysis, elevated liver enzymes and low platelet count. It occurs in 4–12% of women with severe pre-eclampsia. Severe hypertension is not always a feature, and the degree of hypertension rarely reflects overall disease severity. It is more common in multiparous women and is associated with a high perinatal mortality rate.

HELLP syndrome can present with vague symptoms including nausea, vomiting and epigastric/right upper quadrant pain and there is often a delay in diagnosis. Severe epigastric pain not relieved by antacids should raise the index of suspicion. One unique (if somewhat late) feature of HELLP syndrome is 'Coca Cola urine' where small amounts of dark urine are produced, caused by intravascular haemolysis.

The management of HELLP syndrome, as for severe pre-eclampsia, involves evaluating severity, stabilising the mother and delivery. The postnatal course for these women is often complicated by oliguria and slow recovery of biochemical parameters. There is no evidence for the use of high-dose corticosteroids in the management of HELLP syndrome.

27.6 Summary

- Hypertension in pregnancy remains a leading cause of maternal death worldwide and is largely avoidable with good recognition and treatment
- A multisystem disorder, pre-eclampsia can present in varied forms from generally feeling unwell to frontal headaches and abdominal pain
- Recent MBRRACE-UK reports highlight the need to recognise and treat a raised systolic blood pressure of ≥160 mmHg with the risk of intracranial haemorrhage if not stabilised
- Ultimately, treatment of severe pre-eclampsia is delivery of the fetus and placental unit; however, stabilisation of the mother is the priority before considering delivery options

27.7 Further reading

Knight M, Bunch K, Tuffnell D, et al. (eds) on behalf of MBRRACE-UK. *Saving Lives, Improving Mothers' Care – Lessons Learned to Inform Maternity Care from the UK and Ireland Confidential Enquiries into Maternal Deaths and Morbidity 2016–18*. Oxford: National Perinatal Epidemiology Unit, University of Oxford, 2020.

NICE (National Institute for Health and Care Excellence). *Hypertension in Pregnancy: Diagnosis and Management*. NG133. London: NICE, 2019.

Usman S, Foo L, Tay J, Bennett PR, Lees C. Use of magnesium sulfate in preterm deliveries for neuroprotection of the neonate. *Obstet Gynaecol* 2017; 19: 21–8.

Chapter 28: Major obstetric haemorrhage

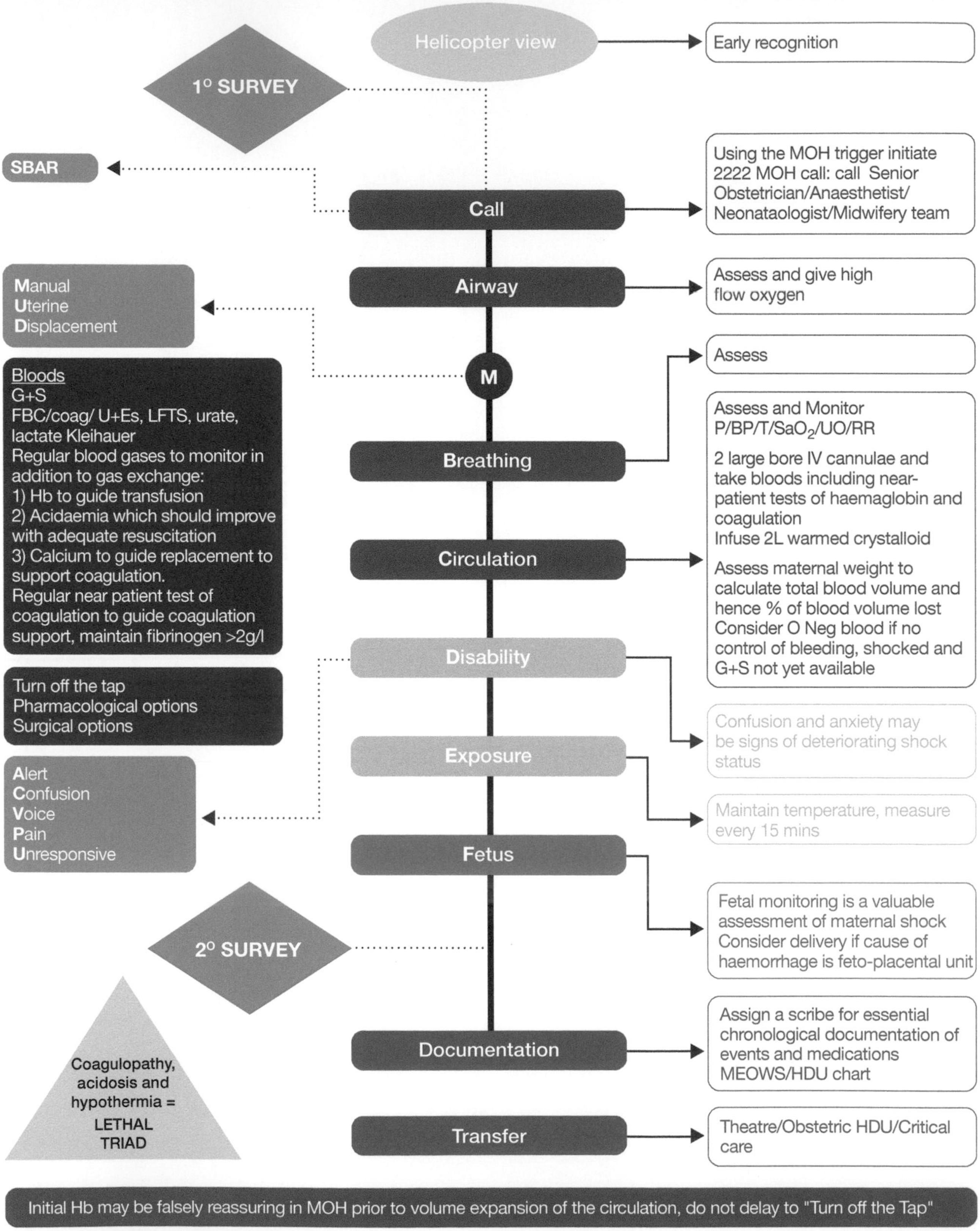

Helicopter view
Early recognition
1° SURVEY
SBAR
Call
Using the MOH trigger initiate 2222 MOH call: call Senior Obstetrician/Anaesthetist/ Neonataologist/Midwifery team
Airway
Assess and give high flow oxygen
Manual Uterine Displacement
M
Assess
Bloods
G+S
FBC/coag/ U+Es, LFTS, urate, lactate Kleihauer
Regular blood gases to monitor in addition to gas exchange:
1) Hb to guide transfusion
2) Acidaemia which should improve with adequate resuscitation
3) Calcium to guide replacement to support coagulation.
Regular near patient test of coagulation to guide coagulation support, maintain fibrinogen >2g/l
Breathing
Assess and Monitor P/BP/T/SaO2/UO/RR
2 large bore IV cannulae and take bloods including near-patient tests of haemaglobin and coagulation
Infuse 2L warmed crystalloid
Circulation
Assess maternal weight to calculate total blood volume and hence % of blood volume lost
Consider O Neg blood if no control of bleeding, shocked and G+S not yet available
Disability
Turn off the tap
Pharmacological options
Surgical options
Confusion and anxiety may be signs of deteriorating shock status
Exposure
Alert
Confusion
Voice
Pain
Unresponsive
Maintain temperature, measure every 15 mins
Fetus
Fetal monitoring is a valuable assessment of maternal shock
Consider delivery if cause of haemorrhage is feto-placental unit
2° SURVEY
Coagulopathy, acidosis and hypothermia = LETHAL TRIAD
Documentation
Assign a scribe for essential chronological documentation of events and medications MEOWS/HDU chart
Transfer
Theatre/Obstetric HDU/Critical care
Initial Hb may be falsely reassuring in MOH prior to volume expansion of the circulation, do not delay to "Turn off the Tap"

Algorithm 28.1 Major obstetric haemorrhage

CHAPTER 28
Major obstetric haemorrhage

Learning outcomes

After reading this chapter, you will be able to:

- Describe the definition and causes of major obstetric haemorrhage
- Recognise and manage maternal collapse caused by obstetric haemorrhage
- Discuss the pharmacological and surgical options for the treatment of major obstetric haemorrhage
- Make a plan to facilitate optimum management in your environment
- Understand the concerns to be discussed with patients declining blood and blood products during pregnancy

28.1 Introduction

Major obstetric haemorrhage remains a leading cause of maternal mortality despite modern improvements in obstetric practice and transfusion services. In addition, all 'near miss' audits, in developed as well as developing countries, show major haemorrhage to be one of the leading causes of severe maternal morbidity.

Complications of haemorrhage associated with first trimester bleeding due to miscarriage or ectopic pregnancy are not within the remit of the mMOET course, although most general principles will apply.

Maternal mortality and the incidence of major obstetric haemorrhage

Obstetric haemorrhage remains an important cause of maternal mortality at the seventh highest cause reported in the most recent MBRRACE-UK report (2020). At an incidence of 0.68/100 000 maternities, there were 14 women who died from haemorrhage-related causes. A review of these cases recognised that there was a failure to have a 'helicopter view' where one senior clinician was not overseeing all the elements of the case to enable them to make a good estimate of blood loss and to spot deterioration in observations that reflected concealed bleeding leading to disseminated intravascular coagulopathy. The 'lethal triad in trauma' of acidosis, coagulopathy and hypothermia were emphasised. A recommendation of temperature checks every 15 minutes in an ongoing major obstetric haemorrhage would highlight this in a resuscitation scenario.

The report also discusses the importance of estimating blood loss in relation to the size and circulating blood volume of the woman as a number of the maternal deaths in this category were due to small quantities of blood lost. A 2 litre loss will have a more catastrophic effect on a woman of 50 kg than 90 kg for example (Table 28.1), and this needs to be taken into account with the management and resuscitation of these different women.

Table 28.1 Estimated blood loss and proportional volumes

Weight (kg)	Total blood volume (ml)*	15% blood volume loss (moderate haemorrhage) (ml)	30% blood volume loss (severe haemorrhage) (ml)	40% blood volume loss (life-threatening haemorrhage (ml)
50	5000	750	1500	2000
60	6000	900	1800	2400
70	7000	1050	2100	2800
80	8000	1200	2400	3200
90	9000	1350	2700	3600
100	10000	1500	3000	4000

* Based on 100 ml/kg blood volume in pregnancy but may overestimate blood volume in obese women (Lemmens et al., 2006).
Source: Knight M, Bunch K, Tuffnell D, et al. (eds) on behalf of MBRRACE-UK. *Saving Lives, Improving Mothers' Care – Lessons Learned to Inform Maternity Care from the UK and Ireland Confidential Enquiries into Maternal Deaths and Morbidity 2016-18*. Oxford: National Perinatal Epidemiology Unit, University of Oxford, 2020

Definition and epidemiology

Major obstetric haemorrhage is defined as the loss of more than 1000 ml blood as either antepartum or postpartum loss. Antepartum haemorrhage is often followed by postpartum haemorrhage (PPH).

Considerable problems are recognised in the accurate measurement of blood loss, and a definition based on volume alone has some shortcomings. Both visual and measured loss can be highly inaccurate, and loss from placental abruption, uterine rupture or after caesarean section (CS) may be partially or completely concealed. Underestimation of blood loss may delay active steps being taken to prepare for or prevent further bleeding. Crucially a woman of *low body weight will have lost a higher proportion of her circulating volume* at the 1000 ml definition than a woman of normal body weight.

Major causes of primary or secondary obstetric haemorrhage

Causes resulting initially in hypovolaemia

- Uterine atony (multiple causes)
- Placenta praevia and placenta accreta
- Retained or adherent placenta or placental fragments
- Genital tract injury including broad ligament haematoma
- Uterine rupture
- Uterine inversion
- Uterine anatomical abnormalities, e.g. multiple fibroids

Causes associated with coagulation failure

- Placental abruption
- Pre-eclampsia
- Septicaemia/intrauterine sepsis
- Retained dead fetus
- Amniotic fluid embolus
- Incompatible blood transfusion
- Existing coagulation abnormalities

28.2 Major obstetric haemorrhage (MOH)

The recommendations of the Royal College of Obstetricians and Gynaecologists (RCOG) Green-top Guideline No. 52, *Postpartum Haemorrhage, Prevention and Management* (updated in 2016) form the basis of this chapter.

Most obstetric units in the UK now have a 'major obstetric haemorrhage' guideline, as recommended by the confidential enquiry and endorsed by the RCOG. This protocol should be readily available on the delivery suite, including details of senior staff to be contacted in obstetrics, anaesthetics and haematology. Its use should also be subject to local audit. Blood loss of greater than 1000 ml or the recognition of maternal signs of shock in the absence of large *visible* loss should prompt the initiation of the protocol set out in the major obstetric haemorrhage guideline.

All detailed advice regarding transfusion of blood products is addressed in Chapter 8.

The cornerstones in the management of major obstetric haemorrhage are early recognition, the restoration of the circulating blood volume and oxygen carrying capacity, and the prevention of further loss. Failure to maintain adequate tissue perfusion leads to loss of vital organ function, and care becomes increasingly more complex.

Recognition of haemorrhage

Not all haemorrhage is revealed, and large volumes of blood can be lost from the circulation while remaining concealed in the peritoneal cavity, uterus, retroperitoneal space or ischiorectal fossa. Clinicians should be aware that the visual estimation of peripartum blood loss is inaccurate and that clinical signs and symptoms should be included in the assessment of PPH. A high index of suspicion should be maintained while assessing patients with abdominal pain, unusual levels of perineal discomfort post delivery, fainting and any signs of shock as listed below. The classes of increasing severity of blood loss are described in detail in Chapter 6 on shock.

Specific situations leading to obstetric haemorrhage

These include the following:

- Bleeding associated with CS (see Chapter 29)
- Placenta praevia and accreta (see Chapter 30)
- Placental abruption

Placental abruption

An abruption results from the separation of the placenta from the uterine wall. Blood is driven into the myometrium (Couvelaire uterus), which interferes with uterine contractility, causing PPH. The associated release of thromboplastins can cause disseminated intravascular coagulopathy.

Classic features of abruption are sudden onset of severe abdominal pain, associated with shock, and a tender, hard uterus. However, with abruption of a posterior placenta, the abdomen may be soft.

Fetal heart sounds may be muffled or absent; abdominal ultrasound is often necessary to establish fetal viability but is not useful for diagnosis of the abruption itself unless the retroplacental clot is large (and this should already be obvious clinically).

If there is fetal death in association with abruption, then the abruption is major, and represents significant maternal blood loss and likely consumptive coagulopathy. The blood loss may be without any vaginal loss (concealed) and may be compensated for in the maternal circulation by the shutting down of the blood supply to the fetoplacental unit. It is therefore frequently underestimated. As a rule of thumb, an abruption resulting in fetal death requires maternal transfusion.

Initial management is:

- ABC
- Send blood samples for tests, including a Kleihauer test
- Deliver the fetus
- Treat coagulopathy; fibrinogen often requires aggressive replacement. Aim to maintain fibrinogen levels a >2 g/l during active haemorrhage

If significant haemorrhage has occurred and the fetus is viable, immediate delivery by CS should be considered. However, labour may progress rapidly in the presence of an abruption; if the cardiotocograph is satisfactory, it may be prudent to aim for a vaginal delivery. If the fetus is dead, induction with a view to a vaginal delivery is usually advisable.

Expect massive PPH. The combination of antepartum and postpartum haemorrhage may result in cardiovascular compromise.

Consider central venous pressure monitoring, involve senior staff and arrange for high-dependency care postoperatively. There is a possibility of caesarean hysterectomy. Senior staff should be involved.

28.3 Maternal signs of shock

Maternal signs of shock include (see also Chapter 6):

- Tachycardia (on occasion a normal pulse rate or bradycardia can be seen – beware the patient on beta-blockers)
- Tachypnoea
- Poor peripheral perfusion
- Confusion or unresponsiveness
- Oliguria
- Hypotension
- Requiring more than 2 litres of crystalloid to maintain blood pressure
- Unexplained metabolic acidosis

28.4 Management of major obstetric haemorrhage

Management involves various elements, all of which need to be undertaken simultaneously:

- Communication, early escalation to senior obstetric and anaesthetic staff and contemporaneous documentation
- Resuscitation and fluid replacement
- Monitoring and investigation
- Management of the haemorrhage
- Anaesthetic management

Communication ('call for help') and documentation

Institute the following:

- Call the senior midwife, obstetric and anaesthetic registrars even if you are the most senior clinician
- Inform the consultant obstetrician and anaesthetist
- Inform the blood bank technician and consultant haematologist (most units will have an agreed form of words, e.g. 'major obstetric haemorrhage' to which the laboratory will respond)
- Call the porter for delivery of specimens and blood products
- Allocate one member of the resuscitation team as team leader and one to record events, fluids, drugs and vital signs
- Ensure a 'helicopter view'

Ongoing written and verbal communication between senior staff is essential. This may involve the assistance of other specialists, such as intensive care specialists, vascular surgeons or radiologists.

Resuscitation and fluid replacement

Assess airway and breathing (see Chapter 10 for details). Conscious level and airway control usually improve rapidly once the circulating volume is restored. If the mother is shocked then administer high-flow oxygen.

Evaluate the circulation (see Chapters 6 and 8 for details).

Correction of the circulation within the primary survey involves the following:

- Establish two large-bore intravenous lines
- Take 20 ml of blood for diagnostic tests including venous blood gas
- Commence the administration of warmed crystalloid intravenously

- The left lateral position should be adopted to minimise the effects of aortocaval compression in an undelivered woman
- A lateral tilt with a wedge (or manual displacement of the uterus by an assistant) should continue to be used when obstetric procedures are in progress
- Stop any epidural infusion pending review by an anaesthetist; compensatory lower limb vasoconstriction will be limited, so the effects of positioning may be more marked
- A head-down tilt can be used as a short-term measure to improve venous return, but this may compromise respiration

Fluid, blood product, cell salvage and clotting factor replacement is all described in detail in Chapters 6 and 8 and is not repeated here.

Diagnostic tests

These include:

- Full blood count and near patient testing of haemaglobin (e.g. Haemacue®)
- Coagulation screen including fibrinogen
- Crossmatch 4–6 units of group-specific blood if urgent
- Baseline renal function
- Blood gas and lactate

Regular reassessment of the haemoglobin, coagulation, blood gases and lactate will help guide resuscitation.

Near patient testing of haemoglobin and coagulation

Caution is required with interpreting the haemoglobin at the start of a haemorrhage emergency. The obstetric team may be falsely reassured by an initial haemoglobin if haemodilution has not yet occurred in an acute haemorrhage.

Many units now have access to thromboelastography (TEG®) or rotational thromboelastometry (ROTEM®) as point-of-care tests of coagulation to facilitate the rapid diagnosis of coagulation failure and enable timely targeted treatment to help 'turn off the tap'.

Monitoring – evaluation of response

A modified early obstetric warning score (MEOWS) chart should be used. This will record the following:

- Pulse
- Blood pressure
- Respiratory rate
- SaO_2
- Temperature
- Urinary output via a urinary catheter
- Detailed fluid balance
- Fetal heart rate should be monitored as appropriate

Healthy women can maintain a normal or even high blood pressure while large volumes of blood are lost intra-abdominally. Most, but not all, women will demonstrate a tachycardia if bleeding significantly, but paradoxical bradycardia has also been observed (peritoneal irritation). This tachycardic response is unlikely to be present in women who have been given labetalol to treat high blood pressure. Additional monitoring by means of arterial lines and central venous monitoring may be indicated. Again, the reader is referred to Chapters 6 and 8.

Management of the haemorrhage

The 'four Ts' acts as an effective aide memoire regarding the causes of PPH:

- *Tone* (poor uterine contraction)
- *Tissue* (retained placenta or placental fragment)
- *Trauma* (of the genital tract)
- *Thrombin* (as a means of remembering coagulation abnormalities)

Tone

Major obstetric haemorrhage is very commonly due to uterine atony. In this situation, the following mechanical and pharmacological measures should be instituted, in turn, until the bleeding stops.

Mechanical measures

- Bimanual uterine compression ('rubbing up the uterus') to stimulate contractions
- Ensuring the bladder is empty by inserting an indwelling Foley catheter

Pharmacological measures

- Syntocinon 5 units by slow IV injection, which may be repeated
- Ergometrine 0.5 mg by slow IV or IM injection (*contraindicated in hypertension*)
- Syntocinon infusion (40 units in 500 ml 0.9% normal saline at 125 ml/h) unless fluid restriction is necessary when a more concentrated solution should be used
- Carboprost 0.25 mg by deep IM injection, repeated at intervals of not less than 15 minutes, to a maximum of eight doses. This drug is contraindicated in asthma. Intramyometrial injection of carboprost is unlicensed and its manufacturer has circulated a warning against its use in this way. The hypervascular and atonic uterus carries a high risk of intravascular drug administration with any direct myometrial injection
- Misoprostol 600 micrograms oral or per rectum is no more effective than oxytocin, but may be of use, particularly in home deliveries or in asthmatics where carboprost is contraindicated
- Tranexamic acid 1 g IV should be given to women with an MOH. The WOMAN Trial demonstrated that intravenous tranexamic acid was safe and effective when given when blood loss exceeds 500 ml after vaginal delivery, and 1000 ml after CS

Advanced techniques

If the above measures fail to control the haemorrhage, invasive advanced haemostatic techniques must be initiated. This will invariably require an examination with some form of anaesthesia in an operating theatre.

The UK Obstetric Surveillance System (UKOSS) reported on 272 women who required second line therapy for the management of PPH. Compression sutures were used in 161 women and were successful in 121 (75%); interventional radiology was used in 14 women with success in 12 (86%). Overall 71 (26%) women required a hysterectomy.

Intrauterine tamponade – Tamponade should be supplemented with some adjustment to uterine tone (e.g. uterotonics).

- Intrauterine balloon tamponade (e.g. Rusch balloon) is an appropriate first line 'surgical' intervention for most women where uterine atony is the only or the main cause of haemorrhage. The balloon should be inflated until bleeding is controlled and then left in place for 6–12 hours. (Condom catheters have been used successfully in developing countries to provide haemostasis.) This technique can also be used to manage an atonic uterus at CS
- Uterine packing may be undertaken if a hydrostatic balloon is not available. A ribbon gauze (bandage rolls securely tied to each other) is inserted into the uterus and snugly packed in a zigzag fashion. This technique can also be used to manage an atonic uterus at CS. The pack should be removed by the vaginal route after 24 hours under the cover of intravenous antibiotics and a syntocinon infusion

If tamponade fails to stop the bleeding, the following conservative surgical interventions may be attempted, depending on clinical circumstances and available expertise.

Haemostatic brace suturing (B-Lynch or modified B-Lynch) – The B-Lynch suture was devised for use at CS. It should only be used if the bleeding is successfully controlled by bimanual pressure. A rapidly absorbable stitch is passed through the anterior wall of the uterus at the level of the uterine incision, over the right cornu, horizontally through the lower posterior wall, over the left cornu, back through the anterior wall at the left side of the uterine incision and tied in front (Figure 28.1). An assistant compresses the uterus manually as the suture is tightened. Various modifications not requiring opening of the uterus have been described.

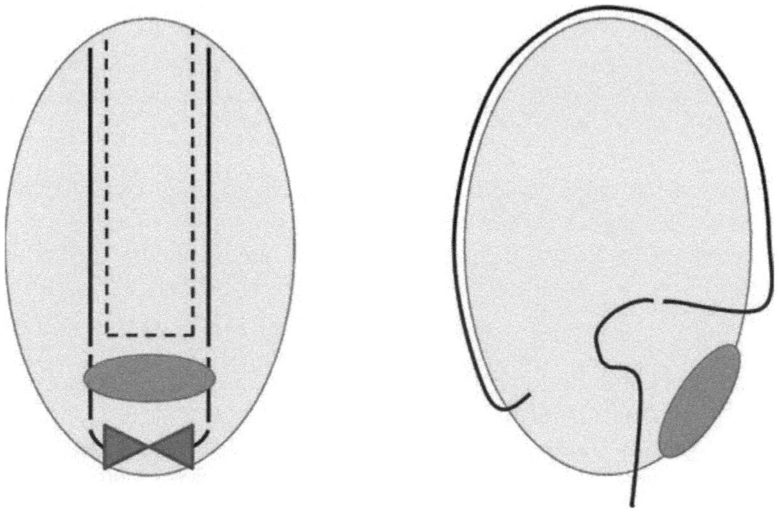

Figure 28.1 B-Lynch brace suture

> **It is recommended that a laminated diagram of the brace technique be kept in theatre**

Stepwise uterine artery ligation or bilateral ligation of the iliac arteries – This procedure is rarely indicated and makes subsequent interventional radiology with embolisation extremely difficult. If needed it is best carried out by a vascular surgeon or one with equivalent experience as it is a hazardous procedure.

Selective arterial embolisation by an interventional radiologist – This may not be possible during an acute bleed as the patient may need to be transported to an imaging suite for the insertion of catheters. Successful use may avert the need for hysterectomy and allow future fertility.

Tissue and trauma

When bleeding persists despite a contracted uterus, or when a uterus fails to contract in response to oxytocic agents, or contracts but then keeps relaxing again, there may be retained tissue or trauma to the genital tract. Once initial resuscitation is effective, the vagina, cervix and uterine cavity need to be explored urgently. Further interventions will depend on the cause found, if any. Interventional radiology techniques may be appropriate.

Hysterectomy should be undertaken sooner rather than later when haemostasis cannot be secured.

Manual compression of the aorta may allow catch-up resuscitation.

Anaesthetic management

The general approach should be the same regardless of the aetiology of the haemorrhage. The anaesthetist needs to be able to assess the patient quickly, to initiate or continue to resuscitate to restore the intravascular volume, and to provide safe anaesthesia.

Important points in the assessment will include:

- Previous medical, obstetric and anaesthetic history
- A working diagnosis as to the likely cause of the obstetric haemorrhage
- Current vital signs and laboratory results
- An examination of the cardiovascular and respiratory systems
- An assessment of the upper airway as regards ease of intubation for rapid sequence induction of anaesthesia

Prophylaxis against acid aspiration is recommended for all patients

Regional or general anaesthesia

The presence of cardiovascular instability and signs of shock are a relative contraindication to regional blockade. The accompanying sympathetic blockade removes compensatory mechanisms and has the potential to worsen hypotension due to haemorrhage.

If cardiovascular stability has been achieved and bleeding has stopped with no evidence of coagulation failure from a consumptive cause or on testing, regional anaesthesia can be used. This may be particularly appropriate where a working epidural has been in place during labour. Continuous epidural block may be preferred to a single injection spinal technique, to allow better control of blood pressure and for prolonged surgery. The height of the block needs to be well maintained to allow intra-abdominal handling of viscera without discomfort.

When bleeding is torrential and cardiovascular stability cannot be achieved and/or a consumptive coagulopathy is possible from the history, rapid sequence induction of general anaesthesia is more appropriate. The anaesthetist should ensure a 'major obstetric haemorrhage (MOH) call' has gone out to mobilise senior help and assistance in addition to alerting the blood bank, labs and portering services that they will be required for emergency management. Sufficient pairs of hands are needed to lead the resuscitation and anaesthetic, to control fluid and blood transfusion ordering and replacement, while simultaneously preparing to site invasive lines and obtaining blood samples (arterial blood gases, haemoglobin, lactate and near patient testing of coagulation). Ideally it requires three anaesthetic team members.

Human factors in such fraught situations can lead to error. The team should ensure effective exchange of information by SBAR (situation, background, assessment and recommendation) and perform a World Health Organization (WHO) surgical pause to ensure all staff involved share the same 'mental model' of the situation. Maintaining communication between the team members during the resuscitation by the use of 'mini pauses' is essential for patient safety. Ensure the team leader maintains a 'helicopter view' of the situation.

Induction agents with minimal peripheral vasodilator action, such as ketamine 1–2 mg/kg (Ketalar®, Parke-Davis) or etomidate 100–300 micrograms/kg (Hypnomidate®, Janssen-Cilag) should be considered. Vasopressors should be ready in case of cardiovascular collapse on induction. Actively warming all fluids and the patient should begin immediately to aid coagulation. Patient temperature should be monitored continuously and documented every 15 minutes. Give tranexamic acid once the blood loss is over 1 litre. Repeat blood gases and coagulation studies every 30 minutes to guide replacement of red cells, platelets and coagulation factors and to optimise ventilation. Replace calcium guided by the blood gases.

Volatile agents have been associated with increased blood loss due to their relaxant effects on uterine muscle. Total intravenous anaesthesia could be considered if uterine atony is a problem.

Cell salvage

The SALVO (Cell Salvage in Obstetrics) trial concluded that the overall reduction observed in donor blood transfusion associated with the routine use of cell salvage during CS was not statistically significant. Therefore, the routine use of cell salvage at the time of CS is not likely to be cost effective. However, in patients who refuse allogenic blood transfusion, cell salvage is the only option to replace oxygen carrying capacity in a haemorrhage emergency.

28.5 Patients declining blood and blood products

Establishing wishes

Patients may decline blood and blood products because of their religious commitment or other personal beliefs. Many Jehovah's Witnesses believe that blood transfusion is forbidden and wish to be treated with effective non-blood alternatives. For all patients, doctors are obliged to deliver the best care in keeping with the patient's wishes. The legal position is that any adult patient (i.e. 16 years of age and over) who has the necessary mental capacity to do so is entitled to refuse treatment, even if it is likely that refusal will result in the patient's death. No other person is legally able to consent to treatment for that adult or to refuse treatment on that person's behalf and the patient should be seen alone at some point in her pregnancy to clarify their exact wishes and ensure they are not being coerced in any way. Having a witness at these discussions is helpful and should be clearly documented.

Generally speaking, Jehovah's Witnesses decline the transfusion of whole blood, packed red blood cells, white blood cells, fresh frozen plasma and platelets. However, when it comes to derivatives of blood components (e.g. cryoprecipitate, fibrinogen concentrate, prothrombin factor concentrate, albumin and immunoglobulins) the use of these products is variably acceptable. Cell salvage is usually acceptable but it should be explained that it will not enable endogenous clotting factors to be returned (see Chapter 8).

Obtaining consent

Document the content of discussions clearly, including the persons present. Obtain from the patient a clear statement of what products and techniques she understands and will accept and what she refuses. Complete a 'no blood' consent form (featured as an appendix in the Royal College of Surgeons of England's 'Caring for patients who refuse blood': www.rcseng.ac.uk; last accessed January 2022).

Explain the risk of refusal of allogenic blood frankly but not dramatically. Discuss earlier surgical intervention, including the possibility of an earlier decision to proceed to CS for antepartum haemorrhage or hysterectomy in uncontrolled PPH.

Most Jehovah's Witnesses will carry with them a clear advance directive prohibiting blood transfusions and including information relating to the patient's view of blood products and autologous transfusion procedures. The advance directive should be lodged with the patient's GP, as well as with family and friends. If the patient is not in a condition to give or withhold consent but has expressed a wish at an earlier date (advance directive or healthcare advance directive), respect the patient's instructions.

If such instructions do not specifically apply to the patient's current condition, if the patient's instructions are vague and open to interpretation or if there is good reason to believe that the patient has had a change of mind since making the declaration, the doctor's duty is to exercise good medical judgement and treat the patient in her best interests as determined by a responsible body of medical opinion.

Allow the patient the opportunity to speak with the hospital liaison committee for Jehovah's Witnesses and, if requested, join their discussion.

A verbally expressed change of mind should be honoured. Again, it should be given in the presence of a witness and recorded in the notes. It is relevant to ensure that women are given an opportunity to change their minds at any stage, but they will eventually become unconscious as they lose blood and will be unable to affect the decision-making process from this point.

Plan antenatal and intrapartum care

Major obstetric haemorrhage is often unpredictable and can become life threatening in a short time. Delivery should be planned in a unit that has the facilities to cope with major obstetric haemorrhage, including appropriate surgical expertise, interventional radiology and the option of cell salvage. Management should be geared to anticipating, preventing or stopping bleeding early. If any complications are noted during the antenatal period, the consultant obstetrician must be informed.

Optimise physiological variables in the antenatal period. The woman's blood group and antibody status should be checked in the usual way and the haemoglobin and serum ferritin should be checked regularly and optimised with oral iron supplementation from the booking appointment. Haematinics should be given throughout pregnancy to maximise iron stores, including intravenous iron if required if ferritin remains low despite oral iron. Treat any complications that could give rise to bleeding.

Manage delivery routinely by experienced staff. The consultant obstetrician and consultant anaesthetist should be informed when a woman who will refuse blood transfusion is admitted in labour. The labour should be managed by experienced staff and prolonged labour should be avoided. If an operative delivery is needed it should be conducted by a senior obstetrician. Oxytocics should be given when the baby is delivered. The woman should not be left alone for at least an hour after delivery and there should be early intervention to stem any postpartum bleeding.

When the mother is discharged from hospital, she should be advised to report promptly if she has any concerns about bleeding during the puerperium.

If unusual bleeding occurs at any time during pregnancy, labour or the puerperium, the consultant obstetrician, anaesthetist and haematologist should be informed and standard management should be commenced promptly. The principle of management of haemorrhage in these cases is to avoid delay. Rapid senior decision making may be necessary, particularly with regard to surgical intervention, and the threshold for such intervention should be lower than in other patients. Extra vigilance should be exercised to quantify any abnormal bleeding and to detect complications, such as clotting abnormalities, as promptly as possible. Give tranexamic acid early. Use cell salvage if acceptable to the patient and the abdomen is open. Optimise physiological variables (oxygenation, temperature, calcium) to reduce the effect of blood loss. If the patient is anaemic below the transfusion threshold refer early to critical care for organ support. Continue iron replacement and consider recombinant erythropoietin. Hyperbaric environments can protect against the physiological effects of anaemia, but are not easily accessible.

28.6 Summary

- Major obstetric haemorrhage is common and all units must have clear guidance and protocols for its management
- Early recognition is essential
- There should be prompt resuscitation (ABC) and volume replacement
- 'Turn off the tap' (the 'four Ts')
- Close monitoring
- Plan for the care of women refusing blood products

28.7 Further reading

Khan KS, Moore PAS, Wilson MJ, et al.; SALVO study group. Cell salvage and donor blood transfusion during caesarean section: a pragmatic, multicentre randomised controlled trial (SALVO). *PLoS Med* 2017; 14(12): e1002471.

Klein AA, Bailey CR, Charlton A, et al. *Guidelines: Anaesthesia and Peri-operative Care for Jehovah's Witnesses and Patients who Refuse Blood.* London: Association of Anaesthetists, 2018.

Knight M, Bamber J, Lucas S, Paterson-Brown S, Tufnell D, on behalf of the MBRRACE-UK Haemorrhage Chapter Writing Group. Messages for prevention and treatment of morbidity from major obstetric haemorrhage. In: Knight M, Bunch K, Tuffnell D, et al. (eds) on behalf of MBRRACE-UK. *Saving Lives, Improving Mothers' Care – Lessons Learned to Inform Maternity Care from the UK and Ireland Confidential Enquiries into Maternal Deaths and Morbidity 2014–2016*. Oxford: National Perinatal Epidemiology Unit, University of Oxford, 2018, pp. 23–33.

RCOG (Royal College of Obstetricians and Gynaecologists). *Postpartum Haemorrhage, Prevention and Management*. Green-top Guideline No. 52. London: RCOG, 2016. https://www.rcog.org.uk/en/guidelines-research-services/guidelines/gtg52/ (last accessed January 2022).

WOMAN Trial Collaborators. Effect of early tranexamic acid administration on mortality, hysterectomy, and other morbidities in women with postpartum haemorrhage (WOMAN): an international, randomised, double-blind, placebo-controlled trial. *Lancet* 2017; 389(10084); 2105–16.

CHAPTER 29

Caesarean section

Learning outcomes

After reading this chapter, you will be able to:

- Discuss how to anticipate and, to some extent, avoid difficulties encountered at caesarean section
- Appreciate the techniques that can help with such difficulties

29.1 Introduction

Caesarean section (CS) may be required on fetal grounds or on maternal grounds. Rates vary enormously, not only between countries but also between hospitals, but trends are generally increasing worldwide. The CS rate for 2018–20 in England was 29%, according to the NHS Maternity Statistics report (May 2020). The caesarean rate continues to rise in developing countries as well, and has now reached 50% in China. This procedure has become one of the most (if not *the* most) commonly performed operations in the world. The decision to perform a CS can appear obvious in some circumstances, whilst in others it can be extremely difficult. Decision making requires experience and clinical judgement, and a CS should never be seen as the easy option. All risks of CS, in comparison to vaginal delivery, should be considered and balanced in each individual circumstance, considering both maternal and fetal interests.

This chapter is not designed to list the indications or arguments for CS, nor to give intricate detail into surgical technique, but rather to highlight the difficulties that can be encountered (both anticipated and unexpected) and to suggest ways in which they can be predicted, recognised and dealt with in the acute situation.

Prerequisites for caesarean section

- The woman should understand the indications for the procedure and agree to it, ideally giving written informed consent
- Anaesthesia should be achieved (either regional or general)
- As with all operative interventions, the World Health Organization (WHO) checklist procedure must first be carried out. This is especially important in the emergency situation, and each unit must devise a way to ensure a succinct and efficient process
- The patient or operating table should be tilted laterally 30° to minimise aortocaval compression during the procedure
- The bladder should be kept empty with a urethral catheter
- Someone who is capable of performing neonatal resuscitation should be present
- The surgical team must have appropriate experience and competence
- Prophylactic antibiotics should be used and appropriate thromboprophylaxis considered
- Blood may need to be grouped and saved or crossmatched, depending on the clinical situation at hand and local arrangements

Managing Medical and Obstetric Emergencies and Trauma: A Practical Approach, Fourth Edition. Edited by Rosamunde Burns and Kara Dent.

29.2 Surgical technique for caesarean section

Before embarking on any surgery, rehearse the principles of good and safe surgical technique:

- Maintain a sterile operative field
- Achieve good exposure with an appropriate incision
- Keep tissue handling to a minimum and avoid unnecessary dissection and trauma
- Treat the tissues with respect
- Achieve meticulous haemostasis
- While operating, positively consider and avoid the common problems that could turn a straightforward procedure into a complex one

Skin incision

A low transverse skin incision is usually adequate for all uterine incisions except the true high classic incision extending up to the fundus. Make sure that the skin incision used affords adequate access.

Entry

Entry to the peritoneal cavity should be careful and safe. Special care is needed if there has been previous surgery, as bowel can be tethered or the bladder can be high and adherent.

Elevating a fold of the peritoneum with two forceps and incising between them with scissors or a knife is preferable to poking the fingers through the peritoneum.

The surgeon and the assistant should avoid hooking fingers under the rectus muscle (between the rectus muscle and the peritoneum), as this can seriously threaten the inferior epigastric vascular bundle, leading to bleeding and to the development of subrectus haematoma.

Before extending the peritoneal incision by tearing or by scissors, check that there are no adhesions hidden from view, and remember to be gentle.

Assess the lower uterine segment

The uterovesical peritoneal reflection identifies the upper limit of the lower uterine segment, and is invaluable in planning the uterine incision in difficult circumstances, such as CS at full dilatation, preterm delivery or abnormal lie.

Always check the degree of uterine rotation, and correct it, or allow for it, prior to making the uterine incision, to reduce the likelihood of angle extension into the broad ligament.

Exposure

Make sure that the peritoneum is reflected well clear of the proposed angles of the uterine incision, as failure to do this can compromise access, haemostasis and closure of the angles if they have extended during delivery.

Uterine incision

Do not do this until you have checked and confirmed that there is a presenting part in the pelvis, or you have felt for the fetal lie and made a plan with your assistant regarding how to conduct the delivery.

In making the uterine incision, always try to leave the membranes intact, as this will make it less likely that you will cut the baby. The membranes can then be carefully nicked just prior to delivery.

Remember that the thicker the uterine lower segment (as in in preterm delivery, placenta praevia, a high presenting part or an abnormal lie), the less space it affords you in terms of access to the fetus. Make sure that the incision is big enough.

Be careful during this stage of the surgery to get your assistant to keep the lie of the fetus longitudinal – this is especially important if the lower segment is poorly formed or full of fibroid or placenta. The last thing you need in this difficult situation with compromised space is for the fetus to drift off into an oblique or transverse lie.

Delivery

The fetus's head delivers into the wound in the occipitotransverse position by lateral flexion. This procedure should be conducted gently and slowly to avoid trauma to, and extension of, the uterine angles.

Fundal pressure during the delivery should be sustained and should follow the distal end of the fetus on its way out (like squeezing toothpaste from a tube).

Placenta

While the placenta is attached, the placental site will not bleed and there is no need to hurry this process. Wait for separation to occur rather than precipitating a problem. Hospital guidelines include delayed clamping of the cord if there is no emergency. If there is bleeding, then Green-Armytage clamps can be placed on the bleeding sinuses or angles as needed.

Check that all placenta and membranes have been removed.

Check the patency of the internal cervical os and that it is not covered with membrane.

Closure of the uterus

Both uterine angles need to be secured carefully and accurately, with each stitch passing full thickness into the uterine cavity. Failure to achieve this full-thickness suturing can leave a bleeding vessel within the cavity, which will remain hidden from the surgeon's view and produce vaginal bleeding later.

If there are placental bed bleeders (commonly seen with placenta praevia), then attention should be given to these before closing the uterus, as once closed such bleeding is hidden from the surgeon's view. These can be dealt with by systemic uterotonics, but may also need an under-running suture. Persistent placental bed bleeding can also be dealt with using tamponade with a balloon catheter, such as a Rusch or Bakri balloon, once the uterus is closed. This allows direct observation of the uterine suture whilst blowing up the balloon to ensure it remains intact.

The uterus should routinely be closed with a double layer suture. Occasionally, the lower segment is so thin that a single layer is all that is possible.

Haemostasis

Once the uterus is closed, the suture line and both angles should be checked for haemostasis while exposed without tension.

Great care should then be taken checking for haemostasis before the sheath is closed, including the peritoneal edges, the subrectus space and, if exposed, the inferior epigastric bundles. Where the peritoneum is not closed, this process of haemostasis is even more important as there is no tamponade effect on bleeding vessels in this layer, potentially leading to significant haemorrhage.

Drains

Anyone who claims never to need drains because they 'never close if everything isn't perfectly dry' paints an enviable but rather naïve picture. Whilst haemostasis should always be the aim, occasionally drains can be useful if there has been extremely difficult surgery with extensive dissection and raw surfaces, or if there is likely to be a postpartum clotting problem (e.g. fulminating pre-eclampsia, HELLP (haemolysis, elevated liver enzymes, low platelet count), disseminated intravascular coagulation, sepsis). Blood pressure may be lower than normal during surgery and give a false sign of haemostasis.

It is important to remember that drains do not reduce bleeding, but rather they alert us to the fact that bleeding is occurring. Any drain placed within the peritoneal cavity should be soft and large bore (such as the Robinson drain) and not suctioned. If a suctioned drain is placed in the rectus space then the peritoneum should be closed (otherwise the drain is effectively intra-abdominal).

Closure

Close the sheath, then check for haemostasis before closing the fat layer and skin.

Postoperative procedure

If the neonate is delivered in good condition, they should be handed to the mother as soon as possible to encourage skin-to-skin contact. The midwife can facilitate this during surgery.

After surgery, the abdomen should be palpated to check that the uterus is well contracted, and the vagina should be swabbed out to check that there is no continued bleeding. The mother should not leave theatre until the uterus is contracted and any bleeding has stopped.

The swabs and instruments should be counted, and the final step of the WHO checklist process should be undertaken.

Every aspect of the delivery should be documented. Most particularly, the findings, including the position of the fetus's head, should be clearly described, as should any problems that were encountered.

Prior to leaving theatre, the estimated blood loss, the urine output and colour, as well as the amount and type of fluids the anaesthetist has given, should all be clearly noted. They can be summarised on a fluid/recovery chart, and discrepancies noted and managed. The VTE score should be recalculated and recorded.

Supervision

The supervisor is responsible for the quality and safety of the surgery. They must be comfortable that the procedure is within the scope of the trainee, and they must be able to stop unsafe hands quickly, effectively and subtly if indicated. Conversation needs to maintain calm and demonstrate control, and frank feedback may have to wait until after the procedure is over.

During the delivery of the head, there needs to be communication as to whether progress is being made or not. This is usually what trainees find most difficult, and talking them through the process of rotation and flexion of the fetal head, followed by lateral flexion into the wound, can be helpful.

29.3 Specific difficulties encountered at caesarean section

Difficulty delivering the head in advanced labour

Caesarean section in the second stage of labour is associated with high maternal morbidity and can be extremely difficult. In the UK, there have been some instances of severe fetal trauma caused by difficulty in delivering an impacted fetal head at CS. There is some work that suggests that this is due to decreasing skill in effecting instrumental vaginal delivery, making CS necessary when forceps or ventouse would have been more appropriate and successful previously. CS at full dilatation is not straightforward and should be decided upon in conjunction with a senior obstetrician, and conducted or supervised by the same (i.e. year 6/7 specialty trainee or consultant).

Do not fight the uterus! If the head is deeply impacted in the pelvis in advanced labour, then once the uterus is opened at CS and the hand inserted into the pelvis, a uterine contraction will follow. This can be felt as huge pressure on the operator's hand. Struggling to manipulate the fetal head against uterine activity in this situation should be avoided – it will prolong the uterine contraction and is highly likely to fail or will cause extension of the uterine angles. Wait with the hand unmoving until the contraction eases off, and the hand no longer feels so squashed. Then proceed with disimpaction, flexion with or without rotation (depending on the position), lateral flexion and delivery, which can usually be achieved gently without force. Consider using your left hand to disimpact the head as it places minimal pressure against the lower segment and allows easy deflexion, minimising damage to the uterus.

Pushing the head up from below, or pushing up on the fetal shoulder, is common practice, but if the uterus is contracting, this can also be unhelpful and patiently awaiting uterine relaxation is the key. If you do need disimpaction from below, be sure your assistant is clear in what you are trying to achieve and does not deflex the head further. Equally, trying to apply one blade of the forceps to try to scoop the head up is illogical and potentially dangerous.

In the rare circumstances when, despite doing the above, the head still cannot be disimpacted, then the uterus can be further relaxed by the anaesthetist administering a tocolytic (either 250 micrograms of terbutaline subcutaneously or 250 micrograms of glyceryl trinitrate sublingually) with circulatory support and intensive monitoring.

Techniques such as the fetal pillow have been introduced to disimpact the head before attempted delivery manually, although the evidence is not there to support it as a recommendation by the National Institute for Health and Care Excellence (NICE). The MIDAS study, being undertaken by the UK Obstetric Surveillance System (UKOSS), is looking specifically at the impacted fetal head at CS and its consequences as well as techniques used in these scenarios.

The uterine incision can be extended (in either an inverted 'T' or a 'J') to improve access if it is inadequate, although this is rarely needed. Patwardhan's procedure can also be used (see 'Shoulder presentation' later in this section).

Access to the uterine cavity

When performing a CS in the second stage of labour, the lower segment will have stretched and its upper limit can extend much higher than initially thought. The danger in this situation is to enter the 'lower segment' too low and inadvertently go straight into the vagina. To avoid such inadvertent laparoelytrotomies, the uterovesical fold should be positively identified and then the uterine incision should be made approximately 3 cm below it.

Fibroids can seriously hamper access to the uterine cavity, and antenatal ultrasound scans, however descriptive of the fibroids, are not conducted with surgical access in mind. For this reason, an ultrasound scan performed immediately before surgery, by the surgeon, can check the thickness of the anterior wall over the proposed incision site and the relative positions of the fibroids to this, as well as the fetal lie. This can be of enormous benefit in planning the most accessible route of entry and how best to conduct the delivery. Another problem regarding fibroids relates to the degree of uterine rotation that they can cause, so checking the position of the fibroids in early pregnancy can help anticipate potential problems.

Access to the fetus

A fetus with an unstable or abnormal lie can cause problems with delivery at CS. The question 'why is this fetus lying abnormally' should be asked and answered prior to surgery. An experienced surgeon should be present in all such 'unexplained' cases in nulliparous women, as the technical problems encountered, if they are due to amniotic bands or uterine anomaly, can be demanding.

Placenta praevia

Placenta praevia is now seen in 1/200 pregnancies and these can be complicated caesareans requiring senior involvement. Access to the uterine cavity and the fetus is hampered by a thick vascular lower segment as well as by the placenta itself. The assistant should maintain the longitudinal lie of the fetus while the uterus is being incised and not get distracted by the bleeding. Interrupting the continuous pressure on the abdomen should be avoided as it can allow the fetus to drift away from a longitudinal lie if the placenta is filling the lower segment. Preparation is vital, ensuring that there is a source of blood readily available for transfusion. Cell salvage is useful if available.

The two recent MBRRACE reports highlight nine and three maternal deaths due to placenta preaevia and/or placenta accrete, respectively, as a cause.

If a woman has had a previous CS and has an anterior, low-lying placenta, imaging and multidisciplinary team (MDT) planning is vital to optimise delivery. Ultrasound and MRI are used to ascertain the degree of parametrial invasion. This can vary and is probably the reason for the large incidences reported of 1/300 to 1/2000 pregnancies. With an MDT approach, these elective cases should take place at 35–36 + 6 weeks if symptomatic, or between 36 + 0 to 37 + 0 weeks if asymptomatic. Interventional radiology may be available. As an emergency and unexpected finding at CS, there are cases described where the placenta has been left with conservative management as an option, if there is no bleeding. There is, however, no evidence for methotrexate in these cases.

Anterior placenta

Depending on where the placenta is lying, it may be possible to incise the uterus down to the placenta and then separate it from the uterine wall to expose membranes without dividing the placenta itself. Planning this preoperatively is aided by an ultrasound scan by the surgeon just prior to surgery (to decide which direction to work towards). Sometimes it is necessary to go through the placenta. In such cases, avoiding the cord insertion site (again helped with a preoperative scan) is important. The cord should be clamped as soon as possible on delivering the neonate, to minimise any fetal blood loss from the torn placenta. The neonatologist in attendance should also be warned that this is what is expected so they are prepared in case the neonate experiences acute haemorrhage.

Breech delivery

Many obstetricians believe that a breech fetus is much more at risk of being cut by the scalpel at uterine incision than with a cephalic presentation, but studies have shown no difference, with a rate of around 1%. This reiterates the previous advice: always take care, and try to leave the membranes intact until the uterine incision is complete.

Make the incision big enough, and all the principles of vaginal breech delivery hold true at CS. Apply pressure from above, do not pull and do not lift the body until the nape of the neck is visible. In most cases, manipulation can be kept to a minimum if the initial incision is adequate.

A trapped fetal head during a breech delivery at CS is particularly stressful for the obstetrician, and it can be helpful if the anaesthetist administers a uterine relaxant.

In anticipation of an entrapment, always ensure that both abdominal and uterine incisions are adequate. If problems are still encountered and tocolysis does not resolve the problem, consider converting the uterine incision to a 'J' shape, by extending upwards from one angle of the incision.

Wrigley's forceps can be applied to assist in the delivery of the aftercoming head at CS. Care still needs to be taken to avoid hyperextension of the neck during the application of the blades. The direction of traction must then flex the neck.

Premature delivery

Assessment at the time of delivery will enable you to decide if there is sufficient lower segment. If not, a classic section is indicated. Delivery of the fetus needs to be very gentle with no unnecessary force, ideally in the sac of membranes if possible. Timing of these sections may have to take into account the administration of magnesium sulphate if below 30–32 weeks for a minimum of 4 hours, for the purposes of cerebral protection for the baby. This and the administration of steroids is if timing allows.

Shoulder presentation

If a fetal arm is prolapsed through the vagina, consider ***Patwardhan's procedure,*** which involves delivering the fetal breech first. Usually, a transverse incision in the uterus is adequate, although the incision can be extended by converting it to a 'J' shape. The operator's hand is passed upwards until a leg is reached and either the leg or the breech is delivered. The rest of the delivery is as for a caesarean breech delivery. This technique can also be used if the head is deeply engaged and disimpaction is unsuccessful.

Extreme prematurity

With extreme prematurity, especially if the fetus is lying transversely or presenting breech, a classical incision should be considered to avoid any extra manipulation of the neonate on delivery.

Uterine trauma

The uterine incision may extend into the broad ligament, tearing uterine vessels and leading to brisk bleeding. After consultation with the anaesthetist, it may be helpful to exteriorise the uterus, so that the posterior aspect of the uterus and broad ligament can be examined. In addition, traction to elevate the uterus may slow the blood loss and help to identify the bleeding areas requiring attention. The proximity of the ureter must be borne in mind and an effort made to sweep the bladder down and with it the ureter. This will enable better access to the uterine vessels. If bleeding is heavy it may be very difficult to identify the ureter. The priority is to control haemorrhage, and subsequent expert urological help should always be requested if damage is suspected.

Troublesome haemorrhage from the angle of the uterine incision may be controlled by the insertion of a suture to control the uterine artery. Again, every effort should be made to identify the ureter.

Thromboprophylaxis

The need for thromboprophylaxis should be considered in all women following CS. The widespread application of thromboprophylaxis protocols following CS is likely to be the cause of the significant reduction in the rate of maternal deaths from venous thromboembolism, as documented in MBRRACE-UK reports. It should be remembered that risk factors are additive, and include advanced maternal age, caesarean in labour, pre-eclampsia, sepsis or other inflammatory conditions, haemorrhage and maternal obesity.

29.4 Audit standards

The following should be audited routinely:

- Rates of CS, especially in different groups of women (e.g. Robson groups)
- Incidence of massive blood loss associated with CS
- Returns to theatre
- Wound infections
- Standard of documentation (including operative findings)

29.5 Summary

- Caesarean section is common, and attention to detail is essential in order to minimise morbidity
- Anticipation of problems and an awareness of the techniques described in this chapter, together with senior experienced help when appropriate, are most likely to lead to the best outcomes

29.6 Further reading

Boatin AA, Cullinane F, Torloni MR, Betrán AP. Audit and feedback using the Robson classification to reduce caesarean section rates: a systematic review. *BJOG* 2018; 125(1): 36–42.

Knight M, Nair M, Tuffnell D, Shakespeare J, Kenyon S, Kurinczuk JJ (eds) on behalf of MBRRACE-UK. *Saving Lives, Improving Mothers' Care – Lessons Learned to Inform Maternity Care from the UK and Ireland Confidential Enquiries into Maternal Deaths and Morbidity 2013–15.* Oxford: National Perinatal Epidemiology Unit, University of Oxford, 2017.

NICE (National Institute for Health and Care Excellence). *Caesarean Section Overview*. London: NICE, last updated July 2017. http://pathways.nice.org.uk/pathways/caesarean-section (last accessed January 2022).

RCOG (Royal College of Obstetricians and Gynaecologists). *Magnesium Sulphate to Prevent Cerebral Palsy following Preterm Birth*. Scientific Impact Paper No. 29. London: RCOG, 2011.

RCOG (Royal College of Obstetricians and Gynaecologists). *Placenta Praevia and Placenta Accreta. Diagnosis and Management*. Green-top Guideline No. 27a. London: RCOG, 2018.

CHAPTER 30

Abnormally invasive placenta and retained placenta

Learning outcomes

After reading this chapter, you will be able to:

- Recognise risk factors for an abnormally invasive placenta
- Describe the need for a multidisciplinary plan of management where abnormally invasive placenta is suspected
- Describe the technique for manual removal of retained placenta

30.1 Introduction

Postpartum haemorrhage (PPH) is a major cause of maternal morbidity and mortality. Chapter 28 covered the management of major obstetric haemorrhage; this chapter will look at the management of problems where there is an abnormally invasive placenta or an adherent placenta, where separation does not occur and manual removal is required.

30.2 Abnormally invasive placenta

Definition and incidence

The normal placenta does not penetrate deeper than the decidua basalis and usually separates spontaneously after uterine contraction at delivery. Abnormally invasive placenta (AIP) is a clinical term used to describe a placenta that does not do so and cannot be removed without causing abnormally high blood loss. The term includes the histopathological diagnoses of placenta accreta, increta and percreta and describes a spectrum disorder, ranging from placentae containing a small area of abnormally adherent tissue (focal accreta) to those which have invaded into the adjacent viscera (percreta) and is potentially life threatening, as forced removal of an AIP can lead to catastrophic maternal hemorrhage.

In developed countries rates of PPH are increasing, with a near-doubling of the maternal death rate from haemorrhage. This is almost entirely due to the increase in the numbers of women dying in association with AIP, itself the commonest indication for caesarean hysterectomy. The incidence of AIP has risen from 1/25 000 deliveries in the 1950s to around 1/500 at present, following the rise in caesarean section (CS) rates. The risk of AIP rises with previous CS, other uterine surgery, assisted reproduction techniques and placenta praevia – the prevalence of all of which has increased in recent decades. It is particularly rising in line with the number of previous CS and especially in the presence of placenta praevia. If a woman having her third CS has a placenta praevia, she has a 40% chance of AIP. In the 2005–2006 UK Obstetric Surveillance System (UKOSS) study of peripartum hysterectomy, 39% of women having this operation had an AIP, and the main risk factor was a previous CS.

Managing Medical and Obstetric Emergencies and Trauma: A Practical Approach, Fourth Edition. Edited by Rosamunde Burns and Kara Dent.

The UKOSS data published in 2013 showed that only 50% of cases of placenta accreta/increta or percreta in the UK were identified antenatally. These were associated with significantly reduced levels of haemorrhage (2750 versus 6100 ml) and reduced the need for blood transfusion as expected. The most recent MBRRACE-UK data show a static rate of maternal death in association with haemorrhage of 0.63/100 000 maternities.

Diagnosis of abnormally invasive placenta

Maternal morbidity and mortality are reduced when AIP is diagnosed antenatally and those women deliver in a specialist centre, with care provided by a multidisciplinary team, consisting of obstetricans, obstetric anaesthetists, urological and vascular surgeons and interventional radiologists and appropriate support staff. All women who have had a previous CS should be advised to have ultrasound assessment of the placental site at 20 weeks, even if they decline an anomaly scan. If the placenta is anterior and appears to cover the scar (i.e. reaches or covers the internal cervical os), the scan should be repeated at 32 weeks. If the placenta remains anterior and low, the woman should be referred for assessment at a specialist centre. Standard ultrasound descriptors of AIP have recently been proposed:

- A loss of the hypoechoic retroplacental zone
- Multiple vascular lacunae, some large and irregular, often with turbulent flow detectable on greyscale imaging
- Bladder wall interruption
- Retroplacental myometrial thickness <1 mm or undetectable
- Blood vessels or placental tissue bridging the uterine–placental margin, the myometrial–bladder interface or crossing the uterine serosa
- Placental bulge
- Focal exophytic mass
- Uterovesical hypervascularity
- Subplacental hypervascularity
- 'Bridging vessels' from the placenta into the bladder or other organs
- Placental lacunae feeding vessels
- Intraplacental hypervascularity on 3D power Doppler

Studies suggest that colour Doppler has the high sensitivity and moderate specificity. Magnetic resonance imaging (MRI) is recommended in cases where the scan is inconclusive, or where there is suspicion that the placenta has invaded adjacent organs.

The features which suggest accreta are:

- Uterine bulging
- Heterogenous signal density within the placenta
- Dark intraplacental bands on T2-weighted imaging

Measurement of cell-free placental messenger RNA (mRNA) in the maternal plasma has been described as a means of improving the accuracy of the diagnosis, but is not clinically available. Elevated levels of alpha-fetoprotein, free beta-human chorionic gonadotrophin (beta-hCG) and creatinine kinase have also been associated with placenta accreta, but are not advocated as screening or diagnostic tests.

Despite these investigations, it is not possible to diagnose or exclude placenta accreta with certainty in the antenatal period, and if the placenta still appears to overlie the scar at 32 weeks' pregnancy the management plan for a woman with a previous CS should assume that there is a risk of accreta.

Management of abnormally invasive placenta

Any pregnant woman with a low anterior placenta or a placenta praevia and a previous CS is at risk of major obstetric haemorrhage and should have a regular assessment of full blood count (give iron supplements where appropriate). Care should be consultant based and follow the 'placenta praevia after CS' care bundle:

- Consultant obstetrician planned and directly supervising the delivery
- Consultant anaesthetist planned and directly supervising anaesthesia at delivery
- Blood and blood products available on site
- Multidisciplinary involvement in preoperative planning

- Discussion and consent including possible interventions (such as hysterectomy, leaving the placenta in situ, cell salvage and interventional radiology)
- Local availability of level two critical care bed

The optimal timing of delivery depends on the clinical features but is generally advocated around 37 weeks to reduce the risks of an emergency procedure should labour start spontaneously or heavy antepartum haemorrhage occur. It is advisable to administer steroids to improve fetal lung maturity.

Multidisciplinary discussion should involve:

- Theatre staff to plan equipment required, such as cell salvage and additional instruments for hysterectomy and balloon tamponade
- Interventional radiologists to decide if preoperative placement of femoral balloons is required, advise on imaging modalities required in theatre or to be on standby should the need arise
- Anaesthetists to plan anaesthesia technique and equipment required, and to liaise with critical care
- Haematologist to alert laboratory staff to possible need for large amounts of blood and clotting factors
- Consideration of the need for other surgical support: gynaecologist, vascular surgeon, urologist
- Neonatal team, especially if surgery has to take place away from the normal theatre to allow access for interventional radiology

It is advisable to draw up a checklist with the names and contact details of all involved in the case. This should be in the patient's notes in case labour starts prior to the planned date.

The consultant obstetrician should discuss plans thoroughly with the woman and her partner antenatally, and document these in the notes. If their family is complete and the placenta does not readily separate, then immediate hysterectomy leaving the placenta in place is the best course of action. If the woman wishes to preserve her fertility, then it may be possible to leave the placenta in situ and close the uterus. She must understand that hysterectomy may still be required, and she will have to attend for prolonged follow-up; there is also a risk of infection to consider.

With a placenta praevia that is asymptomatic, delivery is recommended between 36 + 0 and 37 + 0 weeks. If it is a symptomatic placenta praevia or known placenta accreta, delivery should be considered earlier between 35 + 0 and 36 + 6 weeks (if there are no other risk factors for preterm delivery). This is considered the best balance between an unplanned emergency delivery and fetal maturity. Steroids are recommended for a known placenta praevia between 34 + 0 and 35 + 6 weeks in preparation to aid fetal lung maturity and unplanned delivery.

A retrospective, multicentre study in France from 1993 to 2007 reviewed 167 cases of placenta accreta treated conservatively. Management was successful in 78%, with spontaneous placental resorption occurring in 75% of these women – taking a median of 13.5 weeks (range 4–60 weeks). One woman died of complications related to administration of methotrexate. There were 21 successful subsequent pregnancies, but placenta accreta reoccurred in six pregnancies.

Surgical considerations

Ideally, the uterus should be opened avoiding the placenta; a vertical skin incision may be required. It is good practice to confirm the placental position by ultrasound scan immediately prior to the operation. If necessary, a scan probe can be covered with a sterile sleeve and used directly on the uterus intraoperatively. Exteriorisation of the uterus and a posterior uterine wall incision have been performed in cases where the placenta covered the entire anterior uterine wall. If the placenta is incised on entry to the uterus, immediately clamp the cord once the baby is delivered to avoid excessive fetal blood loss.

If the placenta does not separate following administration of syntocinon, the cord should be unclamped and drained of blood, and the cord ligated close to the placenta and cut short, and the uterine incision should be closed. Depending on the patient's wishes and clinical needs, hysterectomy or conservative treatment follows as appropriate. Prophylactic antibiotics are needed for a few days if the placenta is left in situ. Serum beta-hCG levels should be checked twice weekly, together with full blood count and C-reactive protein levels to look for signs of infection, and the woman kept under close review. Methotrexate has been used with varying degrees of success. As it precludes breastfeeding it should not be routinely used, but may be considered if the beta-hCG levels do not fall.

In the situation where placenta accreta was not anticipated, surgical entry has failed to avoid the placenta or the placenta partially separates and bleeding ensues, the situation is more hazardous and is associated with heavy bleeding. In these situations, it is advisable to remove the placenta as best possible, small portions of myometrium can be removed/sutured to reduce bleeding and local infiltration of uterotonics or balloon tamponade may be helpful. Hysterectomy is, however, likely to be needed in up to 50% of such cases and recognising this and performing it in a timely fashion, before the patient is in extremis, can be life saving.

Anaesthetic considerations

The operation is likely to be prolonged; if regional techniques are used, it may be necessary to convert to general anaesthesia. Large-bore intravenous access and invasive blood pressure monitoring will be required, anticipating a large blood loss. Particular attention should be paid to positioning the patient to avoid nerve compression, and measures taken to reduce thromboembolism and hypothermia. Measure temperature with a temperature probe and document every 15 minutes. Cell salvage should be set up. Regular arterial blood gases and near patient tests of coagulation should be taken from the arterial line to guide resuscitation with red cells and coagulation support. If embolisation is required, it may be necessary to transport the patient from theatre to an imaging department

30.3 Retained placenta

National Institute for Health and Care Excellence (NICE) intrapartum care guidelines define a placenta as retained if it is not delivered within 30 minutes of birth when the third stage is actively managed, or longer than an hour when physiologically managed, without signs of PPH or maternal collapse. The longer the placenta remains undelivered, the greater the risk of haemorrhage. The common risk factors for retained placenta are:

- A previous retained placenta
- Multiparity
- Preterm labour
- Induced labour
- Uterine fibroids and uterine anomaly, such as a bicornuate uterus
- Uterine scar

The placenta may be retained due to ordinary adherence, in which case there is not usually much bleeding until separation occurs, or due to abnormal adherence with accreta as discussed earlier in this chapter. It may also be retained due to a contraction ring in the uterine body or corneal region; in these cases bleeding is heavier as the placenta has partially separated but the uterus cannot contract down fully.

Management of retained placenta

Large-bore intravenous access should be secured, and blood taken for cross-matching as there is a risk of major obstetric haemorrhage. It is likely that the midwife will have already catheterised the patient, but if not an indwelling catheter should be inserted.

The patient should be moved to theatre, and a check made prior to anaesthesia that the placenta has not separated, before undergoing a manual removal. Once the placenta is delivered, IV syntocinon should be considered.

Anaesthesia for manual removal of the placenta

If the patient is haemodynamically stable and not actively bleeding, regional anaesthesia is safer for the mother. If there is active bleeding a general anaesthetic may be required. Regular 'time outs' optimise communication between the anaesthetist and surgical team to ensure shared mental models and agreed goals for care.

This also provides an opportunity to use inhalational agents to relax the uterus. Prophylactic antibiotics should be given, and an oxytocin infusion will be commenced after the placenta has been removed.

Technique of manual removal

Full aseptic precautions are used in theatre. It is advisable to wear gauntlet-length gloves and a non-permeable gown as the operator's arm will usually need to go high into the uterus.

1. If the cord is still attached, the operator's well-lubricated, dominant hand should follow this through the cervix with the fingers held in a cone shape. The other hand is placed on the patient's abdomen to steady the fundus and push it downwards. If there is a constriction ring, steady pressure should allow the hand to pass, but if not uterine relaxation may be required.
2. The fingers and thumb should be kept together and the edge of the placenta identified, the placenta can then be steadily detached by sweeping movements. Clawing should be avoided as it may lead to rupture of the uterus and retention of placental cotyledons.
3. The abdominal hand maintains pressure on the fundus and pushes it down onto the internal hand to facilitate the detachment of the placenta.
4. Once the placenta is separated, it is grasped in the hand and removed slowly to prevent inversion, which may occur if there is still some placenta attached to the uterus. If the cord is still attached, the abdominal hand moves to the cord to apply traction, or grasps the edge of the placenta as it emerges in the vagina.
5. The hand in the uterus should remain there after the placenta is removed to check the cavity to ensure there are no remaining pieces of placenta and that the uterine wall is intact.
6. Bimanual compression may be necessary to reduce blood loss until the uterus contracts in response to oxytocin.

30.4 Summary

- Abnormally invasive placenta remains uncommon, although its incidence is rising. The condition carries significant risks for morbidity, mortality and subsequent fertility. Management requires senior multidisciplinary preparation and involvement and should be undertaken in a specialist centre. Up-to-date guidelines should be used
- Retained placenta is relatively common and can be managed with little difficulty in most cases, although preparation for significant blood loss must be made

30.5 Further reading

Fitzpatrick KE, Sellers S, Spark P, Kurinczuk JJ, Brocklehurst P, Knight M. The management and outcomes of placenta accrete, increta and percreta in the UK: a population-based descriptive study. *BJOG* 2014; 121: 62–71

RCOG (Royal College of Obstetricians and Gynaecologists). *Placenta Praevia and Placenta Accreta: Diagnosis and Management*. Green-top Guideline No. 27a. London: RCOG, 2018.

CHAPTER 31

Uterine inversion

Learning outcomes

After reading this chapter, you will be able to:

- Recognise and describe the management of uterine inversion

31.1 Introduction

Without prompt management of acute uterine inversion, the mother can become profoundly shocked which is potentially fatal. Reported incidence ranges according to geographical location and use of active management of the third stage. On average in the UK, it may present at least once a year in most units, at around 1:4000 births. This may be higher with physiological births.

Although it has often been thought to be related to mismanagement of the third stage, uterine inversion was found even in an institution that did not use Credé's manoeuvre, where they strongly discourage vigorous cord traction and where oxytocin was not given until after placental separation. Brar et al. (1989) found a fundal placenta in the majority of women. Other associated obstetric conditions include a short cord, a morbidly adherent placenta, connective tissue disorders (such as Marfan's syndrome or Ehlers–Danlos syndrome) and uterine anomalies. Remember, however, that in half of cases, no risk factors are identified.

Inversion of the uterus can be puerperal and non-puerperal. Chronic non-puerperal uterine inversions are rare. In a study by Mwinyoglee et al. (1997), only 77 cases were reported; 75 (97.4%) were produced by a tumour and 20% of these tumours were malignant.

Puerperal uterine inversions can follow vaginal delivery or occur at caesarean section. Usual causes are cord traction before the uterus has contracted, but especially when there is a short umbilical cord, fundal insertion of the placenta or an adherent placenta. Prompt understanding and repositioning by manual replacement will prevent further complications.

Immediate, non-surgical measures are successful in the majority of cases of uterine inversion. The pooled experience of Brar et al. (1989) and Watson et al. (1980) demonstrated only three laparotomies requiring surgical reposition out of a total of 102 uterine inversions.

31.2 Recognition of uterine inversion

Early recognition of uterine inversion is vital to enable prompt treatment and to reduce morbidity and mortality. It may present with neurogenic shock, where a bradycardia and hypotensive picture is seen initially, before evidence of haemorrhage.

Managing Medical and Obstetric Emergencies and Trauma: A Practical Approach, Fourth Edition. Edited by Rosamunde Burns and Kara Dent.

In the 2020 MBRRACE-UK report, two of the 14 women who died from haemorrhage did so following unrecognised uterine inversion and a resultant delay in correcting the condition. In both cases controlled cord traction was continued even though there was no evidence of separation. The report makes a clear recommendation that signs of possible uterine inversion should be looked for (rapid deterioration of maternal condition and a loss of fundal height without successful delivery of the placenta) including pain.

Symptoms and signs

These include:

- Severe lower abdominal pain in the third stage
- Shock that is out of proportion to the blood loss, owing to parasympathetic stimulation
- Haemorrhage (present in 94% of cases)
- Placenta may or may not be attached
- Uterine fundus not palpable per abdomen (in milder degrees there may be a dimple in the fundal area)
- Pelvic examination showing a mass in the vagina (in milder degrees) or at/outside the introitus; if the placenta is still attached then it is palpable/visible

Prevention

Mismanagement of the third stage should be avoided, and cord traction should not be applied until the signs of placental separation are apparent.

31.3 Management of uterine inversion

1. Call for help (experienced obstetrician/anaesthetist/midwives).
2. Arrange replacement of the uterus concurrently with antishock measures as resuscitation may not be successful until the inversion is corrected. Sometimes the delivering attendant may be successful at immediate replacement, within seconds of the inversion.
3. Insert two wide-bore intravenous cannulae.
4. Collect blood for full blood count, coagulation studies and group and crossmatch (4–6 units).
5. Start fluid replacement immediately.
6. Continuously monitor blood pressure, pulse, respiratory rate, urine output, and O_2 saturation.
7. If the bradycardia is pronounced, atropine can be administered.
8. Arrange appropriate analgesia.
9. Transfer to theatre.
10. If oxytocin has been running it should be stopped as replacement requires the uterus to be relaxed.
11. If the placenta is still attached, it should be left as such until after repositioning. Attempts to remove the placenta may result in major bleeding as there will be no uterine muscular contraction to constrict blood vessels in the placental bed.
12. Attempt to reposition the uterus; the earlier the restoration, the more likely the success.
13. Anticipate a postpartum haemorrhage once you have been successful.

Replace the uterus using one of the following techniques:

- Manual replacement (Johnson's manoeuvre)
- Hydrostatic repositioning (O'Sullivan's technique)
- Medical approach
- Surgery (laparotomy and Haultain's procedure or Huntingdon's operation)

Manual replacement

Manual replacement should be performed preferably under general anaesthesia. The uterus may require relaxation for manual replacement to succeed, and the aim should be to reduce the uterus in the order of 'last out, first back in', gradually progressing such that the first bit out (the fundus) is replaced last. Once the replacement is complete the hand should be left inside the uterus while a uterotonic is administered, and only when the uterus has contracted should a manual removal of the placenta ensue, with precautions for and treatment of postpartum haemorrhage.

Hydrostatic repositioning (O'Sullivan's technique)

Uterine rupture must be excluded first. Warm saline is infused into the posterior fornix of the vagina under gravity, from a height of about 2 metres while the vaginal orifice is closed. The water distends the vagina gradually so that it stretches, the cervical constriction relaxes and the uterus gradually returns to its correct position.

The process takes about 10–12 minutes and 5–6 litres of warm saline may be required to deliver up to 2 litres internally.

The fluid is best given by attaching the intravenous giving set to a silicone ventouse cup inserted into the vagina; this tends to produce a good seal facilitated by holding the vulva closed over the intravaginal cup.

A hard, black, rubber anaesthetic facemask can be used, which may fit over the vulva. The oxygen inlet allows access for fluid input.

Medical approach

Drugs are used to relax the cervical ring to facilitate replacement. Agents include:

- Terbutaline 0.25 mg subcutaneously
- Glyceryl trinitrate (GTN) 2 puffs sublingually

Surgery

Surgery is only used if all other attempts fail. In Huntingdon's procedure, Allis forceps are placed within the dimple of the inverted uterus and gentle upward traction is exerted on the clamps, with a further placement of forceps on the advancing fundus.

Haultain's technique involves incising the cervical ring posteriorly (where the incision is least likely to involve the bladder or uterine vessels) with a longitudinal incision. This facilitates uterine placement by Huntingdon's method. After replacement has been completed, the hysterotomy site is repaired.

Oxytocics should be administered after repositioning to keep the uterus contracted and prevent recurrence. The attendant's hand should remain in the uterine cavity until a firm contraction occurs.

31.4 Summary

- Prompt replacement of the inverted uterus has the best chance of success; shock must be treated concurrently and, once in place, the uterus must be allowed to, or stimulated to, contract before active placental delivery
- Consider appropriate antibiotic cover following reinversion to avoid infection
- Careful debrief and documentation are essential

31.5 Further reading

Bhalla R, Wuntakal R, Odejinmi F, Khan RU. Acute inversion of the uterus. *Obstet Gynaecol* 2009; 11: 13–18.

Knight M, Bunch K, Tuffnell D, et al. (eds), on behalf of MBRRACE-UK. *Saving Lives, Improving Mothers' Care – Lessons Learned to Inform Maternity Care from the UK and Ireland Confidential Enquiries into Maternal Deaths and Morbidity 2016–18*. Oxford: National Perinatal Epidemiology Unit, University of Oxford, 2020.

CHAPTER 32
Ruptured uterus

Learning outcomes

After reading this chapter, you will be able to:
- Discuss the risk factors for uterine rupture
- Recognise a ruptured uterus early
- Plan and manage a ruptured uterus

32.1 Introduction

Complete rupture of the uterus can be a life-threatening emergency. Fortunately, however, the condition is rare in modern obstetrics, despite the increase in caesarean section (CS) rates, and serious sequelae are even more rare.

32.2 Incidence and predisposing factors

Uterine rupture is more likely in multigravid women, especially those who have undergone previous CS, but spontaneous rupture of the unscarred uterus can occur. A careful history should ensure that there was no previous uterine surgery of any kind that may predispose the uterus to rupture.

Risk factors for the rupture of an unscarred uterus include:

- Grand multiparity
- Undiagnosed cephalopelvic disproportion or malpresentation
- Oxytocin administration
- Macrosomic fetus
- Placenta percreta
- Prior uterine surgery
- External cephalic version
- Uterine abnormalities (e.g. rudimentary horn)

Previous caesarean section

National Institute for Health and Care Excellence (NICE) and Royal College of Obstetricians and Gynaecologists (RCOG) guidance support a planned vaginal birth after a previous lower segment CS in a singleton cephalic presentation at 37 weeks' pregnancy or beyond. With an increase seen in CS rates in the UK (29% of deliveries in 2018–2020 (May 2020 digital NHS)), a rise in the incidence of uterine rupture would be expected. A UK Obstetric Surveillance System (UKOSS) study reported in 2012 that showed the incidence of complete uterine rupture to be lower than expected, at 1.9 per 10 000 maternities. The

Managing Medical and Obstetric Emergencies and Trauma: A Practical Approach, Fourth Edition. Edited by Rosamunde Burns and Kara Dent.

main risk factor for this occurrence is a previous CS with an incidence estimated at 11 per 10 000 maternities as opposed to 0.3 per 10 000 maternities in woman without a previous section.

This study also showed that the risk of uterine rupture was independently increased if the woman had had more than one previous CS, a section less than 12 months before the start of their next pregnancy, those women with a placenta praevia and those with induction/augmentation of labour.

Morbidity and mortality from uterine rupture

Whilst uterine rupture is a rare event, it is accepted that the consequences are significant for both the mother and fetus. There was a national case–control study that took place between April 2009 and April 2010 comprising of 159 women with uterine rupture (448 in the control group). Two of the women who sustained a uterine rupture died (1.3%), with 18 perinatal deaths. This resulted in a perinatal mortality rate of 124 per 1000 total births (NPEU, 2012). These factors need to inform counselling regarding labour in women with a previous section.

Practice and training issues

All involved in intrapartum care of women must be aware of the factors that may lead to uterine rupture. In particular, they must recognise that women with a uterine scar are 'high risk' and should be managed appropriately.

- Antenatal management needs to include plans for delivery and induction, with a documented discussion with a senior obstetrician
- Induction of labour with prostaglandins has a 2–3-fold increased risk of uterine rupture whilst augmentation carries a 1.5-fold increase
- Attentive intrapartum fetal and maternal surveillance should occur in a setting where a CS can be performed within 30 minutes
- Raise awareness of the warning signs:
  - Fetal heart rate anomalies
  - Fetal bradycardia
  - A change in presenting part, being higher than expected or previously found
  - Scar pain and/or tenderness
  - Vaginal bleeding
  - Concealed bleeding (shoulder tip pain)
  - Poor progress in labour

Findings at the time of laparotomy

Lower uterine segment dehiscence is the most common finding. The rupture of the lower segment may extend anteriorly into the back of the bladder or laterally towards the region of the uterine artery, or even into the broad ligament plexus of veins, causing extensive haemorrhage and damage. Posterior rupture of the uterus is uncommon and would usually be seen in relation to previous uterine surgery or intrauterine manipulation, but can occur spontaneously.

32.3 Management of ruptured uterus

Resuscitation of the woman, with expedient delivery of the fetus, is the priority. Fluid and blood transfusion are led by the observations and findings at the time of laparotomy. There is often less bleeding than anticipated as the dehiscence from the scar is less vascular. If there is extension of the scar, this may result in a greater haemorrhage.

Three options exist in terms of surgically managing uterine rupture. Two experienced obstetricians should be present.

Simple repair

This depends on the extent of the injury and on the wishes of the mother. In one series of 23 cases of ruptured uterus, hysterectomy was undertaken in 15 (65%) cases and repair in the other eight. Five successful further pregnancies were reported without repeat rupture (all delivered by CS).

Subtotal hysterectomy

The choice of subtotal hysterectomy may be dictated by the individual situation, the anatomy and the extent of the trauma.

Total hysterectomy

There should be particular concern about the ureters when the rupture has extended laterally into the broad ligament or inferolaterally towards the vagina (and there may be value in obtaining postnatal imaging to check).

32.4 Summary

- Constant vigilance, antenatal as well as intrapartum, is required to diagnose and manage uterine rupture
- Listen to the woman
- Anticipate complications
- Monitor carefully
- Respond quickly
- Follow national recommendations

32.5 Further reading

Al-Zirqi I, Stray-Pedersen B, Forsén L, Vangen S. Uterine rupture after previous caesarean section. *BJOG* 2010; 117: 809–20.

Fitzpatrick KE, Kurinczuk JJ, Alfirevic Z, Spark P, Brocklehurst P, Knight M. Uterine rupture by intended mode of delivery in the UK: a national case control study. *PLoS Med* 2012; 9(3): e1001184.

RCOG (Royal College of Obstetricians and Gynaecologists). *Birth after Previous Caesarean Section*. Green-top Guideline No. 45. London: RCOG, 2015.

CHAPTER 33
Ventouse and forceps delivery

Learning outcomes

After reading this chapter, you will be able to:
- Discuss when an instrumental delivery is appropriate
- Discuss which instrument is most appropriate in a specific circumstance
- Appreciate the techniques required for vacuum and forceps delivery
- Recognise the causes of failure to deliver with the instrument selected
- Describe what to do when the instrumental delivery has failed

33.1 Introduction

Operative vaginal delivery (OVD) aims to expedite the delivery of a baby who is either believed to be at risk of compromise or is in prolonged labour. Worldwide, assisted vaginal delivery remains an integral part of the obstetrician's duties. Rates vary from 1.5% of deliveries (Czech Republic) to 15% (Australia and Canada) and between 10% and 15% regionally in the UK. It is estimated that nearly one in three woman undergo an assisted delivery in their first labours although this incidence is lower in midwife-led settings.

These varying rates reflect not only different clinical practices but also different attitudes. Low OVD rates may reflect high caesarean section (CS) rates, including those performed at full dilatation, because of a reluctance to perform instrumental deliveries. There is evidence of an increasing trend towards using emergency CS directly for delay in the second stage, without resort to a trial of instrumental delivery. This is particularly with occipito-posterior positions at mid-cavity. Although instrumental vaginal delivery can be hazardous and should be undertaken with care, the difficulty of CS at full dilatation should not be underestimated; it can be extremely difficult and is associated with high maternal morbidity. Achieving an assisted vaginal delivery in the first pregnancy means that these women are far more likely to have a successful vaginal delivery in following pregnancies. There is emerging evidence to support the direct supervision of trainees in this situation in order to maximise the appropriate number of OVDs both attempted and achieved.

Women who labour are, by definition, aiming for vaginal delivery and therefore efforts should be focused on helping them to achieve this normally and safely. Various techniques may help in achieving high spontaneous vaginal delivery rates, such as the use of a partogram, companionship in labour, delaying pushing in women who have had epidural anaesthesia, upright posture and active management of the second stage of labour using oxytocin in nulliparae with epidurals.

Managing Medical and Obstetric Emergencies and Trauma: A Practical Approach, Fourth Edition. Edited by Rosamunde Burns and Kara Dent.

33.2 Training and simulation in obstetrics

Simulation has an increasing role in developing appropriate skills for OVD. Use of 'high fidelity' manikins such as the PROMPT pelvic simulator, can allow objective assessment of traction force. Dupuis et al. (2011) have shown that sophisticated simulators can accelerate gaining competence in accurate forceps application (using computer-aided tracking technology).

Importance of non-technical skills in OVD

Bahl et al. (2009) initially described the 'technical skills' required to undertake an operative vacuum delivery and described three 'skills' covering the areas of:

- Assessment and preparation
- Cup application
- Traction with the cup

These are particularly useful in teaching trainees, both on simulators and in early patient contact. In their subsequent paper, Bahl et al. (2010) outlined the vital importance of 'non-technical skills', which includes:

- Situation awareness
- Decision making
- Task management
- Teamwork/communication
- Appropriate professional behaviour
- Cross-monitoring of performance

It is often errors in these areas that compromise patient safety – one example being loss of situational awareness with an inappropriate number of pulls to try and achieve vaginal delivery. The experienced operator should consider how they teach these skills to their trainees.

33.3 Indications for operative vaginal delivery

Indications for OVD are:

- Delay in the second stage of labour
- Fetal compromise in the second stage of labour
- Maternal conditions that require either a short second stage or avoidance of the Valsalva manoeuvre

Prerequisites for OVD

Clinical examination should include both abdominal palpation and vaginal examination.

- Preferably, the fetal head should not be palpable abdominally (i.e. 0/5 palpable); an experienced clinician can consider OVD if the head is no more than 1/5 palpable (this is usually associated with mid-cavity arrest and malposition)
- The cervix should be fully dilated
- The vertex (bone, not caput) should be at or below the ischial spines
- The exact position of the fetal head should be established
- The pelvis should feel adequate clinically

Informed consent is needed: check that the mother understands and agrees with your plan. The Royal College of Obstetricians and Gynaecologists (RCOG; Edozien, 2010) has produced advice on consent for OVD and this guideline paper outlines which risks should ideally be discussed (within the constraints of the individual clinical situation). A model consent form is provided in the guideline.

Adequate analgesia is needed but this will vary according to the type of delivery proposed.

Make sure the woman is sitting up and tilted as far as practicable to minimise aortocaval compression during the procedure – ideally this should be towards her left side (this is best achieved by placing a wedge underneath her right hip).

Someone should be in attendance who is capable of performing neonatal resuscitation.

The operator must be appropriately experienced and skilled.

Safety matters and choice of instrument

When an assisted vaginal delivery is contemplated, careful clinical assessment is vital in order to confirm whether it is appropriate to proceed and to select the most suitable instrument. The different types of ventouse and forceps instruments both have their advantages and disadvantages. Promoting one type over another is inappropriate, as the instrument most suited for the situation at hand, with which the operator is experienced and skilled, is what matters to each individual mother and baby. The advantage of the ventouse cup over forceps relates to it being associated with significantly less maternal trauma and requiring less analgesia, but it is more likely to cause fetal cephalohaematoma and retinal haemorrhage. In addition, ventouse deliveries are significantly more likely to fail than forceps deliveries. Both forceps and vacuum deliveries are associated with an increased risk of shoulder dystocia, but the risk is highest with vacuum (3.5% versus 1.5%). Using a combination of instruments is associated with increased complications. It is best to choose one likely to achieve success.

Different types of ventouse and forceps instruments are available to deal with lift out and rotational deliveries, but rotational deliveries require particular skills, especially when using forceps. Use of Kielland's forceps has declined because of concerns about the risks of increased neonatal and maternal morbidity. However, in skilled hands and following appropriate training and supervision, the overall rates of morbidity are low and can avoid the trauma associated with CS at full dilatation. Recent observational data suggest that the risk of a third/fourth degree tear is no higher with Kielland's forceps than with non-rotational forceps (although both have a higher risk than vacuum delivery). Whichever instrument is selected, the operator must be experienced and skilled in its use (or be supervised directly by someone who is).

In all cases, the exact position of the baby's head must be established before proceeding. There have been many publications over the past 5 years confirming that ultrasound assessment in the second stage of labour allows more accurate confirmation of fetal position and it is now recommended in the latest RCOG guidance (2020) that ultrasound is used where 'uncertainty exists following clinical examination'. This technique is particularly useful when there is marked caput and can be used as an adjunct (rather than as a replacement) to careful abdominal and vaginal assessment. The operator should place the ultrasound probe suprapubically and seek to delineate the prominent orbital ridges. Ultrasound has also been used in labour to measure the degree of asynclitism and descent, as well as predicting the likelihood of achieving a vaginal delivery.

It is universally acknowledged that the tendency to put a ventouse on a baby because the position is not clear is totally unacceptable and dangerous. One study demonstrated that 17 of 64 (27%) fetal head positions diagnosed clinically on digital vaginal examination were incorrect when checked with ultrasound. Continued vigilance, training and supervision in this area are urgently needed.

Conditions where ventouse should be preferred to forceps

- Where urgent delivery is required for a mother who has had no previous analgesia and when a low lift out, easy delivery is anticipated
- A low lift out delivery, especially if there has been no prior analgesia
- Rotational delivery if the operator has inadequate experience with Kielland's forceps
- Operator or maternal preference, when either instrument would be suitable

Conditions where forceps should be preferred to ventouse

- Face presentation (an absolute contraindication to ventouse)
- Aftercoming head of the breech (ventouse is not an option)
- Marked active bleeding from a fetal blood sampling site
- Gestation of less than 34 weeks (between 34 and 36 weeks the ventouse is 'relatively' contraindicated)
- Large amount of caput
- Certain fetal or maternal haematological conditions (e.g. immune thrombocytopenia, haemophilia)
- Mother who is unable or unwilling to push
- Operator or maternal preference when either instrument would be suitable

33.4 Ventouse/vacuum cup

There are a number of *soft cups* in common use which are smoothly applied to the contour of the fetus's head and do not develop a 'chignon'. The vacuum achieved is particularly poor when soft cups are applied to moderate or severe caput (as adhesion to folds of oedematous skin is poor). In addition, they have limited manoeuvrability and cannot be correctly placed when the head is deflexed. Consequently, soft cups have a poorer success rate than metal cups, but are less likely to be associated with scalp trauma. Being soft, they are easy to apply and unlikely to injure the mother. As they are cleaned and sterilised as one item, they present no problems with assembly or leakage.

The *hard cups* are traditionally made of metal, the most widely used being the 'Bird-modification' cups. These have a central traction chain and a separate vacuum pipe. The anterior cups come in 4, 5 and 6 cm sizes. The posterior cup is 5 cm in diameter and has either the standard chain or the new cord for traction. The posterior cup is designed to be inserted higher up in the vagina than the anterior cups, to allow correct placement when the head is deflexed. Many units will use the 'kiwi' omnicup cup (a light, disposable, hard plastic cup with an integrated vacuum mechanism). A variant has an additional display which allows semiobjective estimation of the traction force applied. These cups are useful for both rotational and non-rotational deliveries, but operators should be aware that two studies have suggested a higher failure rate compared with standard metal ventouse cups. Experienced operators usually recommend use of the largest metal cup available when trying to achieve delivery from transverse or posterior positions at the pelvic mid-cavity level (i.e. from 0 to +2 cm below the ischial spines).

It has been shown that successful delivery is most likely with ventouse when the cup is applied over the flexion point, which lies in the midline about 2 cm in front of the posterior fontanelle. It is symmetrically placed over the sagittal suture and should not be directly over the posterior fontanelle. A well-placed cup will result in a well-flexed head (Figure 33.1), while failure to put the cup far enough back will result in deflexion and a higher chance of detachment and failure.

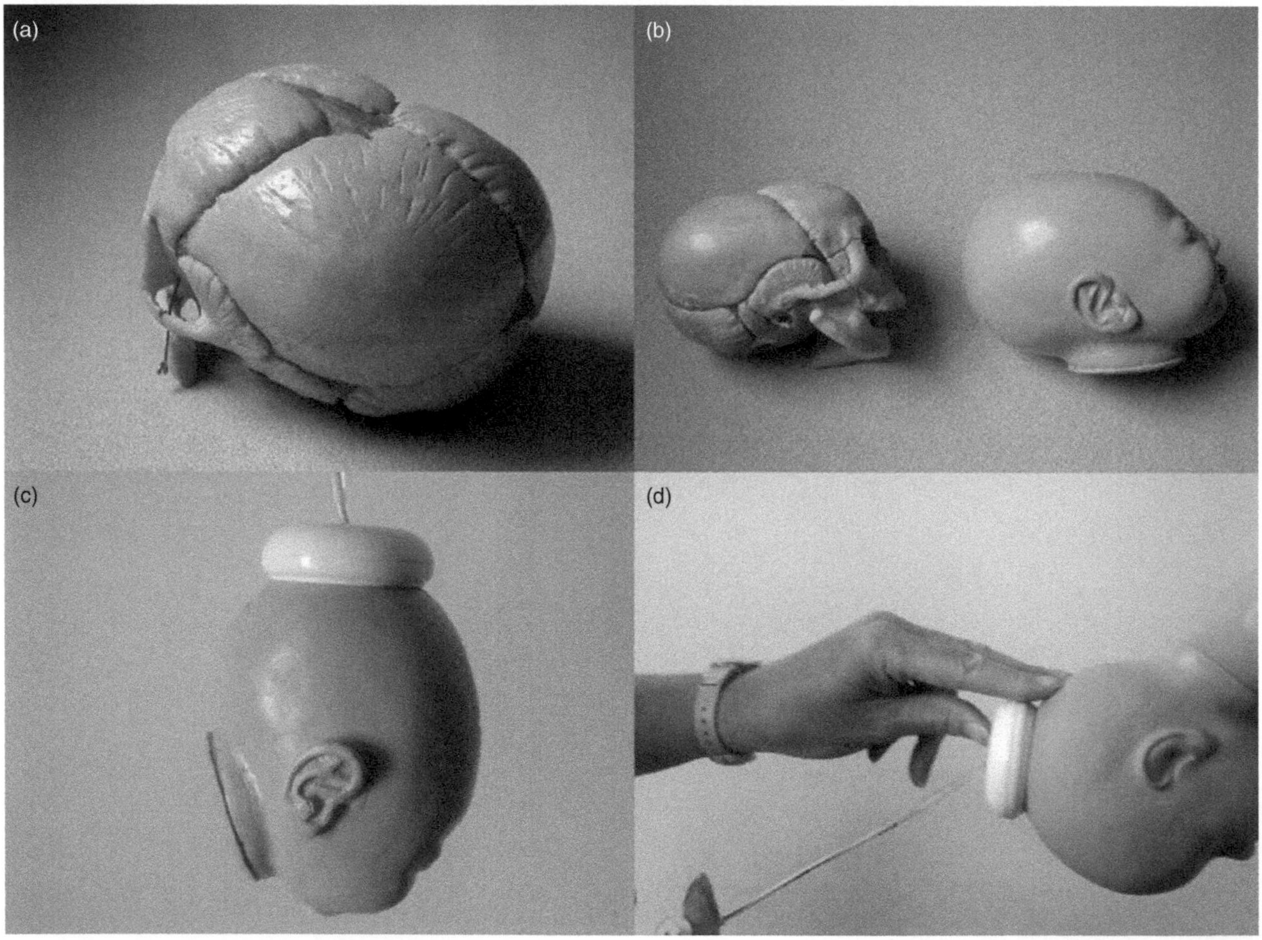

Figure 33.1 Ventouse delivery. (a) Note how far back the posterior fontanelle is. (b) Note the axis through the flexion point, which results in the smallest presenting diameter. (c) The ventouse cup applied over the flexion point. (d) Traction (along the pelvic axis) and the three-fingered grip of the ventouse cup with the second hand

Safe delivery with ventouse

To minimise the chances of any fetal damage, the basic rules for delivery with the ventouse should be followed (Box 33.1). Overall, the risks of perinatal trauma using the vacuum extractor correlate with the duration of application, the station of the fetal head at the commencement of the delivery, the degree of difficulty of the delivery and the condition of the baby when commencing the procedure. When contemplating using the ventouse, in addition to the factors mentioned earlier, it is particularly important that there are good uterine contractions and that the mother is fully cooperative and able and willing to push. The increasing tendency to perform operative deliveries in theatre as 'trials' (which are conducted under dense regional blockade with associated significant compromise to maternal efforts) may be increasing the likelihood of failures with these instruments.

Box 33.1 Basic rules for safe use of the ventouse

- The delivery should be completed within 15 minutes of application of the vacuum (15 minutes is given as the maximum time allowed for application but the average time from insertion of the cup to delivery in over 400 deliveries was 6 minutes)
- The head, not just the scalp, should descend with each pull
- Delivery should be complete within three pulls (if the head is crowning on the perineum, three additional gentle pulls can be used to deliver the head)
- Keep the hands steady during traction – do not waggle, as this increases scalp trauma
- The cup should be reapplied no more than twice (and after one detachment an experienced operator should be summoned)
- If failure with the ventouse occurs despite good cup placement and good traction, do not try forceps as well

Method of delivery with ventouse

1. Lithotomy is the most common position used (and should be used with lateral tilt) but delivery may be possible in dorsal, lateral or squatting positions.
2. Examine the woman carefully. Estimate the size of the baby by abdominal examination and ensure that the head is fully engaged (less than one-fifth of the head should be palpable). Confirm vertex presentation, position and amount of caput through vaginal examination. Describe the attitude of the presenting part as 'flexed' or 'deflexed' (any situation where the anterior fontanelle can be felt easily) and take note of any asynclitisim.
3. The appropriate cup should be chosen:
   - The *kiwi or silicone rubber cup* can be used with any well-flexed vertex presentation, as long as the mother is cooperative, the baby is average sized and there is minimal caput (i.e. when pressing firmly all details of the cranium should be felt, the skin will not be deep and will feel only slightly spongy). This cup is rarely suitable for occipito-lateral positions, as the asynclitism associated with them tends to make placement of this cup over the posterior fontanelle difficult
   - The *anterior metal cup* should be chosen if the baby is big, if the second stage is prolonged or if there is a moderate degree or more of caput (the skin may feel deep, may be folded and will definitely be spongy). It may also be used if the head is only slightly deflexed or slightly rotated, provided correct cup placement can be achieved. The 6 cm cup is preferable to the 5 cm cup because it allows greater traction without increasing the risk of scalp trauma. Only where the vagina is narrow should the 5 cm cup be used. The small 4 cm cup is reserved for use with the second twin, particularly if the cervix is no longer fully dilated
   - The *posterior metal cup*, if it is available on the labour ward, is used for occipito-posterior positions, but also for occipito-lateral positions. It is particularly useful in situations with significant asynclitism and/or deflexion
4. Once the correct cup has been chosen and connected to its pump as required (electric or hand), a check should be made for leakages prior to commencing the delivery. Common problems include suction bottles not tightly screwed in or tubing loosely attached to the metal cups (not locked with the small plastic ring). The metal cups should have a meshed bottom plate, which functions to maintain a clear space between the scalp and the cup so that an effective vacuum can be applied.

Silicone rubber cup

Few units now have the silicone cup on their labour suites as the kiwi cup is the most frequently used type. However, overseas this may be the only option available. The silicone rubber cup is used in the following manner: it is folded and gently inserted into the vagina with one hand from above downwards, while the other hand parts the labia. A gentle twist may help it to unfold into place in the vagina and thereafter it is essentially non-manoeuvrable, being larger in diameter than the metal cup and having a relatively inflexible handle.

Take the pressure up to 0.2 kg/cm^2, check that no maternal tissue is caught under the cup and then continue directly to 0.8 kg/cm^2, beginning traction with the next contraction after this pressure has been achieved. In a recent randomised controlled trial (RCT), there was no significant difference in successful vaginal delivery rates where this method was used as opposed to sequential pressure increases of 0.2 kg/cm^2 (Suwannachat et al., 2011). There were significant reductions in the mean application/maximum negative pressure time (–4.6 95%CI (–4.4 to –4.8) minutes) and in mean application/delivery time (–4.4 95%CI (–4.8 to –4.0) minutes). Where gentle to moderate traction is required, it is reasonable to take the pressure to 0.6 kg/cm^2 and in those rare situations where deliveries are undertaken between 34 and 36 weeks, it may suffice to stop at 0.4 kg/cm^2.

Traction should be along the pelvic axis for the duration of the contraction. One hand should rest on the bell of the cup (see Figure 33.1d) while the other applies traction. Malmstrom, who developed the ventouse, said: 'Vacuum extraction is a matter of cooperation between the traction hand and the backward-pressing hand'. The hand on the cup detects any early detachment and also indicates whether the head moves downwards with each pull. The fingers on the head can promote flexion and can help to guide the head under the arch of the pubis by using the space in front of the sacrum. As the head crowns, the angle of traction changes through an arc of over 90°, but the fetal head should guide the hands, not the other way around: raising the hands too early causes extension of the fetal head, increasing the diameter of the presenting part. This, in turn, increases the risk of trauma to the perineum and can cause cup detachment.

At this point, if necessary, an episiotomy can be made but if the perineum is stretching as normal, it is simply supported with the hand that was on the bell. Occasionally, an edge of the cup might lift off at the introitus (this is more likely to happen if there is caput present or if the hands have been raised too early). If this occurs, you must be careful not to catch maternal tissue under the cup as it reattaches, and thus this should be rechecked before final delivery of the head.

Anterior metal cup

The metal cup is lightly lubricated and then inserted sideways into the vagina. To orientate the cup, make sure the chain and vacuum pipe lie centrally over the posterior fontanelle. Check that no maternal tissue is included at low pressure, then traction can commence once a negative pressure of 0.8 kg/cm^2 has been achieved. Otherwise, the controlled two-handed manner of delivery is similar to that described for the soft cup, classically using the 'three-finger grip' for the fingers on the cup and head (see Figure 33.1d). This not only helps to confirm that the fetal head and not just the scalp is descending, but also that the fingers apply a force which opposes the lifting tendency of the upper edge of the rigid cup when pulling downwards earlier in the delivery and which oppose the lifting tendency of the lower edge when pulling upwards at the end of the delivery.

Posterior metal cup

When confronted with a deflexed head in an occipito-posterior position, the 'OP' cup should be used. It is applied as far back on the head as possible, again aiming to lie in the midline 2 cm from the posterior fontanelle, on the flexion point. To allow good placement of the cup, it sometimes helps to try to flex the head, with two fingers of the left hand pressing on the sinciput, while the right hand inserts the cup behind the head. Once correctly placed, the vacuum can be started and taken directly to the required level (because the cup lies parallel to the vagina it is unlikely to catch any maternal tissue).

The first pull will be in the direction required to flex the head and with this flexion the presenting diameter immediately becomes smaller. Thereafter, traction should be along the pelvic axis. The delivery may be completed simply by a standard spontaneous rotation with maternal effort and gentle assistance. It is important not to try to twist the cup to rotate the fetus as this can increase scalp injuries.

Difficulty is sometimes encountered once the head flexes, as the suction pipe can tend to kink, making it more likely to detach. If the cup detaches at this point (after flexion and rotation), it may be simplest to change to an anterior cup or, if speed is essential, to perform a lift out with forceps.

Avoiding failure with ventouse delivery

Failure rates reported in the literature vary enormously but studies report rates from 6% to as much as 20–30%. There is increasing concern that failure rates are rising and with the evidence that CS in the second stage is associated with significant morbidity, attention to technique is vital. The following factors contribute to ventouse failure:

- Inadequate initial assessment of the case: the head is too high. A classic mistake is to assume that because caput can be felt below the ischial spines the head must be engaged: always palpate the abdomen carefully
- Misdiagnosis of the position and attitude of the head: attention to simple detail will minimise the occurrence of this problem
- Incorrect instrument selected: failures with the silicone rubber cup will be common if it is used inappropriately such as when there is deflexion of the head, excess caput, a big baby, a prolonged second stage of labour or an uncooperative mother
- Anterior or lateral placements of the cup: these will increase the failure rate; anterior placements are also more likely to be associated with fetal injury. In this respect, preterm babies are more vulnerable (even greater care should be taken to check position before application in these cases). If the cup placement is found to be incorrect, it may be appropriate to begin again with correct placement or change to forceps.
- Failures due to traction in the wrong direction: these may be amenable simply to a change in angle of traction
- Excessive caput: rarely, even with metal cups, adequate traction is not possible because of excessive caput and forceps may be more appropriate
- Poor maternal effort: there is no doubt that maternal effort can contribute substantially to the success of the delivery. Adequate encouragement and instruction should be given to the mother

The incidence of cephalopelvic disproportion (true failure) is low.

Special indications for ventouse delivery

In the hands of an experienced operator, the ventouse can also be used to expedite delivery complicated by a prolapsed cord at full dilatation and for delivery of the second twin with fetal distress (thereby avoiding a CS).

33.5 Forceps

There are over 700 makes of forceps. Most authors subscribe to a classification system that divides forceps into classic and specialised subtypes. Classic subtypes that are traction in design include Simpson, Anderson and Neville-Barnes forceps, while specialised forceps include Kielland (for rotation) and Piper (for the aftercoming head of the breech). Variations in cephalic curvature, fenestration and design of shank allow selection to be made on the basis of individual circumstances. There have been no RCTs comparing different types of forceps and it is recognised that the choice is often subjective. One RCT was identified; in this study decreased facial marking was found when soft blade pads were used.

Safe delivery with forceps

It is important that the practitioner is comfortable with and skilled in the use of the instrument selected and that adequate supervision is available as required. To minimise morbidity, the prerequisites for any instrumental delivery should be followed and particular points of safety for forceps delivery should be respected (Box 33.2).

Box 33.2 Basic rules for the safe use of forceps

- Check the forceps are a pair before starting. This is done by locking them together and checking that they produce a symmetrical neat fit. It is also useful to check the maximum diameter between the two blades (a pair that is not true will have a maximum diameter of as little as 7 or 7.5 cm; the maximum diameter should be at least 9 cm)
- If there is resistance when trying to apply the blades or if, when applied to the fetal head, the blades do not sit correctly or lock together, this is usually due to misdiagnosis of the position of the vertex and the blades should be removed and the situation reassessed with senior aid
- The head should descend with each pull
- Traction should be steady and the hands should not waggle, as this risks fetal injury
- The delivery should be completed within three contractions
- If failure occurs, abandon the procedure and proceed to CS

Method of delivery with traction forceps

1. The woman is placed in lithotomy and tilted by means of a wedge under the right hip. An in–out catheterisation is required to empty the bladder prior to forceps delivery. Check that the forceps are a pair.
2. The blades should be applied in turn when the uterus is relaxed between contractions with one hand guiding the blade in (while following in from the line of the contralateral femur) while the other protects the maternal soft tissues. If the blades do not insert easily then they should be removed and the situation reassessed with senior aid; there is no place for forcing the blades.
3. Once applied, the blades should lock together easily (no force should be needed to achieve this) and their position should be checked relative to the fetal landmarks (Figure 33.2).
4. Traction during a contraction attempts to follow the pelvic curve by using Pajot's manoeuvre, which involves two separate components: the dominant hand applies traction while the other hand gently presses downwards on the shank of the forceps (Figure 33.3). The strength of the left hand is crucial to successful and safe delivery: too strong a left hand increases perineal trauma and too weak a left hand means the traction is transmitted too anteriorly – i.e. up against the bladder – causing inefficiency, possible failure and possible bladder trauma. This latter effect is also produced if the direction of traction is too vertical.
5. The timing of the episiotomy should be when the perineum has thinned out and once the operator is totally confident the delivery is going to be completed successfully.
6. As the head crowns, the hands will need to rise up but, as for ventouse delivery, they should follow the head, not lead it, to minimise perineal trauma.

(a) (b)

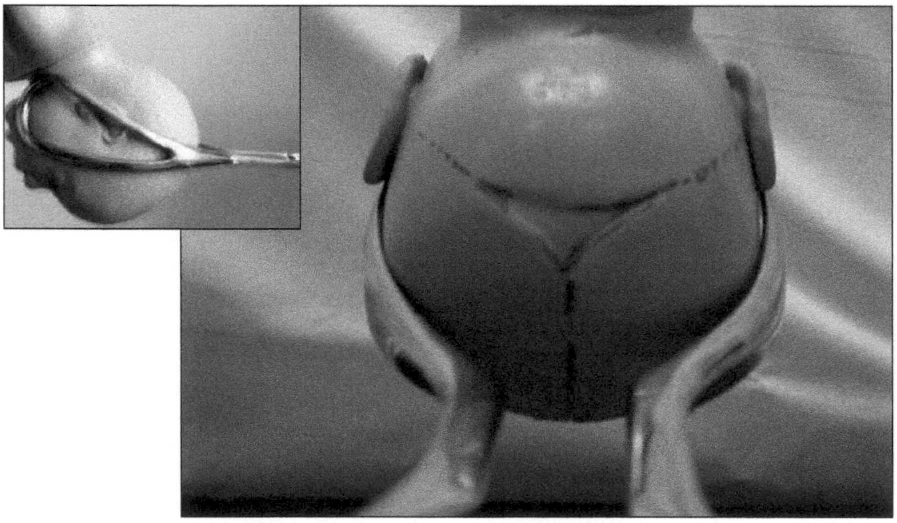

Figure 33.2 Forceps delivery. (a) Forceps blades correctly applied – lying along the mentovertical axis. (b) The forceps blades should lie *parallel* to the sagittal suture and *equidistant* from the lambdoidal suture on each side – always check these bony landmarks after forceps application *before* traction is applied

(a) (b)

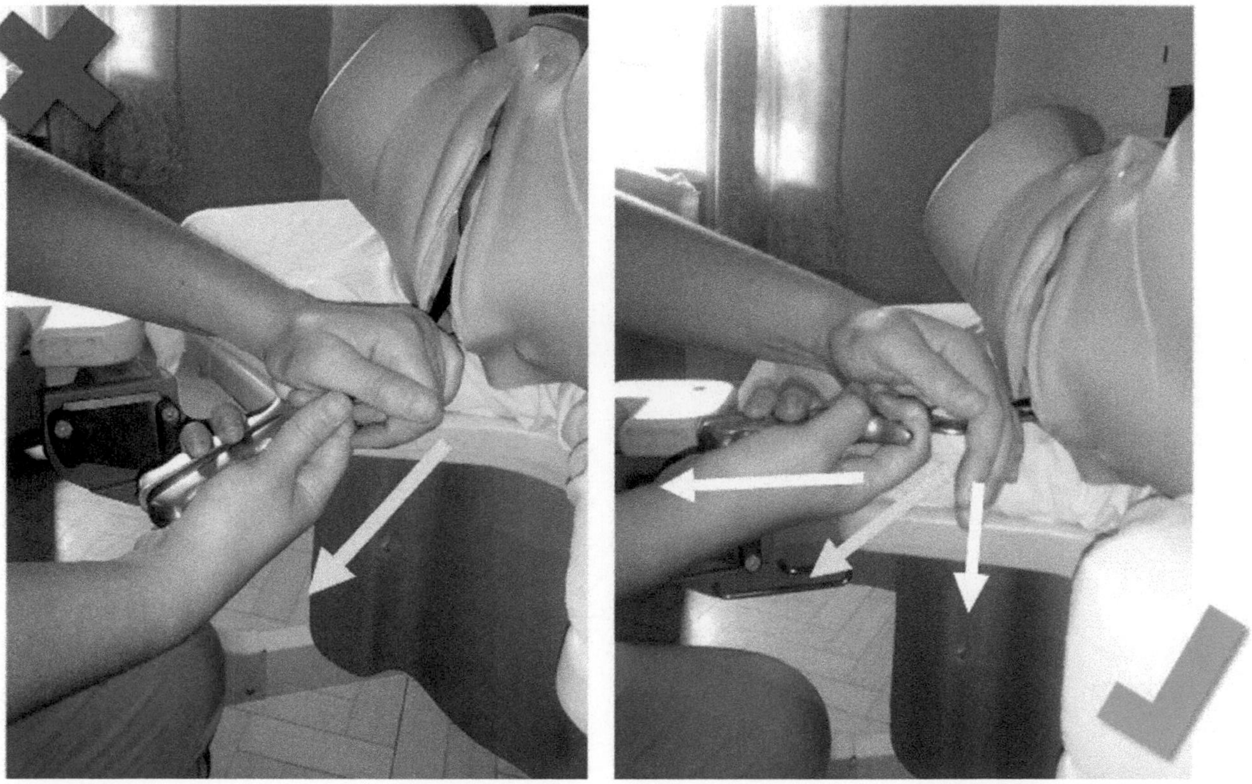

Figure 33.3 Pajot's manoeuvre. (a) Incorrect interpretation – the forceps handles have been dropped to about 45° below the horizontal. (b) Correct application – the dominant hand applies traction along the long axis of the forceps horizontally, while the other hand applies downward pressure on the shanks. This produces a resultant vector (yellow arrow) with direction of traction in line with the pelvic axis until the head passes under the symphysis pubis

Special indications for forceps delivery

Rotation

Rotational delivery for occipito-transverse or occipito-posterior positions can be effected following manual rotation or using a suitable ventouse cup as described earlier. However, Kielland's forceps still have an important place in operative obstetrics for rotational deliveries, but they do require special expertise.

Be especially careful in the abdominal palpation to identify which side of the mother the baby's back is lying, as this will define which direction (clockwise or anticlockwise) that the baby's head should be rotated. When occiput and fetal back are on the same side, the direction of rotation is obvious, but when they lie on opposite sides (sometimes seen with occipito-posterior positions), the occiput should be rotated towards the fetal back to avoid traction on the fetal neck (e.g. left occipito-posterior and fetal back on maternal right then rotation should occur clockwise, i.e. the long way round).

Check that the blades are a pair. The blades are applied ensuring that the nipple on the shank is facing towards the occiput.

Blade application is achieved during uterine relaxation between contractions:

- With occipito-posterior positions the blades are usually applied directly
- With occipito-transverse positions, the blade destined to lie anteriorly is applied first and usually wandered over from the lateral position across the brow. It should not be inserted so far that it ends up wandering over the face. Particular attention to this point should be made in training and supervising this technique. (In some cases, it may be possible to insert the anterior blade 'directly' by careful insertion under the pubic bone. This may not be possible when the head is lower in the pelvis.) The posterior blade is then applied directly and negotiating the coccyx is usually the technically demanding part of this step

Once the blades are applied they should be gently approximated and the lock engaged, but rather than clasping the handles together as with other types of forceps (which compresses the Kielland blades) they should be held with the thumb between the handles, which serves to fix the blades together without squashing them (Figure 33.4). Their position relative to the fetal landmarks should be confirmed.

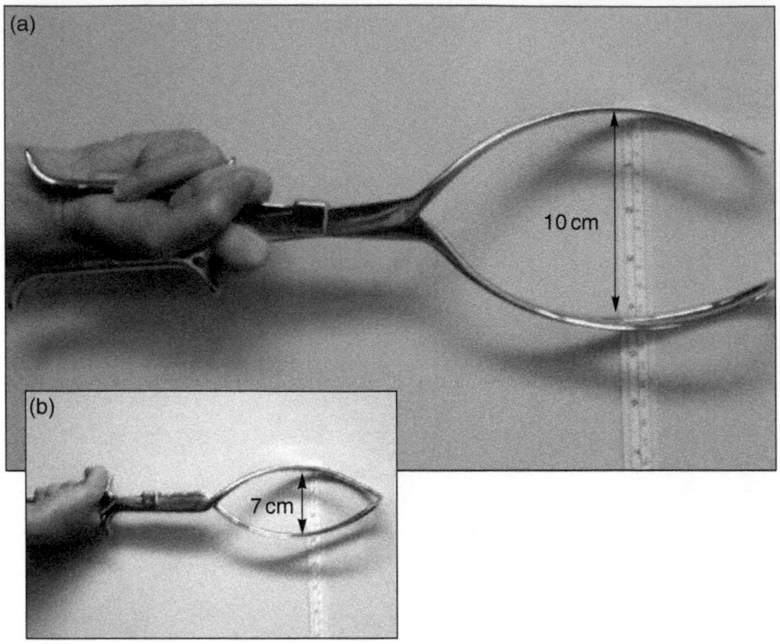

Figure 33.4 Kielland's forceps showing: (a) correct grip (10 cm diameter) and (b) incorrect grip (7 cm diameter)

Once locked together, the handles are very likely to lie slightly removed from each other (enabled by the sliding lock on Kielland's forceps) due to asynclitism. This is normal and attempts should not be made to force them to correct, as this should occur naturally as rotation is completed and asynclitism resolved.

Rotation should be attempted between contractions when the uterus is relaxed and the force required should be minimal. This is a 'feeling' technique and it should never be forced. It is vitally important, at this point, that the operator lowers the handles by lowering the hands. The aim is to angle the forceps to lie in the true axis of the pelvis and to encourage flexion of the head at the same time. The commonest reason for unsuccessful rotation (in terms of technique) is the failure to have the handles moved low enough to allow the forceps blades to lie in the line of the true pelvic axis. This can be facilitated by the operator kneeling down between the patient's legs.

Rotation should only be attempted between contractions. Rotation can first be attempted at the level at which the blades are lying after application. If an initial attempt at rotation is unsuccessful, first recheck that the handles have been pushed downwards adequately. If so, the operator can gently try and move the fetal head either marginally upwards (by no more than 1 cm) or marginally downwards (again by no more than 1 cm). Rotation may be easier at the slightly higher or lower levels. *Attempts should never be made to 'disimpact' the head back into the upper pelvis*. If a contraction develops during rotation, further movement should cease until it relaxes again, but keep gentle hold of the handles of the forceps otherwise they tend to drift.

Once rotation is complete, it is imperative that the fetal head is palpated to check its position and to confirm it is now occipito-anterior. The blades can slip round the fetal head and traction must not be applied until the operator is confident that this has not occurred.

Traction with Kielland's forceps requires the handles to be kept in a low position as there is no pelvic curve (as in standard non-rotational forceps). Traction is then applied in the line of the true pelvic axis and therefore Pajot's manoeuvre is not required. The operator should take care to maintain the safe Kielland grip during traction. An episiotomy will be required (in nearly all cases) as the lack of pelvic curve means that the Kielland shafts cause additional perineal stretch.

As the fetal head crowns, delivery is completed by raising the handles as in a standard forceps delivery. However, because of the absence of a pelvic curve, the Kielland handles will not end up as high over the symphysis pubis as occurs with standard forceps.

Face presentation

Face presentation is covered in Chapter 36, but it is important to reiterate that it is essential to judge the station of the head prior to embarking on a forceps-assisted mentoanterior delivery. The head in these circumstances is always higher than one thinks and not only is careful abdominal palpation crucial, but a careful vaginal examination is mandatory. If vaginal examination reveals a hollow sacrum, then the head is not fully engaged and vaginal delivery is not appropriate.

Aftercoming head of a breech baby

Piper's forceps were designed for this manoeuvre but any traction forceps can be used. If the operator is familiar with Kielland's forceps, these may be used. The absence of a pelvic curve has the advantage that the forceps are easier to apply because they lie away from the baby's body. Breech delivery is covered in Chapter 37 and, as mentioned, forceps may not be needed but, if required, their principle of application and direction of traction is similar to that described in this chapter. Safety points are listed in Box 33.3.

Box 33.3 Safety points for forceps delivery of the aftercoming head of a breech

- Forceps are not appropriate for delivery of the head of a breech that has not entered the pelvis. The nape of the neck/base of the occiput must be seen before the baby's body is lifted up
- When conducting forceps delivery for the aftercoming head of the breech, an assistant is needed and coordination between operator and assistant must be maintained, as one is in control of the baby's body, the other the head
- The baby should be lifted into the horizontal position but, as the arms tend to fall into the way, interfering with the forceps application, the assistant is advised to wrap the baby, including its arms, into a towel to keep things clear
- Hyperextension of the neck should be avoided at all times and the operator should keep strict control of the elevation of the baby provided by the assistant
- An episiotomy is required for delivery in this circumstance and, if not already cut when the breech distended the perineum, it should be cut after the application of the forceps

The place of trial-of-instrumental delivery

If there is uncertainty about whether an instrumental delivery is appropriate because the operator is uncertain about the position or degree of engagement of the head, good analgesia should be achieved to allow adequate examination. If uncertainty remains, someone of greater experience should be called to assess and assist prior to attempting delivery. Any trial-of-instrumental in theatre must be sanctioned and/or supervised by a consultant or experienced registrar. It is important that written consent is obtained with a trial-of-instrumental in theatre.

The place of forceps after failure to deliver with ventouse

There is no place for an attempt at forceps delivery if:

- The position of the fetal head was correctly diagnosed
- The cup was applied correctly
- Adequate traction was applied and there was no descent with the ventouse

If these were not the case and there was a misdiagnosis, misapplication of a cup or traction was inadequate (e.g. due to caput, leaking equipment, no maternal assistance) it may be justified to change to forceps. Murphy et al. (2011) showed that use of sequential instruments is more commonly associated with fetal malpositions (OR 1.8, 95%CI 1.3–2.6). It is associated with increased maternal and neonatal morbidity compared with 'single instrument use':

- Anal sphincter tear: 17.4% versus 8.4% (OR 2.1, 95%CI 1.2–3.3)
- Umbilical artery pH <7.10: 13.8% versus 5.0% (OR 3.3, 95%CI 1.7–6.2)

This decision must therefore be made at an experienced level and will require a formal clinical assessment to be made by the senior clinician.

The situation may also arise that after rotation of the head and good descent into the lower pelvis (i.e. more than 2 cm below the ischial spines), the ventouse cup detaches. In such cases what might have been a difficult Kielland's delivery has now become a potentially straightforward 'lift-out' forceps delivery. Double instrumentation in this last circumstance is acceptable after careful reassessment by the operator.

33.6 Following on from any instrumental delivery

- If the baby is delivered in good condition they should be handed to the mother as soon as possible to encourage skin–skin contact
- After delivery, perineal damage should be assessed carefully with particular attention given to check for anal sphincter and anal mucosa integrity
- After repairing any tear or episiotomy, the swabs and instruments should be counted
- A vaginal and rectal examination should be performed at the end of the procedure to confirm restoration of anatomy, exclude any stray sutures having entered the rectum and confirm no swabs have been retained
- Every aspect of the delivery should be documented
- Examine the baby's head, when you get a chance, to confirm the positioning of the instrument used relative to where you thought it was, and where it should have been. This is important in self-audit of your technique and in teaching and feedback for trainees
- Recent evidence from the ANODE trial (2019) recognises that up to 16% of women following an operative delivery – as opposed to 20–25% of women undergoing a lower segment CS without prophylactic antibiotics – have an infection. This RCT included 3427 women randomly assigned to a placebo arm or treatment with one dose of antibiotics (amoxicillin and clavulanic acid) following an instrumental delivery. There was a significant decrease in suspected or confirmed infection in the group given a single dose of antibiotics with a risk ratio of 0.58 (*P* <0.0001). Future practice should reflect this, with the use of antibiotics as standard. Recent RCOG guidance recommends a single dose of amoxicillin and clavulanic acid IV (if no allergies). Venous thromboembolism risk should then be reassessed following an instrumental delivery

33.7 Supervising an instrumental delivery

The supervising obstetrician must make a full clinical assessment, otherwise they have no way of knowing whether the operative delivery is appropriate or the instrument selected is suitable for the task.

During traction, the supervisor needs to be confident that descent is occurring with each traction and, if in doubt, they should feel for themselves to confirm this fact. Leaving the trainee to pull for three contractions before assessing the situation leaves an almost impossible decision of whether and how to continue and risks inappropriate excessive attempts at delivery.

After delivery, a careful examination of the extent of perineal trauma should be conducted together. This is not only important in identifying third or fourth degree tears (which are often underdiagnosed clinically), but can also provide useful feedback on instrument technique: tears or episiotomies that have extended may have been due to lifting the hands too early on crowning, or too strong a left hand with forceps deliveries.

33.8 Documentation and debriefing

After completion of the delivery, the operator should complete a detailed and (ideally) contemporaneous delivery note for the clinical records. A model example is appended to the RCOG OVD Green-top Guideline (RCOG, 2011).

Despite the problem of continuity of care related to shift systems in obstetrics, it is mandatory (and good clinical practice) to ensure that the operator meets up with the patient to offer a formal debrief before she is discharged home. If that is not possible, the operator should specifically ask a colleague to undertake the debrief on their behalf. This does not usually require more than a few minutes, but should include positive psychological support by confirming with the woman that her own efforts helped the operator to complete the delivery. Confirmation that a normal delivery in the future is most likely can also be very reassuring for the patient.

33.9 Summary

- OVD must be performed by an experienced practitioner or under direct supervision
- Correct assessment of the fetal position is paramount; ultrasound is a useful adjunct to careful examination
- Informed consent and counselling is needed with good documentation of the procedure and timings
- A single dose of amoxicillin and clavulinic acid IV is recommended after the ANODE trial, if there are no allergies

33.10 Online resources

There are several excellent online resources and these are listed here. The RCOG resource is open access.

Garrison A, Ramus RM (chief ed.). *Vacuum Extraction*. Medscape, 2017. http://emedicine.medscape.com/article/271175-overview (last accessed January 2022).

RCOG (Royal College of Obstetricians and Gynaecologists). *eLearning and Simulation for Instrumental Delivery (EaSi)*. RCOG, 2021. https://elearning.rcog.org.uk/tutorials/technical-skills/elearning-and-simulation-instrumental-delivery-easi (last accessed January 2022).

Ross MG, Isaacs C (chief ed.). *Forceps Delivery*. Medscape, 2020. http://emedicine.medscape.com/article/263603-overview (last accessed January 2022).

33.11 Further reading

Edozien LC. *Operative Vaginal Delivery*. Consent Advice No. 11. London: Royal College of Obstetricians and Gynaecologists, 2010.

Knight M, Chiocchia V, Partlett C, et al. Prophylactic antibiotics in the prevention of infection after operative vaginal delivery (ANODE): a multicentre randomised controlled trial. *Lancet* 2019; 3939(10189): 2395–403.

Murphy DJ, Strachan BK, Bahl R, on behalf of the Royal College of Obstetricians Gynaecologists. Assisted vaginal birth. *BJOG* 2020; 127: e70–e112.

CHAPTER 34
Shoulder dystocia

Learning outcomes

After reading this chapter, you will be able to:
- Describe the aetiology and complications of shoulder dystocia
- Discuss the risk factors for shoulder dystocia
- Be aware of strategies that can be tried to prevent shoulder dystocia
- Be confident in understanding the variety of obstetric manoeuvres used to overcome shoulder dystocia
- Appreciate the benefits of formal skills/drills training on maternal and fetal outcomes in cases of shoulder dystocia

34.1 Introduction

Shoulder dystocia remains one of the most dreaded obstetric complications and one that is often unanticipated. It is associated with significant perinatal mortality and morbidity, maternal morbidity and is a costly source of litigation. In this chapter, a number of matters will be addressed.

Definition and incidence

Shoulder dystocia describes difficulties encountered with delivering the shoulders after the fetal head is born. Discrepancies in the definition have resulted in differences in the reported incidence of this obstetric emergency from 0.15% to 2% of all vaginal deliveries. mMOET considers shoulder dystocia to be a condition requiring special manoeuvres to deliver the shoulders that have been arrested due to impaction of the anterior shoulder above the symphysis pubis.

34.2 Clinical risks and outcomes of shoulder dystocia

Fetal mortality and morbidity

Shoulder dystocia is still a significant cause of term fetal mortality. In the Confidential Enquiry into Stillbirths and Deaths in Infancy (CESDI) annual report for 1993, shoulder dystocia was responsible for 8% of all intrapartum fetal deaths. A later, focused report (1998) critically reviewed 56 cases of death associated with shoulder dystocia: 47% of the babies had died despite delivery within 5 minutes and, in 37 (66%) cases, the level of substandard care offered by professionals was graded at 'level 3' (i.e. a different management would have likely resulted in an improved outcome). The babies were delivered by both midwives and medical staff, emphasising the need for all professionals involved in delivery to be aware of appropriate drills.

Managing Medical and Obstetric Emergencies and Trauma: A Practical Approach, Fourth Edition. Edited by Rosamunde Burns and Kara Dent.

Shoulder dystocia can result in:

- Cerebral hypoxia
- Cerebral palsy
- Fractured clavicle and/or humerus
- Brachial plexus injuries

Following delivery of the head, the umbilical cord pH falls by 0.04 units/min. In addition, cranial venous congestion occurs, which exacerbates the fetal insult. As a result, delay in completing the delivery may result in asphyxia and, if the interval between head and trunk delivery is prolonged, permanent neurological deficit may occur. Delivery should occur within 5 minutes and permanent injury is progressively more likely with delays above 10 minutes.

Brachial plexus injuries can occur in shoulder dystocia due to downward traction with excessive lateral flexion of the neck, which stretches its soft tissues. Erb's palsy is the most common of these. A study in 2000 (Wolf et al., 2000) found 62 cases of brachial plexus injury in 13 366 deliveries (incidence 0.46%): 22 recovered completely within a month, while a further 23 had delayed but complete recovery. Of 17 with residual paresis, 11 underwent surgery but only three had severe paresis. The most significant marker to predict the likelihood of 'non-recovery' was birth weight greater than 4000 g.

It has been suggested that intrauterine maladaptation may play a role in brachial plexus impairment, implying that brachial plexus impairment should not be taken as prima facie evidence of birth process injury. The mechanism of damage may not always be clear, as brachial plexus injury has also been reported in the opposite arm to the trapped shoulder and also without any recorded dystocia. Furthermore, it has also been reported after delivery by caesarean section (CS), although clearly injudicious traction on the fetal head and neck can also occur during this delivery.

Bony injuries in the form of a fractured clavicle or humerus can also occur. These fractures usually heal quickly and have a good prognosis.

Maternal morbidity

Postpartum haemorrhage and genital tract trauma are common following shoulder dystocia. Uterine rupture may also occur, especially if undue abdominal force is used.

Antenatal risk factors

Antenatal risk factors are so common that they lack sensitivity and specificity, and the majority of cases of shoulder dystocia occur without any risk factors. There is a strong correlation between fetal weight and shoulder dystocia (Table 34.1). Increasing maternal obesity, diabetes and gestational diabetes all increase the likelihood of macrosomia; however, shoulder dystocia occurs with a normal fetal weight therefore all professionals need to be prepared for unexpected shoulder dystocia at all deliveries.

Table 34.1 Risk factors for shoulder dystocia

Antepartum factors	Intrapartum factors
Fetal macrosomia	Prolonged first stage
Maternal obesity	Prolonged second stage
Diabetes	Assisted delivery
Prolonged pregnancy	
Advanced maternal age	
Male gender	
Excessive weight gain	
Previous shoulder dystocia	
Previous big baby	

Intrapartum risk factors

Secondary arrest and slow progress in the first stage of labour can be associated with an increased incidence of shoulder dystocia (Table 34.1), but many studies have shown labour abnormalities to be similar in both the shoulder dystocia and the control groups, making clinical predictors for subsequent development of shoulder dystocia imprecise.

Shoulder dystocia is more frequently encountered in assisted vaginal deliveries. Boekhuizen et al. (1987) analysed 256 vacuum extractions and 300 forceps deliveries. They found an incidence of 4.6% of shoulder dystocia compared with 0.17% of all cephalic vaginal deliveries. This emphasises the importance of particularly careful abdominal and vaginal assessment before performing assisted deliveries for clinically macrosomic fetuses.

Training and teaching

In the CESDI report of 1993 it is stated that: 'There should be regular rehearsals of emergency procedures and training sessions in the management of rare or troublesome complications for obstetricians and midwives involved in care.' Such complications include obstructed delivery and shoulder dystocia.

There is now clear evidence of benefit from the work of the research team led by Draycott and Crofts. In a randomised trial (Crofts et al., 2008) of 450 clinicians, formal skills/drills training in shoulder dystocia resulted in an increase in successful delivery rate (72% prior to training versus 94% post-training), with a reduction in total force applied. Of even greater importance is the improvement in neonatal outcomes following the introduction of training (Draycott et al., 2008). In an analysis of >29 000 births, the use of correct manoeuvres was significantly increased. This resulted in a significant reduction in neonatal injury at birth after shoulder dystocia.

Prevention

Antenatal estimates of fetal weight are notoriously unreliable (especially at the extremes). Many cases of shoulder dystocia occur in fetuses of average weight, and most macrosomic fetuses delivered vaginally do not suffer from shoulder dystocia. Most cases of shoulder dystocia can be overcome without trauma to mother or neonate if proper precautions are taken. Abdominal delivery is not 100% safe to the neonate and causes morbidity to the mother. Thus, a blanket policy of elective CS for all clinically big babies will not be effective in reducing the incidence of shoulder dystocia and subsequent brachial plexus injuries. However, the Royal College of Obstetricians and Gynaecologists (RCOG) guidelines advocate considering an elective CS for those pregnancies complicated by diabetes (pre-existing or gestational) when the fetus is estimated to weigh more than 4.5 kg. In non-diabetic pregnancies, this cut-off is increased to 5 kg.

Induction of labour for suspected macrosomia

Induction of labour has been considered as an option for managing mothers with suspected macrosomic babies to try to reduce the incidence of shoulder dystocia and subsequent birth trauma. One study (Friesen et al., 1995) reviewed 186 mothers with suspected macrosomic fetuses at term. Labour was induced in 46 cases and 23.9% of them needed CS while, with spontaneous onset of labour in 140 cases, the CS rate was 14%. This difference was statistically significant, regardless of parity or gestational age. The frequencies of shoulder dystocia, a 1 minute Apgar score of less than 7 and abnormal umbilical blood gas were not different. The authors concluded that spontaneous labour is associated with a lower chance of CS than induced labour when the birthweight is 4 kg and above.

The situation in women with diabetes is different, for reasons mentioned earlier. Various authorities recommend CS for babies with an estimated fetal weight of 4 kg or above. Induction of labour is also recommended for women with pre-existing diabetes at 37–38 weeks' gestation, especially if their diabetic control has not been ideal, not only to avoid intrauterine death but also shoulder dystocia and birth trauma.

Documentation

Risk factors should be documented in the notes, especially if there are multiple factors. It is also recommended that an experienced clinician is present during the second stage. It is strongly recommended that events, manoeuvres and accurate times are documented in the notes. Using a proforma for this ensures all important facts are noted.

Early detection

The following events may be early signs of shoulder dystocia:

- 'Head bobbing' (the head coming down towards the introitus with pushing but retracting well back between contractions)
- 'Turtle' sign at delivery (the delivered head becomes tightly pulled back against the perineum)
- Failure of restitution

34.3 Management of shoulder dystocia

As shoulder dystocia is infrequently predictable, every clinician should be armed with a plan of action – that is, a sequence of manoeuvres. All manoeuvres result from one (or a combination of) the following three mechanisms:

- Increase in the available pelvic diameter
- Narrowing of the transverse (bisacromial) diameter of the shoulders by adduction
- Movement of the bisacromial diameter into a more favourable angle relative to the pelvic inlet (oblique diameter is larger than the anteroposterior pelvic diameter)

Sequence of management

1. Call for help.
2. Draw the buttocks to the edge of the bed.
3. Consider episiotomy.
4. McRoberts' manoeuvre plus moderate traction.
5. Suprapubic pressure plus moderate traction.
6. Episiotomy (if not already cut) to allow space to insert the hand for internal manoeuvres.
7. Deliver posterior arm and shoulder or internal rotational manoeuvres (including Wood's screw manoeuvre).
8. Repeat manoeuvres or try:
   - Digital axillary traction
   - Posterior axillary sling traction (PAST)
9. Change of position ('all fours' or Gaskin's manoeuvre).
10. If all the above fail, try symphysiotomy, cleidotomy or Zavanelli's manoeuvre.
11. Ensure comprehensive and contemporaneous written records.

Call for help

This includes calling the most experienced obstetrician available, a paediatrician and an anaesthetist, and other nursing and ancillary staff as available.

Episiotomy

An episiotomy is recommended to allow more room for manoeuvres such as delivering the posterior arm or internal rotation of the shoulders. Although it has been suggested that episiotomy does not affect the outcome of shoulder dystocia, there is strong evidence to suggest that the incidence of vaginal lacerations with shoulder dystocia is high and performing an episiotomy to reduce the chance of severe lacerations is recommended. The main reason for recommending an episiotomy is to allow the operator more space to use the hollow of the sacrum to perform the different internal manoeuvres.

McRoberts' manoeuvre (with or without moderate traction)

Both thighs are sharply flexed, abducted and rotated outwards (knees to shoulders) (Figure 34.1a). The bed should be flat and the legs should not be in lithotomy poles, as this would limit the amount of flexion obtained. This position serves to straighten the sacrum relative to the lumbar vertebrae and causes cephalic rotation of the pelvis to occur, which helps to free the impacted shoulder. McRoberts' reduces the amount of traction needed and the likelihood of subsequent brachial plexus injuries or fractured clavicle. For this reason, patients should be put in McRoberts' position before applying appropriate traction on the fetal neck. McRoberts' manoeuvre is associated with the least neonatal trauma.

The traction applied during delivery can be measured objectively using the PROMPT Trainer, with studies showing a mean maximum applied traction force of 106 Newtons (a range varying from 6 to >250 N). Computer modelling suggests that the maximum traction force should not exceed 100 N in order to reduce the risk of neonatal brachial plexus injury.

(a) (b)

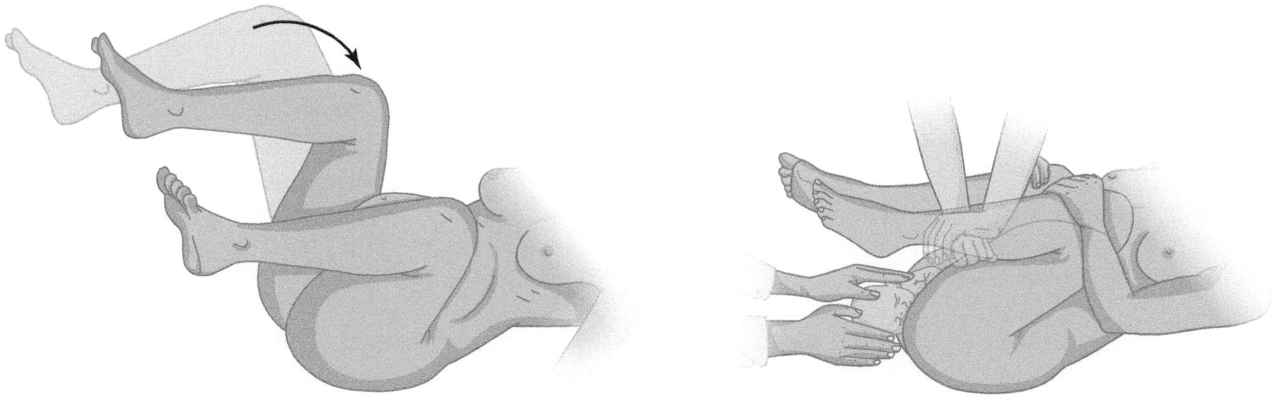

Figure 34.1 (a) McRoberts' manoeuvre. (b) McRoberts' manoeuvre with suprapubic pressure

In theatre to avoid injury to staff use Lloyd Davis stirrups to achieve McRobert's manoeuvre.

Suprapubic pressure (with moderate traction)

Suprapubic pressure (Figure 34.1b) is applied to adduct and internally rotate the anterior shoulder and thus reduce the bisacromial diameter and push the anterior shoulder underneath the symphysis pubis into the pelvis. A 'cardiac massage' grip is used, with pressure applied to the posterior aspect of the shoulder with the heel of the hand. It is important to know where the fetal back lies so that pressure is applied in the right direction. If continuous pressure is not successful, a 'rocking' movement may be tried. This is also known as the Rubin I manoeuvre. At this stage, only moderate traction is applied; strong traction, as well as fundal pressure, should always be avoided. Strong pushing may have similar effects to fundal pressure and maternal efforts should be discouraged until shoulder displacement is achieved, as these could increase the impaction of the shoulders and increase the neurological and orthopaedic complications.

Deliver the posterior arm and shoulder

The hand of the operator should move up to the fetal axilla and the shoulder hooked down. There is always more room in the hollow of the sacrum. Traction on the posterior axilla usually enables the operator to bring the posterior arm within reach.

The posterior arm can then be delivered or, if the cubital fossa is within reach, backwards pressure on it will result in disengagement of the arm, which will then be brought down. This is achieved by getting hold of the hand and sweeping it across the chest and fetal face. This process is similar to Pinard's method for bringing down a leg in breech presentation. This procedure is usually successful.

Internal rotatory manoeuvres

Internal rotatory manoeuvres, such as Rubin II, Wood's screw and reverse Wood's screw, are often confused with each other and are often incorrectly described in the literature.

Rubin II

The operator inserts the fingers of one hand vaginally, positioning the fingertips behind the anterior shoulder. The shoulder is pushed towards the fetal chest (adducting the shoulders and rotating the bisacromial diameter into the oblique). If unsuccessful, this can then be combined with the Woods' screw manoeuvre.

Wood's screw

This manoeuvre was described by Woods in 1943. The fingers of the opposite hand are inserted vaginally to approach the posterior shoulder from the front of the fetus, aiming to rotate the shoulder towards the symphysis pubis. The Rubin II and Woods' screw can be combined to rotate the shoulders through 180° ('like a thread on a screw'). It is important not to twist the fetal head or neck.

Reverse Wood's screw

If the above fail, an attempt is made to rotate in the opposite direction to the original Woods' screw. If successful, the shoulders will rotate 180° in the opposite direction and deliver.

Hoffman et al. have confirmed that delivery of the posterior arm achieved the highest rate of delivery compared with other manoeuvres (84.4% versus 24.3–72.0%, P <0.005 to P <0.001), but with no differences in rates of neonatal injury (8.4% versus 6.1–14.0%, P = 0.23 to P = 0.7). However, it was clear that the total number of manoeuvres performed correlated significantly with the rate of neonatal injury. Other papers have confirmed increased success rates with use of multiple manoeuvres (72% rising to 79% then 95% with two then three manoeuvres), but higher rates of neonatal injury with removal of the posterior arm relative to internal rotatory methods.

Overall, the literature supports the judicious use of multiple manoeuvres to achieve successful delivery and the accoucheur should be familiar with the different approaches. Which to use first will depend on training and familiarity.

Finally, using computer modelling, Grimm et al. confirmed that **all** manoeuvres *reduce the amount of force and resultant brachial plexus stretch required to achieve delivery*. The greatest effect using the modelling technique was with delivery of the posterior arm, with a 71% decrease in nerve stretch and an 80% reduction in traction force.

'Sling' or posterior axillary sling traction

These techniques to deliver the posterior arm are described in two case series (Menticoglou, 2006; Cluver and Hofmeyr, 2009). The approach may be particularly helpful when the posterior shoulder is held up on the sacral promontory, and other standard manoeuvres are unsuccessful. Menticoglou describes insertion of the clinician's hand along the sacral hollow and delivery of the *posterior shoulder* before delivering the posterior arm. Cluver and Hofmeyr describe the use of a soft silastic suction catheter that is looped around the posterior shoulder and under the axilla using the index fingertip. The loop is retrieved with the opposite index finger and withdrawn to create a sling around the shoulder that can be used for downward traction (again aiming to deliver the *posterior shoulder* itself first). The techniques are associated with a high risk of humeral fracture.

'All fours' position (Gaskin's manoeuvre)

In this position the maternal weight lies evenly on the four limbs and this increases the anteroposterior diameter of the inlet and facilitates other manoeuvres. The posterior shoulder (with respect to the maternal pelvis) may be delivered first in this position. Midwives will often use this manoeuvre early in the management of shoulder dystocia. In a series of 82 cases of shoulder dystocia among 4452 deliveries (incidence 1.8%), all neonates were delivered successfully with this manoeuvre in a mean time of 2.3 minutes (range 1–6 minutes). There were no cases of mortality and no cases of brachial plexus injury. One neonate suffered a fractured humerus. Obstetricians should consider the merits of this alternative approach if it is practicable (i.e. no dense epidural blockade).

Other measures

Zavanelli's manoeuvre (cephalic replacement)

This method is been named after the physician who first performed the manoeuvre in 1978. It describes reversal of the delivery process by rotating, flexing and reinserting the head into the vagina, followed by CS; that is, after failure of all manoeuvres to overcome shoulder dystocia, restitution and neck extension are reversed and the head recoils into the vagina. It may be of particular use when both shoulders remain in the abdomen (double shoulder dystocia) where cephalic replacement is relatively easier as the pelvis does not contain the posterior shoulder.

One study reported 59 women who underwent cephalic replacement. All but six were successfully replaced and delivered by CS without excessive maternal or fetal morbidity. The study described the need for a tocolytic and used 0.25 mg subcutaneous terbutaline, depressing the posterior wall and using firm and constant pressure on the head. Those who have had experience of applying this technique have reported very good outcomes.

Descriptions in the literature report an almost automatic ease in performance of Zavanelli's manoeuvre and a complication-free procedure. However, it has also been reported how difficult the process can be. One author reported three cases of hysterectomies necessitated by uterine rupture during the procedure. There have also been cases of severe perinatal hypoxia, which ultimately resulted in brain damage and/or death. It has been recommended that it should only be used as a last resort.

Symphysiotomy

Symphysiotomy is described in Chapter 40. The procedure requires inserting a urethral catheter to move the urethra to one side, which is extremely difficult, if not impossible, to achieve when the head has been born. Two assistants support the legs after taking them out of the stirrups. An incomplete midline cut in the symphyseal joint is made. This, in addition to an episiotomy, will increase the space available and facilitate the delivery of the shoulders. Performance of this uncommon procedure, in an emergency situation, by an operator who has never performed it before, must carry a considerable risk. However, the successful use of the technique has been described. The importance of supporting the woman's legs when the incision is made must be emphasised, in order to prevent sudden abduction.

Intentional fracture of the clavicle (cleidotomy)

The clavicle may fracture spontaneously with the above manoeuvres. Whilst surgical cleidotomy may feel like a last resort, the clavicle can be bent by the operator's finger and this may be viewed as the preferable choice by some clinicians in what is by then an extremely adverse situation.

Approaches advocated by other authors

Several authors have advocated the use of similar systematic approaches to the hands-on management of shoulder dystocia. They vary in the order in which manoeuvres may be recommended, but the more important principle of having an orderly, logical and calm approach is advocated by all. The Advanced Life Support in Obstetrics (ALSO) approach uses the mnemonic **HELPERR** (the order of manoeuvres is not mandatory):

- **H** Help (call for plenty)
- **E** Evaluate for episiotomy
- **L** Legs (McRoberts' manoeuvre)
- **P** Pressure (suprapubic)
- **E** Enter (rotational manoeuvres)
- **R** Remove the posterior arm
- **R** Roll (Gaskin's manoeuvre)

Guidelines may differ at the point where internal manoeuvres are required. Should one 'enter and rotate' (the shoulders) first or 'enter and remove' (the posterior arm) first? There is no scientific evidence on which to base this choice. Therefore, it should be left to the attending professional to use the manoeuvre with which they are most familiar and most comfortable. In a survey of obstetricians, it was found that 56% would attempt delivery of the posterior arm first and 36% would attempt the internal rotatory manoeuvres first. mMOET instructs in both techniques as each may be invaluable in any specific case.

34.4 Following delivery

As stated at the beginning of this chapter, shoulder dystocia is a dreaded obstetric emergency, and successful delivery of the neonate is naturally accompanied by an overwhelming sense of relief. However, the team must remain alert and prepared for the associated maternal complications of genital tract trauma, including third and fourth degree tears, and postpartum haemorrhage. In addition, cord pH should be checked, accurate documentation is essential, including which shoulder was anterior, and parents and staff should be debriefed.

34.5 Medicolegal aspects

Courts have found in favour of the professionals involved when the allegations have been that shoulder dystocia 'should have been predicted' and CS offered in order to avoid the complication. It is accepted that the majority of cases are unpredictable and that professionals cannot be expected to predict this catastrophe antenatally. However, in many cases, there were no departmental guidelines available for the management of shoulder dystocia once it had occurred. Inappropriate manoeuvres such as excessive lateral traction and fundal pressure would not be acceptable and, indeed, would be difficult to defend in present-day practice. Between 2000 and 2009 the NHS Litigation Authority paid more than £100 million in litigation for cases due to shoulder dystocia.

Units should continually review and revise their management guidelines with reference to changing evidence-based practice. It is accepted that it is not possible to produce grade A (randomised controlled trial) evidence in this field. Therefore, the manoeuvres recommended by 'expert' opinion will be the basis of best practice.

34.6 Summary

- Although shoulder dystocia is usually an unpredictable obstetric emergency, having guidelines and a plan of action and being vigilant to the possibility of shoulder dystocia should minimise fetal and maternal trauma
- There is now grade A evidence that simulation with skills/drills training can result in improved operator technique and a reduced incidence of brachial plexus injury
- It is important that every institution has a guideline and documentation proforma, with which all staff are familiar and comfortable
- Simulation training
- Confidence with this rare emergency can be enhanced with the use of 'fire drills' and by completing structured skills training courses

34.7 Further reading

NHS Litigation Authority. *Ten Years of Maternity Claims: an Analysis of NHS Litigation Authority Data*. London: NHS Litigation Authority, 2012.

RCOG (Royal College of Obstetricians and Gynaecologists). *Shoulder Dystocia*, 2nd edn. Green-top Guideline No. 42. London: RCOG, 2012.

CHAPTER 35
Umbilical cord prolapse

Learning outcomes

After reading this chapter, you will be able to:

- Describe how to safely and efficiently manage prolapse of the umbilical cord to improve perinatal outcome whilst minimising maternal risk

35.1 Introduction

Cord prolapse occurs when a loop of umbilical cord descends below the presenting part and the membranes are ruptured. Umbilical cord prolapse occurs in approximately 0.1–0.6% of all births, and can be as high as 1% with breech births.

A high percentage of mothers are multiparous. The incidence of prolapsed cord was 0.6% of all births in 1932. The reduction in frequency of the complication probably reflects a decrease in family size, as well as changes in obstetric practice. These include the increased use of elective and intrapartum caesarean section (CS) for a non-cephalic, or an unengaged, presenting part with a more active approach to intrapartum management of the very preterm fetus.

Significance

In cord prolapse, the fetal perinatal mortality has been reported to be as high as 25–50% from asphyxia due to:

- Mechanical compression of the cord between the presenting part and bony pelvis
- Spasm of the cord vessels when exposed to cold or manipulation

The perinatal mortality rate associated with umbilical cord prolapse has also fallen over the years. A large study (Murphy and MacKenzie, 1995) found a perinatal mortality rate of 91/1000. The cause of death for infants born after umbilical cord prolapse now seems to be related more to the complications of prematurity, associated congenital malformations and low birth weight, rather than intrapartum asphyxia as such.

It is considered that part of the fall in perinatal mortality is due to the more rapid and frequent use of CS once a prolapsed cord has been diagnosed. However, given the association between umbilical cord prolapse and preterm birth, improvements in neonatal intensive care are probably at least as important.

Managing Medical and Obstetric Emergencies and Trauma: A Practical Approach, Fourth Edition. Edited by Rosamunde Burns and Kara Dent.

35.2 Clinical management of umbilical cord prolapse

Aetiology

Umbilical cord prolapse tends to occur when the presenting part does not snugly fit in the lower pelvis and this, in turn, could be due to *fetal causes* such as:

- Malpresentations (e.g. footling breech, transverse and oblique lie)
- Prematurity/preterm labour
- Low birth weight (<2.5 kg)
- Polyhydramnios
- Multiple pregnancy
- Congenital malformations

Or it could be due to *maternal causes* such as:

- Multiparity
- Unstable lie
- Unengaged presenting part
- Low-lying placenta

Other risk factors

In one series, obstetric interventions preceded 47% of umbilical cord prolapse; interventions included amniotomy, scalp electrode application and intrauterine pressure catheter insertion; fetal manipulation during external cephalic version, internal podalic version and manual rotation; and expectant management of premature rupture of membranes.

Diagnosis of umbilical cord prolapse

Clinical suspicion

A high presenting part can raise suspicions of a problem with cord presentation or prolapse especially if the fetal heart rate is showing decelerations suggestive of cord compression.

Vaginal examination

This should be performed carefully and thoroughly to check if cord is palpable. If membranes are intact and the cord is felt this is termed cord presentation, but if the membranes are ruptured, the term is cord prolapse. Examination should be gentle, with minimum pressure on the cord, to avoid further compression or even spasm.

Ultrasound

An ultrasound scan can be performed to confirm a fetal heartbeat if this facility is rapidly available. Fetal heart monitoring should be started/continued with whatever tools are to hand (Pinard/Doppler/cardiotocography). Colour flow Doppler can be useful if there is reason to suspect cord presentation.

Obstetric management of umbilical cord prolapse

Obstetric management of umbilical cord prolapse has largely been unchanged since the 1950s. The approach if the fetus is alive and of a viable gestation continues to be elevation of the presenting part and rapid delivery, usually by CS (unless the cervix is fully dilated and vaginal delivery can be expedited quickly). Any oxytocin infusion should be turned off immediately.

Early diagnosis is important and continuous electronic fetal monitoring may be of assistance as fetal heart rate changes frequently occur. The speed required to expedite delivery will vary according to whether there is a bradycardia that does not respond to the following measures, or whether the fetal heart remains normal. In either situation, if the cervix is fully dilated and the presenting part well down in the pelvis, rapid vaginal delivery can be effected.

Measures to reduce cord compression and improve the fetal heart rate

A number of manoeuvres have been described to reduce cord compression, including manual elevation of the presenting part of the cord, tocolysis, bladder filling, placing the patient in the knee–chest position and funic reduction (manual replacement of the umbilical cord).

Traditionally, management of umbilical cord prolapse has included knee–chest or Trendelenburg positioning and manual elevation of the presenting part of the fetus above the pelvic inlet, to relieve cord compression. Provided that delivery is not imminent and the fetus is viable, this traditional management occurs while preparations for emergency CS are made.

Measures to perform intrauterine fetal resuscitation are indicated if there is concern about the fetal heart rate: increasing the intravenous fluid rate, administering oxygen by facemask and discontinuing the oxytocin infusion are indicated. If the umbilical cord visibly protrudes through the introitus, it should be replaced in the vagina with the minimum of handling. If this is not possible it can be laid carefully between sterile gauze *soaked* in *warm,* physiological saline, although this is of unproven benefit in reducing the risk of vasospasm.

If the cord is non-pulsatile or the fetal heart is not audible the importance of prompt ultrasound assessment is vital and urgent as it has been demonstrated that fetal heart movements can be visualised in such circumstances and fetal resuscitation, as described above, should be carried out urgently.

An advance in the management of umbilical cord prolapse has been the development of bladder filling (unless rapid vaginal delivery is planned). Bladder filling was first proposed by Vago, in 1970, as a method of relieving pressure on the umbilical cord. Bladder distension raises the presenting part of the fetus off the compressed cord for an extended period of time, thereby eliminating the need for an examiner's fingers to displace the presenting part. A number 16 Foley catheter is placed into the urinary bladder. The bladder is filled, via the catheter, with physiological saline by a standard infusion set. The quantity of saline needed is determined by the fetal heart rate response and the appearance of the distended bladder above the pubis, with 500 ml usually being sufficient. The balloon is then inflated, the catheter is clamped and the drainage tubing and urine bag are attached and secured, ready for when the fluid is released prior to CS.

Bladder filling has an additional advantage in that the full bladder may decrease or inhibit uterine contractions. In a series by Chetty and Moodley (1980), there were no cases of perinatal mortality. All the neonates had Apgar scores of 6 or more and the mean elapsed time from diagnosis to delivery was 69 minutes. Eight women in their study delivered after an elapsed time of 80 minutes or more. If successful, this will allow time for a spinal rather than a general anaesthetic, reducing maternal complications and risk.

Tocolysis may be initiated to reduce contractions and improve bradycardia by using terbutaline 0.25 mg subcutaneously. If there is no evidence of fetal distress, it may be reasonable to proceed with a regional block (conducted in left lateral, not sitting, position). The bladder is emptied by unclamping the catheter at the time of the skin preparation.

Vaginal delivery can be conducted when the umbilical cord prolapse occurs at full dilatation with either the vacuum extractor or forceps, but only if the delivery is anticipated as being straightforward and easy. This is no time to embark on a complicated or protracted instrumentation that will exacerbate cord compression and potentially worsen the fetal condition.

The evidence relating to the interval between diagnosis and delivery being associated with stillbirth and neonatal death is conflicting. Neonatal condition, assessed by Apgar scores and paired cord blood gas analysis, is more likely to be influenced by the condition of the neonate during the acute event, rather than the time interval itself, and fetal mortality has been more consistently attributed to prematurity and congenital anomalies. Birth asphyxia is important and when this condition occurs outside of hospital (approximately 25% of patients), it carries a perinatal mortality rate as high as 86.4%.

35.3 Documentation

Careful contemporaneous documentation is essential as with all obstetric emergencies; remembering to assign a scribe to note manoeuvres and timing is vital. The guidelines from the Royal College of Obstetricians and Gynaecologists (RCOG) have an example of a cord prolapse proforma that local units can adopt.

35.4 Summary

- Umbilical cord prolapse is an infrequent obstetric emergency that requires prompt recognition and rapid action
- Perinatal outcome is improved with attention to fetal resuscitation while preparing to expedite delivery
- Occasionally vaginal delivery can be achieved, but most patients need a CS and the urgency of this depends on the condition of the fetus as assessed by the fetal heart rate
- Regular drills on an annual basis, at least, should be mandatory for staff involved in maternity services, each being aware of their specific role in such an emergency
- It is vital to debrief staff, women and partners after such an emergent situation

35.5 Further reading

RCOG (Royal College of Obstetricians and Gynaecologists). *Umbilical Cord Prolapse*. Green-top Guideline No. 50. London: RCOG, 2014.

CHAPTER 36
Face presentation

Learning outcomes

After reading this chapter, you will be able to:

- Describe the mechanics of delivery of the neonate presenting by the face
- Discuss the importance of the positioning of the face in labour and prior to delivery
- Identify how to assess the situation when contemplating operative vaginal delivery

36.1 Introduction

Face presentation occurs in approximately 1/600 to 1/800 deliveries at term.

Aetiology

Predisposing causes are characteristics that reduce cephalic flexion, and include the following:

- Multiparity
- Prematurity and birth weight <2.5 kg
- Multiple pregnancy
- Loops of cord around neck
- Fetal neck tumours
- Uterine abnormalities
- Cephalopelvic disproportion
- Fetal macrosomia
- Platypelloid pelvic anatomy

36.2 Clinical approach to face presentation

Diagnosis

A primary face presentation might be detected on a late ultrasound scan. The majority of face presentations are secondary, however, and arise in labour.

Abdominal examination

Before the head has entered the pelvis a large amount of head is palpable on the same side as the back, with no cephalic prominence on the same side as the limbs.

Managing Medical and Obstetric Emergencies and Trauma: A Practical Approach, Fourth Edition. Edited by Rosamunde Burns and Kara Dent.

Vaginal examination

In early labour, the presenting part will be high. At vaginal examination, landmarks are the mouth, jaws, nose, malar and orbital ridges. The presence of alveolar margins distinguishes the mouth from the anus, distinguishing a face presentation from that of a breech. In addition, the mouth and the maxillae form the corners of a triangle, while in a breech presentation the anus is on a straight line between the ischial tuberosities. During vaginal examination, avoid inadvertently damaging the eyes by trauma or antiseptics.

Management

Follow these steps:

1. Make a diagnosis.
2. Check for cord presentation or prolapse.
3. Continuously monitor the fetal heart rate.
4. Examine regularly to check that progress is adequate.
5. Give oxytocin if contractions are poor and progress is not satisfactory.
6. Do not use scalp electrodes or perform fetal blood sampling.
7. If the position is mentoanterior, vaginal delivery should be possible (rotation from other positions can occur during labour).
8. Perform an episiotomy.
9. If the fetus is persistently presenting mentoposteriorly, deliver by caesarean section (CS).

Intrapartum considerations

Face presentation

In early labour, minor deflexion attitudes are common, especially with occipito-posterior positions and multiparity. In such cases, uterine contractions often cause increased flexion. Occasionally, extension will increase, producing successively a brow presentation and, finally, the fully extended face. Most face presentations are thus secondary, becoming evident only in established labour. Diagnosis is notoriously difficult. In approximately 50% of cases the diagnosis is not made until delivery is imminent.

Descent is usually followed by internal rotation, with the chin passing anteriorly; thus, as with other labours, progress is assessed by dilatation, rotation and descent. If contractions are inadequate, they can be augmented with oxytocin if signs of obstruction have been excluded.

It must be remembered that the biparietal diameter is 7 cm behind the advancing face, so that, even when the face is distending the vulva, the biparietal diameter has only just entered the pelvis. Descent is thus always less advanced than vaginal examination would suggest, even when one allows for the gross oedema that is usually present. The value of abdominal examination in such cases cannot be overstressed. However, when the chin is anterior and the occiput is posterior, it can be difficult to feel the fetal head abdominally even when it is still in the abdomen – 'the head is always higher than you think with a face presentation'. The key is feeling posteriorly on vaginal examination – check the sacral hollow, which should be filled up by the occiput – if the sacral hollow is empty, the occiput is still intra-abdominal.

Mentoanterior position

Anterior rotation of the chin usually occurs during descent and this brings the neck behind the symphysis pubis. The head is born by flexion, with the occiput following behind and causing considerable perineal distension in the process, hence the recommendation to cut an episiotomy in most cases.

With satisfactory uterine action and a mentoanterior position, spontaneous delivery or easy 'lift out' with forceps (*never* ventouse) assisted delivery will ensue in 60–90% of patients. The shoulders and body are born in the usual way.

Mentoposterior position

Even with mentoposterior positions diagnosed in labour, anterior rotation will occur in the first or second stage in most cases, so that persistent mentoposterior position or mentotransverse arrest is encountered in only 10% of face presentations.

In cases of persisting mentoposterior position, the neck is too short to span the 12 cm of the anterior aspect of the sacrum. Additionally, to complete delivery, the neck would have to be extended even further, to allow the occiput to pass under the symphysis, and this is not possible as the neck is already maximally extended. Delivery in the direct mentoposterior position is thus impossible unless, as can happen with a very small fetus, the shoulders can enter the pelvis at the same time as the head. Persistent mentoposteriorly presenting fetuses are therefore delivered by CS to reduce fetal and maternal morbidity.

Vaginal manipulation in face presentations

Vaginal manipulation, including forceps delivery and Thorn's manoeuvre to convert the mentoposterior fetal head to the occipito-anterior position, were reported historically and are contraindicated in modern obstetrics due to the high risk of fetal injury. However, it is worth noting a report by Newman et al. (1994) who reported on 11 cases of intrapartum bimanual conversion of mentoposterior to occipito-anterior position in orthodox Jews who refused CS delivery. In the 10 patients where ritodrine was administered, the manoeuvre was successful and vaginal delivery was achieved. A ritodrine bolus was administered, with concurrent upward transvaginal pressure, and the fetal head was disengaged. Bimanual fetal head flexion was then attempted using ultrasound guidance and transabdominal palpation of the occiput with gentle flexion towards the maternal pubis. Once the occipito-anterior presentation was achieved, oxytocin infusion was started. The one failure in this report was the author's initial case, in which ritodrine was not employed. Maternal and neonatal outcomes were good in all cases.

After birth, oedema and bruising of a neonate's face is inevitable and the parents should be warned of this in advance. In some cases, it may persist for some days and can make feeding difficult.

36.3 Summary

- Face presentation is not common but when it does occur, it is often identified late
- Accoucheurs should be prepared for this eventuality and be aware that a persistent mento-posterior position will need a CS

36.4 Further reading

Shaffer BL, Cheng YW, Vargas JE, Laros RK, Caughey AB. Face presentation: predictors and delivery route. *Am J Obstet Gynecol* 2006; 194: e10–e12.

CHAPTER 37
Breech delivery and external cephalic version

Learning outcomes

After reading this chapter, you will be able to:

- Discuss the risks and benefits of external cephalic version
- Understand the techniques of external cephalic version
- Discuss the risks and benefits of vaginal breech delivery
- Understand the techniques to manage normal and complicated vaginal breech births

37.1 Introduction

The incidence of breech presentation is about 20% at 28 weeks but has dropped to 3-4% by term as most fetuses turn spontaneously. Breech presentation can be a consequence of fetal or uterine abnormality, but mostly occurs by chance. It is commoner preterm. It has been widely recognised that there is higher perinatal mortality and morbidity with breech presentation, principally associated with prematurity, congenital anomalies and birth asphyxia. Breech presentation, whatever the mode of delivery, is a signal for potential fetal handicap and this should inform antenatal, intrapartum and neonatal management.

Caesarean section (CS) for breech presentation has been suggested as a way of reducing the associated fetal problems and in many countries in northern Europe and North America CS has become the most common mode of delivery in this situation. However, it remains vitally important to maintain the technical skills required to manage breech presentation both antenatally and intrapartum. External cephalic version (ECV) will be described and the various techniques to manage straightforward and complex breech delivery are reviewed.

37.2 External cephalic version

External cephalic version, the manipulative transabdominal conversion of the breech to cephalic presentation, has been practiced since the time of Hippocrates and through the European Middle Ages up to modern times. In the late 1970s and 1980s, the procedure fell into disrepute but subsequent trials and the decline in women choosing a vaginal breech birth has led to its wider reintroduction. The Royal College of Obstetricians and Gynaecologists (RCOG) has set an audit standard to reinforce the recommendation to offer ECV to women with a diagnosed breech presentation at term.

Managing Medical and Obstetric Emergencies and Trauma: A Practical Approach, Fourth Edition. Edited by Rosamunde Burns and Kara Dent.

Efficacy

The use of ECV at term has been subjected to rigorous scientific appraisal in a number of randomised controlled trials (RCTs). There is significant reduction in the risk of CS in women where there is an intention to undertake ECV (OR 0.52, 95%CI 0.4–0.7) with no increased risk to the baby (RCOG, 2017). When ECV was attempted at term, in comparison with no ECV attempted, a Cochrane review of eight studies (n = 1308) showed a statistically significant and clinically meaningful reduction in: (i) non-cephalic presentation at birth (average RR 0.42, 95%CI 0.29–0.61; eight trials, 1305 women); (ii) vaginal cephalic birth not achieved (average RR 0.46, 95%CI 0.3–0.62; seven trials, 1253 women); and (iii) CS being performed (average RR 0.57, 95%CI 0.40–0.82; eight trials, 1305 women) (Hofmeyer et al., 2015). There were no differences in perinatal outcome.

The perceived reduction in success rates in nulliparous women has led to an examination of ECV before term. A systematic review of three older studies involving 900 women showed no reduction in CS rate (RR 1.1, 95%CI 0.78–1.54). The Early ECV 2 Trial (Hutton et al., 2011) showed an increase in cephalic presentation at birth but no reduction in CS rate. Furthermore, early ECV possibly increased the risk of premature birth.

ECV can be carried out in early labour (if the membranes are intact) with success but no randomised trials exist and studies are too small to assess safety.

ECV has been introduced successfully into practice in the UK. Although the success rate (conversion to cephalic presentation) found is less than that quoted in some trials (e.g. over 80% in Africa), others have found similar success rates. Generalisation of these results in the UK would result in a significant reduction in the numbers of CS. With case selection, it is possible to achieve higher success rates and operators improve with experience. Among published US studies, an overall success rate of 65% was found.

Reversion to breech can occur after successful ECV, with between 3% and 7% being reported for term ECV. Rates of over 20% have been reported for preterm ECV.

Factors affecting success

Parity is the main factor that affects success, with nulliparous success rates around one in three and multiparous success rates around two in three or greater. Amniotic fluid volume may affect success, although there is no consensus on whether there should be an absolute cut-off for attempting the procedure. Maternal weight and height affect success and fetal weight (both macrosomia and small for gestation) may be a factor. Even within the 'term' period, length of gestation may matter, and the degree of engagement of the fetal breech has an effect. Attempts to produce a predictive algorithm have not been helpful.

Techniques to improve success

Tocolysis and anaesthesia have been advocated to improve success rates. A Cochrane review (Cluver et al., 2012) confirmed that tocolytic drugs were effective in increasing cephalic presentation in labour (average RR 1.38, 95%CI 1.03–1.85; eight studies, 993 women) and in reducing the number of CSs (average RR 0.82, 95%CI 0.71–0.94; eight studies, 1177 women). Regional analgesia in combination with tocolysis was more effective than tocolytics alone in terms of successful version (assessed by the rate of failed ECVs: average RR 0.67, 95%CI 0.51–0.89; six studies, 550 women) but with no difference identified in cephalic presentation in labour (average RR 1.63, 95%CI 0.75–3.53; three studies, 279 women) nor in CSs (average RR 0.74, 95%CI 0.40–1.37; three studies, 279 women).

Alternative methods of producing cephalic version

Various postural methods, such as knee–elbow, knee–chest, Indian and Zilgrie positions, have been advocated. A review of clinical trials has shown no increase in the rate of cephalic births.

The technique of moxibustion involves the use of burning herbs at acupoint BL 67 beside the outer corner of the fifth toenail. Although an early trial suggested an increase in cephalic presentations, a subsequent larger and better-conducted study has shown no benefit.

Complications

Systematic reviews of safety of ECV have been carried out. Transient fetal heart rate abnormalities occur in 5.7%, with persisting abnormal cardiotocography (CTG) in approximately 1/300. Placental abruption was rare, occurring in 1/1000 patients. A detailed examination of perinatal deaths in a series of ECV births suggests a perinatal mortality of 1.6/1000. This is not different from the perinatal mortality of pregnancies between 37 and 40 weeks.

There is a growing body of evidence that the CS rate for women who have successful ECV is around twice that of cephalic-presenting pregnancies and that the vaginal operative delivery rate may also be increased. The data are sufficiently consistent that women undergoing ECV should be informed of this.

Most women are still prepared to choose ECV to allow a subsequent vaginal delivery. However, some surveys have suggested that a substantial minority of eligible women would decline ECV, instead opting for CS. In part, this may be a failure of education and uptake can be increased by well-constructed information packages.

Technique of external cephalic version

There are no studies comparing different methods of performing ECV. Training is largely 'hands-on' and may vary slightly between different practitioners. Whilst the RCOG guidance does not promote a specific technique, it acknowledges that use of tocolysis with beta-mimetics has been show to improve the success rate of ECV.

Preparation

1. Inform the woman fully of the risks, national and local success rates and about the procedure itself.
2. Perform a CTG, which should be normal.
3. Ultrasound examination should be carried out by a practitioner with appropriate training. The examination should determine:
   - Fetal position
   - Position of the legs
   - Liquor volume
   - Exclude head extension
   - Exclude nuchal cord
4. A prior formal scan assessment to exclude both small for gestational age (SGA) and fetal macrosomia is useful.
5. Ideally, written rather than verbal consent should be obtained.
6. Although serious complications are rare, the practitioner should ensure that there is immediate access to an obstetric operating theatre and that the obstetric anaesthetist is immediately available.
7. Tocolysis should be given at this stage. If there are no contraindications to beta-mimetic drugs, give terbutaline 250 micrograms by subcutaneous injection. The woman should be warned of the potential side effects.

Procedure

1. Lay the woman flat ensuring she does not suffer from significant supine hypotension. If necessary, arrange for lateral tilt using a folded pillow or a wedge. Some practitioners also tilt the head of the bed downwards, placing the woman slightly head down.
2. Disengagement of the breech from the pelvis can be achieved by a number of methods. Most practitioners use the palmar surfaces of the fingers of both hands to gradually pull up the breech (Figure 37.1). Others use a modification of Pawlik's grip to push up the breech. An assistant may help to push the breech up whilst the obstetrician concentrates on flexing the head and encourages rotation.
3. Some use talc or various oils. There is no evidence that the use of these influences success or comfort rates and choice depends on individual preference.
4. Once disengaged, the breech is slowly pulled or pushed upwards and laterally towards the side of the fetal back. Further manipulations aim to encourage fetal flexion. Some practitioners rely totally on achieving disimpaction, allowing the fetus to perform a forward somersault in their own time while maintaining the breech free and to the side. Others use one hand to grasp the now mobilised breech, with the other hand gently flexing the fetal head with pressure on the occiput and nape of the neck (Figure 37.2). The hands follow the fetus as it rotates. The main aim is to encourage the fetus to move into the transverse plane. At that point, the head often moves quickly and easily without further effort to lie over the pelvic brim.

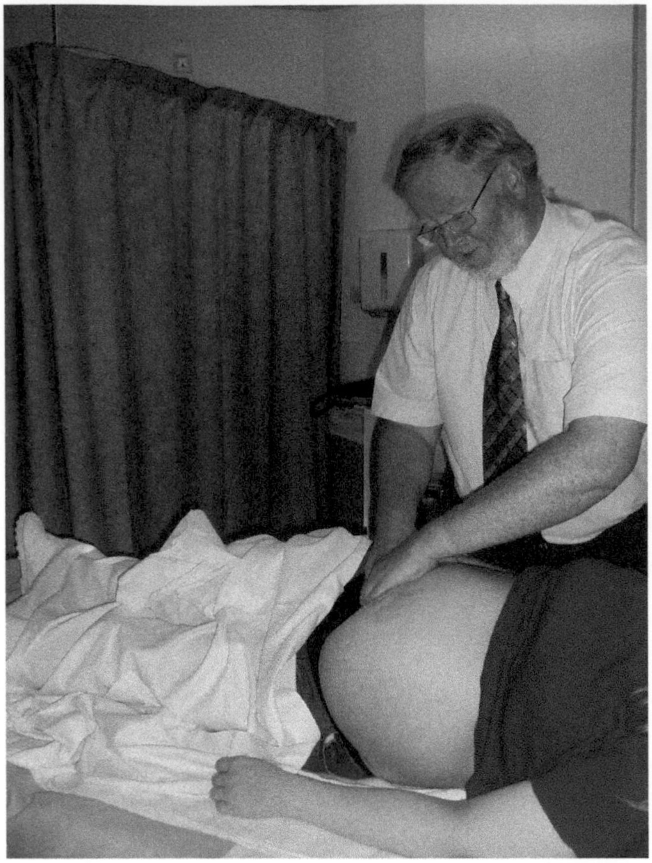

Figure 37.1 Disimpaction of the fetal breech

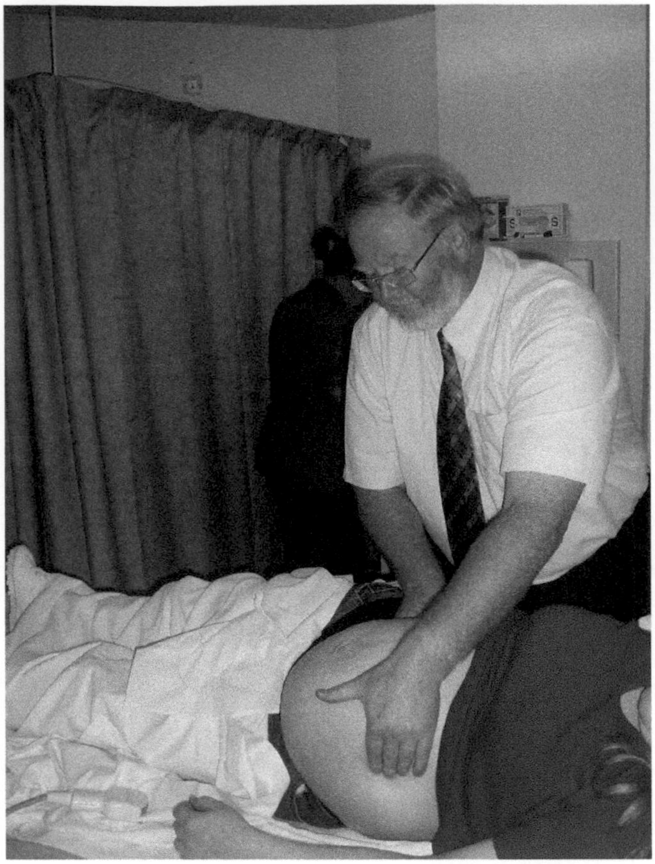

Figure 37.2 Flexion of the fetal head

5. The procedure should not be lengthy and there should be constant feedback between the obstetrician and the woman, which not only keeps her informed about progress, but acts as a distraction to the inevitable discomfort felt. The fetal heart should be intermittently monitored by external CTG or observed by scan, especially if the procedure takes more than 2–3 minutes to complete. A maximum of three attempts should be made. A 'forward somersault' is usually the best direction to aim for, but a backward somersault approach can be considered if a third attempt is to be undertaken. The fetal heart should always be observed or auscultated between attempts.

Post-procedure

- A continuous CTG should be performed for 15–20 minutes post-procedure, whether successful or not
- If the woman is Rhesus (Rh) negative, blood for Kleihauer's estimation should be taken and a minimum of 500 units of Rh immunoglobulin given (final dose to be directed by the laboratory results)
- If successful, spontaneous labour is awaited with advice given to report any bleeding, ruptured membranes or reduction in fetal movements. A clinic review may be offered to allay maternal anxiety about the possibility of spontaneous reversion to breech
- If unsuccessful, then the reasons for this should be discussed. In some circumstances, the woman may request a further attempt on another day, but more usually discussions will move on to decide the final chosen mode of delivery

37.3 Vaginal breech delivery

Term birth

The use of CS as a primary choice of delivery mode for breech presentation at term has increased in the developed world after the publication of the Term Breech Trial (Hannah et al., 2000) which demonstrated clear fetal and neonatal short-term advantages for elective CS. However, 2-year follow-up data showed no significant difference between the planned CS group and the trial of labour group for combined perinatal death and abnormal neurological outcomes. Furthermore, the children born in the trial of labour group reported fewer medical problems, although the significance of this is unclear.

Dutch data (Verhoven et al., 2005; Schutt et al., 2007) have shown that the alteration in practice to a higher CS rate resulted in the predicted reduction in perinatal mortality, but at a cost of an increased maternal mortality rate and increased maternal morbidity in the short and long term. The recommendation in the Netherlands and some other countries remains that the preferred mode of delivery for breech presentation at term is vaginal, if that is maternal preference and with appropriate case selection. Data from the retrospective French PREMODA study suggested that with careful case selection, close monitoring in labour and an experienced accoucheur, neonatal outcomes are not significantly different (Goffine et al., 2006). Selection of cases included assessment of the type of breech, attitude of the fetal head and estimated fetal weight.

There are maternal disadvantages to a policy of routine CS for breech. Therefore, it is imperative that clinical skills of the accoucheur should be such that the option of vaginal breech delivery is available. Currently, in the UK setting, the vast majority of women are having an elective CS for breech, although this practice continues to be questioned.

As a consequence of these concerns, and of breech presentations being diagnosed for the first time in labour (a group which the Term Breech Trial did not address), the need to undertake vaginal breech birth will still occur and skills in delivering the vaginal breech must be maintained.

Many of the manoeuvres used during an assisted breech delivery or Bracht's manoeuvre can and should be used to deliver the breech at CS and this, as well as formal manikin training, can be used to teach and maintain the necessary skills.

Preterm birth

A Cochrane review (Alfirevic et al., 2013) found only four studies that contributed data to the analysis ($n = 116$). The optimum mode of delivery for the preterm breech fetus remains unclear. There was no significant difference between planned immediate CS and planned vaginal delivery with respect to birth injury to the infant (RR 0.56, 95%CI 0.05–5.62; one trial, 38 women) or birth asphyxia (RR 1.63, 95%CI 0.84–3.14; one trial, 12 women). There were no significant differences in perinatal death (RR 0.29, 95%CI 0.07–1.14; three trials, 89 women).

Women should be informed that planned CS may be recommended for preterm breech presentation where delivery is due to maternal and/or fetal compromise, but at present is not routinely recommended for spontaneous preterm labour with a breech presentation at the thresholds of viability (22–25 + 6 weeks of gestation). A recent cohort trial ($n = 390$) confirmed no neonatal benefit of planned CS for preterm breech singletons born at 26–34 weeks of gestation after preterm labour or preterm pre-labour rupture of membranes (Lorthe et al., 2019). Overall, management of labour with a preterm breech involves close monitoring of fetal well-being and labour progress. Care should be taken to avoid early pushing which may result in the rare complication of head entrapment in an incompletely dilated cervix. Epidural analgesia should be considered in *preterm* breech labour to reduce the risk of this complication.

Conduct of labour

Where vaginal breech birth is being considered, ultrasound examination should be carried out to establish the type of breech presentation, the degree of flexion of the fetal head and the estimated fetal weight. If the presentation is footling (at term), if the head is hyperextended or if the estimated weight is less than 2500 g or more than 4000 g, then the woman should be advised to consider delivery by CS and must be made aware of the additional risks should she decide to continue with a planned vaginal birth. Women near to or in the active second stage of labour should not be routinely offered CS. Indeed, women in labour with a breech presentation at term were excluded from the Term Breech Trial and the results of that trial are not directly relevant to this group of women. Retrospective data suggest that this group has a relatively high chance of achieving vaginal delivery without affecting perinatal outcome adversely. Good outcome requires skilled supervision and the direct presence of a skilled accoucheur.

The following description of vaginal breech delivery is what the majority of obstetricians will follow. The 'all fours' delivery technique is also now used, particularly by midwifery colleagues for women who request vaginal breech birth outside obstetric units. This will be described later in the chapter.

First stage management

1. On admission, senior midwifery, obstetric and anaesthetic staff should be alerted and the conduct of the labour should be supervised by the most experienced obstetrician available.
2. One-to-one midwifery care with an experienced midwife should be ensured.
3. If there is spontaneous labour, then maternal and fetal surveillance should follow the guidance as for any labour. The breech baby requires particularly close monitoring and labour progress should be normal.
4. Analgesia, as requested by the woman in consultation with her midwife, should be provided. There is no evidence that epidural analgesia is of specific benefit for breech labour and delivery.
5. Labour can be accelerated using the normal doses of oxytocin where there is good evidence of poor uterine activity as a cause for poor progress in the first stage of labour. Evidence for and against augmentation is not robust and the decision to augment is best made at consultant level. *This is particularly so when there is arrest of progress in the late first or second stages of labour.*
6. Continuous electronic fetal monitoring is generally recommended unless the woman specifies that she does not wish this to be used. Care must be taken when the CTG is suspicious or pathological. Although fetal buttock blood sampling can be performed there is little evidence to support its reliability in breech presentation. It is recommended that significant CTG abnormalities in breech labour should be discussed with the consultant to ensure appropriate decisions are made.
7. As soon as the second stage is diagnosed, a practitioner experienced in vaginal breech birth should be present to undertake or supervise the delivery. The anaesthetic resident on call should be available on the delivery suite and the obstetric operating theatre must be available.

Conduct of delivery

There are no recent data comparing safety or efficacy of the various techniques used in breech birth. Therefore, debates on whether classic techniques are superior to Bracht manoeuvres or whether forceps are superior to the Mauriceau–Smellie–Veit (MSV) technique are simply personal. The last detailed comparison of Bracht's technique versus classic techniques was carried out in 1953 and actually recommended Bracht's technique. A study in 1991 showed no difference in neonatal outcomes, comparing classic and Bracht's techniques. The techniques used by midwifery practitioners are essentially derived from Bracht. *In all techniques, the avoidance of traction on the breech is the key.*

Second stage management – assisted breech delivery

The following describes an assisted breech delivery with the woman in a semirecumbent position (often formally in a lithotomy position). This is the one that obstetricians are most familiar with. The 'all fours' position is also being used more commonly, particularly by the midwifery profession and is described later.

1. Delay active pushing until the breech is distending the introitus. Look for maternal anal dilatation, with the fetal anus visible during pushing as it 'rises' over the distended maternal perineum.
2. The woman who is lying semirecumbent is usually placed in lithotomy at this point. Ensure the maternal bottom is over the edge of the delivery bed. An episiotomy will be required for nulliparous breech deliveries and is often needed for multiparous deliveries. This is a decision to be made individually by the experienced accoucheur. At delivery the breech will usually present in a left or right sacrotransverse position.
3. *A 'hands-off' approach is to be encouraged throughout a vaginal breech delivery.* The stool of the operator is best placed at a distance from the maternal buttocks to encourage this approach. The only exceptions to the 'hands-off' approach are where the fetal back appears to be rotating backwards to lie sacroposterior, or when assistance is required to deliver the legs or arms. If posterior rotation occurs, then it must be corrected. Hold the fetus using a 'pelvic grasp' (Figure 37.3) – the accoucheur wraps both hands around the pelvis, with the thumbs lying parallel to the lower fetal spine and *the index fingers placed on the anterior superior iliac spines*. This avoids injury to the internal organs. Again – only handle the fetus when absolutely necessary and otherwise allow it to descent under its own weight.

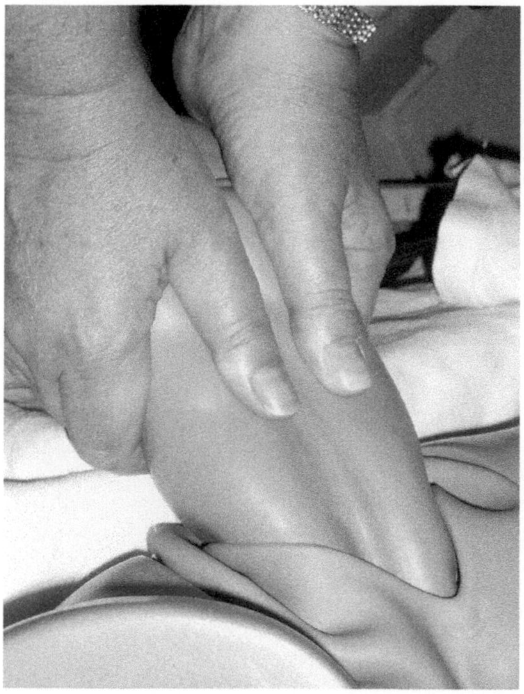

Figure 37.3 The pelvic grasp or grip

4. Allow maternal effort to expel the breech to the level of the umbilicus. The back will arch towards the maternal symphysis. There is no evidence that pulling a loop of cord down at this point is of any benefit and should be avoided, as handling of the cord may produce arterial spasm.
5. Once the umbilicus is reached, there is inevitably some cord compression. The woman should be encouraged to continue pushing between contractions. This can aid steady descent.
6. If flexed, the legs will usually deliver spontaneously. If extended, Pinard's manoeuvre may be required: simply flex the hip by placing one or two fingers behind the thigh, along the length of the femur (with the fingertips in the popliteal fossa). The femur is 'hyperflexed' at the hip joint around the side of the fetal abdomen. The knee will flex and the foot will drop downwards and can be grasped. Gentle traction downwards on the foot will complete delivery of the leg.
7. If the second leg does not deliver spontaneously, use the pelvic grip and rotate the fetus so the leg lies anteriorly. Repeat the manoeuvres above to deliver the leg. *No outward traction should be applied when rotating the fetus as this may lead to extension of the arms (making subsequent delivery more difficult).* Further expulsive efforts will continue to arch the fetal back.
8. The next 'marker' of good descent is when the tip of the anterior scapula appears outside of the introitus. At that point, the arms are ready to deliver. The arms are usually flexed in front of the fetal chest and will usually deliver spontaneously. If not, they can be assisted out by passing the index and middle fingers over the shoulder to lie along the length of the humerus (with the fingertips in the antecubital fossa). In a similar way to that described for delivering the legs, apply pressure and gently deliver the arm around the side of the fetal chest. If the second arm does not deliver spontaneously, rotate the fetus using the pelvic grip (without traction) to bring the arm anterior and deliver as before.
9. If the arms are extended upwards and cannot be reached, then Løvset's manoeuvre should be employed. This situation usually only arises when inappropriate traction has been applied during delivery. The anterior arm cannot be reached as it will be behind or above the symphysis pubis. With the fetus lying in a sacrotransverse position, grasp the breech using a 'pelvic grip'. Start by gently flexing the body **laterally upwards** about 20° above the horizontal. This draws the posterior arm further down the sacral curve *where it will lie lower in the pelvis relative to the extended anterior arm*. Next rotate the body through 180° to bring the posterior arm anterior – ***keep the back uppermost during rotation***. Halfway through rotation when the back is uppermost, **start to apply gentle traction and lower the fetus**, flexing the body **downwards** until it lies 20–30° below the horizontal as rotation is completed. At that point, the arm that was posterior will now lie anterior and will appear from under the symphysis pubis, and can be delivered as described before. Reapply the 'pelvic grip' and repeat the manoeuvres rotating the body through 180° in the opposite direction to deliver the second arm. *Careful flexion and subsequent traction downwards during the latter part of rotation are important elements of this manoeuvre.*

10. After delivery of the arms, allow further descent of the head within the pelvis and await the appearance of the nape of the neck (i.e. the base of the occiput). Allowing the fetus to hang under its own weight for 15–20 seconds promotes flexion and head descent to the appropriate level. Delivery of the head can be achieved manually or with use of forceps. The MSV manoeuvre allows the accoucheur to deliver the fetus without an assistant (Figure 37.4). The fetus is draped over one arm, with two fingers placed alongside the nose on the malar bones (usually the index and middle fingers). Take care to avoid pressure on the eyeballs. Avoid inserting the middle finger into the fetal mouth as this can result in inappropriate traction being applied to the fetal jaw. The other hand is inserted anteriorly with the middle finger placed on the fetal skull below the occiput. The index and ring fingers are hooked over the fetal shoulders. Both hands are used to brace the fetal neck and promote flexion during delivery of the head. Ask the mother to push during traction, delivering the head in an upwards arc, following the pelvic curve. As assistant may apply suprapubic pressure if needed, but this is not usually required.

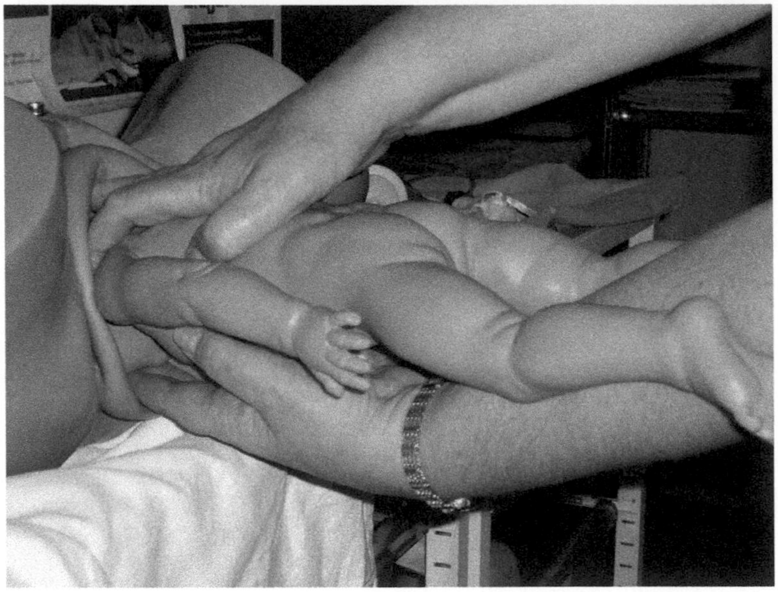

Figure 37.4 Mauriceau–Smellie–Veit manoeuvre

11. If forceps are applied, use a type with long handles such as Neville–Barnes. Wrigley's forceps are not suitable. An assistant carefully grasps the fetus by the ankles and lifts the body just above the horizontal plane. Care must be taken not to hyperextend the neck. The forceps are applied from below the fetus. Each blade should be carefully inserted along the side of the fetal head, with the accoucheur's second hand protecting the lateral vaginal wall. In the USA, Piper's forceps are used. These have very long shanks which have an exaggerated curve 'downwards' which keeps the handles away from the fetus's body during insertion. When forceps with a pelvic curve are used (e.g. Neville–Barnes), the handles will lie close to the fetal body during and after application (Figure 37.5). Kielland's forceps lack a pelvic curve and are a useful instrument to consider for delivering the aftercoming head. Ensure that the handles are not compressed together after application or during traction.
12. Complete third stage management and undertake a systematic check of the vagina and perineum. Repair any perineal or vaginal trauma. Document the delivery carefully and consider when to debrief the mother and her partner.

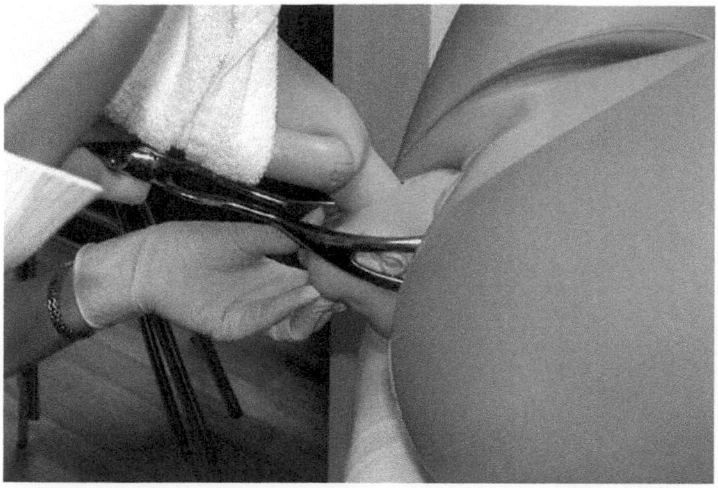

Figure 37.5 Application of non-rotational forceps to the aftercoming head (Kiellands' forceps are a good alternative)

Alternative delivery techniques

Bracht's technique

This technique allows spontaneous delivery of the fetal head as the legs and trunk of the fetus are extended over the symphysis pubis.

1. Delay active pushing until the presenting breech is distending the introitus.
2. Place the woman in lithotomy and perform an episiotomy at the appropriate point.
3. Allow spontaneous delivery to the umbilicus.
4. Grasp the fetus with the thumbs pressing the fetus's thighs against its stomach and the hands wrapped around the pelvic girdle (Figure 37.6). This is known as a 'pelvi-femoral' grip and is essentially the reverse of the pelvic grip described earlier. While the woman is pushing, gently lift the fetus 'up and around' the maternal symphysis, maintaining upwards movement with minimal traction.

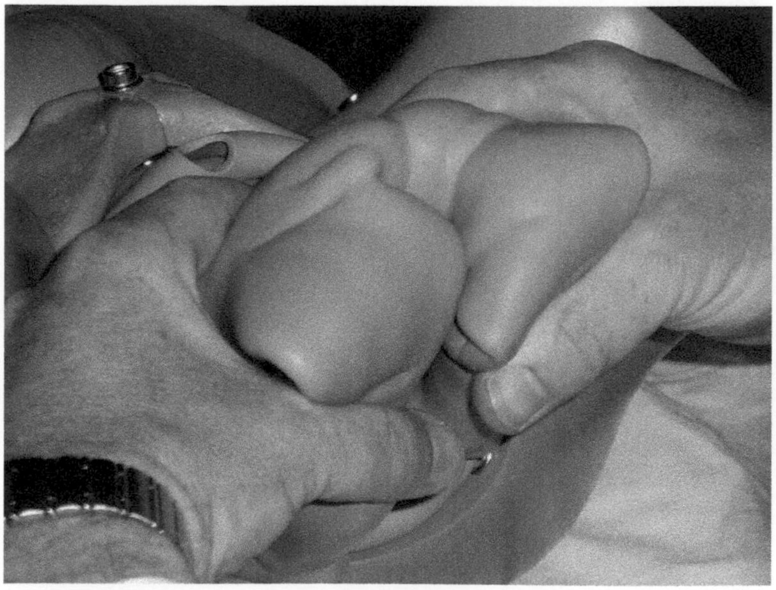

Figure 37.6 Placement of the hands for delivery using Bracht's technique

5. The legs will deliver and as the upwards rotation continues, the arms will follow.
6. Most practitioners of this technique advise using an assistant to provide gentle suprapubic pressure on the maternal abdomen to encourage head flexion and descent.
7. If the arms do not deliver spontaneously, revert to the manoeuvres described in the previous section.
8. With continued upwards rotation, the head will usually deliver spontaneously (Figure 37.7). The assistant should support the perineum during head delivery to reduce the chance of anal sphincter injury. If the head does not deliver then either forceps or the MSV manoeuvre can be used.

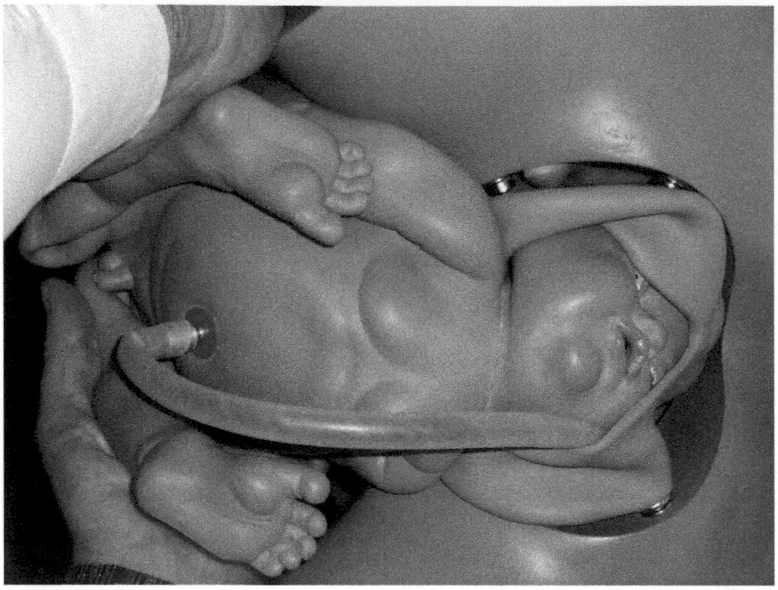

Figure 37.7 Delivery of the head using Bracht's technique (an assistant should support the perineum to avoid obstetric anal sphincter injury)

'All fours' technique

This technique is often used by midwifery colleagues. It can also be a useful technique for unexpected breech delivery managed out of hospital by ambulance personnel who will be unfamiliar with the relatively 'complex' manoeuvres sometimes required for vaginal breech delivery in the standard semirecumbent position. RCOG guidance suggests either position as suitable, dependent on maternal wishes and the experience of the accoucheur. Women should be advised that if the 'all fours' position is used, recourse to a semirecumbent position may become necessary, depending on progress, etc.

1. The mother will be in an 'all fours' (or elbows–knees) position on the bed.
2. The fetus will usually deliver spontaneously onto its bottom, ending up in a 'sitting position' on the bed as the rest of the body and head follow.
3. Obstetricians will be less familiar with this position – i.e. with the fetal abdomen facing them during delivery! It is useful to remember that in *all* delivery positions, **only one back should be facing the accoucheur**. In the 'all fours' position it is the '*mother's back* and fetal abdomen'. In the semirecumbent position, it is the '*fetal back* and mother's abdomen'.
4. Encourage spontaneous delivery. In general the approach during an 'all fours' breech delivery is to encourage *some maternal movement*. Also encourage *continuous, gentle pushing during and between contractions*. Ensure steady descent and progress.
5. Support the perineum as appropriate and consider episiotomy as clinically indicated. 'All fours' breech delivery does not routinely require an episiotomy.
6. The legs usually deliver without intervention. Encourage continuous pushing. As the umbilicus and lower chest deliver, the fetus will 'sit' on the delivery bed.
7. With further pushing, the upper chest will appear and the clavicles will come into view. **The arms will usually deliver spontaneously.**

8. If the arms do not deliver spontaneously – assist delivery. **The anterior arm should always be brought down first by 'sweeping' it across the fetal face**. *This is the one closer to the maternal pubic bone – i.e. the one further away from the accoucheur.* This will potentially restore the physiological mechanism and the other arm will then follow (or can be swept down if required).
9. The head will usually descend and deliver by flexion with maternal effort. If there is failure to flex and deliver, **use the 'shoulder press' technique**:
   - Wrap both hands around the shoulders – fingers on the fetus's back with the thumbs on the fetus's sternum
   - Push the fetus backwards whilst maintaining the shoulder grip
   - The fetal head should flex and distend the posterior perineum before delivering
   - If flexion and delivery do not occur – **try the 'rocking shoulder press' technique** (i.e. gently rocking the fetal body backwards and forwards while maintaining the shoulder grasp)
10. Delivery is complete and the neonate assessed as he/she is passed over to the mother.
11. **At any point if there is delay and these simple manoeuvres are not effective, ask the mother to move into a semirecumbent position, supporting the fetus as she turns over**.
12. Ensure the maternal buttocks are over the edge of the delivery bed to allow access for any necessary manoeuvres (e.g. Løvset's or MSV techniques).
13. Complete delivery as described earlier.

37.4 Failure to deliver

The greatest fear of vaginal breech delivery is head entrapment or nuchal arms that significantly delay delivery. Most experienced obstetricians will have dealt with each of these, but experience is decreasing. Like any rare, unpredictable obstetric emergency, clinicians should have a plan or drill that they follow. There is no literature other than case reports or small series, to guide practice.

Nuchal arms

Nuchal displacement is a rare complication whereby one or both arms are displaced *behind the fetal head/neck.*

1. The accoucheur must picture the situation 'in the mind's eye'. For a **left arm** which is nuchally displaced, the accoucheur uses the pelvic grip to rotate the body and 'unwrap' the arm from behind the neck – **rotate the fetus in a clockwise direction**. For a nuchally displaced **right arm**, rotate the fetus in a **counter-clockwise** direction. You are turning the fetus in the direction of the fingers of the nuchal arm – the baby is guiding you!
2. Once the arm (or arms) have moved from behind the fetal neck, Løvset's manoeuvre may be required to complete delivery (see detailed description earlier).
3. If this fails, grasp the fetal feet. Rotate (swing) the fetus towards the hand of the posterior nuchal arm and *above the level of the maternal symphysis*. This may result in delivery of the posterior arm but, if not, it allows room for the occiput to slip below the elbow. A hand can be placed over the shoulder and behind the humerus to allow pressure on the humerus, with delivery in front of the face.
4. If the other arm does not deliver after this, the procedure can be repeated.
5. If this manoeuvre fails, then time is vitally important. It may be possible, with the back anterior, to insert a hand to grasp the elbow of one arm and exert sufficient pressure to correct the shoulder extension, allowing subsequent use of Løvset's manoeuvre. If this attempt fails, then it is legitimate to force the arm across the face to deliver.
6. Humeral or clavicular fractures are very likely with these later manoeuvres, but will not cause long-term harm; perinatal hypoxia does.

Head entrapment

Intriguingly, few recent texts mention how to deal with this when it occurs, merely providing advice on how to avoid it.

Ensure adequate midwifery and anaesthetic support and prepare for an immediate CS. If expertise is available, call for symphysiotomy equipment.

Fetal back anterior (cervix fully dilated)

1. Start by using McRoberts' position to increase pelvic diameters and apply suprapubic pressure to flex the fetal head and encourage descent.
2. If unsuccessful, lift and rotate the fetal body into a sacrolateral position. Apply suprapubic pressure to flex and rotate the head and apply traction to draw the head into the pelvis. Finally, rotate the back to sacroanterior and complete delivery by forceps or use the MSV technique.
3. If the head has rotated to occipito-anterior but remains high, attempt mid-cavity forceps application if analgesia allows.

Fetal back posterior (cervix fully dilated)

This is a consequence of an unsupervised delivery or failure to correct malrotation of the fetus as it descends. *The fetal chin may be caught behind the symphysis pubis.*

1. Insert a hand along the sacral curve, aiming to rotate the fetal head into the transverse to disimpact. Alternatively, try to reach the fetal chin directly to rotate and disimpact.
2. Apply traction with suprapubic pressure and manage as earlier to complete delivery.

Final options

1. Perform a symphysiotomy if you have adequate training.
2. If not, then you will need to carry out a category 1 CS if the fetus is still alive. When anaesthesia is in place, the fetus will need to be manipulated back into the vagina, starting with the shoulders – this will not be easy, so consider the following recommendations:
   - Consider tocolysis
   - Use a 'classic' uterine incision to maximise access
   - Consider using a vacuum cup applied to the head via the uterine incision to help elevation from deep in the pelvis

Failure of the head to descend (incompletely dilated cervix)

This is a rare emergency which can occur when pushing has started too early. It is more likely with a preterm vaginal breech delivery. The cervix will be felt as a constricting ring around the fetal neck, under the chin.

1. Attempt to dilate the cervix manually (more likely to be successful in parous women). If required, forceps may then be carefully applied to expedite delivery.
2. Use Duhrssen's incisions – carefully guide scissors into the vagina taking care to avoid maternal and fetal trauma. Incise the cervix at **2, 6 and 10 o'clock**. Repair the incisions post-delivery under appropriate anaesthesia.
3. If unsuccessful and the fetus is still alive – consider performing a category 1 CS as described earlier.

Breech extraction

Breech extraction is most commonly used for the delivery of the second twin and is covered in Chapter 38. This technique is also used for delivery of an abnormal lie at CS.

37.5 Medicolegal matters

Medicolegal concerns are increasingly rare for the singleton breech in the UK as most women with breech presentation who decline or have an unsuccessful version, choose CS. However, if proper delivery techniques are not employed at CS, trauma can still result and this may lead to litigation.

Where vaginal breech delivery is to occur at any gestation, consultant or experienced specialist input at every point in the decision process is vital. Although the literature is not supportive of absolute rules on use of oxytocin, continuous electronic monitoring or epidural analgesia in labour, these can be contentious and discussion should take place at consultant level if there is any doubt.

For UK trained practitioners, competence in management of vaginal breech delivery is now an issue. Even consultant or specialist-level staff may have little experience or confidence at conducting a vaginal breech birth and they should ensure the availability of other colleagues where necessary.

37.6 Summary

- Offer and encourage ECV after 36 weeks' pregnancy
- There is no simple algorithm for predicting ECV success
- Tocolysis with a beta-mimetic drug appears to increase ECV success rates
- Audit success rates for ECV
- Where vaginal breech birth is chosen, ensure early involvement of consultant staff in labour and the presence of the most experienced accoucheur for delivery
- Delivery in the lithotomy position is most familiar for obstetricians – they should develop knowledge and skills in the 'all fours' technique
- Ensure familiarity with Løvset's manoeuvre for displaced arms
- Use simulation and ensure drills are used to familiarise teams with management of nuchal arms and the entrapped head
- Maintain competences through the practice of techniques for breech delivery at caesarean section and with regular manikin training

37.7 Further reading

RCOG (Royal College of Obstetricians and Gynaecologists). *External Cephalic Version and Reducing the Incidence of Breech Presentation*. Green-top Guideline No. 20a. London: RCOG, 2017.

RCOG (Royal College of Obstetricians and Gynaecologists). *Management of Breech Presentation*. Green-top Guideline No. 20b. London: RCOG, 2017.

CHAPTER 38
Twin pregnancy

Learning outcomes

After reading this chapter, you will be able to:
- Discuss how to assess suitability for vaginal delivery
- Describe how to safely manage appropriate vaginal twin deliveries

38.1 Introduction

Monozygous twinning rates are relatively constant, with an incidence of 3.5/1000 births. However, dizygous twinning rates vary enormously depending on age, parity, racial background and use of assisted conception techniques. The incidence of twin pregnancies continues to increase, largely due to assisted reproduction techniques. The Office of National Statistics quotes a multiple birth rate of 15.4/1000 maternities in England and Wales in 2018. Overall maternal and perinatal mortality and morbidity are higher in multiple gestations than in singletons. Premature delivery and the complications of prematurity are the main contributors to adverse outcomes. Other factors contributing to the risk are: intrauterine growth restriction, congenital anomalies, malpresentation, cord prolapse and premature separation of the placenta.

The use of routine antenatal ultrasound assessment has facilitated the diagnosis of multiple gestations. Women with multiple fetuses who attend for antenatal care should have the chorionicity of the pregnancy determined early in pregnancy and then have serial growth scans as specified in the recent National Institute for Health and Care Excellence guideline (NICE, 2019) on the antenatal care of multiple pregnancies. It is recommended that uncomplicated monochorionic diamniotic twins are delivered between 36 + 0 and 36 + 6 weeks following a course of antenatal steroids, and dichorionic twins are delivered between 37 + 0 and 37 + 6 weeks. A meta-analysis of the management of twin delivery did not find significant differences in outcome, in terms of mortality or neonatal morbidity, when comparing policies of planned vaginal delivery against planned caesarean section (CS). A cohort study of 2890 twin pairs delivered after 36 weeks of gestation found that there were no deaths in those twins delivered by CS, but found nine second-twin deaths in those delivered vaginally. An international, multicentre, randomised controlled trial (RCT), the Twin Birth Study (Barrett et al., 2013), of 2400 women randomly delivered by CS and planned vaginal birth has now been completed, and shows that vaginal delivery is safe. However, some aspects of twin delivery remain controversial.

38.2 Clinical approach to a twin pregnancy

Twin 1 vertex

Suitability for vaginal delivery must be assessed, allowing for the fact that, even if twin two is cephalic pre-labour, it is difficult to predict its eventual presentation at the time of delivery. If the second twin is breech, vaginal delivery is considered safe, and may be undertaken by assisted breech delivery or breech extraction. If the second twin remains transverse, then delivery can be with either external cephalic version (ECV) or internal podalic version and breech extraction.

Twin 1 non-vertex

When twin one is breech, current opinion favours CS. This is the case despite a large, multicentre, retrospective study of breech first-twin births, which showed no increased risk attributable to vaginal delivery. One of the main concerns quoted about vaginal delivery in this situation is the risk of locked twins, the incidence of which is very low, at 1/645. The Term Breech Trial was a singleton study, and the results should not be extrapolated to twins. However, any decision to proceed with vaginal birth where the first twin presents by breech should be made at consultant level. When twin one is transverse, CS is indicated.

Intertwin delivery interval

The ideal time interval between the delivery of the first and second twins is not agreed. Undue haste with rupture of the membranes before the presenting part of twin two has entered the pelvis can cause problems, whilst undue delay is not without hazards either. In one report, umbilical cord arterial and venous pH and base excess were shown to deteriorate with increasing twin-to-twin delivery interval. There were no second twins with an umbilical pH less than 7.00 when delivered within 15 minutes of twin one. If the intertwin delivery interval was greater than 30 minutes, 27% had an umbilical artery pH of less than 7.00. Among those with an intertwin delivery interval of more than 30 minutes, 73% had evidence of fetal distress that required operative intervention.

Studies have previously suggested that no specific time interval needs to be set, providing that there is progress and continuous electronic fetal heart rate monitoring of twin two is reassuring.

External cephalic version versus internal podalic version for transverse twin two

Both techniques are reasonable, but whilst many investigators report success with an attempt at ECV in the first instance, other authors have reported lower success rates with ECV with increased maternal complication rates compared with proceeding straight to internal podalic version. Nevertheless, given that ECV is less invasive, it is reasonable to consider this in the first place, if the operator is more comfortable with that technique. The experience of the operator is probably the most important factor, and more senior practitioners may choose to go straight to internal manoeuvres.

Higher multiples

Even though the incidence of triplets is rising, most obstetricians have relatively little experience of delivering triplets, and even less of delivering them vaginally. Although a study from the Netherlands reported more favourable outcomes for triplets delivered vaginally when compared with CS delivery, the unit was particularly experienced at this type of delivery. For most obstetricians, the safer option would almost certainly be CS.

Previous caesarean section

The scarce evidence available suggests that a trial of labour is a safe option for twins in the absence of a contraindication to vaginal birth. Scar dehiscence rates have been reported to be 0–3%. Clearly, vaginal delivery is most suitable when both twins are longitudinal (both cephalic or cephalic/breech). Employing ECV or internal podalic version for the transverse lie is more controversial.

Preterm/very low birth weight twins

There seems to be little difference in outcome between vaginal and caesarean delivery in very low birth weight gestations, and little difference in terms of perinatal outcome. However, fetal monitoring of both twins must be accurate and continuous.

Indications for caesarean section in twin pregnancy

As well as the general indications for CS, such as placenta praevia, these include:

- Conjoined twins
- Monoamniotic twins (with possible interlocking or cord entanglement), where delivery is advised between 32 and 34 weeks
- Certain congenital anomalies

38.3 Intrapartum management of vaginal twin deliveries

Management of the first stage

1. Admit to the delivery suite.
2. Set up an intravenous line.
3. Do blood tests – full blood count, group and save serum.
4. Perform continuous cardiotocography on a twin monitor.
5. If there are fetal heart rate abnormalities in twin one, take a fetal scalp blood sample.
6. Ideally, a fetal scalp electrode should be applied to twin one for monitoring to distinguish clearly between the twins.
7. If there are fetal heart rate abnormalities in twin two, perform CS.

If, at any stage, either twin cannot be monitored, then CS may be the only safe option. It is imperative that both twins are monitored and the trace should be scrutinised to ensure that this is the case (i.e. each twin has a distinct rate, and both of these are different from the mother's heart rate). Equally, it is crucial to be sure which recording relates to which twin, as this has, on occasion, been erroneously interpreted and a fetal blood sample performed on twin one for a pathological trace of twin two.

Ultrasound assessment should be performed by an appropriately trained practitioner to determine:

- Presentation of each fetus
- Liquor volume assessment
- Placental site
- Viability of each fetus
- Estimation of fetal weight if not recently performed

Ultrasound can also guide the operator if ECV or internal podalic version is needed for twin two – see later.

The use of epidural analgesia may be justified for possible intrauterine manipulations required for the delivery of the second twin. Inform the:

- Anaesthetist
- Neonatologist
- Neonatal unit

Management of the second stage

1. Provide appropriate analgesia.
2. Prepare oxytocin 40 IU in 500 ml of 0.9% N saline, if not already receiving oxytocin infusion, in case contractions need to be stimulated between delivery of twins one and two.
3. Deliver twin one as if singleton whilst stabilising twin two in a longitudinal lie.
4. Clamp and cut the cord with a labelled clamp.
5. Perform abdominal palpation to determine the lie of the second twin.
6. Confirm lie, presentation and fetal heart rate of twin two, with an ultrasound scan if needed.
7. Monitor the electronic fetal heart rate of twin two continuously.
8. If in transverse lie, perform ECV or internal podalic version (ultrasound can help with this).
9. If there are no contractions within 5–10 minutes, commence oxytocin infusion.
10. When twin two is in longitudinal lie and the presenting part is in the pelvis, perform amniotomy with contraction and proceed with the delivery.

Management of the third stage

1. Give Syntometrine 1 ampoule (or Syntocinon 5 IU if Syntometrine is contraindicated) with the delivery of the second twin.
2. Deliver the placenta.
3. Most obstetric units recommend commencing oxytocin infusion (40 IU oxytocin in 500 ml of 0.9% N saline), as there is a risk of uterine atony following delivery of multiple gestations.

Internal podalic version

A fetal foot is identified by recognising a heel through intact membranes. The foot is grasped and pulled gently and continuously lower into the birth canal. Keep the membranes intact as long as possible as this facilitates movement. They may break spontaneously; otherwise rupture them as late as possible once the rotation is complete. This procedure is easiest when the transverse lie is with the back superior or posterior. If the back is inferior, or if the limbs are not immediately palpable, ultrasound may help the operator identify where they may be found. This will minimise the risk of bringing down a fetal hand. If the foot cannot be safely reached then it may be necessary to proceed to delivery by CS.

Caesarean section for twin two

This is often the consequence of mismanagement of the twin delivery with a lack of stabilisation during delivery of twin one or rupture of membranes of twin two before the presenting part is engaged in the pelvis. The other error is to feel the cervix after twin one has delivered and think that it has contracted down and delivery is no longer possible. The only reason the cervix is palpable at this stage is because the presenting part remains high. Proceeding as described previously will bring the fetal pole down and the cervix will then stretch up over it.

38.4 Communication and team working

In the delivery of twins and higher multiples, team working is essential to optimise the outcome for mother and babies. Obstetricians (including a senior obstetrician), midwives and neonatologists should be present at the delivery. An anaesthetist should be available on the delivery suite in case it may become necessary to perform a CS urgently.

38.5 Summary

- Vaginal delivery of twins is often straightforward, but can be hazardous, and an experienced obstetrician should be on hand to avoid the common pitfalls
- Be diligent in fetal monitoring of both twins accurately
- Do not rupture the membranes of twin two too hastily, but rather wait until the presenting part is in the pelvis and contractions have recommenced

38.6 Further reading

Barrett J, Aztalos E, Wilan A, et al. The Twin Birth Study: a multicenter RCT of planned cesarean section (CS) and planned vaginal birth (VB) for twin pregnancies 320 to 386/7 weeks. *Am J Obstet Gynaecol* 2013; 208: S4–5.

NICE (National Institute for Health and Care Excellence). *Twin and Triplet Pregnancy*. NG137. London: NICE, 2019.

RCOG (Royal College of Obstetricians and Gynaecologists). *Management of Monochorionic Twin Pregnancy*. Green-top Guideline No. 51. London: RCOG, 2016.

CHAPTER 39

Complex perineal and anal sphincter trauma

Learning outcomes

After reading this chapter, you will be able to:

- Recognise and assess first to fourth degree perineal tears
- Understand all techniques of perineal repair
- Manage postoperative care and follow-up of third and fourth degree tears

39.1 Introduction

Perineal trauma resulting from childbirth remains a common problem that is associated with considerable maternal morbidity, and may have a devastating effect on family life and sexual relationships. Following vaginal birth more than 85% of women sustain perineal trauma, up to two-thirds need suturing and up to 30% sustain obstetric anal sphincter injury (OASI). Many OASIs go unrecognised, and there is considerable under-reporting, with incidences quoted as low as 1–2% of vaginal deliveries. Injury increases significantly in the presence of the following risk factors, which often occur in combination: birth weight >4 kg, persistent occipto-posterior position, nulliparity, induction of labour, epidural anaesthesia, prolonged second stage >1 hour, shoulder dystocia, midline episiotomy and forceps delivery. Detection rates are increased by increased awareness and training, but 'occult' anal sphincter injury (i.e. defects in the anal sphincter detected by anal endosonography) from vaginal delivery is common and is most commonly due to lack of recognition, with misclassification as a second degree tear.

Definition

Perineal trauma may occur spontaneously during vaginal birth or as a result of a surgical incision (episiotomy) that is intentionally made to facilitate delivery. It is also possible to have both an episiotomy and a spontaneous tear. The following classification of spontaneous perineal trauma described by Sultan has now been accepted by the Royal College of Obstetricians and Gynaecologists (RCOG) and also internationally by the International Consultation on Incontinence.

- *First degree*: Injury to vaginal or perineal skin only
- *Second degree*: Injury to perineal muscles but not involving the anal sphincter
- *Third degree*: Anal sphincter muscles torn. Further subdivided into:
  - 3a: <50% thickness of external sphincter torn
  - 3b: >50% thickness of external sphincter torn
  - 3c: internal sphincter also torn
- *Fourth degree*: A third-degree tear with disruption of the anal epithelium and tears where the anus and/or rectum are damaged
- *Button hole tear*: An isolated rectal mucosal tear without involvement of the anal sphincter

Managing Medical and Obstetric Emergencies and Trauma: A Practical Approach, Fourth Edition. Edited by Rosamunde Burns and Kara Dent.

Episiotomy

Episiotomy is a surgical incision of the perineum that increases the diameter of the vulval outlet to facilitate delivery. The mediolateral episiotomy (associated with fewer complications than the midline incision) extends from the midpoint of the posterior fourchette at an angle of 60° from the midline at approximately 8 o'clock to avoid the anal sphincter complex.

Episiotomy should not be used routinely, but has a place in facilitating delivery in the following situations:

- Fetal distress
- To allow access for internal manoeuvres during shoulder dystocia
- To minimise severe perineal trauma during an instrumental delivery, particularly forceps
- To aid vaginal delivery when the perineum appears thick and inelastic
- When prolonged 'bearing down' may be detrimental to the mother's health, e.g. severe hypertension or cardiac disease

39.2 Assessment of perineal trauma

The perineum must be examined thoroughly following the birth, with good exposure and lighting. The assessment should include a rectal examination to exclude OASI (Figure 39.1). This is of considerable importance, as 'buttonhole' injuries of the rectum can occur in isolation even with an intact perineum (Figure 39.2). The anal sphincter should be palpated with the index finger in the rectum and the thumb on the perineum or over the posterior fourchette while performing a pill-rolling motion. In the absence of an epidural, the woman could be asked to contract her anal sphincter to accentuate any anal sphincter disruption. The ends of a completely disrupted sphincter can retract (following the circular pattern of the external sphincter) and therefore may not be visible. Care should be taken to explore any defects or 'spaces' at either side of the anus, as the torn free ends of muscle will be found in their depths (often at 8 o'clock and 4 o'clock, respectively). It is essential that, prior to examination or suturing, the procedure is explained to the woman and her partner and consent obtained.

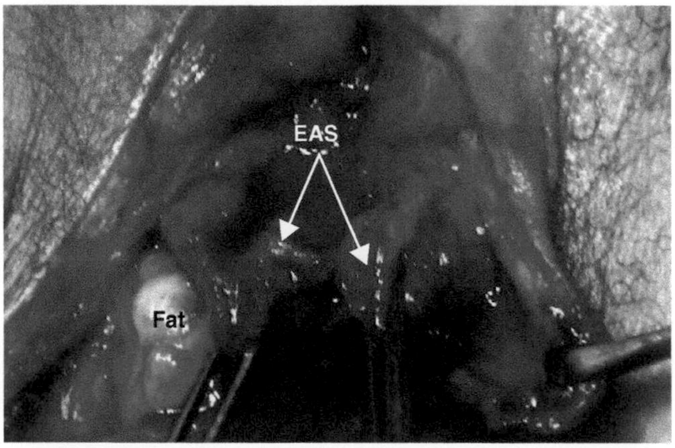

Figure 39.1 Third degree tear (grade 3b) with the external anal sphincter (EAS) grasped by Allis forceps; the ischioanal fat is lateral to the EAS

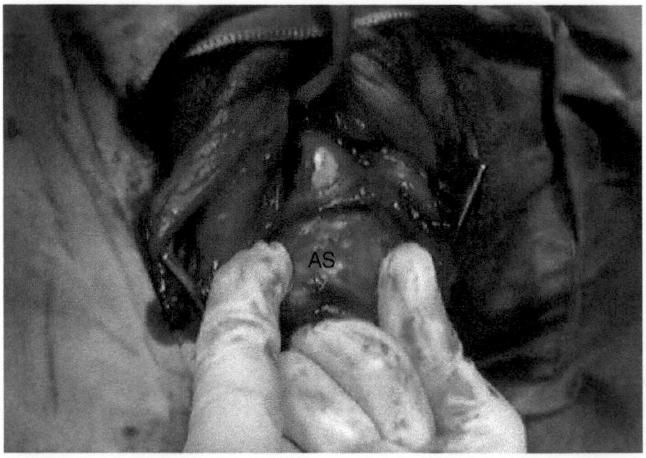

Figure 39.2 'Buttonhole' tear (arrow) in the rectum with an intact anal sphincter (AS)

39.3 Repair of trauma

1. Excessive uterine bleeding should be managed appropriately prior to commencing the perineal suturing.
2. Ensure that the wound is adequately anaesthetised prior to commencing the repair:
   - Local infiltration with 1% lignocaine is adequate for simple trauma, but extensive damage and difficult repairs may need more effective analgesia than the maximum dose of 20 ml will achieve. Always be careful to avoid injecting directly into a vessel
   - Top up an existing epidural or administer regional anaesthesia; this is especially worthwhile for extensive trauma where access is difficult (e.g. high fornices trauma), or where the anal sphincter complex is involved
3. A quick assessment should be made as to whether the operator is capable of completing the repair, as this facilitates an early request for senior assistance rather than struggling for ages before admitting defeat, during which time significant blood loss may have occurred.
4. Current research suggests that perineal trauma should be repaired using the continuous non-locking technique to reapproximate all layers in turn (vagina, perineal muscles and then subcuticular to the skin) with absorbable polyglactin 910 material (Vicryl rapide®).
5. Be careful to identify the apex and check the extent of the trauma, whether the trauma is unilateral or bilateral and how deep it goes. The first stitch is inserted 5–10 mm above the apex of the vaginal trauma to secure any bleeding points that may not be visible, and thence proceeds caudally. Any large bleeding vessels should be secured individually rather than 'hiding them' as continued bleeding can occur, concealed from view, to produce an ischiorectal haematoma.
6. Check that the finished repair is anatomically correct, and complete haemostasis is achieved. Perform a vaginal examination, and check that the vagina is not stitched too tight.
7. A rectal examination should be performed after completing the repair to ensure that suture material has not been accidentally inserted through the rectal mucosa.
8. Check that all swabs, needles and instruments are accounted for.
9. Following completion of the repair, the extent of the injury sustained and the suture technique and materials used must be documented in the case notes in black ink. It is also useful to include a diagram to illustrate the extent of the trauma.

Repair of third and fourth degree tears

A repair should be performed only by a doctor experienced in anal sphincter repair or by a trainee under supervision. If in any doubt about diagnosis, it would be prudent to inform the consultant and await a second opinion (see DVD – www.perineum.net; last accessed January 2022).

Colorectal surgeons are not needed for straightforward third and fourth degree tears but the height of the damage when the tear is fourth degree is vital to assess. If the tear extends beyond the anal canal into the rectum *above the levator plate* then a defunctioning colostomy may be indicated and a surgical colleague should be involved (tears of this severity are rare).

Third and fourth degree tears should repaired in the operating theatre where there is access to good lighting, appropriate equipment and aseptic conditions. The perineal repair pack should contain appropriate instruments (demonstrated in Box 39.1 and Figure 39.3).

General or regional (spinal/epidural) anaesthesia is an important prerequisite, particularly for overlap repair, as the inherent tone of the sphincter muscle can cause the torn muscle ends to retract within the sheath. Muscle relaxation is necessary to retrieve the ends, especially if it is intended to overlap the muscles without tension.

The full extent of the injury should be evaluated by a careful vaginal and rectal examination in lithotomy, and graded according to the classification given earlier in the chapter.

Step 1: suturing the anal epithelium

In the presence of a fourth degree tear, the torn anal epithelium is repaired with polyglactin 3-0 (Vicryl® Ethicon, Edinburgh, UK). Continuous or interrupted sutures can be used (knots tied in the anal lumen).

Box 39.1 Instruments and sutures used for the repair of anal sphincter trauma

Instruments

- Weislander's retractor (or Gilpin's retractor)
- Tooth forceps (fine and strong)
- Needle holder (small and large)
- Allis forceps (×4)
- Artery forceps (×4)
- McIndoe's scissors
- Stitch cutting scissors
- Sims speculum
- Deep vaginal side wall retractors
- Sponge holding forceps (×4)
- Tampon
- Large swabs
- Diathermy

Sutures

- Anal epithelium
  Vicryl 3-0, 26 mm round-bodied needle
- Internal anal sphincter
  PDS 3-0, 26 mm round-bodied needle
- External anal sphincter
  PDS 3-0, 26 mm round-bodied needle
- Perineal muscles
  Vicryl rapide 2-0, 35 mm tapercut needle
- Perineal skin
  Vicryl rapide 2-0, 35 mm tapercut needle

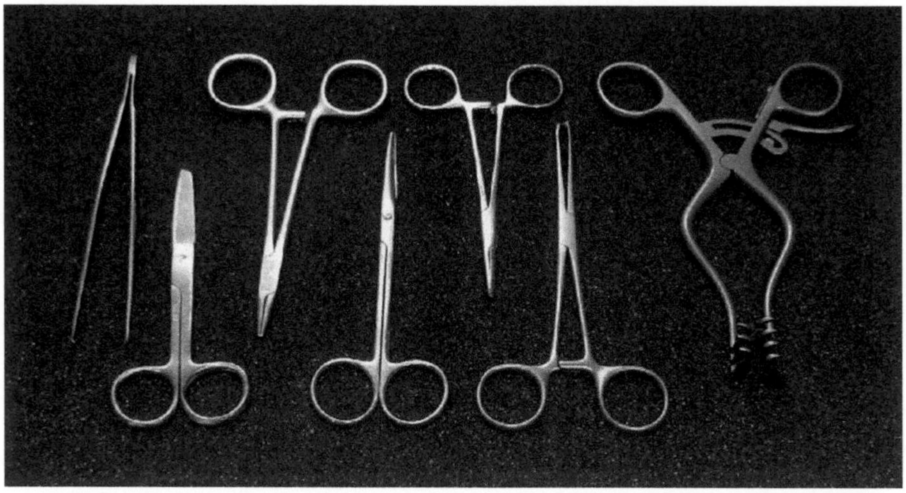

Figure 39.3 Instruments specifically used for repair of anal sphincter trauma. From left to right: tooth forceps; stitch cutting scissors; needle holder; McIndoe's scissors; artery forceps; Allis forceps; Weislander's retractor

Step 2: suturing the anal sphincter

Prior to repairing the anal sphincter it is often worth securing the apex of the vaginal tear while access to it is facilitated by the sphincter tear, and then leave the suture with its needle protected ready to be completed later.

When torn, the internal anal sphincter (IAS) should be identified and sutured separately from the external anal sphincter (EAS). The IAS lies between the EAS and the anal epithelium. It is paler (raw fish-like) than the striated external sphincter (red meat-like) (Figure 39.4) and the muscle fibres run in a longitudinal fashion unlike the circular fibres of the external sphincter. A torn IAS should be approximated (not overlapped) with interrupted or mattress sutures using a fine monofilament suture material such as 3-0 polydiaxanone (PDS) or braided 2-0 polyglactin (Vicryl). It is very important for obstetricians to identify and repair the torn IAS as colorectal surgeons find it almost impossible to identify and therefore repair as a secondary procedure if these women present with faecal incontinence.

Repair of the EAS should be with either monofilament sutures such as PDS or braided sutures such as polyglactin (Vicryl). For partial thickness tears (grade 3a and 3b) an end-to-end technique should be used, while full thickness tears can be repaired with either an end-to-end approximation or an overlap technique. The evidence to date indicates that there is no significant difference in anal incontinence with the end-to-end (Figure 39.5) or overlap (Figure 39.6) technique with full thickness tears.

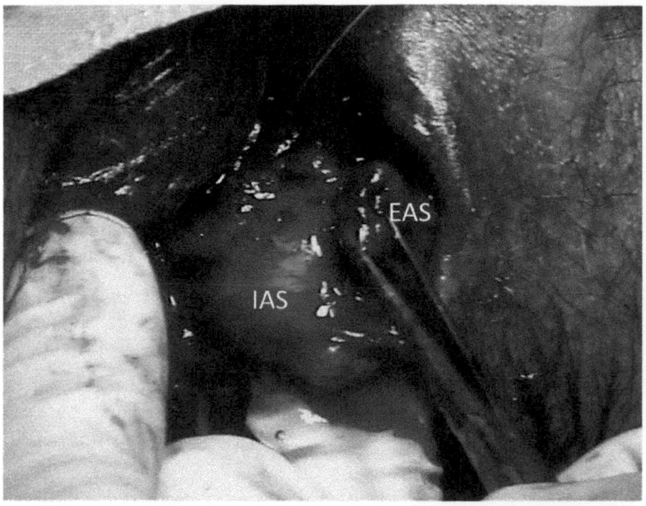

Figure 39.4 Third degree tear (grade 3b) demonstrating an intact internal anal sphincter (IAS) and the torn ends of the external anal sphincter (EAS)

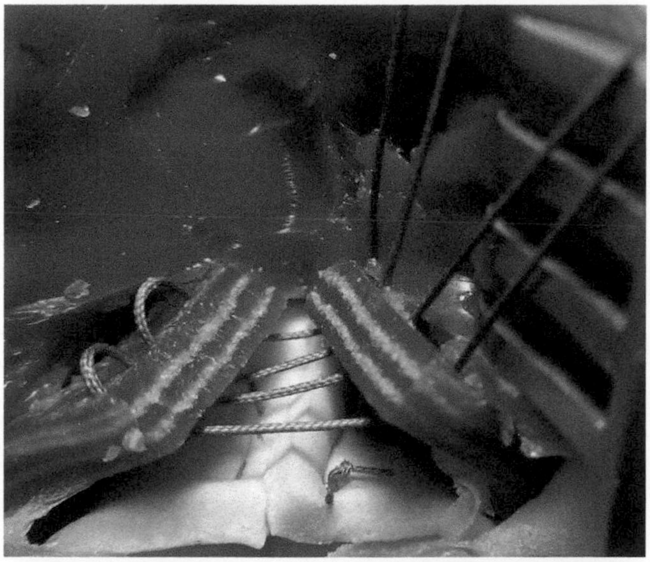

Figure 39.5 Model representation of an end-to-end repair with figure of eight sutures of full thickness tear

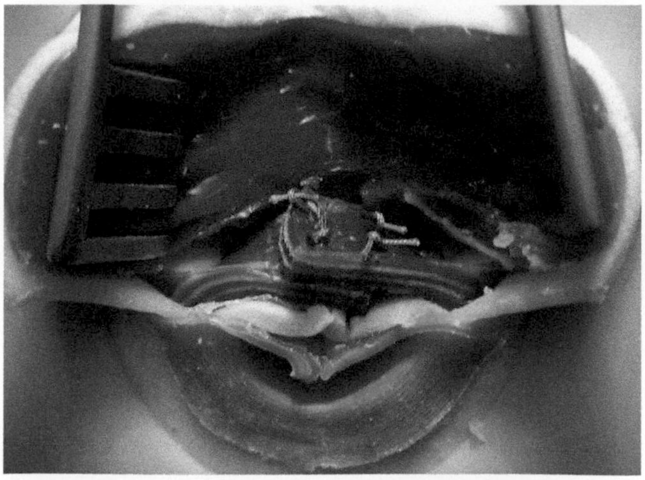

Figure 39.6 Model representation of an overlap repair of full thickness tear

The torn ends of the external anal sphincter are identified and grasped with Allis tissue forceps. Whichever technique is used, care should be taken that the ends of the knots are buried beneath the perineal muscles, particularly when using PDS, in order to minimise the risk of suture migration necessitating removal at a later date.

If an end-to-end repair is being performed, mattress sutures are recommended (as figure of eight sutures may cause more ischaemia). Two sutures are usually sufficient.

For an overlap repair, more extensive dissection is needed:

- The muscle may need mobilisation by dissection with a pair of McIndoe scissors separating it from the ischioanal fat laterally (see Figure 39.1)
- Then the external sphincter should be grasped with the Allis forceps and pulled across to overlap in a 'double-breast' fashion
- The torn ends of the external sphincter can then be overlapped as shown in Figure 39.6
- It is important that the full length of the external sphincter is identified to ensure complete approximation or overlap

The vaginal skin is then sutured, the muscles of the perineal body are reconstructed and the perineal skin approximated (follow as for the repair of episiotomy and second degree tears). Great care should be exercised in reconstructing the perineal muscles to provide support to the sphincter repair and burying the PDS sutures beneath the superficial perineal muscles to avoid migration. A short, deficient perineum would make the anal sphincter more vulnerable to trauma during a subsequent vaginal delivery.

Procedure

- As with all perineal repairs, a rectovaginal examination should be performed afterwards to confirm complete repair, make sure no sutures have inadvertently gone through the anorectal mucosa and to ensure that all tampons or swabs have been removed
- Intravenous broad spectrum antibiotics (e.g. co-amoxiclav) should be commenced intraoperatively and continued orally for 5–7 days. Although there are no randomised trials to substantiate benefit of this practice, the development of infection could jeopardise repair and lead to incontinence or fistula formation
- Severe perineal discomfort, particularly following instrumental delivery, is a known cause of urinary retention and following regional anaesthesia it can take up to 12 hours before bladder sensation returns. A Foley catheter should be inserted for between 12 and 24 hours and midwifery staff should check that spontaneous voiding occurs on its removal
- Good note-keeping of the findings and repair techniques is essential. A pictorial representation of the tears may prove to be useful when notes are being reviewed following complications, audit or litigation

Postnatal care

- Regular, effective analgesia is essential to facilitate early mobilisation
- As passage of a large bolus of hard stool may disrupt the repair, a stool softener (lactulose 10–15 ml twice daily) should be prescribed for 10–14 days postoperatively
- The extent of the tear should be explained to the woman and she should be advised how to seek help if symptoms of infection or incontinence develop
- The woman should be reviewed before she goes home, instructed in perineal care and asked to commence pelvic floor exercises when comfortable
- Follow-up is recommended in a dedicated perineal clinic

39.4 Training

More focused and intensive training is required to improve recognition of anal sphincter trauma. This can be facilitated by establishing hands-on workshops using purpose built models (Figure 39.7) and fresh animal anal sphincters.

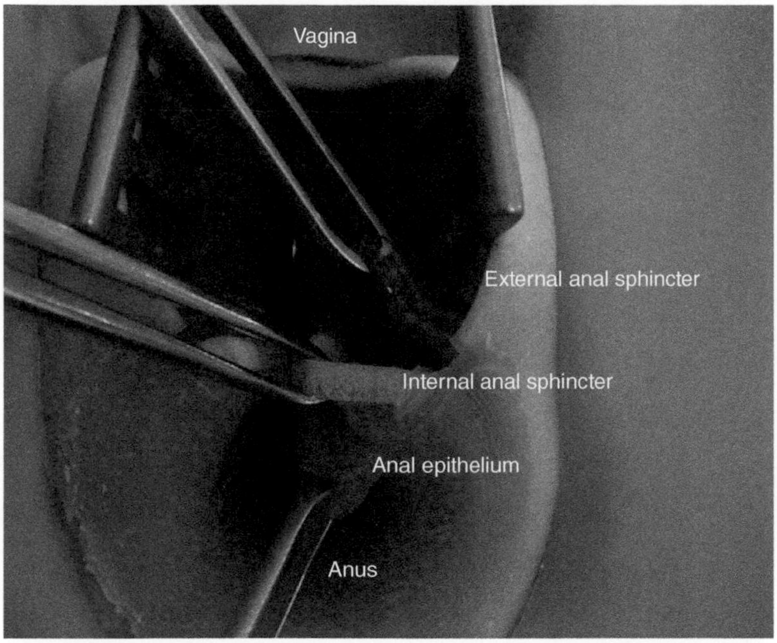

Figure 39.7 Purpose-built teaching model demonstrating anal sphincter anatomy

39.5 Summary

- Perineal trauma is common following vaginal delivery
- A clear explanation of the extent of the injury and consent for repair are necessary
- Practitioner skills should be kept sharp by training
- Third and fourth degree trauma require senior involvement
- Meticulous technique during repair and good aftercare are necessary for a good outcome

39.6 Further reading

Fernando RJ, Sultan AH, Kettle C, Thakar R. Methods of repair for obstetric anal sphincter injury. *Cochrane Database Syst Rev* 2013; 12: CD002866.

RCOG (Royal College of Obstetricians and Gynaecologists). *Third- and Fourth-Degree Perineal Tears, Management*. Green-top Guideline No. 29. London: RCOG, 2015.

CHAPTER 40

Symphysiotomy and destructive procedures

Learning outcomes

After reading this chapter, you will be able to:

- Discuss the indications and technique for symphysiotomy
- Recognise the role of destructive operations
- Describe the procedures involved in destructive operations

40.1 Introduction

Symphysiotomy is rarely used in UK practice but may be useful in dealing with the rare complication of a trapped aftercoming head in vaginal breech delivery. Its use is also described as a method of last resort in severe cases of shoulder dystocia.

Destructive procedures are rarely used in contemporary obstetric practice in the UK, but are still employed regularly in the developing world, often in cases of obstructed labour, where absent prenatal care and poor intrapartum care at peripheral hospitals or in the bush have resulted in fetal demise. Reported incidences range between 0.094% and 0.98% of all deliveries. A destructive procedure is an alternative to an abdominal delivery that may carry considerable risk to the mother. The main reason is to avoid caesarean section (CS) and the associated risk of uterine rupture in future pregnancies when access to monitoring in labour and hospital care may not be available. With the use of prophylactic antibiotics and thromboprophylaxis, CS in the developed world is relatively safe and there is only a limited role in modern practice for destructive procedures. Situations where symphysiotomy or a destructive procedure may be considered in UK practice are described in the following sections.

Symphysiotomy is a relatively common procedure in the developing world, where it is used in situations of cephalopelvic disproportion when CS is not readily available. Symphysiotomy leaves no uterine scar and the risk of a ruptured uterus in future labours is not increased. Van Roosmalen (1987, 1990) illustrated the potential morbidity and mortality of CS operations carried out in rural hospitals in developing countries. Mortalities of up to 5% and an incidence of uterine scar rupture in subsequent pregnancies of up to 6.8% have been reported. Symphysiotomy has a low maternal mortality, with three deaths reported in a series of 1752 procedures. All three deaths were unrelated to the symphysiotomy.

Hartfield (1973) reviewed the cases of 138 women in whom symphysiotomy had been performed. Early and late complications were few and rarely serious, if recommended guidelines were followed. He also reviewed published series of women followed up, for 2 years or more (1975), after symphysiotomy and concluded that *permanent major orthopaedic disability* only occurs in 1–2% of cases.

Managing Medical and Obstetric Emergencies and Trauma: A Practical Approach, Fourth Edition. Edited by Rosamunde Burns and Kara Dent.

Pape (1999) carried out a prospective review of 27 symphysiotomies performed between 1992 and 1994. Five women had paraurethral tears needing suturing, and nine had oedema of the vulva or haematomas tracking from the symphysiotomy. All made a full recovery and severe pelvic pain was not a feature in any woman.

In 2001, the question of legal action against obstetricians in Ireland who carried out symphysiotomies was raised (Payne 2001). Verkuyl (2001) made the point that many symphysiotomies were performed in Roman Catholic countries because contraception was illegal, even for medical reasons, and women were spared repeated operative deliveries.

Symphysiotomy is a useful technique that is occasionally required in UK practice. One report highlighted four cases where it has been used successfully in the UK. Facilitating release of the stuck aftercoming head in a vaginal breech delivery and as an adjunct in shoulder dystocia have been described.

Björkland (2002) published a comprehensive retrospective review of the literature based on papers published between 1900 and 1999; 5000 symphysiotomies and 1200 CS operations were included and the results indicated that symphysiotomy is safe for the mother and potentially life saving for the child. Severe complications were rare.

40.2 Symphysiotomy

Indications

- Trapped aftercoming head of breech fetus due to cephalopelvic disproportion (CPD)
- Severe cases of shoulder dystocia that do not resolve with routine manoeuvres

  Symphysiotomy in the following situations is essentially only used in some areas of the developing world:
- In cases of CPD with a vertex presentation and a living fetus, when at least one-third of the fetal head is still above the pelvic brim (note that the use of forceps is contraindicated with a high head)
- In cases of CPD with a vertex presentation when CS is declined by the mother

Technique

1. Place the woman in the lithotomy position, with her legs supported by two assistants. The angle between the legs should never be more than 60–80° to avoid putting a strain on the sacroiliac joints and tearing the urethra and/or bladder.
2. Inject local anaesthetic into the skin and fibrous part of the symphysis pubis. This step identifies the joint space and the needle can be left in place as a guide wire if the joint has been difficult to locate.
3. Insert a firm urinary catheter. Apply antiseptic solution suprapubically.
4. Push the catheter and urethra laterally with the middle finger, whilst the index finger remains against the posterior aspect of the symphysis pubis under the ligament. Monitor the action of the scalpel, taking care not to injure your index finger under the symphysis by inserting the blade too deeply.
5. Incise the symphysis pubis in the midline, at the junction of the upper and middle thirds. Use the upper third of the uncut symphysis as a fulcrum against which to lever the scalpel to incise the lower two-thirds of the symphysis. Cut down through the cartilage until the pressure of the scalpel blade is felt near the finger in the vagina.
6. Remove the scalpel and rotate it through 180° and cut the remaining upper third of the symphysis. If a solid-bladed scalpel is available, this is better. If not, take great care with the replaceable standard scalpel blade, which is much sharper. The symphysis is cut through very easily; beware of going deeper and injuring the vagina or bladder or the operator's finger.
7. Once the incision is made, pinch it between the finger and thumb – the symphysis should open as wide as the operator's thumb.
8. After this separation of the cartilage, remove the catheter to decrease urethral trauma.
9. Use a large episiotomy to relieve tension on the anterior vagina and pelvis during delivery.
10. After delivery of the baby and placenta, compress the symphysis between the thumb above and index and middle fingers below for some minutes, to express blood clots and promote haemostasis. Consider giving tranexamic acid 1 g IV slowly over 10 minutes.

11. Recatheterise and leave a urinary catheter in place for 5 days or until reasonably mobile.
12. Apply elastic strapping across the front of the pelvis, from one iliac crest to the other, to stabilise the symphysis and reduce pain. The woman needs to be nursed on her side as much as possible, with her knees strapped loosely together for 3 days. After this, mobilisation can begin.
13. Involve the physiotherapist. Consider orthopaedic opinion and follow-up.

40.3 Destructive procedures

Destructive operations may be required where the fetus is dead and where a vaginal delivery is being attempted. It may be the most appropriate method for delivery to minimise maternal risk, or it may be the only route by which the mother wishes to be delivered. Whenever a destructive procedure is being considered, it must only be performed with the mother's consent.

The following are the general principles of destructive procedures:

1. If the mother is unstable, basic resuscitation must be carried out quickly, to avoid undue delay in delivering a dead fetus.
2. Catheterise.
3. Since urinary and genital tract infections are common, antibiotic prophylaxis should be used.
4. General or regional anaesthesia combined with sedation is ideal for the procedure.
5. The cervix should be fully dilated. (Note: destructive surgery may be performed by an experienced operator when the cervix is dilated at least 7 cm.)
6. The genital tract and rectum must be systematically examined after the procedure.
7. A catheter should be left in place for at least 48 hours.

The four most common destructive procedures are:

- Craniotomy
- Perforation of the aftercoming head/drainage of major hydrocephalus
- Craniocentesis
- Decapitation

Background

In resource-poor areas of the world, CS is often unavailable or carries significant risks. Potential problems include haemorrhage from uterine extension, generalised peritonitis and the risk of rupture of the scar in a subsequent pregnancy. Gogoi (1971) showed a much lower morbidity and mortality with craniotomy than with CS in a group of 158 women who were grossly infected. Peritonitis occurred in 66% of women after CS and was nil after destructive operations; the maternal mortality in the CS group was 13/107 (12%) compared with 1/37 (2.7%) in the craniotomy group.

Marsden et al. (1982) described a series of four cases where the Blond–Heidler saw wire was used in the case of a dead fetus in a transverse lie. They had no complications and suggested that, in such situations, this method of delivery is more appropriate than CS, when a classic incision may often be required, which significantly increases risks for the mother.

Reports from the developing world of maternal morbidity and mortality following destructive procedures confirm that most problems encountered can be attributed to prolonged obstructed labour, which resulted in the need to consider a destructive operation in the first place. Ekwempu (1978) reported on a series of 112 patients treated by embryotomy between 1974 and 1975. The only complications that he could attribute to the destructive procedure were seven cases of soft tissue laceration (mainly vaginal and perineal). The procedures themselves have been shown to be relatively simple to perform with little morbidity.

There are several reports from the developing world of postoperative vesicovaginal fistulae. These are often attributed to pressure necrosis in obstructed labour. However, it has been suggested that they could be secondary to the use of sharp instruments or from bony spicules exposed during destructive procedures. Trauma can be minimised by regular training using manikins and with appropriate case selection.

Craniotomy

Indications

Craniotomy is indicated for the delivery of a dead fetus in situations of CPD and hydrocephalus.

Technique

1. Ensure appropriate analgesia/sedation where possible.
2. The fetal head should be no more than three-fifths above the pelvic brim, except in cases of hydrocephalus.
3. Ask an assistant to steady the head from above the pubic symphysis.
4. Perforate the skull via the fontanelle, using a Simpson's perforator, with the instrument at right angles to the surface of the skull to minimise the risk of slipping. If a fontanelle cannot be palpated, the perforator should be inserted through the bone.
5. Push the blades as far as their shoulders and separate first in one direction and then repeat at right angles.
6. Evacuate the cerebrospinal fluid/brain tissue and deliver the fetal head by pulling on the skull edge using vulsellum forceps and countertraction. If delivery is difficult, attach the vulsellum to a 1 kg weight using a bandage (e.g. a 1 litre bag of fluid). This will allow a slower and possibly less traumatic delivery.
7. If the fetus is very large, reduction in the size of the shoulder girdle by cleidotomy may be required after delivery of the head. This can be achieved by cutting the clavicle(s) at their midpoint using heavy scissors.

Perforation of the aftercoming head/drainage

The aftercoming head of a breech can be managed similarly by craniotomy, with perforation of the head through the base of the skull, beginning at the nape of the neck, aiming towards the vertex. If the head is deflexed, perforation of the occiput may be achieved in the region of the posterior fontanelle.

In cases of hydrocephalus, head decompression can be achieved by inserting a curved metal Drew–Smythe catheter (Figure 40.1) via a small perforation as described above. Where the hydrocephalus is associated with spina bifida, cerebrospinal fluid can be withdrawn by exposing the spinal canal, passing the catheter into the canal and up into the cranium. The hydrocephalic head can also be decompressed transabdominally under ultrasound control using a wide-bore spinal needle.

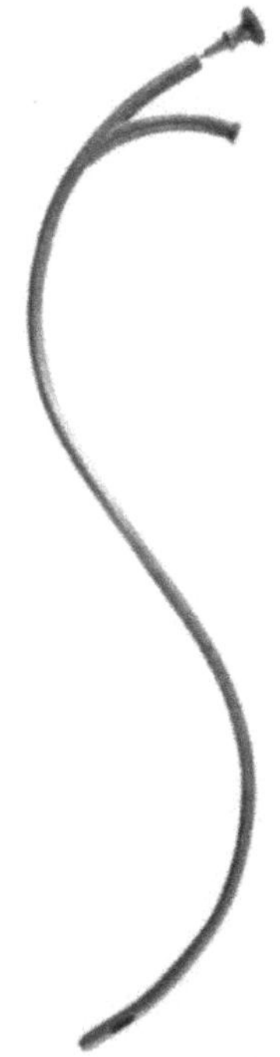

Figure 40.1 Drew–Smythe catheter
Source: Courtesy of Omega Healthcare

Craniocentesis

In developed countries, when severe hydrocephalus with an enlarged head is diagnosed antenatally, CS may be required. In the presence of an underlying lethal condition, transabdominal decompression of the fetal head under ultrasound control may be considered in order to achieve a vaginal delivery. This may need to be combined with feticide. Multidisciplinary team discussion and direct parental involvement are vital in these difficult situations.

Decapitation

Indications

Decapitation is indicated in cases of neglected, obstructed labour with oblique or transverse lie with a shoulder presentation and a dead fetus. In an already emotionally fraught situation, the prospect of explaining this option to parents may be distressing for all. Nevertheless, in terms of minimising harm to the mother, a very early delivery remains optimal. In developed countries, CS will be considered as an alternative option. Delivery can also occur naturally through a process known as 'spontaneous evolution'. The fetus folds up on itself and elongates, the presenting shoulder delivering first. This is more likely at earlier gestations (<26 weeks).

Technique

1. If the fetus is small and the neck can easily be felt, it may be severed with stout scissors. However, for the larger fetus, and especially where the neck is not easily accessible, the Blond–Heidler decapitation tool (Figure 40.2) is the safest instrument.

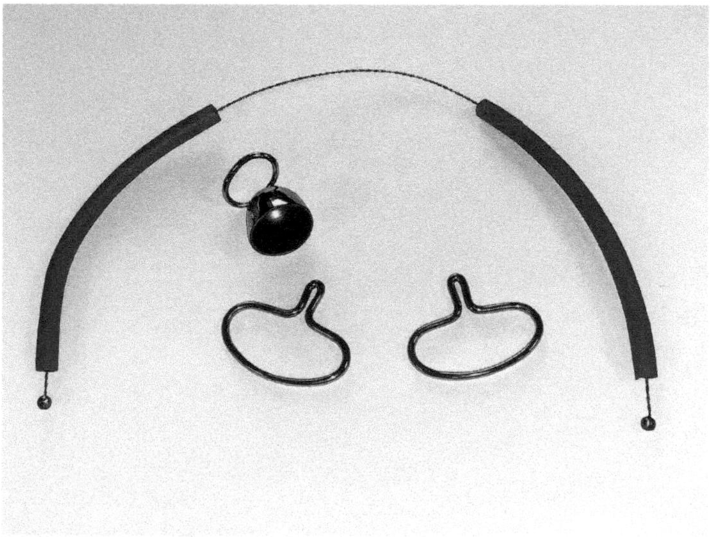

Figure 40.2 Blond–Heidler wire saw

2. If possible, a fetal arm is brought down and firmly pulled on by an assistant, which brings the neck lower to make it more accessible.
3. A modified metal 'thimble' is attached to one end of a flexible wire saw. This is used to thread the saw carefully around the fetal neck. The ends are attached to two handles which are kept close together. This prevents injury to the vagina and the neck is then easily severed with a few firm strokes.
4. Deliver the trunk by traction on the arm, with the operator's hand protecting the vagina from laceration by any bony spicules.
5. Deliver the aftercoming head by grasping the neck/stump with a heavy vulsellum and consider using the Mauriceau–Smellie–Veit manoeuvre.
6. Anatomical continuity can be restored with simple skin sutures around the fetal neck.
7. The fetus should be wrapped respectfully before showing to the parents.

40.4 Summary

- Symphysiotomy is a useful procedure that can be used in certain emergency situations
- Symphysiotomy must only be performed by trained clinicians aware of the potential complications
- Prompt decisions may be required in managing obstructed labour to avoid or minimise fetal morbidity
- Intrapartum and postpartum management are both important to minimise longer term maternal morbidity
- Destructive procedures have a limited, but useful, place in the delivery of a dead fetus in the context of an obstructed labour; their main use is in developing countries

40.5 Further reading

Björklund K. Minimally invasive surgery for obstructed labour: a review of symphysiotomy during the twentieth century (including 5000 cases). *BJOG* 2002; 109: 236–48.

Wykes CB, Johnston TA, Paterson-Brown S, Johanson R. Symphysiotomy: a lifesaving procedure. *BJOG* 2003; 110: 219–21.

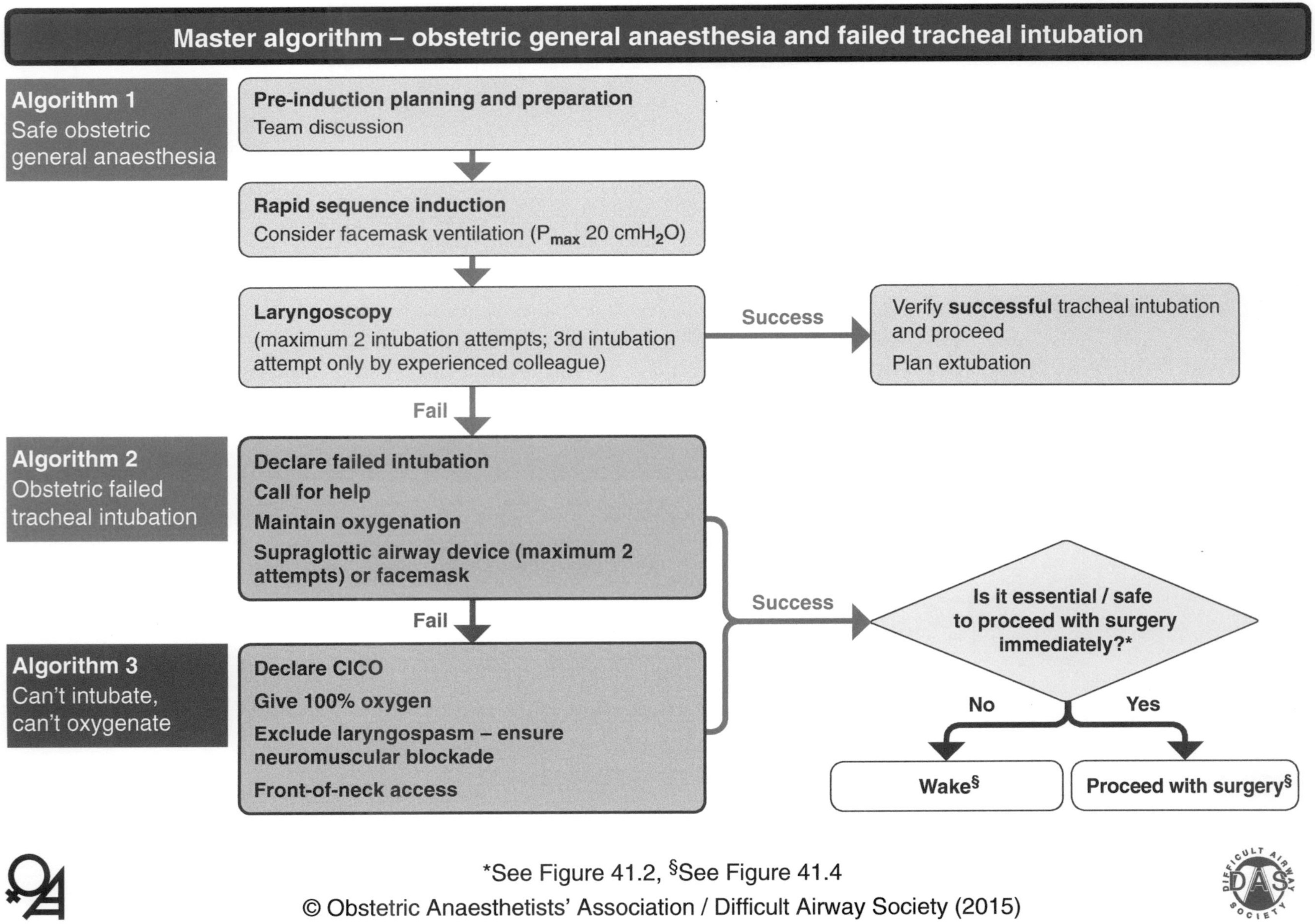

Master algorithm – obstetric general anaesthesia and failed tracheal intubation
Algorithm 1
Safe obstetric general anaesthesia
Pre-induction planning and preparation
Team discussion
Rapid sequence induction
Consider facemask ventilation (P_{max} 20 cmH_2O)
Laryngoscopy
(maximum 2 intubation attempts; 3rd intubation attempt only by experienced colleague)
Success
Verify successful tracheal intubation and proceed
Plan extubation
Fail
Algorithm 2
Obstetric failed tracheal intubation
Declare failed intubation
Call for help
Maintain oxygenation
Supraglottic airway device (maximum 2 attempts) or facemask
Fail
Algorithm 3
Can't intubate, can't oxygenate
Declare CICO
Give 100% oxygen
Exclude laryngospasm – ensure neuromuscular blockade
Front-of-neck access
Success
Is it essential / safe to proceed with surgery immediately?*
No
Yes
Wake§
Proceed with surgery§
*See Figure 41.2, §See Figure 41.4
© Obstetric Anaesthetists' Association / Difficult Airway Society (2015)

Algorithm 41.1 Master algorithm for obstetric general anaesthesia and failed tracheal intubation

Source: Mushambi MC, Kinsella SM, Popat M, et al. Obstetric Anaesthetists' Association and Difficult Airway Society guidelines for the management of difficult and failed tracheal intubation in obstetrics. *Anaesthesia* 2015; 70: 1286–306. © 2015 Obstetric Anaesthetists' Association/Difficult Airway Society

CHAPTER 41

Anaesthetic complications in obstetrics

Learning outcomes

After reading this chapter, you will be able to:

- Appreciate the risks posed to the pregnant women by anaesthetic drugs and techniques
- Describe anaesthetic emergency problems affecting the pregnant woman

41.1 Introduction

The proportion of women dying from complications of anaesthesia has declined markedly over the last 20 years. The risk of death from an obstetric general anaesthetic is now estimated at 1 in 20 000. Deaths from airway-related problems have declined over the last 10 years of Confidential Enquiry reports. A literature review in 2015 showed an incidence of 1 in 390 for failed intubation in obstetric patients, which is about seven times higher than in non-obstetric patients. Maternal, fetal, surgical and situational factors contribute to this increased incidence. Failure to intubate the obstetric patient is related to increasing urgency of the delivery and more frequently occurs out of hours with less experienced staff in attendance and a failure to follow standard practice. The 2015 Obstetric Anaesthetists' Association (OAA) and Difficult Airway Society (DAS) obstetric airway guidelines should reduce the incidence of failed intubation by improved airway assessment and anticipation of problems (Algorithm 41.1).

Box 41.1 lists the recommendations made by the Confidential Enquiry reports specific to anaesthesia.

Managing Medical and Obstetric Emergencies and Trauma: A Practical Approach, Fourth Edition. Edited by Rosamunde Burns and Kara Dent.

Box 41.1 Specific anaesthetic recommendations from Confidential Enquiry reports

Airway
- Management of difficult/failed/oesophageal intubation and severe bronchospasm is a core anaesthetic skill that should be rehearsed regularly
- Capnography must always be used to confirm correct endotracheal tube placement
- 7.0 mm is the default endotracheal tube size for pregnant women; size 6.0 and 5.0 mm tubes should be immediately available

Anaesthetic emergencies
- Subdural haematoma and cerebral venous sinus thrombosis are complications of dural puncture and pregnancy, respectively, and must be included in the differential diagnosis of headache
- Anaesthetists must be ready to deal with the adverse effects of local anaesthetics including accidental intrathecal or intravenous injection
- In sudden onset severe maternal shock (e.g. anaphylaxis), the presence of a pulse may be an unreliable indicator of adequate cardiac output
- In the absence of a recordable blood pressure or other indicator of cardiac output, the early initiation of external cardiac compressions may be life saving
- Aortocaval compression should be suspected in any supine pregnant woman who develops severe hypotension after induction of anaesthesia

Critical care/illness
- Recognition and management of severe, acute illness in a pregnant woman requires multidisciplinary teamwork including an anaesthetist and/or critical care specialist
- Obstetricians and obstetric anaesthetists must remain closely involved in the management of women with obstetric-specific conditions in critical care units

Other
Pregnant or postpartum women require the same standard of intra- and postoperative monitoring as non-obstetric patients

41.2 Difficult intubation

Prevention is better than cure.

Preparation for general anaesthesia

Algorithm 1 (Figure 41.1) of the obstetric airway guidelines by the OAA and DAS helps the team to prepare for a safe obstetric general anaesthetic. There is an emphasis on airway assessment and planning for difficult/failed intubation. The discussion should be facilitated by the use of a World Health Organization (WHO) checklist, which is even more important in urgent and emergency cases than during elective cases.

When planning for an obstetric general anaesthetic it is essential to make a decision on whether to proceed or to wake up a patient in the face of a failed intubation. The obstetric airway guidelines by the OAA and DAS provide a useful tool for the anaesthetist to make this decision (Figure 41.2).

The Fourth National Audit Project (NAP4) of the Royal College of Anaesthetists (RCoA, 2011) looked at major complications of airway management in the UK. Three of the four obstetric cases reported to NAP4 occurred in obese women. Using the 25° 'back up' or ramped position makes it easier to intubate obese patients. It may be useful to employ a specific pillow that allows the woman to be placed in the optimal position (Figure 41.3).

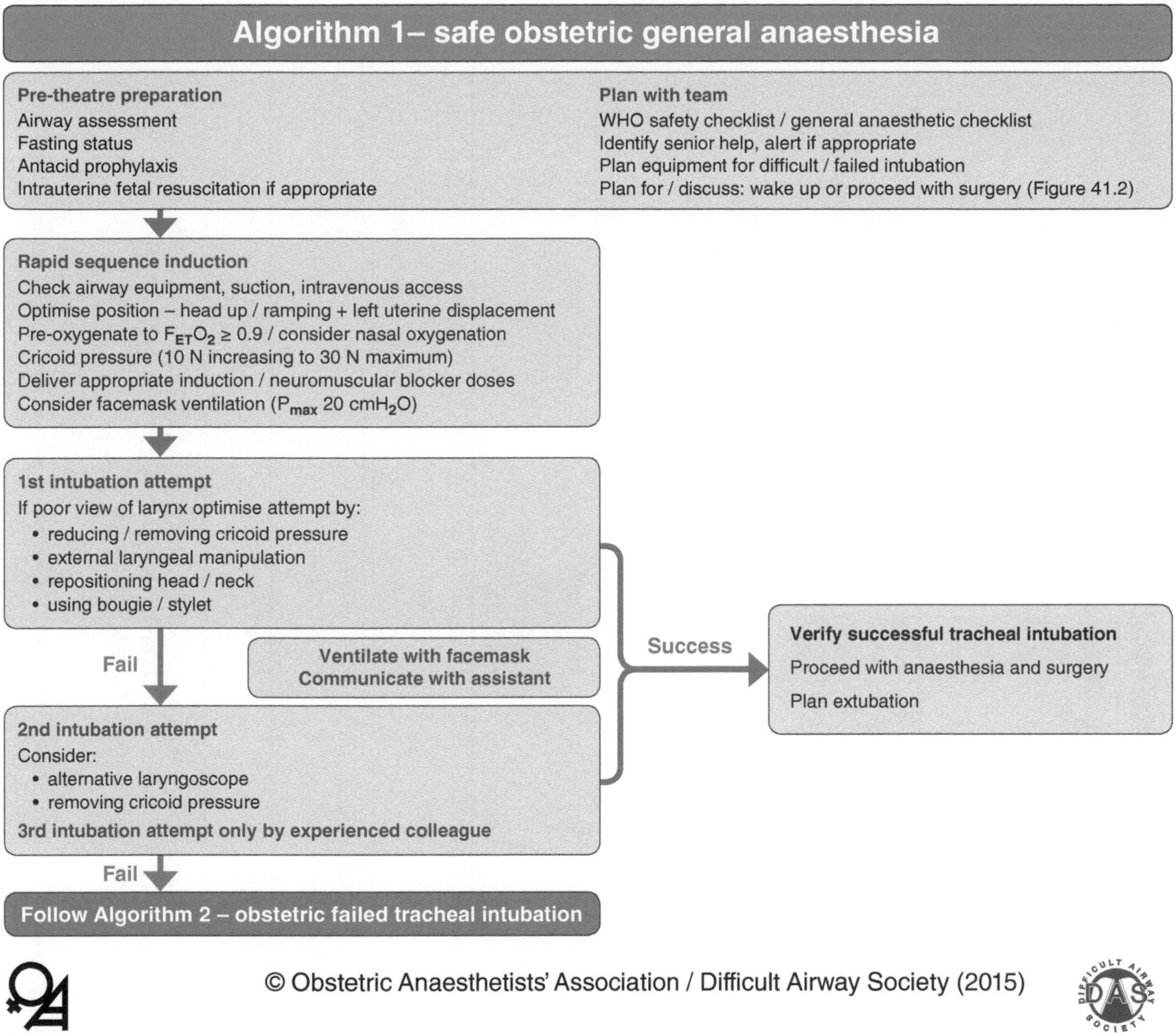
Algorithm 1– safe obstetric general anaesthesia
Pre-theatre preparation
Airway assessment
Fasting status
Antacid prophylaxis
Intrauterine fetal resuscitation if appropriate
Plan with team
WHO safety checklist / general anaesthetic checklist
Identify senior help, alert if appropriate
Plan equipment for difficult / failed intubation
Plan for / discuss: wake up or proceed with surgery (Figure 41.2)
Rapid sequence induction
Check airway equipment, suction, intravenous access
Optimise position – head up / ramping + left uterine displacement
Pre-oxygenate to $F_{ET}O_2 \geq 0.9$ / consider nasal oxygenation
Cricoid pressure (10 N increasing to 30 N maximum)
Deliver appropriate induction / neuromuscular blocker doses
Consider facemask ventilation (P_{max} 20 cmH_2O)
1st intubation attempt
If poor view of larynx optimise attempt by:
• reducing / removing cricoid pressure
• external laryngeal manipulation
• repositioning head / neck
• using bougie / stylet
Fail
Ventilate with facemask
Communicate with assistant
Success
Verify successful tracheal intubation
Proceed with anaesthesia and surgery
Plan extubation
2nd intubation attempt
Consider:
• alternative laryngoscope
• removing cricoid pressure
3rd intubation attempt only by experienced colleague
Fail
Follow Algorithm 2 – obstetric failed tracheal intubation
© Obstetric Anaesthetists' Association / Difficult Airway Society (2015)
DIFFICULT AIRWAY SOCIETY
DAS

Figure 41.1 Safe obstetric general anaethesia

Source: Mushambi MC, Kinsella SM, Popat M, et al. Obstetric Anaesthetists' Association and Difficult Airway Society guidelines for the management of difficult and failed tracheal intubation in obstetrics. *Anaesthesia* 2015; 70: 1286–306. © 2015 Obstetric Anaesthetists' Association/Difficult Airway Society

Table 1 – proceed with surgery?

	Factors to consider	WAKE	⟵	⟶	PROCEED
Before induction	**Maternal condition**	• No compromise	• Mild acute compromise	• Haemorrhage responsive to resuscitation	• Hypovolaemia requiring corrective surgery • Critical cardiac or respiratory compromise, cardiac arrest
	Fetal condition	• No compromise	• Compromise corrected with intrauterine resuscitation, pH < 7.2 but > 7.15	• Continuing fetal heart rate abnormality despite intrauterine resuscitation, pH < 7.15	• Sustained bradycardia • Fetal haemorrhage • Suspected uterine rupture
	Anaesthetist	• Novice	• Junior trainee	• Senior trainee	• Consultant / specialist
	Obesity	• Supermorbid	• Morbid	• Obese	• Normal
	Surgical factors	• Complex surgery or major haemorrhage anticipated	• Multiple uterine scars • Some surgical difficulties expected	• Single uterine scar	• No risk factors
	Aspiration risk	• Recent food	• No recent food • In labour • Opioids given • Antacids not given	• No recent food • In labour • Opioids not given • Antacids given	• Fasted • Not in labour • Antacids given
	Alternative anaesthesia • **regional** • **securing airway awake**	• No anticipated difficulty	• Predicted difficulty	• Relatively contraindicated	• Absolutely contraindicated or has failed • Surgery started
After failed intubation	**Airway device / ventilation**	• Difficult facemask ventilation • Front-of-neck	• Adequate facemask ventilation	• First generation supraglottic airway device	• Second generation supraglottic airway device
	Airway hazards	• Laryngeal oedema • Stridor	• Bleeding • Trauma	• Secretions	• None evident

Criteria to be used in the decision to wake or proceed following failed tracheal intubation. In any individual patient, some factors may suggest waking and others proceeding. The final decision will depend on the anaesthetist's clinical judgement.

Figure 41.2 The decision whether to proceed with surgery

Source: Mushambi MC, Kinsella SM, Popat M, et al. Obstetric Anaesthetists' Association and Difficult Airway Society guidelines for the management of difficult and failed tracheal intubation in obstetrics. *Anaesthesia* 2015; 70: 1286–306. © 2015 Obstetric Anaesthetists' Association/Difficult Airway Society

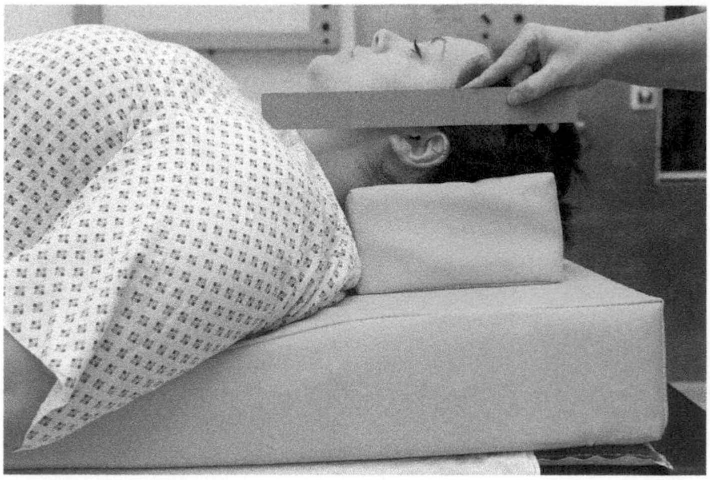

Figure 41.3 The ALMA Medical company version of the head elevation laryngoscopy pillow (HELP) showing the optimum position, with the tragus of the ear in line with the xiphisternum.
Source: Courtesy of Alma Medical, info@almamedical.com

Failed intubation

Management of failed intubation is a core skill that should be rehearsed and practised regularly by the whole team including obstetricians, midwives and theatre staff (Figure 41.4). Algorithm 2 (Figure 41.5) of the obstetric airway guidelines by the OAA and DAS provides an easy to follow decision-making process that focuses on oxygenation of the mother as the most important goal. It is essential for the anaesthetist not to become fixated on intubation. Where intubation has failed, second generation supraglottic airway devices are preferable. These devices have a channel which allows for early identification and drainage of regurgitated gastric contents. Case reports show these have been commonly used since 2003 to achieve successful oxygenation. Obstetricians and midwives can help in this situation by ensuring that additional help is called, oxygen saturation is being monitored and by reminding the anaesthetist of the importance to oxygenate rather than intubate the mother (Figure 41.6). There should be an appreciation of the implications for decision making regarding delivery.

Table 2 – management after failed tracheal intubation	
Wake	**Proceed with surgery**
• Maintain oxygenation • Maintain cricoid pressure if not impeding ventilation • Either maintain head-up position or turn left lateral recumbent • If rocuronium used, reverse with sugammadex • Assess neuromuscular blockade and manage awareness if paralysis is prolonged • Anticipate laryngospasm / can't intubate, can't oxygenate	• Maintain anaesthesia • Maintain ventilation - consider merits of: ▫ controlled or spontaneous ventilation ▫ paralysis with rocuronium if sugammadex available • Anticipate laryngospasm / can't intubate, can't oxygenate • Minimise aspiration risk: ▫ maintain cricoid pressure until delivery (if not impeding ventilation) ▫ after delivery maintain vigilance and reapply cricoid pressure if signs of regurgitation ▫ empty stomach with gastric drain tube if using second-generation supraglottic airway device ▫ minimise fundal pressure ▫ administer H_2 receptor blocker i.v. if not already given • Senior obstetrician to operate • Inform neonatal team about failed intubation • Consider total intravenous anaesthesia
After waking	
• Review urgency of surgery with obstetric team • Intrauterine fetal resuscitation as appropriate • For repeat anaesthesia, manage with two anaesthetists • Anaesthetic options: ▫ Regional anaesthesia preferably inserted in lateral position ▫ Secure airway awake before repeat general anaesthesia	

© Obstetric Anaesthetists' Association / Difficult Airway Society (2015)

Figure 41.4 Management after failed tracheal intubation
Source: Mushambi MC, Kinsella SM, Popat M, et al. Obstetric Anaesthetists' Association and Difficult Airway Society guidelines for the management of difficult and failed tracheal intubation in obstetrics. *Anaesthesia* 2015; 70: 1286–306. © 2015 Obstetric Anaesthetists' Association/Difficult Airway Society

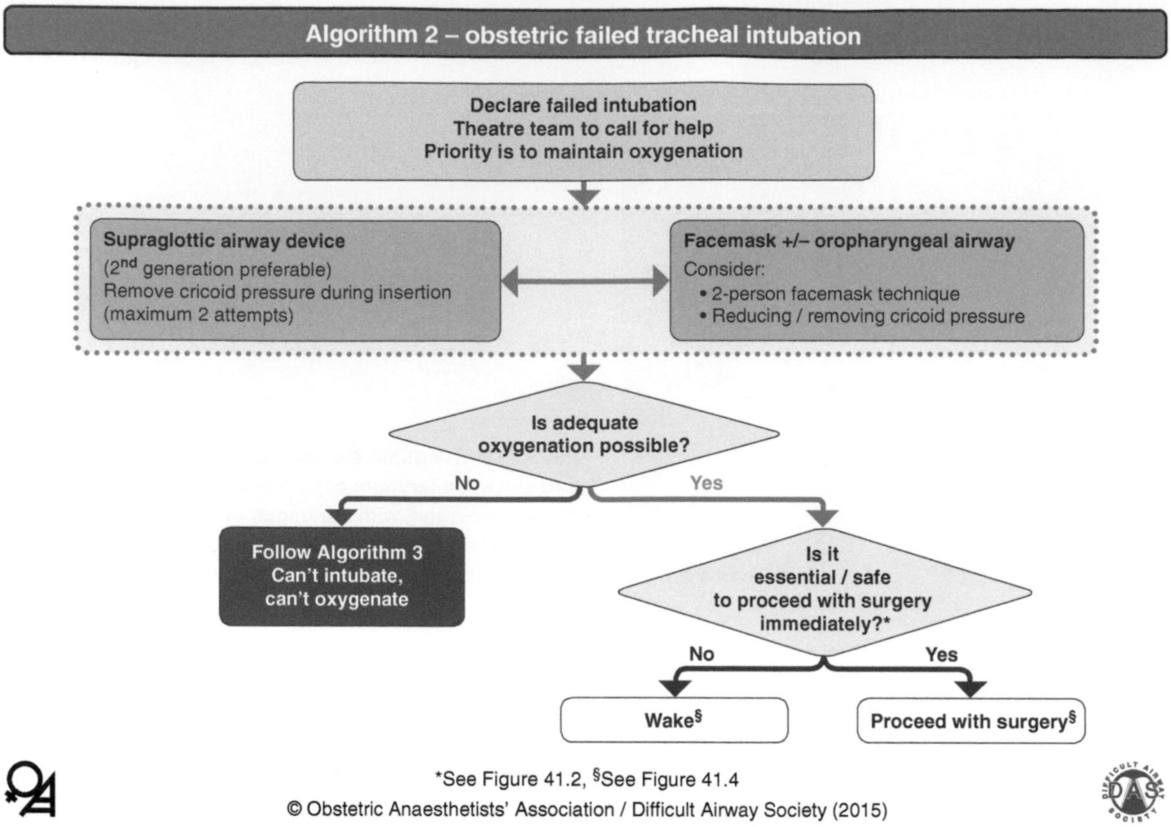
Algorithm 2 – obstetric failed tracheal intubation
Declare failed intubation
Theatre team to call for help
Priority is to maintain oxygenation
Supraglottic airway device
(2nd generation preferable)
Remove cricoid pressure during insertion
(maximum 2 attempts)
Facemask +/– oropharyngeal airway
Consider:
• 2-person facemask technique
• Reducing / removing cricoid pressure
Is adequate oxygenation possible?
No
Yes
Follow Algorithm 3
Can't intubate, can't oxygenate
Is it essential / safe to proceed with surgery immediately?*
No
Yes
Wake§
Proceed with surgery§
*See Figure 41.2, §See Figure 41.4
© Obstetric Anaesthetists' Association / Difficult Airway Society (2015)

Figure 41.5 Obstetric failed tracheal intubation
Source: Mushambi MC, Kinsella SM, Popat M, et al. Obstetric Anaesthetists' Association and Diffiult Airway Society guidelines for the management of difficult and failed tracheal intubation in obstetrics. *Anaesthesia* 2015; 70: 1286–306. © 2015 Obstetric Anaesthetists' Association/Difficult Airway Society

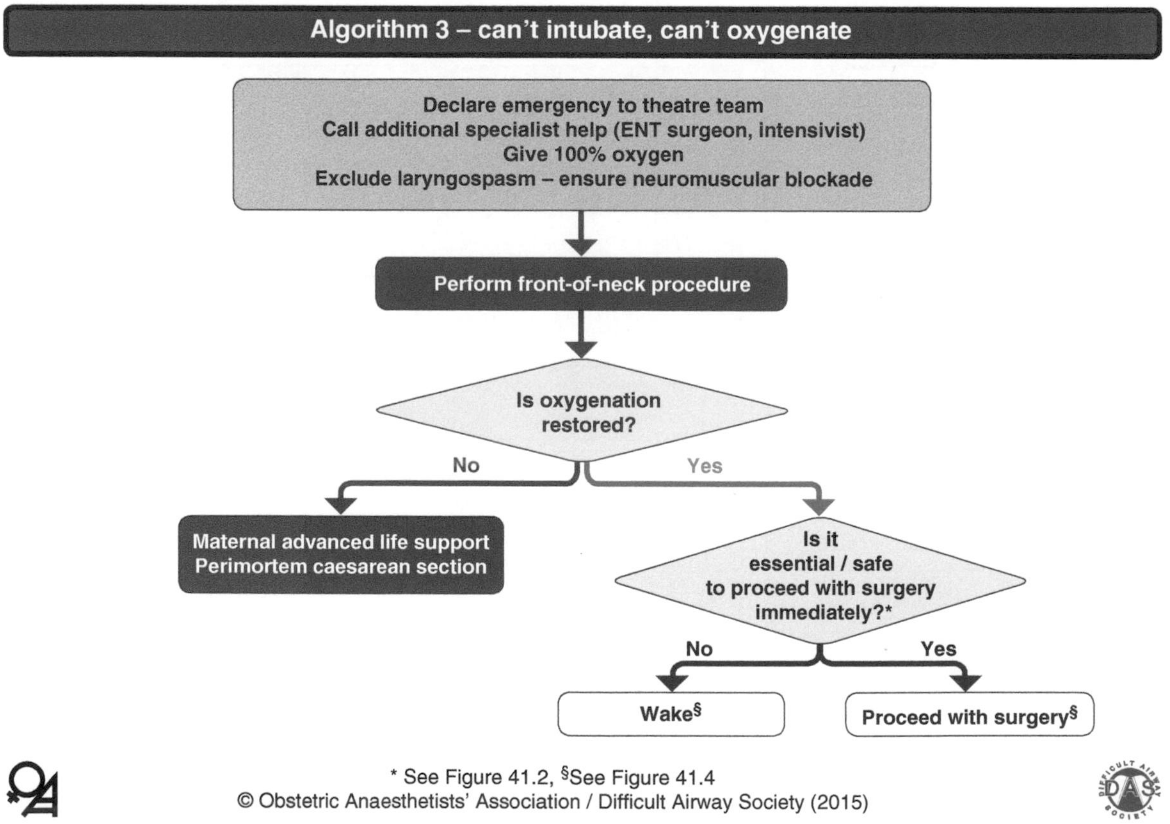
Algorithm 3 – can't intubate, can't oxygenate
Declare emergency to theatre team
Call additional specialist help (ENT surgeon, intensivist)
Give 100% oxygen
Exclude laryngospasm – ensure neuromuscular blockade
Perform front-of-neck procedure
Is oxygenation restored?
No
Yes
Maternal advanced life support
Perimortem caesarean section
Is it essential / safe to proceed with surgery immediately?*
No
Yes
Wake§
Proceed with surgery§
* See Figure 41.2, §See Figure 41.4
© Obstetric Anaesthetists' Association / Difficult Airway Society (2015)

Figure 41.6 Can't intubate, can't oxygenate
Source: Mushambi MC, Kinsella SM, Popat M, et al. Obstetric Anaesthetists' Association and Diffiult Airway Society guidelines for the management of difficult and failed tracheal intubation in obstetrics. *Anaesthesia* 2015; 70: 1286–306. © 2015 Obstetric Anaesthetists' Association/Difficult Airway Society

Other complications

Premature extubation

Before removing the endotracheal tube the woman must be fully awake, able to protect her own airway, breathing adequately and cardiovascularly stable. Most commonly, the anaesthetist will extubate the patient in the left lateral or sitting position in theatre with all monitoring left attached. Premature extubation is associated with aspiration of gastric contents, hypoxia and laryngospasm. Respiratory failure can occur as a result of incomplete reversal from neuromuscular blockade. Drugs, equipment and assistance should be instantly available.

Mortality reports have highlighted that outside theatre respiratory deaths have resulted from the incorrect administration of opioids and insufficient supervision of patients receiving opioids.

Awareness

The RCoA's Fifth National Audit Project (NAP5) looked at accidental awareness during general anaesthesia (AAGA) (RCoA, 2014). AAGA is where a patient becomes or remains conscious when the anaesthetist intends them to be unconscious. With an incidence of 1 in 670 general anaesthetics in obstetric patients, it is 10 times more common compared with non-obstetric patients. In NAP5 12 of 14 obstetric AAGA cases occurred with caesarean section and at induction or early during surgery.

Risk factors for AAGA include emergency surgery, out-of-hours procedures, junior staff, rapid sequence induction, thiopentone as the induction agent, obesity and difficulties in airway management. AAGA may occur due to accidentally swapping the thiopentone syringe with a syringe containing the antibiotic. All of these risks are common in obstetric anaesthesia.

To reduce the risk of AAGA, NAP5 recommends increasing the dose of induction agent, rapidly attaining adequate end-tidal volatile levels, the use of nitrous oxide in adequate concentrations, appropriate use of opioids and maintaining uterine tone with uterotonic agents to allow adequate concentrations of volatile agent to be used.

NAP5 also recommends having an additional syringe of intravenous hypnotic immediately available to maintain anaesthesia in the event of a difficult airway and when it is not appropriate for the mother to return to consciousness.

Patient reports of awareness must always be taken seriously and reported to the anaesthetist for investigation and management, with the aim of avoiding the patient developing a post-traumatic stress disorder.

41.3 Regional blocks (epidural and spinal anaesthesia and analgesia)

The spinal cord starts at the occipital bone and leaves the skull at the foramen magnum. It continues in the central canal, and in adults typically extends to the first or second lumbar vertebrae. The central canal is bordered by the arachnoid and dura mater, extends into the upper part of the sacrum and is filled with cerebrospinal fluid (CSF).

The epidural space is a 'potential' space that extends from the base of the skull to the sacral hiatus and contains nerve roots, fat and blood vessels. The dura and arachnoid mater form the anatomical boundary that divides the subarachnoid or intrathecal space from the epidural space.

In regional blocks a local anaesthetic is used to provide anaesthesia and analgesia in a group of nerves, as opposed to nerve blocks where a single, specific nerve is targeted (e.g. pudendal block). A regional block where the local anaesthetic is delivered into the CSF is called a spinal, subarachnoid or intrathecal block. If the local anaesthetic is injected outside the dura it is called an epidural, extradural or peridural block. In both techniques, the local anaesthetic blocks the transmission of impulses along the nerves.

- In a spinal block a small amount of local anaesthetic is injected into the CSF where it spreads and has a rapid onset of action
- Because nerves in the epidural space have an additional covering, the onset of the action of local anaesthetic is slower and a greater volume of local anaesthetic must be used to account for the larger space
- Epidural analgesia for labour requires a sensory block from T10 to L1 during the first stage and T10 to S4 during the second stage
- Anaesthesia for a caesarean section (CS) requires motor and sensory blockade from T4 to S5

Characteristics of spinal and epidural anaesthetics

Epidurals are most often used for analgesia during labour and vaginal delivery (labour epidural). A labour epidural can be modified (topped up) to provide anaesthesia for operative delivery. Commonly, an epidural involves the placement of a small catheter into the epidural space. Through this catheter drugs can be repeatedly added or continuously infused to provide analgesia for the duration of labour. Epidurals can also be used with the sole intention of providing anaesthesia for a CS. The slow onset of surgical anaesthesia limits their usefulness in routine cases but can be useful in providing safe regional anaesthesia, e.g. for patients with severe cardiac disease.

Spinals are commonly used for surgical procedures, e.g. CS or forceps delivery. With spinals the drug is delivered through the spinal needle and produces surgical anaesthesia for about 2 hours. The duration of spinal anaesthesia cannot be extended as, unlike with epidurals, no catheter remains in the subarachnoid space.

A third technique involves a **combined spinal and epidural** and is called a CSE. Used in labour this technique combines the fast onset of analgesia from the spinal with the ability to provide continuous analgesia for as long as is required by the epidural.

CSEs also have a place in operative obstetrics. The spinal component provides fast onset surgical anaesthesia while the epidural may be used to extend surgical anaesthesia if the operation is prolonged or may be used to provide postoperative analgesia.

A spinal anaesthetic provides a rapid onset of block over a continuous area supplied by the spinal cord. The block has three modalities: sensory, motor and autonomic. The latter is responsible for the undesired effect of spinal anaesthesia – hypotension secondary to vasodilatation. This is treated prophylactically using phenylephrine as a vasopressor and positioning the patient to prevent aortocaval compression. Ephedrine, metaraminol and adrenaline can be used as second and third line alternatives.

The height of a spinal block, as measured in dermatomes, is influenced by the dose/volume of drug injected, patient height and body habitus but is not accurately predictable. To a degree, block height can be influenced by patient positioning: head up to prevent a further rise in block and head down to increase block height. For a CS the desired block height is the T4 dermatomal level, and blocks higher than T2 are called high spinals (see later in this chapter). Insufficient height of block will result in the patient experiencing pain during surgery.

Typical doses

Anaesthetists will usually use a combination of a local anaesthetic and an opioid. For both drugs, epidural blocks require a 5–10-fold higher dose compared with spinals.

Spinal block

The dose for a spinal block for a CS typically ranges between 2.2 and 2.7 ml of 0.5% hyperbaric ('heavy') bupivacaine. In most cases an opioid will be added to this, e.g. 15–25 micrograms fentanyl, 300–400 micrograms diamorphine or 100 micrograms morphine. Opioids improve the intraoperative quality of the block and provide prolonged postoperative analgesia. Hyperbaric bupivacaine is a solution that is denser than CSF, which helps to prevent excessive cephalad spread. Fentanyl and diamorphine improve the intraoperative quality of the block and diamorphine and morphine provide prolonged postoperative analgesia.

Epidural block

The most common local anaesthetic used for labour epidurals is 0.1% levobupivacaine with fentanyl 2 micrograms/ml. A typical dose of this immediately after siting the epidural would be 15–20 ml. The addition of an opioid to the local anaesthetic improves the quality of analgesia and allows a lower concentration of local anaesthetic to be used, minimising side effects such as motor block.

To provide ongoing analgesia the same mixture can be given by intermittent bolus injection, continuous infusion or by a patient-controlled analgesia device.

41.4 Complications of regional anaesthesia

Complications of regional blocks can be related to the technique itself or caused by drugs, e.g. local anaesthetics, opioids or vasopressors, as discussed in the following sections.

41.5 Complications due to local anaesthetic drugs

Local anaesthetic drugs can cause a number of complications, which include hypotension, motor block, urinary retention, high block, total spinal and local anaesthetic toxicity. Of these the latter two are extremely rare but immediately life threatening.

Hypotension

No universal definition of hypotension exists and whilst mean arterial pressure would be the most meaningful indicator for organ perfusion, insufficient data exist in obstetrics for its use. The most common definition used is that of systolic arterial pressure (SAP) of <80% of baseline or <100 mmHg. The 2017 'International Consensus Statement on the Management of Hypotension with Vasopressors' during caesarean section under spinal anaesthesia makes the following recommendation (Kinsella et al., 2018):

> The aim should be to maintain SAP ≥90% of baseline until delivery, with the intention of reducing the frequency and duration of episodes of significant hypotension <80% baseline. Systolic arterial pressure values <80% should be treated expeditiously.

Hypotension occurs more frequently following spinal than epidural block and is often heralded by nausea and vomiting. It is caused by the blockade of sympathetic innervation to the cardiovascular system. Maternal hypotension can cause changes in fetal heart rate and fetal acidaemia.

The treatment of hypotension following spinal block should be prophylactic, whereas after epidural block it is reactive. For prophylactic treatment a phenylephrine infusion of 25–50 micrograms/min is recommended. For reactive treatment, a bolus of 50–100 micrograms of phenylephrine or 3–6 mg of ephedrine may be used, bearing in mind that ephedrine may worsen fetal acidosis.

In pregnant women with pre-eclampsia or cardiac disease, vasopressors must be used cautiously and expert advice should be sought on the optimal vasopressor and dose before undertaking regional blockade.

Management of hypotension

- ABC approach
- Manual uterine displacement or left lateral tilt
- Fluid loading: increase rate of crystalloid infusion; but be cautious in pre-eclampsia and cardiac disease
- Vasopressors:
  - The vasopressor of choice in pregnant women is phenylephrine
  - If there is maternal bradycardia an alternative vasopressor with beta-agonist action may be more appropriate, e.g. ephedrine
  - For spinal-induced hypotension the use of prophylactic infusions of phenylephrine at a rate of 25–50 micrograms/min should be considered
  - The bolus dose of phenylephrine ranges from 50 to 100 micrograms
  - 6 mg of ephedrine is an equipotent dose to phenylephrine 75 micrograms
  - Women with pre-eclampsia or cardiac disease require special consideration regarding choice and dose of vasopressor

Motor block

Motor block is required for CS under spinal anaesthesia. When providing labour analgesia, motor block is unwanted as it is associated with maternal dissatisfaction, pressure sores and an increase in instrumental delivery rate.

Maternal dissatisfaction and pressure sores are caused by the mother's relative immobility and loss of sensation. Labouring women must be encouraged to change position regularly and the bedsheet should be kept as dry as possible.

The incidence of motor block from labour epidurals can be reduced by using less concentrated local anaesthetics, supplementing them with opioids and avoiding the use of continuous infusions to maintain labour analgesia.

Urinary retention

The combination of sensory and parasympathetic block can cause urinary retention that is unnoticed by the patient. It is important that a bladder voiding protocol is followed for all women with labour epidurals and women after operative delivery under regional block.

41.6 Serious immediate complications of local anaesthetic drugs

Local anaesthetic systemic toxicity

Local anaesthetics cross plasma and intracellular membranes quickly and can have a variety of toxic effects on the heart, central nervous system (CNS) and skeletal muscle. Systemic toxicity of local anaesthetics is dose related. Recommended safe doses for common local anaesthetics are given in Table 41.1.

Table 41.1 Recommended safe doses for common local anaesthetics

Drug	Maximum safe dose (mg per kg body weight) given in any 4 hour period
Lidocaine	3
Lidocaine with 1:200 000 adrenaline	7
(Levo)bupivacaine	2
Ropivacaine	3
Prilocaine	6

Most local anaesthetics are labelled as relative concentrations, e.g. 1% lidocaine. To calculate the dose in milligrams (mg):

$$\text{Dose (mg)} = \text{percentage} \times 10 \times \text{volume (ml)}$$

For example, if a labour epidural is topped up with 20 ml of 2% lidocaine with 1:200 000 adrenaline, the dose is calculated as:

$$2\% \times 10 \times 20\text{ml} = 400\text{mg}$$

Systemic toxicity resulting from bupivacaine is thought to be the most treatment resistant. Levobupivacaine is a single isomer variety of bupivacaine and thought to be less cardiotoxic. Nevertheless due to a lack of data, both drugs have the same maximum safe dose. Ropivacaine is another newer local anaesthetic thought to be less cardiotoxic.

Local anaesthetic toxicity can occur from any route of administration but is very unlikely after spinal block as the dose used is very small. Following epidural block, toxicity may occur due to absorption from the epidural space or as a result of inadvertent injection into a blood vessel. The latter can occur when the epidural is sited and is sometimes not recognised as the epidural catheter is very thin and may not allow the aspiration of blood. It can also occur with a previously normally working epidural where the catheter has migrated into an epidural vein.

CNS toxicity

Central nervous system toxicity is characterised by two phases, the excitatory phase followed by a depressive phase.

The excitatory phase is characterised by:

- Perioral tingling
- Metallic taste in mouth
- Tinnitus
- Slurred speech
- Light-headedness
- Tremor
- Confusion
- Agitation

The depressive phase is characterised by:

- Generalised convulsions
- Coma
- Respiratory depression

Cardiovascular toxicity

There are three phases to cardiovascular toxicity.

Symptoms and signs in the initial phase include:

- Hypertension
- Tachycardia

The intermediate phase is characterised by:

- Hypotension
- Myocardial depression

The terminal phase may include:

- Peripheral dilatation
- Severe hypotension
- Cardiac dysrhythmias including:
  - Sinus bradycardia
  - Conduction blocks
  - Asystole
  - Ventricular tachyarrhythmias

Management

If systemic local anaesthetic toxicity is suspected the definitive treatment is the intravenous administration of a 20% lipid emulsion which should be instituted as soon as possible. The AAGBI guideline for this emergency can be accessed online and is summarised in Figure 41.7. As help arrives this task should be delegated to one person.

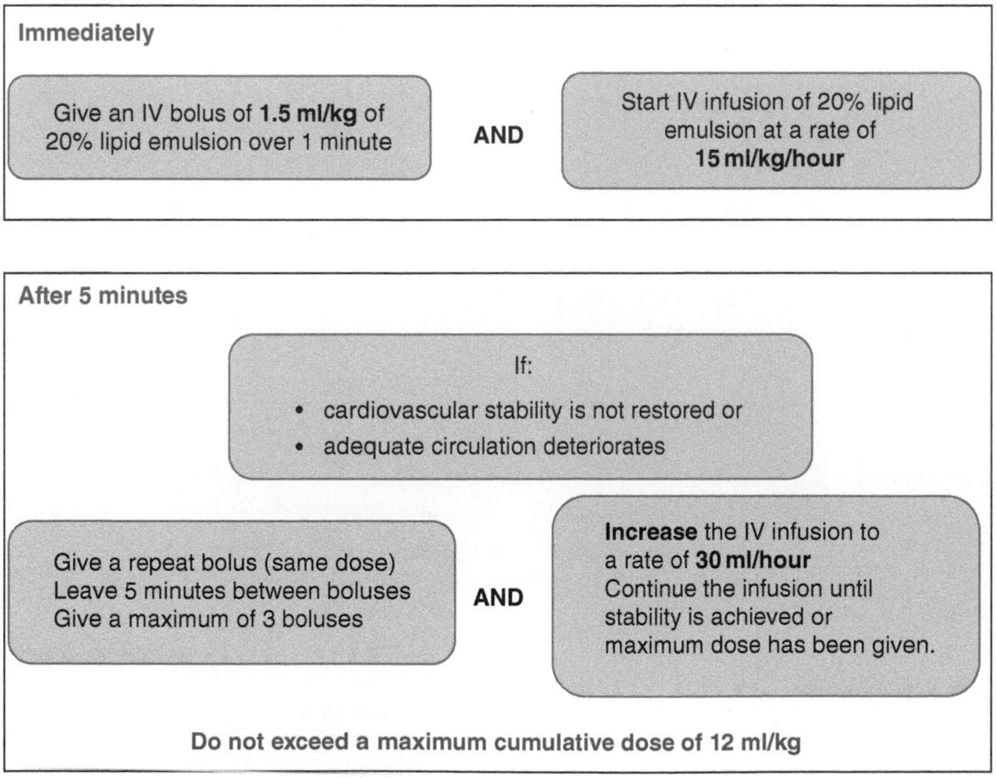

Figure 41.7 Antidote to local anaesthetic

Immediate management

- Stop administration of local anaesthetics
- Call for senior help: anaesthetic, critical care, obstetric, neonatal
  - Designate one helper to get 20% lipid emulsion and administer it according to protocol
- ABC approach as for any resuscitation in a pregnant woman
  - Left lateral tilt if conscious, or manual uterine displacement if not
- Treat hypotension with IV fluids and vasopressor titrated against blood pressure
- If in cardiac arrest, use adrenaline as dictated by the cardiac arrest protocol and prepare to empty the uterus
- Increased amounts of adrenaline may be required as there will be a profound vasodilatation

Treat peri-arrest arrhythmias

- Local anaesthetic-induced VT and VF are often resistant to electrical defibrillation
- Amiodarone 300 mg is the antiarrhythmic drug of choice
- Prolonged cardiopulmonary resuscitation may be required and consideration of cardiopulmonary bypass should be made if available

Control seizures

- Control seizures with small incremental doses of benzodiazepine, thiopental or propofol
- Intubation may be required to protect the airway
- Check fetal heart and consider timing and method of delivery if not required in response to maternal cardiac arrest, once immediate resuscitation steps are complete

High spinal block

A high spinal block is a block that extends above the level of T4 and can cause respiratory and cardiovascular compromise. It may be caused by unpredictably excessive spread of the local anaesthetic or an inappropriately high dose for the patient. High spinals may result from epidurals where the epidural catheter has migrated through the dura into the CSF. Therefore, the epidural catheter must be aspirated prior to the administration of a large volume top-up for theatre delivery to rule out migration of the catheter into the CSF or a blood vessel.

A high spinal block should be suspected if the patient becomes bradycardic and hypotensive and/or if they report tingling or weakness in their hands, and complain of difficulty in breathing and talking. Reduced sensation at the level of the sternal notch confirms a high spinal block. The signs and symptoms reflect the height of the block (Table 41.2).

Table 41.2 High spinal block signs and symptoms

Height of block	Signs and symptoms
T4–T1 Causing: block of sympathetic innervation of the heart block of motor fibres to accessory respiratory muscles	Bradycardia Severe hypotension Difficulty coughing Difficulty to take deep breath
C8–C6 Causing: block of ulnar, radial and median nerves	Paraesthesia of hands Weakness in hands and arms Breathing difficulties Only able to whisper Anxiety/distress
C5–C3 Causing: block of phrenic nerve paralysis of the diaphragm	Severe respiratory distress Hypoxia Respiratory arrest

Figure 41.8 outlines the management procedure for high and total spinal blocks.

Call for help! (2222 obstetric emergency)
anaesthetist, obstetrician, resuscitation trolley
consider: neonatologist, intensivist

↓

Immediate management

- Stop epidural (if running)
- Left lateral tilt (if conscious)
- Manual uterine displacement (if unconscious)
- Consider placing patient in head-up position
- Explain to birthing partner

Airway

- Assess
- Open and maintain airway
- Consider oral airway
- Oxygen at 15 l/min

→

Breathing

- Assess
- Assist with bag–mask–valve if required
- Oxygen at 15 l/min
- Record every 5 minutes

→

Protect airway by intubation if patient unconscious

Circulation

- Assess pulse and blood pressure
- Large bore IV access
- Take bloods for FBC and U&Es
- Commence CPR if patient arrests
- Perform perimortem caesarean section within 5 minutes of arrest

→

Bradycardia?
Give atropine 600 micrograms IV bolus

→

Hypotension?

- rapid IV fluid infusion
- phenylephrine 75 micrograms IV bolus but not if bradycardic
- ephedrine 6 mg IV bolus
- severe/unresponsive hypotension consider adrenaline

Other

- Check fetal heart
- Consider need for delivery
- Exclude other causes of unconsciousness

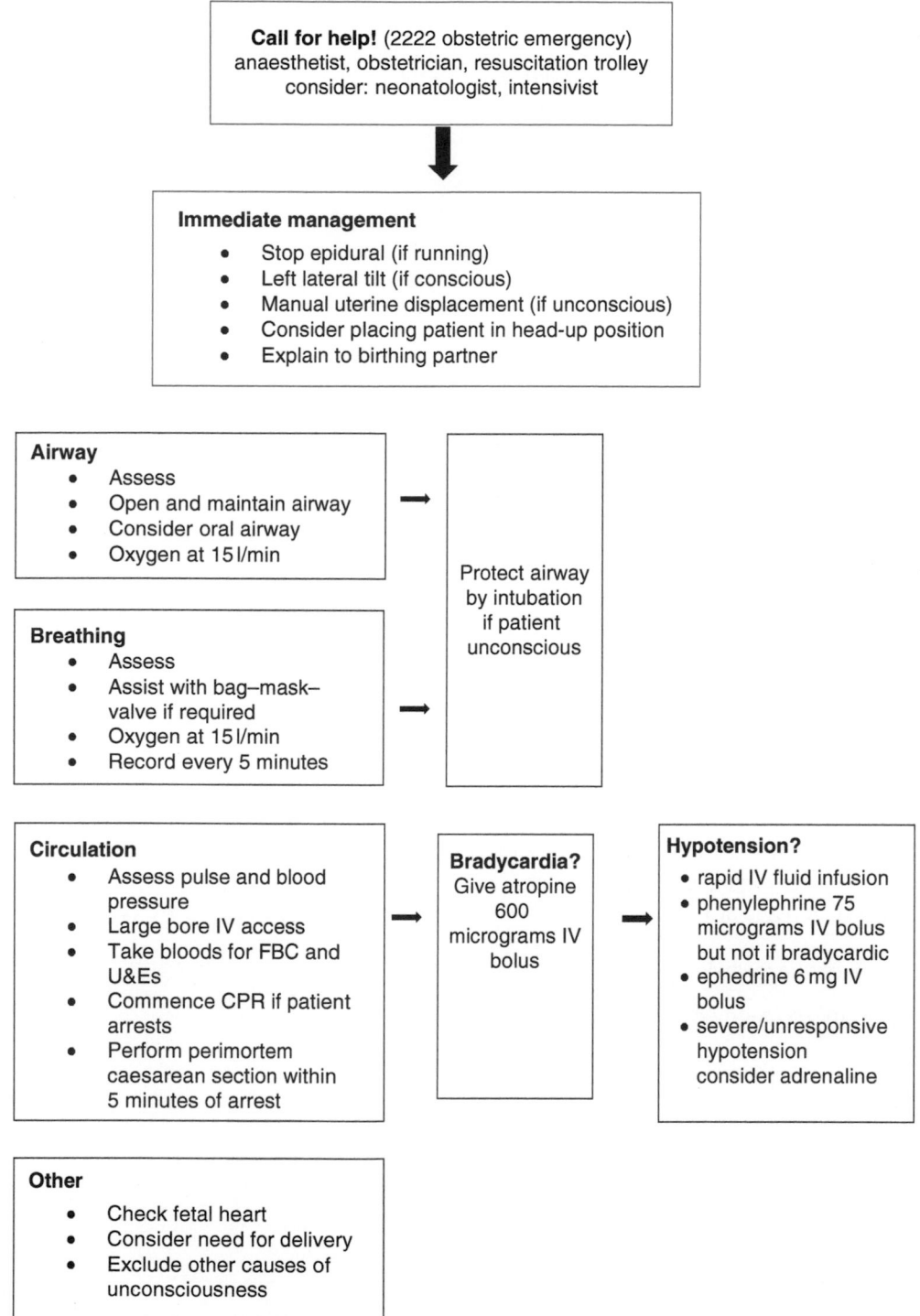

Figure 41.8 Management of high and total spine block

Total spinal block

A total spinal block is an extension of the high spinal block where the local anaesthetic has spread intracranially. As a total spinal block develops the signs and symptoms are those of a high spinal block but are more severe and loss of consciousness will occur. Depression of the medulla and the brain stem vasomotor centres can lead to cardiac arrest.

The 2017 CAPS UK Obstetric Surveillance System (UKOSS) study showed that maternal cardiac arrest is rare. However, 25% of arrests were caused by anaesthesia alone and of these two-thirds were due to a total spinal. Three-quarters of women with an anaesthetic cause of cardiac arrest, all of whom survived, were obese. The 100% survival rate in the anaesthetic group emphasises the importance of correct and timely treatment (Figure 41.8). There is an opportunity to further reduce the incidence of maternal cardiac arrest.

41.7 Complications of opioids

Complications of opioids include:

- Pruritus
- Urinary retention
- Late respiratory depression in absence of overdose, especially with long-acting opioids

Pruritus secondary to intrathecal or epidural opioids is not related to histamine release, making antihistamines ineffective in its treatment. Ondansetron at a dose of 0.1 mg/kg has been suggested as a treatment.

Urinary retention can be caused by neuroaxial blockade itself but also by opioids. There must be a bladder care protocol in place in every obstetric unit.

Respiratory depression following intrathecal or epidural opioids is relatively uncommon, with morphine being the drug most likely to cause this. Treatment is by ventilatory assistance and naloxone. Naloxone should be given intravenously in increments of 100 micrograms and titrated to response. Due to its shorter half-life it may have to be administered repeatedly. Any woman who has had long-acting spinal or epidural opioids must be closely monitored for late respiratory depression. Naloxone is also effective against opioid-induced pruritus.

41.8 Complications of technique

The RCoA's Third National Audit Project (NAP3) looked at major complications of central neuraxial blockade (RCoA, 2009). Approximately 140 000 epidurals are performed each year in obstetric patients. The incidence of permanent harm after obstetric central neural blockade was estimated at 1 in 80 000 judged pessimistically and 1 in 320 000 judged optimistically.

Complications due to technique include the following:

- Failure to locate the correct site, missed segment and unilateral block
- Postdural puncture headache
- Neurological damage – temporary and permanent
- Migration of catheter causing relative intrathecal overdose
- Epidural/intrathecal haematoma
- Epidural abscess
- Meningitis

Failure of block

Failure to identify the intrathecal and/or epidural space is relatively uncommon and occurs more often in morbidly obese patients. The incidence of failed spinal block varies widely in the literature but with experienced practitioners should be 1% or less. Insufficient height of spinal block can sometimes be remedied by putting the patient into a head-down position to encourage cephalad spread of the local anaesthetic. Alternatively, the spinal block may have to be repeated or a general anaesthetic may be required.

Failure of epidural block occurs in approximately 12% of patients, of which almost half can be made functional by simple manipulations. Missed segments and unilateral blocks occur in 5–8% of epidurals. The management options for failed epidurals include withdrawing the epidural catheter a small amount, repositioning the patient, the use of a more local anaesthetic, the use of additional epidural opioids and the use of epidural clonidine. Approximately 7% of patients will require a repeat epidural. Epidural blocks that have failed to provide adequate analgesia in labour are unlikely to provide anaesthesia for operative delivery when topped up.

For operative procedures the extent of the block must be carefully assessed and documented before surgery can start.

Postdural puncture headache

Postdural puncture headache (PDPH) is a low-pressure headache caused by leakage of CSF through the hole in the dura created by a spinal needle or, accidentally, by an epidural (Tuohy) needle. In extreme cases the traction on intracranial structures caused by the low pressure can lead to a posterior fossa intracranial haemorrhage. The incidence of PDPH is about 1 in 200 following spinal anaesthesia using a 25 G or smaller needle of pencil point design. Accidental puncture of the dura with a Tuohy needle causes PDPH in about 70% of cases.

The onset of PDPH is often delayed by 24–48 hours. Typically the headache is frontal and/or occipital and relieved when the patient lies down. It is often accompanied by other symptoms including tinnitus, nausea and vomiting, visual disturbances and photophobia. A headache requiring opioid analgesia is unlikely to be PDPH and should raise suspicion of other serious and urgent intracranial pathology. If the diagnosis is in any doubt, neuroimaging must be performed as soon as possible and a neurological opinion should be sought.

Management

- Inform the anaesthetic team
- Advise the patient to remain supine
- Initial conservative management includes:
  - Ensuring appropriate hydration
  - Simple analgesics
  - Caffeine
- Definitive treatment is an epidural blood patch:
  - Approximately 20 ml of the woman's own blood are injected into the epidural space under aseptic conditions
  - This may need to be repeated
  - Success is increased by delaying the procedure until >48 hours after puncture of the dura
- Consider the differential diagnoses, which can include:
  - Migraine
  - Meningitis
  - Cerebral venous sinus thrombosis
  - Subarachnoid haemorrhage
  - Subdural haematoma

41.9 Neurological damage

Peripheral neurological signs and symptoms in the postpartum period are common and may be caused by regional anaesthesia or nerve compression/injuries during labour and delivery.

Neuropraxia

Neuropraxia secondary to regional blocks can be caused by irritation of or direct injury to a nerve with a needle. Short-lived nerve root damage occurs in 1 in 3000 and permanent neuropathy develops in about 1 in 15 000 obstetric blocks. When a patient reports pain on injection of local anaesthetic through the spinal needle or epidural catheter, the injection should be stopped immediately.

Obstetric neuropraxia intrinsic to the mechanics of labour or fetal pressure on nerves occurs *much more commonly,* approaching 1 in 100 deliveries. The most common complaint is that of meralgia paraesthetica which is caused by compression of the lateral cutaneous nerve of the thigh.

Treatment of neuropraxia is usually conservative and referral for physiotherapy can be helpful. More complex pathology may require investigation with electrophysiological studies, and referral to a neurologist may be indicated.

Neuraxial blocks do not cause back pain other than local discomfort at the site of needle insertion nor do they worsen pre-existing lower back pain. Patients complaining of severe back pain following central neuraxial blockade whose pain is resistant to routine analgesia may require urgent investigation. The differential diagnosis in these patients includes epidural and intrathecal haematoma, epidural abscess and acute disc prolapse. Patients with signs and symptoms of spinal cord compression (i.e. severe pain, sensory and motor deficit and bowel/bladder dysfunction), require urgent magnetic resonance imaging (MRI). In these cases, urgent spinal cord or nerve root decompression may be required to avoid permanent neurological deficit.

Infection (epidural abscess, meningitis or discitis) and haematoma

These are extremely rare but potentially devastating complications. Epidural abscess formation occurs in around 0.2–3.7 per 100 000 obstetric epidurals. Bacterial meningitis is a complication of spinal or combined spinal and epidural blocks with an incidence of <1.5 per 10 000 patients. Signs and symptoms include severe backache, neurological deficit including bowel/bladder dysfunction and unexplained fever. CNS infection may cause signs of cerebral excitation or depression.

A suspicion of any of these pathologies should lead to immediate investigation as delay may lead to irreversible loss of neurological function. The patient's vital signs and temperature as well as their neurological status must be monitored regularly. Bloods should be sent including a white cell count, C-reactive protein and blood cultures. If there is the slightest likelihood of these pathologies, patients should be treated as per sepsis protocols. Radiologists will advise on the most appropriate form of imaging which, depending on the suspected pathology, may be a computed tomography (CT) scan or MRI. An urgent referral to a neurologist may be required.

The signs and symptoms of an epidural or intrathecal haematoma are similar to those of an epidural abscess but without any of the features of sepsis. The risk of epidural haematoma is estimated as 1 in 168 000 patients.

41.10 Effects of complications on the fetus

Maternal compromise such as hypoxia and cardiovascular instability will result in fetal distress causing fetal bradycardias, abnormal cardiotocographic recordings and pathological fetal blood gases. Intrauterine resuscitation should be instituted immediately in these cases, recognising that resuscitation of the mother will improve conditions for the fetus.

Opioids readily cross the placental barrier and can cause respiratory failure in the neonate. This is more likely where opioids have been given intravenously or by intramuscular injection and the paediatrician should be advised of this as respiratory support may be required.

41.11 Summary

- There is ample evidence in the literature that with prompt and correct treatment of anaesthetic emergencies in pregnant women the outcome for mothers and their babies is often good
- Anaesthetists, obstetricians and midwives must work as a team on the labour ward and in theatres. Their shared care of the mother and fetus requires close cooperation and good communication. This is never more important than in high-risk obstetrics, obstetric emergencies and anaesthetic complications
- The simulation of anaesthetic emergencies in multidisciplinary drills in the obstetric unit will lead to an appreciation of the importance of teamwork and human factors for a successful outcome

41.12 Further reading

AAGBI (Association of Anaesthetists of Great Britain and Ireland). *Quick Reference Handbook 3-10 Local Anaesthetic Toxicity, 2019.* https://anaesthetists.org/Home/Resources-publications/Safety-alerts/Anaesthesia-emergencies/Quick-Reference-Handbook/PDF-version (last accessed January 2022).

Beckett VA, Knight M, Sharpe P. THE CAPS Study: incidence,management and outcomes of cardiac arrest in pregnancy in the UK: a prospective, descriptive study. *BJOG* 2017; 124(9): 1374–81.

Kinsella JM, Carvalho B, Dyer RA, et al. International consensus statement on the management of hypotension with vasopressors during caesarean section under spinal anaesthesia. *Anaesthesia* 2018; 73(1): 71–92.

OAA/DAS (Obstetric Anaesthetists' Association/Difficult Airway Society). *Obstetric Airway Guidelines 2015.* https://www.oaa-anaes.ac.uk/OAA_DAS_Obstetric_Airway_Guidelines (last accessed January 2022).

CHAPTER 42
Triage

Learning outcomes

After reading this chapter, you will be able to:
- Describe the systematic approach advocated for prioritisation when casualties exceed resources available
- Explain why prioritisation is essential in emergency situations including obstetrics

42.1 Introduction

The word 'triage' is derived from the French *trier*, to sort or to sift as through a sieve. The word was originally used to describe the process of selecting coffee beans. Triage was first described in modern times by Baron Dominique Jean Larrey, who was Napoleon's Surgeon Marshal. He introduced a system of sorting casualties presenting to field dressing stations to ensure that soldiers with only minor wounds could be returned quickly to the battlefield with minimum treatment. In more recent times, triage has become a daily management tool within civilian emergency departments.

The aim of triage in civilian practice, wherever it is carried out, is not only to deliver the right patient to the right place at the right time so that they receive the optimum treatment but also to treat the most urgent ahead of the less urgent. Triage principles should be applied whenever the number of patients exceeds the skilled help immediately available.

Triage can be applied to acute medical and obstetric workloads. It can take place formally, as in the management of major incidents, or as a routine approach to our day-to-day practice in resuscitation rooms or on delivery suites. It must reflect the changing state of the patient and is therefore a dynamic, rather than a static, process; *regular reassessment of priorities across patients is vital.*

The endpoint of the triage process is the allocation of a priority. This priority is then used in conjunction with other factors to determine optimum care. Most triage systems have four categories of patients. There has to be a method of assessment to determine the category (Figure 42.1).

The triage priorities given in Table 42.1 are used in major incidents and reflect the need for clinical intervention, not the severity of injury. For example, a shocked patient bleeding from a simple scalp wound may need urgent intervention (priority red) but the injury itself may be relatively minor. By prioritising such a patient in a high category, a simple manoeuvre (application of pressure dressing) may save the casualty's life. Similarly, a patient with a large burn to the extremities clearly has a severe, possibly life-threatening anatomical injury, certainly worse than the patient with the scalp laceration. However, their prognosis may not be altered by receiving care within the first few hours rather than the first minutes.

Managing Medical and Obstetric Emergencies and Trauma: A Practical Approach, Fourth Edition. Edited by Rosamunde Burns and Kara Dent.

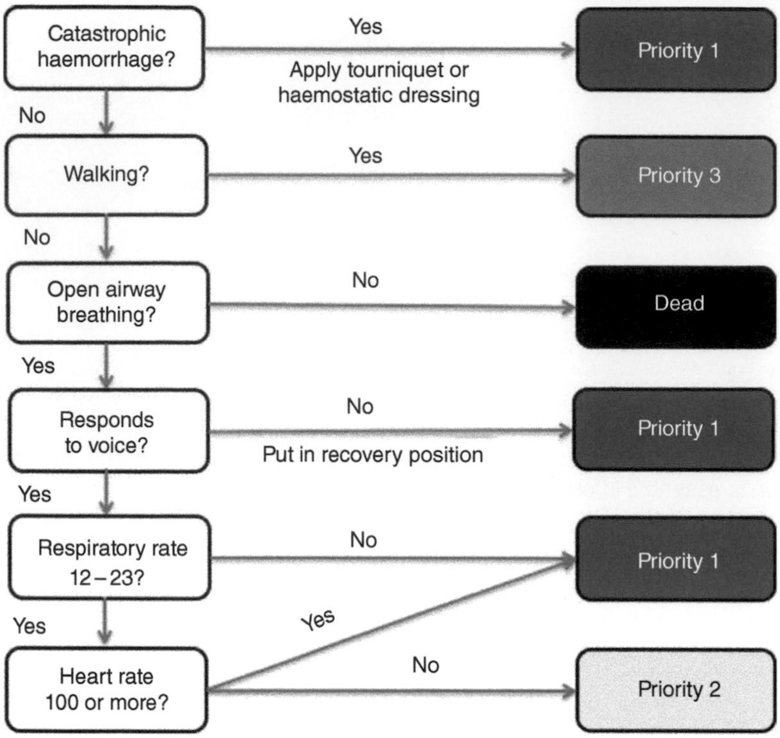

Figure 42.1 The Modified Physiological Triage Tool 24 (MPTT-24) triage sieve
Source: Vassallo J, Smith JE, Wallis LA. Major incident triage and implementation of a new triage tool, the MPTT-24. *J Roy Army Med Corps* 2017; 164(2): 103–6. Licensed under CC by 4.0

Table 42.1 Major incident triage categories

Treatment system	Priority system	Category	Colour	Description
T1	P1	Immediate	Red	Casualties who require immediate life-saving treatment
T2	P2	Urgent	Yellow	Casualties who require surgical or medical intervention within 2–4 hours
T3	P3	Delayed	Green	Less serious cases whose treatment can safely be delayed beyond 4 hours
T4	P4	Expectant	Blue (not standard)	Casualties who (i) cannot survive treatment; (ii) require such a degree of intervention that in the circumstances their treatment would seriously compromise the provision of treatment for others
Dead	Dead	Dead	White or black	Dead

Source: From Major incident triage categories. © Advanced Life Support Group

If the 'P' system is in use during a major incident then the use of the fourth category is very much a decision for the senior personnel involved. The decision must be based on an overall assessment of the situation: it must take into account both the patient load and the resources available. If the category is used, patients must be only considered to be within the category after assessment by senior medical personnel.

In the third trimester pregnant woman, assessment of the fetus would immediately follow assessment of the mother.

42.2 Assessment of the pregnant woman

Obstetric triage

Triage tools are commonly used in the emergency department, many of which are based on the Manchester Triage System, otherwise known as MTS. Obstetric triage is now an accepted field that remains more specialised than other triage systems simply because it has to take into account the mother, the fetus and/or stage of labour if appropriate. It is necessary to triage appropriately in order to deliver the right care in the right time in order to keep patients safe. An obstetric triage tool has to differ to standard tools to allow for the different physiology of pregnancy (relative hypotension, tachycardia and tachypnoea).

To date, there are no standardised obstetric triage tools in the UK although work has been done in Birmingham to develop the Birmingham Symptom-specific Obstetric Triage System (BSOTS). This works by each patient being triaged by a midwife within 15 minutes of admission, using a four tier colour-coded system. This colour coding allows the staff to see and understand the severity of the condition clearly. It acknowledges that it requires training but allows standardised care based on assessment of observations, history, pain and examination (including fetal heart). BSOTS has been launched online for free via the Meridian Health Innovation Exchange (March 2021).

Obstetric trauma triage

The principles of obstetric trauma triage are the same, involving the ability to identify immediately life-threatening conditions and to deal with them in the correct order. The priority category is determined by the identification of problems that are likely to kill and the order in which they are likely to kill: the ABCs. In the pregnant woman, the triage category is determined firstly by threats to maternal life and then presence of threats to the fetus (Figure 42.1).

- Think ABC
- Assess before treating but treat each problem before moving on
- Assess mobility then assess ABC
- Is the patient walking?
  - If so, the patient has a patent airway, is breathing and has sufficient circulating blood volume to allow locomotion

Move on:

- Is the patient talking?
  - If so, the airway is open, the patient is breathing and there is sufficient circulating blood volume to allow oxygenation of the brain

Move on:

- Is the patient breathing but unconscious?
  - If so, they have a potentially urgent airway problem
- Is the patient not breathing?
  - Open the airway
- Is the patient still not breathing?
  - Probably dead, especially in the trauma scenario
- If the patient is breathing, check their respiratory rate
- If the respiratory rate is normal, check the circulation and the capillary refill
- Assess fetal well-being and viability

42.3 Scenarios

Scenario 1

You are the on-call registrar for obstetrics. You are on the labour ward reviewing a cardiotocograph (CTG) when you hear a horn blaring, followed by a loud crash and then splintering noises. A lorry transporting a magnetic resonance imaging scanner has crashed into the building, demolishing a wall. You run towards the affected room to find student midwife A covered in debris, walking out in a dazed way bleeding from a scalp wound. As you enter the labour room, you find that the lorry has gone through the window, the driver is still in his cab, which has stoved inwards and the windscreen has shattered. He is grasping the steering wheel and breathing very rapidly. He was not wearing a seat belt.

Mrs B is on the bed in established labour, her legs are in lithotomy as the junior doctor was about to perform a ventouse delivery for prolonged second stage. The CTG machine is still running: the fetal heart appears to be normal. Mrs B is panting and saying she needs to push. The junior doctor is on the floor groaning, with a large piece of masonry on his pelvis. Midwife C is lying on top of Mrs B, motionless, with an obvious injury to the back of her head.

Mr B appears unscathed but grabs you on entry telling you that you must immediately deliver his baby.

Now take a few minutes to write your own order of priority . . .

Order of priority

1. *Midwife C* may have an airway problem; she may be unconscious or dead. Quickly assess her airway, breathing and the presence of circulation. If she is not breathing, after checking her airway is not obstructed, there is nothing further that can be done.
2. The *lorry driver* has a breathing problem, there is likely to be a chest injury, which will need early assessment. He may be trapped in the cab and may also have a circulatory problem secondary to fractured long bones. He must have early attention.
3. The *junior doctor* is groaning and therefore does not have an airway or breathing problem. He is likely to have a significant circulatory problem.
4. *Student midwife A* has a circulation problem. Her confusion may be secondary to cerebral hypoxia/hypovolaemia, or due to concussion from a blow to the head.
5. *Mrs B* appears not to have an airway or breathing problem, the midwife has shielded her from injury although her fall onto Mrs B's abdomen may have caused some trauma. There is no immediate urgency to deliver the baby.
6. *Mr B* does not require any immediate medical attention.

Scenario 2

You are the registrar arriving for your shift at 08:00 hours on a Sunday morning on the labour ward. The midwife in charge tells you it has been a very busy night. The previous team has recently gone to theatre with a patient who had an anterior placenta praevia and was bleeding heavily; the consultant is with them. She goes through the labour ward board with you (Table 42.2). Just as you finish the report, the support worker comes in with an urgent message from the midwife in room 7, who is unable to hear the fetal heart. The buzzer then goes off in room 1 where the midwife has recently given her patient intravenous penicillin, she is complaining of itching and is now very breathless.

Now take a few minutes to write your own order of priority . . .

Table 42.2 Labour ward board

Room	Parity	VE	Epidural	Syntocinon	Comments
1	1 + 0	07:30 5 cm	No	No	Group B *Streptococcus* carrier
2	5 + 1	06:30 del.	No	No	Retained placenta: cord snapped, PPH 600 ml, continues to trickle
3	0 + 0	05:00 4 cm	Yes	Yes	38 weeks, induced for marked oedema and protein ++++, poor urine output, BP 160/95
4	2 + 0				Term + 14 for induction
5	0 + 0	07:30 9 cm	Yes	No	CTG late decelerations, FBS pH 7.21 at 07:30
6	2 + 1	06:00 fully	No	No	
7	1 + 0		No	No	34 weeks, c/o decreased FM and abdominal pain, previous SB at 38 weeks

BP, blood pressure; c/o, complains of; CTG, cardiotocograph; FBS, fetal blood sampling; FM, fetal movement; PPH, postpartum haemorrhage; SB, stillbirth; VE, vaginal examination.

Order of priority

1. *Room 1* has a breathing problem that could become an airway problem, as she may be having an anaphylactic reaction and needs urgent attention.
2. *Room 3* could be developing a breathing and airway problem; her blood pressure is inadequately controlled, she needs early review.
3. *Room 2* has a circulation problem, ensure intravenous access and crossmatched blood; she will need to go to theatre for a manual removal of placenta as soon as possible.
4. *Room 7* may have a circulatory problem as she has probably had an abruption. She will need intravenous access, crossmatched blood and clotting studies.
5. *Room 5* has a fetal concern; the CTG should be reviewed and a decision made if further fetal blood sampling is necessary.
6. *Room 6* should have delivered and will need review if there is delay in the second stage.
7. *Room 4* is not a problem and induction should be deferred until there are sufficient staff to safely care for her.

As there are several major problems requiring attention, it will be necessary to divide the resources available. If there is an anaesthetist and a junior doctor also coming on duty they could be sent to rooms 1 and 3. Theatre should be made aware that there are other problems so that a speedy turnaround is encouraged if possible and the consultant can be freed to help as soon as the bleeding is under control.

42.4 Summary

- Triage is the key component whenever the number of casualties/patients to treat exceeds the available resources
- More details on the process of triage are outside the scope of this manual, but are covered in the mMOET course and other Advanced Life Support Group (ALSG) training courses, such as Hospital Major Incident Medical Management and Support (HMIMMS) and Manchester Triage

42.5 Further reading

ALSG (Advanced Life Support Group); Carley S, Mackway-Jones K (eds). *Major Incident Medical Management and Support: The Practical Approach in the Hospital*, 2nd edn. Oxford: Wiley Blackwell, 2018.

ALSG (Advanced Life Support Group); Mackway-Jones K, Marsden J, Windle J (eds). *Emergency Triage: Manchester Triage Group*, 3rd edn. Oxford: Wiley Blackwell, 2013.

Kenyon S, Hewison A, Dann S-A, et al. The design and implementation of an obstetric triage system for unscheduled pregnancy related attendances: a mixed methods evaluation. *BMC Pregnancy Childbirth* 2017; 17: Article 309.

CHAPTER 43
Transfer

Learning outcomes

After reading this chapter, you will be able to:
- Outline an overview of the principles of the safe transfer or retrieval of critically ill patients
- Describe the systematic ACCEPT approach for managing such patients

43.1 Introduction

Due to the complexity of healthcare provision arising from the reconfiguration, consolidation and centralisation of specialist hospital services, patients increasingly require transfer between hospitals. Such transfers can be highly complex logistical undertakings with journeys ranging from a few miles and a few minutes in major cities, to several thousand miles over many hours in countries with vast geographical areas and scattered rural and remote communities, like Australia, Canada and the USA. Interhospital transfer of the pregnant woman and/or newborn may be indicated when their clinical care needs either exceed the resource capacity, or expertise, of the current facility.

This chapter will deal with the approach needed for any type of transfer, both ex-uterine and intrauterine, and outline the principles needed to make these successful and safe. These principles can then be applied to your own practice, whether in the UK, or overseas.

Common reasons for needing to transfer a pregnant/recently pregnant woman to another hospital include:

- Clinical reasons:
  - Need for enhanced care for the mother, either pre-delivery or postpartum, for either an obstetric problem (e.g. preterm labour, pre-eclampsia toxaemia, fetal growth retardation) or for a problem not directly related to the pregnancy
  - Need for a specialist neonatal services (e.g. high risk of spontaneous or iatrogenic birth of an extremely preterm fetus within the next 7 days or a fetus with a known abnormality)
- Operational reasons:
  - Neonatal intensive care unit closed (staffing/capacity)
  - Neonatal request (staffing/workload)
  - Delivery suite capacity (staffing/workload)

Being transferred out of the local area is a significant source of stress, inconvenience and expense for the woman and her family, as well as having a resource and operational impact on the transferring unit. The aim of a transfer and retrieval policy is to ensure the safe, timely and appropriate transfer of a woman and/or neonate to facilities with optimal capabilities for their needs, whilst minimising the number of unnecessary and costly transfers and subsequent back transfers.

Managing Medical and Obstetric Emergencies and Trauma: A Practical Approach, Fourth Edition. Edited by Rosamunde Burns and Kara Dent.

To achieve a successful transfer or retrieval, both clinical and transport expertise are required. The right patient has to be taken at the right time, by the right personnel, with the right equipment, to the right place - first time, by the right form of transport, receiving the right care throughout. Transfer is not an alternative to diagnosis and treatment.

43.2 ACCEPT approach

Preparation and planning for transfer begins as soon as the decision to transfer has been made. The coordination and facilitation of a transfer should follow local network guidelines. Arranging a transfer requires effective communication between the referring, transporting and receiving teams. The added complexity in obstetrics of dealing with 'two patients' demands that a highly systematic approach to this process is adopted. One such approach is the ACCEPT method developed by the Advanced Life Support Group (ALSG).

A	Assessment
C	Control
C	Communication
E	Evaluation
P	Preparation and packaging
T	Transportation

Following ACCEPT ensures that assessments and procedures are carried out in the right order. This method also correctly emphasises the preparation that is required before the patient is transported.

Assessment

The clinician involved in the transportation may have been involved in the care given up to that point. However, the transporter may have been brought in especially for that purpose and will have no prior knowledge of the patient's clinical history. It is the responsibility of the person undertaking the transfer to become fully appraised of the clinical situation.

For a woman to be suitable for transfer, staff at the referring hospital need to balance the risks of transfer against the potential benefits.

Clinical circumstances where transfer may be considered inappropriate or unsafe include:

- Known fetal or maternal compromise requiring immediate delivery
- Significant risk of delivery occurring during the transfer (i.e. in active labour where the cervix is more than 3 cm dilated)
- Unstable maternal or fetal condition that could deteriorate during the transfer
- Refusal of the patient
- In the absence of maternal concerns, pregnancy less than/at 22 weeks (i.e. below the threshold of viability), or of a pregnancy complicated by the presence of a potentially lethal fetal condition where active intervention of the fetus is not being considered, even if live born
- Parents at risk of having an extremely preterm birth (at 23 + 0 to 24 + 6 weeks and/or <500 g) who, after appropriate counselling (i.e. in conjunction with a neonatologist they have been informed about the prognosis and morbidity and mortality figures relevant to their pregnancy), do not wish active resuscitation of their newborn to occur, should be given the option of not transferring
- Low probability of delivery in a woman presenting with symptoms of threatened preterm labour

If a woman refuses, she cannot be transferred against her wishes. The woman needs to be counselled of the risks that refusal may bring to both herself and her baby, and details of this conversation should be documented carefully within the medical records. The woman should also be informed of the chance, and implications, of transfer after birth. There is clear recognition in the literature that a premature neonate will have a significantly better outcome if born in the unit that has the neonatal facilities required rather than as an ex-utero transfer.

Preterm delivery (before 37 weeks' pregnancy) occurs in 7.1% of pregnancies in the UK (>50 000 deliveries per annum), with the majority the result of preterm labour. Of the births that are preterm, 5% are extremely preterm (before 28 weeks), 11% are very preterm (between 28 and 32 weeks) and 85% are moderately preterm (between 32 and 37 weeks). Prematurity remains the leading cause of neonatal morbidity and mortality, but timely interventions – such as antenatal steroids to promote lung maturity, magnesium sulphate for neuroprotection and delivery in a unit with appropriate neonatal care facilities – can improve neonatal outcome

Place of birth. Marlow et al. (2014), using the EPICure 2 data, considered the effect of place of birth and perinatal transfer on survival and neonatal morbidity within a prospective cohort of births of extremely preterm babies in England. Within this cohort of neonates (born with a gestation between 22 and 26 weeks), the study found a significantly reduced mortality for those born within a level 3 neonatal unit when compared with birth in a level 2 or less setting (adjusted OR 0.73, 95%CI 0.59–0.90). This was attributed to both a reduction in fetal deaths and a reduction in deaths in the first week of life and may therefore be related to both obstetric and neonatal care.

Establishing an accurate diagnosis of preterm labour is, however, challenging. Clinical signs are non-specific and false positive diagnoses are common, with up to 80% of women with signs and symptoms of preterm labour remaining pregnant after 7 days, and the majority going on to deliver at term. Such diagnostic uncertainty means a large proportion of women with symptoms of preterm labour are treated unnecessarily to ensure benefits to the small proportion of babies that do actually deliver preterm. Current overintervention of threatened preterm labour results in many women being hospitalised and/or transferred unnecessarily out of their local hospital. This also prevents appropriate transfers as neonatal cots become 'blocked' in order to accept a preterm neonate just in case delivery occurs – negatively impacting the efficiency of already stretched neonatal units and networks. This frequently has knock-on effects to other women and babies, who may need transfer to another unit due to lack of cot availability despite an empty, but 'blocked', cot. It may also increase the number of more dangerous ex utero transfers.

Bedside point-of-care diagnostic tests for preterm labour are available and should be used to help improve the prediction of impending preterm delivery before a decision to transfer is made. Biochemical tests available include: (i) fFN® (Hologic, Marlborough, MA, USA), which measures fetal fibronectin in samples of cervicovaginal secretions collected at speculum examination; (ii) Actim® Partus (Medix Biochemica, Espoo, Finland), which measures phosphorylated insulin-like growth factor binding protein-1; and (iii) PartoSure™ (Parsagen Diagnostics, Boston, MA, USA), which measures placental alpha-microglobulin-1. The available data for fetal fibronectin are considerably greater than for the other markers. Within the UK the most widely utilised test is the fFN. Fetal fibronectin is not normally found in cervicovaginal secretions after 22 weeks' gestation until towards the end of pregnancy after 35–37 weeks. Detection is a good predictor of spontaneous preterm birth in both asymptomatic and symptomatic women. Quantitative testing improves the positive predictive value and likelihood ratios of the test, whilst maintaining the high negative predictive value over qualitative testing.

An alternative approach (which can be combined with quantitative fetal fibronectin) is to measure the cervical length using transvaginal ultrasound, as the longer the cervix is, the less likely a preterm delivery. Precise thresholds for intervention will depend on the overall clinical picture, but it is recommended that where the risk of delivery in the next 7 days is predicted to be low, transfer may be withheld.

The median latency between the rupture of membranes occurring between 24 and 31 weeks and delivery is 7–10 days. This an indication for in utero transfer to a unit with appropriate neonatal facilities should perhaps not be because of preterm premature rupture of the membranes alone, but because of evidence of associated uterine activity or signs suggestive of chorioamnionitis.

Control

Once assessment is complete, the transport organiser needs to take control of the situation. This requires the following:

- Identifying the clinical team leader
- Identifying the tasks to be carried out
- Allocating tasks to individuals or teams

The lines of responsibility must be established urgently. In theory, ultimate responsibility is held jointly by the referring consultant clinician, the receiving consultant clinician and the transfer personnel at different stages of the transfer process. There should always be a named person with overall responsibility for organising the transfer.

The organiser needs to display leadership whilst at all times taking a systems perspective and avoiding tunnel vision or task fixation.

In many cases coordination is typically undertaken by specialist regional network coordinators, who usually utilise sophisticated communication technologies such as multiparty conference calls, telehealth videoconferencing, case recording and comprehensive data management systems.

Coordination of a transfer requires an ongoing process of communication and feedback with the team about case progress, estimated response time and patient status changes. During the response and transfer phase, the coordination centre maintains communication with response teams providing logistic support and oversight.

Communication

The single most important aspect of conducting a successful and safe retrieval is communication. Moving ill patients from one place to another requires cooperation and the involvement of several people. Therefore, key personnel need to be informed when transportation is being considered.

The neonatologists in the referring and receiving units should communicate directly. Who to involve in maternal care depends on whether the mother is being transferred for an obstetric problem or a non-obstetric problem. If the transfer is for a non-obstetric problem, obstetric care also has to be continued in the receiving unit and has to be transferred to an obstetric team at the receiving unit.

The mother and her relatives must be kept informed.

Consider informing the following people, as appropriate:

- Consultant responsible for current maternal clinical care
- Consultant responsible for current obstetric care if different from above
- Consultant responsible for current neonatal clinical care
- Special care unit staff in the transferring unit
- Consultant responsible for transfer of the patient (if different from above)
- Consultant responsible for maternal intensive care if appropriate
- Senior midwife in the transferring unit
- Consultant responsible for maternal clinical care in the receiving unit
- Consultant responsible for obstetric care in the receiving unit
- Consultant responsible for neonatal care in the receiving unit
- Special care unit staff in the receiving unit
- Senior midwife in the receiving unit
- Ambulance control or special transportation controls (as appropriate)

If anaesthetists have been involved in the obstetric care, they should communicate directly.

Communication may take a long time to complete if one person does it all. It is therefore advisable to share the tasks between corresponding teams, taking into account expertise and local policies. Team-to-team communication is imperative. In all cases it is important that information is passed on unambiguously. This is particularly the case when talking to people over the telephone.

The **ISBAR** tool should be utilised as it provides a framework to ensure the safe, timely and structured exchange of clinical information.

I Introduction
S Situation
B Background
A Assessment
R Recommendation

Information needs to be relayed slowly and clearly. It is useful to plan what to say before telephoning. It is important to identify who are you are (name, role and facility you are telephoning from) and identify the patient (with at least three identifiers).

The steps involved are:

1. Situation:
   - What is going on with the patient (main diagnosis/presenting problem(s)); reason for transfer)
   - If pregnant, what is the pregnancy gestation/expected delivery date?
   - Is the woman in confirmed labour?
   - If postpartum, details of labour and birth/third stage
   - What the hospital level of capability/capacity is at this time
   - Is medical/midwifery support currently available?
2. Background:
   - Provide relevant clinical history and background
   - State briefly what has been done to date to address the problem
   - Medications/allergies
   - Weight (this is needed for air transfers)
   - Highlight any safeguarding issues
3. Assessment:
   - What is the current clinical assessment of the situation?
   - Convey concerns, uncertainties and urgency. (Is the patient haemodynamically unstable? Is the situation time critical?)
   - Describe your assessment and investigation results (have details of labour assessment, MEOWS (modified early obstetric warning score) chart, imaging findings and blood results to hand).
4. Recommendation:
   - Discuss what is needed from the listener (e.g. clinical advice, assistance in finding a bed, organisation of transport and staff for a transfer)
   - Be clear about what you are requesting and the timeframe

Clarification and assuring comprehension as part of the 'recommendation' step is vital. The risks of inadequate communication, or even worse a misunderstanding of conveyed information, are high. The request for immediate and direct assistance should be clear, so there is no misunderstanding. Details of the conversation need to be documented in the patient's medical notes. Some units utilise specific forms or checklists to aid this process.

The decision to refuse acceptance of an appropriate transfer should be made at consultant level. There should be recognition by the receiving neonatal unit that unless delivery is likely to occur imminently after transfer, there will not necessarily need to be a vacant neonatal cot to accept the transfer. Likewise, the receiving maternity unit should consider both their antenatal and labour ward capacity. Many pregnant women can be managed on the antenatal ward after transfer, and the immediate acuity of the labour ward may not impact on the ability to accept the referral as transfers often take a few hours to complete.

Even in emergency situations, it is important not to neglect the principles of family-centred care. Care providers need to be attentive to the emotional needs of the woman and her family. The need for transfer must be sensitively communicated and discussed with the woman and her family, with adequate opportunity provided, as circumstances permit, for the woman's questions and concerns to be addressed. Information provided to the woman and her family should include:

- Reasons for transfer
- Scheduled date, time and duration of transfer
- Destination
- Names of staff members who will accompany her
- Visiting hours and telephone number of the receiving hospital
- Anticipated length of hospital stay
- Travel directions to the receiving hospital for cars or information on other modes of transportation for family members
- Accommodation options for family members

Evaluation

The dual aims of evaluation are to assess whether transfer is appropriate for the patient and, if so, what the degree of urgency for the transfer is. Often, it is only when the first phase of ACCEPT (that is, ACC) has been completed that enough information will have been gathered to make an evaluation. Evaluation is a dynamic process which starts from first contact with the patient, and includes continuous reassessment of the patient to assess the effectiveness of the resuscitation and stabilisation process.

Is transfer appropriate for this patient?

The reasons for transfer should be justifiable, preferably by demonstrating direct benefit to the woman and/or her fetus.

The risks involved in transfer must be balanced against the risks of staying and the benefits of care that can only be given by the receiving unit.

Clinical urgency?

With the indication for transfer clear, the urgency must be evaluated. The severity of illness and natural history of the condition (which may be known or unknown, predictable or unpredictable), together with an assessment of patient stability can be used to rank the urgency for transfer. This hierarchy also helps determine both the personnel and the mode of transportation required. Senior staff should be involved in this decision and it should be based on the risks and benefits of immediate versus delayed transfer. Guidelines have been published to help the decision-making process, for example of the brain-injured patient (by the Association of Anaesthetists and the Neuro Anaesthesia and Critical Care Society (NACCS) of Great Britain and Ireland), but in other situations can be more difficult.

Transfer categories

- Intensive/life-threatening emergency
- Time critical
- Ill and unstable
- Ill and stable
- Unwell
- Well/elective transfer

Preparation and packaging

Preparation and packaging both have the aim of ensuring that the patient transport proceeds with the minimum change in the level of care provided and with no deterioration in the patient's condition.

'Scoop and run' versus 'stay and play' has long been a point of difference between many retrieval medicine experts. In essence, there are patients who will benefit most from a rapid assessment, minimal stabilisation and prompt transfer to definitive care. Others will deteriorate significantly en route without the initiation of further stabilisation prior to transfer. The decision regarding which of these principles is most appropriate in any given circumstance is complicated, varying not just with patient and illness factors, but also with local skill, transport team skill, logistics and time to definitive care.

The first stage (preparation) involves completion of patient stabilisation and preparation of transfer team personnel and equipment. The second stage (packaging) involves the final measures that need to be taken to ensure the security and safety of the patient during the transportation itself.

Patient preparation

To ensure the best outcome for the mother and fetus, and to reduce the likelihood of complications during the journey, meticulous resuscitation and stabilisation should be carried out prior to transfer. This may involve carrying out procedures requested by the receiving hospital or unit (maternal or fetal). Adequate preparation for transport should follow the standard ABCDE approach, and examples of issues to address include the following.

Airway

- A patent airway is the goal
- The use of non-invasive positive pressure ventilation during transfers (especially by air) is controversial
- If it is deemed likely that airway intervention will be needed in transit, this should be achieved prior to transportation
- Tracheal intubation during transfer is difficult

Breathing

- Maintain adequate oxygenation
- All patients requiring oxygen on the ground will require more oxygen at altitude if transported by air
- If indicated, intercostal chest drains should be inserted prior to transfer, especially if being transferred by air

Circulation

- Volume status should be assessed and normalised prior to departure as hypovolaemic patients tolerate movement and inertial forces of transportation very poorly
- Ensure good venous access
- An interosseous needle is acceptable as reliable access
- A urinary catheter should be considered, for comfort, or in cases where strict input and output monitoring is required

Disability

- Document level of consciousness and exam pupils prior to transfer
- An uncooperative, combative or disturbed patient can put the safety of themselves and staff at risk
- A fear of flying and of heights are well recognised phobias that can be very challenging to manage if not considered and dealt with prior to transfer
- Fractures and suspected fractures must be immobilised with attention paid to the prevention of pressure damage
- If diabetic, aim for normoglycaemia

Exposure

- Expose and examine the patient as appropriate
- Consider the implications of a long transfer
- Positioning: the patient should be transferred onto the transport trolley and should be properly secured with due regard paid to any possible spinal injury. The patient should be tilted to prevent aortocaval compression
- Medications: rationalise therapies and minimise the number of infusions. Ensure adequate analgesia and/or sedation and antiemetics. The need for steroids, magnesium and toccolysis should be considered if the woman is preterm
- Thermal control: the patient should be well covered and kept warm during the transfer
- Venous thromboembolism (VTE) prevention: immobility during long transfers increases the risk of a VTE event

Inadequate resuscitation or missed illnesses and injuries will result in instability during transfer and will adversely affect outcome.

Moving the patient is only part of the job. The medical and treatment records (or photocopies) should accompany the patient. If there has been haemorrhage, ensure the estimated blood loss has been clearly documented. If the blood results are not available by the time of departure, they should be telephoned through as soon as available. Major trauma patients will also have had imaging; ensure both the images (and/or PACS access) and reports are sent to the receiving unit.

Have a plan for the patient's belongings.

Equipment preparation

All equipment must be functioning and be fitted with appropriate auditory and visual alert systems. Transfer equipment should only be used for transfers. It must be serviced in accordance with the manufacturer's guidance and checked regularly, with a further test immediately before transfer. Particular care should be taken to ensure an adequate supply of batteries for portable electronic equipment.

Retrieval teams typically have access to the following equipment: a complete range of airway management equipment including a difficult airway kit, cardiac monitor defibrillator pacer, multiple infusion pumps appropriate for inotrope infusions, a transport ventilator capable of complex respiratory support, invasive pressure monitoring, temperature monitoring, capnography and oximetry.

Supplies of oxygen, essential drugs (paying particular attention to inotropes and sedative drugs) and fluids should be more than adequate for the whole of the intended journey, including an allowance for unforeseen delays.

Specialist equipment may also be required for particular patients; for example, those patients who might be at risk of delivering (although a high risk of this would preclude transfer until post-delivery) and those with spinal injuries.

The transfer team should be in possession of a mobile phone with a fully charged battery or radio for urgent communication during transportation. Relevant contact telephone numbers should be preprogrammed into the mobile phone.

Personnel preparation

The transfer team also need to be prepared, with attention to warm clothing, suitable footwear, food if the journey is long, mobile phones and sufficient money to enable them to get home if needed. They should know the name and contact details of the receiving doctor and the exact location at the receiving unit at which they are expected.

The number and nature of staff accompanying patients during transport will reflect the patient's transfer category. For example, a sick, pre-eclamptic patient would normally be escorted by an anaesthetist and midwife.

Whatever category the patient, all personnel should be competent in the transfer procedure and be familiar with the practical aspects of working in an ambulance or aircraft, they should have knowledge of the equipment and drugs used in transfer, as well an understanding of adverse physiological changes that may occur with moving an unwell patient.

All staff must practice within their areas of competence. For an intensive care transfer, the Intensive Care Society recommends that the accompanying physician, 'should have received training in intensive care and transport medicine, had involvement in previous transfers and preferably have at least 2 years' experience in anaesthesia, intensive care medicine or other equivalent specialty.' In addition, they should be accompanied by another experienced doctor, nurse, paramedic or technician familiar with intensive care procedures and with all transport equipment.

Employers must ensure there is appropriate medical indemnity insurance for such patient transfers. Additionally, adequate death and accidental personal injury insurance must also be provided for the members of the transfer team.

Packaging

Correct packaging of the patient is very important and involves the physical preparation of the patient for transfer and aims to minimise the risk of disconnecting IV lines, tubes and equipment. Endotracheal tubes and venous access lines should be fixed securely, be visible and accessible with extension sets applied as necessary. In ventilated patients, placement of a nasogastric tube is recommended. Drains and catheters should be fixed securely and freely draining. Chest drains should be secured and unclamped with any underwater seal device replaced by an appropriate commercial drainage valve and bag system.

Upon departure, the receiving unit should be provided with an estimated time of arrival. The referring unit is responsible for arranging a safe, efficient and rapid transfer. Realistically, some transfers can take longer to arrange. In this situation, given that the transfer time itself can be lengthy, a reassessment of the clinical status of the woman and/or well-being of the fetus, including a repeat vaginal examination if appropriate, should occur prior to departure. A change in clinical status may make the planned transfer now impractical or unsafe. If this is the case, the receiving unit and the transport team need to be updated.

Transportation

Mode of transport

A number of transport platforms can be utilised including road ambulance, rotary and fixed wing aircraft and, occasionally, boats. Each of these has specific benefits and limitations to use. When deciding on the best mode of transportation, several factors need to be taken into account:

- Nature of the illness
- Patient size
- Urgency of transfer
- Availability of transport and the the priorities and demands on resources
- Civilian aviation restrictions
- Medical and transport team fatigue limitations (safe working hours)
- Number of retrieval personnel and volume of accompanying equipment
- Possible clinical impact of transport equipment on patient access to perform acute medical interventions
- Mobilisation time
- Geographic factors (location of patient, distances involved and transit times, need for refuelling)
- Terrain (including proximity of landing strip, availability of helipad, road access and road conditions)
- Weather conditions
- Traffic conditions
- Cost

Minimising the number of patient transfers and the total out-of-hospital time for the patient are important principles. Heightened risk for patients in transit is experienced during platform transfers (from bed to trolley to ambulance to aircraft stretcher and so on).

Road ambulances are by far the most common means of transportation used in the UK. They have a low overall cost, have a rapid mobilisation time and are less affected by adverse weather conditions. They also give rise to less physiological disturbance and make patient access and monitoring easier.

The aim is for the road journey to be smooth and steady rather than fast and rocky. The transporting team should dictate the road speed the vehicle travels at. The speed will reflect both the clinical urgency and the availability of limited resources such as oxygen.

Air transfer may be used for journeys over 80 km, or 2+ hours in duration, or if road access is difficult. The perceived speed of the air transport itself must be balanced against organisational delays and the need for intervehicle transfer at the beginning and end of the journey.

The physiological effects of flying must also be taken into account. Increasing altitude results in a reduction in barometric pressure and an associated reduction in the partial pressure of oxygen and an expansion of gas within enclosed spaces. Expansion of gas (such as in an undrained pneumothorax, or in a distended bowel) may result in pain or significant worsening of the underlying pathology. Relative hypoxia (either due to altitude or inadequate pressurisation of the aircraft) is common. In a normal person with sea-level SpO_2 of 98%, and without supplemental oxygen, SpO_2 decreases to about 90% at 3000 m altitude (10 000 feet). Potential effects include myocardial ischaemia, syncope, impaired mental performance and loss of consciousness.

Most fixed-wing aircraft routinely pressurise cabins to around 2450 m (8000 feet) above sea level. However, some aeromedical platforms may be able to be pressurise to sea level, whilst some (including most helicopters) cannot be pressurised at all. When pressurised to sea level, aircraft cannot reach their normal cruising altitudes. They need to carry higher fuel loads, and fly lower and slower, which will reduce their flying range and may expose them to increased turbulence and adverse weather conditions.

Care during transport

The patient should be positioned to provide maximum access. Sufficient space should be available at the head to allow monitoring and management of the airway, with equipment readily available that is required to deal with dislodged lines or tubes.

During transfer, everybody's safety is important. Both the patient and accompanying personnel need to be restrained (seat belts on at all times) and all equipment needs to be securely stowed. This can limit rapidity of access in the event of a problem en route. Likewise, communication with the patient and other personnel may be limited due to noise and isolation.

Basic minimum standards of monitoring need to be followed during transport as far as possible. Oxygen saturation, electrocardiogram (ECG) and non-invasion blood pressure may need to be monitored in all patients. In mechanically ventilated patients, the oxygen supply inspired oxygen concentration, end-tidal CO_2, ventilator setting and airway pressure should also be monitored. Fetal monitoring may be appropriate.

Physiological problems that occur during transportation may arise as a result of the effects of the transport environment on the deranged physiology of the patient. Careful preparation can minimise the deleterious effects of inertial forces, such as tipping, acceleration and deceleration, as well as changes in temperature and barometric pressure.

With adequate preparation, the transportation phase is usually incident free. The single most feared complication when transporting the gravid female is in-flight delivery and the subsequent resuscitation of a distressed and often preterm infant. Fortunately, this is a rare event with very few in-flight births occurring. However, untoward events do occur. Should this be the case, the patient needs to be reassessed using the ABC approach.

Appropriate corrective measures should then be instituted. Clinical intervention in a moving vehicle is almost impossible and special consideration should be given to stopping at the first available place. Following any untoward events, communication with the receiving unit is important and should follow the ISBAR framework described previously.

Handover

At the end of the transfer, direct contact with the receiving team must be established so that a succinct, systematic summary of the patient can then be provided. Following which, the receiving unit assumes responsibility for the patient's care. Medical notes and a copy of the transfer record should be left with the receiving staff. This should be accompanied by a written record of the patient's history, vital signs, therapy and significant clinical events during transfer. All the other documents that have been taken with the patient should also be handed over. While this is going on, the rest of the transferring team can help in moving the patient from the ambulance trolley to the receiving unit's bed. The transfer team can then retrieve all equipment and personnel and make their way back to their home unit.

43.3 Common coordination problems

Problem 1

The transport platform is unavailable due to one of the following:

- Weather conditions
- Currently on another transfer
- Tasked to do something else

Solutions

- Consider halfway meet with road vehicles for time critical conditions (may need an escort from the hospital or local paramedics)
- Can other tasks be done another way or deferred?
- Staged road retrieval (transfer to larger centre than later transfer to definitive care)

Problem 2

There is conflict with the referrer because, for example:

- They feel that the retrieval should occur sooner than has been arranged
- Referrer refuses to perform the intervention advised by the coordinator
- Referrer refuses to give information to the coordinator

Solutions

- Explain reasoning behind decisions
- Involve third party, e.g. receiving hospital clinician
- Use videoconferencing to enhance communication

Problem 3

There is conflict with receiving hospital staff because, for example:

- They are unable to confirm they can accept the case due to key personnel being uncontactable
- The receiving facility states they are full so cannot take the patient
- Conflict over management; receiving hospital staff feel the patient should be treated at the referral site or that the patient should stay and be palliated

Solutions

- Retrieval services should advocate for and be aware of policies that make certain hospitals responsible for patients in their area or who have certain conditions, e.g. severe trauma, acute ST segment elevation myocardial infarction (STEMI) or acute stroke
- Policies should be in place when hospitals are at capacity, e.g. defined transfer
- Retrieval service arrangements with local respected specialist advisors, e.g. receiving intensivist, are invaluable to give independent advice when conflict regarding management and disposition occurs
- Multiparty teleconference or videoconferencing can assist in problem solving
- Escalation of problem within retrieval organisation and hospital executive if all else fails

Problem 4

The referral centre is requesting transfer for an unstable surgical patient prior to surgical intervention.

Solutions

- Communicate directly with the surgical consultant at the referral hospital. Examine the risk of surgical intervention versus 4–6 hours out-of-hospital transfer time in a patient who is likely to deteriorate with no prospect of surgical intervention en route
- Consider as a rare option the transfer of the surgical team with an unstable patient to provide intervention

43.4 Summary

- The safe transfer and retrieval of a patient requires a systematic approach
- By following the ACCEPT method important activities will be carried out at the appropriate time
- A holistic approach to patient preparation that includes addressing psychological and social issues as well as the critical care elements of resuscitation and stabilisation should be adopted
- A poorly organised and hastily done patient transfer can significantly contribute to morbidity and mortality
- Specific training is available for staff undertaking transfers on the Neonatal, Adult and Paediatric Safe Transfer and Retrieval Course (NAPSTaR) delivered by the Advanced Life Support Group (ALSG)

43.5 Further reading

ALSG (Advanced Life Support Group); Mackway-Jones K, Marsden J, Windle J (eds). *Neonatal, Adult and Paediatric Safe Transfer and Retrieval: A Practical Approach to Transfers*. Oxford: Wiley Blackwell, 2019.

Marlow N, Bennett C, Draper ES, Hennessy EM, Morgan AS, Costeloe KL. Perinatal outcomes for extremely preterm babies in relation to place of birth in England: the EPICure 2 study. *Arch Dis Child Fetal Neonatal Ed* 2014; 99(3): F181–8.

CHAPTER 44

Consent matters

Learning outcomes

After reading this chapter, you will be able to:

- Outline when and why consent is required
- Appreciate the concepts of validity, capacity, autonomy and responsibility
- Define the legal status of the fetus

44.1 Introduction

When is consent required?

Consent is required before any treatment, investigation or physical contact with a patient is undertaken. Consent is also required before involving patients in research, teaching or disclosure of confidential information (which may be written, pictorial or auditory).

In England and Wales there is no statute, as in some countries, stating the principles of consent. Failure to obtain informed consent may give rise to civil or criminal proceedings as any touching of the person, no matter how well intentioned, is a trespass. However, to protect against a claim of battery, consent only in the broadest terms has to be obtained.

By contrast, a much more demanding obligation to obtain informed consent arises from a duty of care to the patient by the health professional. Failure to provide sufficient information prevents a patient making an informed choice. If, as a result, the patient agrees to a procedure she would have refused had she been fully informed and harm arises as a result, there would be grounds for a claim of negligence (even if the harm is a recognised hazard of the procedure rather than the product of poor management).

The case of Chester versus Afshar (2004) suggests that failing to provide relevant information to a patient and ensuring that information is understood in a timely manner, could lead to a successful claim, even if the patient would have chosen the treatment had they been informed of the risk. In this case, the patient developed cauda equina syndrome following discectomy (a recognised complication of this procedure). She claimed that her surgeon had not warned her of this complication. The court accepted this. She admitted that it was likely that she would have chosen to undergo surgery by the same surgeon, even if she had known, but she had been deprived of the ability to make an informed choice in the matter. The majority view, when this case was appealed in the House of Lords, was that being denied the opportunity to make a properly informed decision about whether to undergo surgery constituted the injury. The implications for English case law as a result of this ruling are profound and the NHS Litigation Authority (NHSLA, 2004) has issued an alert on this subject.

Managing Medical and Obstetric Emergencies and Trauma: A Practical Approach, Fourth Edition. Edited by Rosamunde Burns and Kara Dent.

Obtaining consent should be a process begun as far in advance of a procedure as possible, but the doctor should recheck immediately prior to the procedure that the patient still consents. In obstetrics, information about potential complications and possible treatment options should be made available in the antenatal period. It is recognised that this will not be possible in the emergency situation and that those most at risk may not be accessible antenatally.

The General Medical Council (GMC) suggests that obtaining informed consent is a process, not an isolated event. It suggests that, 'When providing information you must do your best to find out about patients' individual needs and priorities. You should respond honestly to any questions the patient raises.' A whole section is devoted to withholding information: 'You should not withhold information necessary for decision making unless you judge that disclosure of some relevant information would cause the patient serious harm. In this context serious harm does not mean the patient would become upset, or decide to refuse treatment.' Guidance is currently being updated by the GMC.

Why is consent required? The legal and ethical considerations

The need for valid consent is not just a legal requirement but also an ethical principle that reflects respect for an individual's autonomy and is a fundamental part of good practice. This is the view of both the Department of Health and the GMC.

The traditional model of consent is the 'harm avoidance model', in which the patient is informed of the risks of a procedure, described in general terms, but is otherwise excluded from the decision-making process. The patient is dealt with, 'In an authoritarian but benevolent way (e.g. by supplying all their needs but regulating their conduct)' (Switankowsky, 1998). This was considered acceptable in the case of Sidaway versus Board of Governors of the Bethlehem Royal Hospital (1985). As the judge put it: 'When telling a patient about an operation, the doctor has to decide what ought to be said and how it should be said.'

The increased emphasis on the rights of individuals has led to the requirement for a more demanding form of consent. This is the so-called 'autonomy enhancing model of consent', in which the patient must be given all the information they require to make their own fully informed decision about a proposed course of action.

Consent may be implied or express. An example of implied consent is the action of a patient holding out an arm for venepuncture to be performed. Such implied consent would usually protect against a charge of battery. This might be difficult to evidence however.

Express consent is required for a procedure carrying a 'material' risk (see later in this chapter). The validity of consent does not depend on the form in which it is given: a signature on a form will not necessarily make consent valid. Equally, if consent has been validly given, the absence of a signed consent form is no bar to treatment. Written consent is considered advisable when the procedure involved is complex or risky, where research or screening rather than clinical care is involved, or there may be 'significant consequences for the patient's employment, social or personal life' (GMC, 2008).

The most recent guidance from the GMC (2020) acknowledges that 'although a patient can give consent verbally (or non-verbally) you should make sure this is recorded in their notes'.

Principle of decision making and consent

The most recent guidance published by the GMC in 2020 outlines the 'Seven Principles' that should be applied when gaining consent and making decisions with a patient regarding their care:

1. All patients have the right to be involved in decisions about their treatment and care and be supported to make informed decisions if they are able.
2. Decision making is an ongoing process focused on meaningful dialogue: the exchange of relevant information specific to the individual patient.
3. All patients have the right to be listened to, and to be given the information they need to make a decision and the time and support they need to understand it.
4. Doctors must try to find out what matters to patients so they can share relevant information about the benefits and harms of proposed options and reasonable alternatives, including the option to take no action.
5. Doctors must start from the presumption that all adult patients have capacity to make decisions about their treatment and care. A patient can only be judged to lack capacity to make a specific decision at a specific time, and only after assessment in line with legal requirements.

6. The choice of treatment or care for patients who lack capacity must be of overall benefit to them, and decisions should be made in consultation with those who are close to them or advocating for them.
7. Patients whose right to consent is affected by law should be supported to be involved in the decision-making process, and to exercise choice if possible.

What makes consent valid?

1. The patient must have sufficient information.
2. The patient must have the capacity to make a decision.
3. The patient must be allowed to make the decision voluntarily.
4. Consent is obtained by a suitably qualified and trained individual.

44.2 Sufficient information

This is an area of uncertainty with considerable changes occurring over time and between countries. Only the case in the UK will be discussed in detail.

In the UK in 1957, in the case of Bolam versus Friern Hospital (1957), it was established that a doctor's practice would be judged against that of his medical peers – the Bolam principle or 'reasonable doctor test' – and this was specifically applied to what information to give a patient. This was challenged in 1985 in the case of Sidaway, when it was opined that there might be occasions when information about a particular risk was so obviously necessary that the court would decide that its omission was negligent even if this was not the opinion of a 'responsible body of medical opinion'. In the cases of Bolitho (1997) and Pearce (1999), the Bolam principle was overturned. The courts made it clear that the court itself would be the final arbiter of what was a reasonable amount of information to give a patient and not the medical profession. The reasonable doctor has been replaced by what the reasonable patient would expect to be told. The situation is different in the USA where, in some states, the policy of 'full disclosure' is advocated (the patient is told as much as possible).

Material risk is a risk to which a person in the patient's position would be likely to attach significance. Rogers versus Whitaker (1992) showed that a risk cannot be judged material on the basis of frequency alone. The severity must be taken into account. The individual circumstances of the patient are also pertinent. For example, the risk of infertility following a procedure may be more significant to the primiparous woman than one who has completed her family. The type of information that patients should be told includes a description of the procedure and the incidence and severity of the risks involved (which should be mentioned even if they have not occurred in the practice of the particular doctor involved). There should be discussion on the likely or possible outcome of following or declining to follow a particular course of action and what the alternatives are (if any exist).

The Association of Anaesthetists (Yentis et al., 2017) suggests that factors that might influence what the patient is told could include 'the estimated capacity' (see next section) 'of the patient to want to know and to be able to understand the risks' and 'the degree of urgency of the proposed treatment'.

The Bolam test has now been upturned by the Supreme Court ruling regarding the Montgomery versus Lanarkshire case of March 2015. This was a landmark case regarding a type 1 diabetic, Nadine Montgomery. She was known to be of a small stature and carrying a large baby, and had voiced her concerns regarding delivery. She underwent a vaginal delivery with a shoulder dystocia, resulting in her son consequentially suffering from cerebral palsy. Despite her concerns being voiced antenatally, the consultant had not disclosed the risk of shoulder dystocia and possible option of a caesarean section (CS). She was adamant that if she had known the risk, she would have opted for a CS and the Supreme Court upheld in her favour. This case has changed our approach to what informed consent means in that it was decided that a patient should be told whatever they need to know, rather than what a doctor wants to tell them. It requires a doctor to tell the risks where a reasonable person in the patient's position would be likely to attach significance to the risk, or the doctor should reasonably be aware what significance that particular patient would be likely to attach to it.

Occasionally, a patient might wish to know very little, or request that a relative make decisions for them (commonly the partner in obstetrics). In law, no-one may make decisions on behalf of an adult. In this situation, the GMC suggests trying to explain the importance of knowing what is happening to the patient and the Department of Health considers it 'good practice' to record in the notes if information is offered but declined. A relative of an adult cannot choose to withhold information; the patient must be consulted.

In obstetrics, the problem of how much to tell the patient can be particularly demanding. Obstetric patients are usually young and fit, and younger patients often want more information. Women and their partners are often highly motivated to become informed. Several studies (Pattee et al., 1997; Kelly et al., 2004; Plaat and McGlennan, 2004) show that obstetric patients want more information than they are receiving. There is evidence to suggest that providing more information does not increase anxiety levels, which is a common concern among the medical profession (Inglis and Farnhill, 1993).

Adversely influencing the opportunity to provide information that women want, is a lack of time: the majority of medical interventions in childbirth are unplanned, such as augmentation of labour, assisted vaginal delivery, episiotomy or manual removal of the placenta. Two-thirds of CS operations are non-elective. In a national audit by the Royal College of Obstetricians and Gynaecologists (RCOG), 16% of CS operations were considered to be category 1: when there is immediate threat to the life of the woman and her fetus and delivery within 30 minutes is considered mandatory (RCOG, 2001). When trauma is involved, time is invariably at a premium. Most authorities suggest that women are given information about all the obstetric complications that might arise in the antenatal period. One trial showed that a combination of printed material with face-to-face question and answer sessions appear to be the most effective way of informing patients (Webber et al. 2001).

In a true emergency situation, where time is of the essence, the RCOG guidelines on consent advise that verbal consent should be obtained where it can be witnessed by another care professional and documented accordingly (Re T 1992).

Our awareness of gaining good consent since the Montgomery ruling has led to many units introducing the **BRAIN** concept to help parents approach the process of making informed consent by asking themselves the following questions:

B	Benefits	'How is this going to help me and my baby?'
R	Risks	'What are the risks to me and my baby with this procedure?'
A	Alternatives	'Are there any alternatives for me?'
I	Intuition	'What does my gut, my instincts, say I should do?'
N	No change	'What happens if I do nothing in this instance?'

44.3 Capacity

For a patient to have capacity (to be competent) to make a decision concerning medical treatment the following criteria must be met:

1. The patient must be capable of comprehending the information.
2. They must be able to retain the information long enough to use it as a basis for decision making.
3. They must be able to evaluate/weigh the information as part of the decision-making process.
4. They must be able to communicate their decision (not necessarily verbally).

In the UK, anyone over the age of 18 years is assumed to be competent to choose or refuse treatment unless shown not to be (for 16–18-year-olds, see below). This is not a question of the degree of intelligence or education of the adult concerned. In order for a patient to be able to comprehend information, it must be presented in a form comprehensible to that patient (e.g. in a language they can understand or avoiding written material in the case of illiteracy). The Department of Health warns not to underestimate the capacity to consent by a patient with learning disabilities. Extra effort should be made to present information in a form comprehensible to such patients. Furthermore, the patient need not come to a decision that is seen as rational by others: 'The patient's right of choice exists whether the reasons for making that choice are rational, irrational, unknown or even non-existent' (Lord Donaldson (Re T 1992)).

No other person can consent to treatment on behalf of any adult, including incompetent ones, unless they are legally appointed with power of attorney.

Since 1969, those aged 16 or 17 years are entitled to consent to medical intervention (Section 8, Family Law Reform Act 1969). Unlike adults, however, their refusal of medical treatment may sometimes be overturned by an adult with parental responsibility. The power to overrule is based on the paramount importance of the welfare of the child. Refusal of treatment by a child or those with parental responsibility can be overruled by a court in the interests of the child's welfare. This has obvious implications in the case of children of Jehovah's Witnesses (this is not the case in Scotland, where a competent child's refusal cannot be overturned).

Children under the age of 16 years *may* have the capacity to consent to medical treatment if they are judged to have capacity by their doctor, taking into account the complexity and risk of the procedure and the child's state of health and mind. This process was known as assessing the child to be 'Gillick competent'. The doctor should ensure that all relevant considerations pertaining to their decision are documented.

In the case of obstetrics, it is worth noting that, in the UK in 2000, over 41 000 girls under the age of 18 years became pregnant, of whom 8000 were under 16 years old. A high proportion of young girls seek to terminate their pregnancy. In such circumstances, there is potential for conflict between parents and children over whether to terminate the pregnancy and it is vital to establish whether the girl is 'Gillick competent'.

Lack of capacity for consent: incompetence

The range of ability among patients follows a continuum from incompetence through to competence (Maybury and Maybury, 2003). Where capacity is absent, so that valid consent cannot be obtained, the underlying principle guiding treatment is that of the person's best interests (the 'welfare of the child' in the case of minors). Treatment can and should be given on the legal grounds of necessity. The best interests of an individual do not refer only to their physical health but must depend on:

- The risks and benefits of available options
- Whether the patient had been previously competent and evidence of previously held views, e.g. advance statement (see later)
- Knowledge of the patient's views or beliefs
- Views of the patient's preferences given by a third party
- The treatment option that gives the patient most chance of choice in the future

The Mental Capacity Act

This Act came into force in England and Wales in 2007 and is designed to protect people who lack capacity. It is based on five fundamental principles:

1. A person must be assumed to have capacity unless it is established that they lack capacity.
2. A person should not be deemed to lack capacity until all practicable steps to regain capacity have been taken without success.
3. A person cannot be judged to lack the capacity to make a decision merely because they make an unwise decision.
4. Any decision made under this Act for, or on behalf of, a person who lacks capacity must be made in their best interests.
5. Before the procedure is done, or the decision is made, regard must be had to whether the purpose for which it is needed can be as effectively achieved in a way that is less restrictive of the person's rights and freedom of action.

The Act requires assessment of capacity to be a two-stage process (Box 44.1).

Box 44.1 Two-stage assessment

Stage one

Does the person have an impairment of the mind or brain, or is there some sort of disturbance affecting the way their mind or brain works? (It does not matter whether the impairment or disturbance is temporary or permanent.)

Stage two

If so, does that impairment or disturbance mean that the person is unable to make the decision in question at the time it needs to be made?

Capacity may be decision specific (the patient may have capacity to make some decisions but not others), and may fluctuate over time. Psychiatric illness does not necessarily mean lack of capacity (Tameside and Glossop Acute Services Trust versus CH; www.medicalprotection.org/uk/articles/assessing-capacity; last accessed January 2022).

The Act entitles any patient of 18 years or over with capacity to refuse specific medical treatment at a time in the future when they may lack capacity. This is known as an **advance decision**:

- The individual was competent when drawing up the directive
- The directive expresses *refusal* of a treatment (a doctor is not obliged to undertake any particular course of action and cannot be required to undertake an illegal course of action)
- The specific *circumstances* in which the question of treatment arises are those anticipated by the patient when drawing up the directive and the proposed treatment explicitly stated
- There is no evidence that the patient may have changed her mind, while she retained capacity

Advance decisions can be verbal unless they refer to life-saving treatment when they have to be written and signed by the patient. The Act does not dictate the format of verbal advance decision and it will be up to the treating clinicians to decide if they exist and are valid at the time.

A doctor cannot choose to ignore a valid advance directive on terms of conscience or belief.

Examples of advance directives include refusal of heroic surgery or resuscitative measures in the case of progressive, debilitating disease and statements that Jehovah's Witnesses may carry, refusing the use of blood or blood products. In the case of obstetrics, the birth plan may fulfil the criteria of an advance directive. In such circumstances, what is paramount is to determine if the patient had anticipated the circumstances (e.g. more severe pain than ever previously experienced), if she had changed her mind and whether the present circumstances have rendered her currently incompetent.

If there are concerns about the validity of an advance directive, it may be necessary to consult the courts. Article 9 of the Human Rights Act 1998 (freedom of thought, conscience and religion) may have an impact in this area in the future.

Under the safeguards of the Mental Health Act 1983, patients who are mentally incapacitated may be treated compulsorily, but only for the mental disorder from which they are suffering. In Norfolk and Norwich NHS Trust versus W (1996), a parturient with schizophrenia was forced to undergo a CS against her will on the grounds that the caesarean formed part of the treatment for her schizophrenia, not because it would save her life or that of her child. The judge was of the opinion that delivery would halt further deterioration to the patient's psychiatric state; psychiatric opinion was that a live birth was necessary to make schizophrenia treatment successful, and finally that the patient could not be given strong enough medication until after delivery as it might harm the fetus (but see 'Status of the fetus' later).

In the case of the child who lacks capacity, the Children Act 1989 sets out who can assume parental responsibility. These include the following:

- The children's parents if married at the time of birth or conception; this responsibility is not lost on divorce
- The child's mother if unmarried but not the father, unless they subsequently marry or he is granted parental responsibility by a court. However, in England and Wales for births registered from December 2003 (different dates in Scotland and Northern Ireland), an unmarried father, as long as he is named on the child's birth certificate, has parental responsibility
- A legally appointed guardian or adoptive parents
- A person in whose favour a court has made a residence order for the child
- A local authority if the child is under its care (usually shared with parents)
- A local authority or person holding an authorised emergency protection order for the child.

One person with parental responsibility may give consent to essential treatment in the face of refusal by another; in this case, if practical, such decisions should be referred to a court. In an emergency, a child who lacks capacity may be treated without consent from the person with parental responsibility.

The question of capacity and temporary incapacity is a particular dilemma in obstetrics. This has been highlighted by a series of cases in which applications were made to courts to allow an emergency CS to be performed against the will of the woman. In the case of CH, the surgery was allowed under the Mental Health Act 1983 because the surgery itself was deemed to be an essential part of the treatment of the woman's mental illness. In subsequent cases, the decision whether to allow surgery was based on the question of capacity of the labouring woman. In one case (Norfolk and Norwich NHS Trust versus W), the 'pain and acute emotional stress' of labour combined with the patient's history of mental illness (she did not believe she was pregnant) were the grounds on which the judge concluded that she was incapable of weighing up the information presented to her. However, in a second case (Rochdale NHS Trust versus C), later the same day, the same judge concluded that the patient was 'unable to make any valid decision about anything of even the most trivial kind' due to the emotional stress and pain of labour. This was a woman whose obstetrician considered to be competent and who had no history of mental illness.

A third case involved a patient (Re MB, 1997) with a severe needle phobia who required a CS for breech presentation. In this case it was judged that the woman's capacity was temporarily diminished by the panic and fear induced by her needle phobia.

Factors that may temporarily erode capacity include shock, confusion, fatigue, pain and drugs. All these may be pertinent when considering the capacity of a woman in labour.

The Human Rights Act 1998 incorporates the European Convention on Human Rights into UK law. It is likely that it will serve to strengthen protection of individuals against treatment they refuse (Article 3, prohibition of torture; Article 5, right to liberty and security; Article 6, right to a fair trial) and emphasise their right to be fully informed (Article 8, right to private and family life).

Status of the fetus

The Abortion Act 1967 gave statutory status to the principle that the fetus does not have a legal right to life. The Act sets out clearly the circumstances when termination of pregnancy is allowable, which extends far beyond the physical well-being of the woman. The grounds for an abortion are:

- That the pregnancy has not exceeded its 24th week and that the continuance of the pregnancy would involve risk, greater than if the pregnancy were terminated, of injury to the physical or mental health of the pregnant woman or any existing children of her family
- That the termination is necessary to prevent grave permanent injury to the physical or mental health of the pregnant woman
- That the continuance of the pregnancy would involve risk to the life of the pregnant woman, greater than if the pregnancy were terminated
- That there is a substantial risk that if the child were born it would suffer from such physical or mental abnormalities as to be seriously handicapped

If, 'the termination is immediately necessary to save the life or to prevent grave permanent injury to the physical or mental health of the pregnant woman', the pregnancy may be terminated if one registered medical practitioner is of the opinion, formed in good faith, that an abortion is justified within the terms of the Act.

The fetus's lack of legal right was demonstrated in a case in which a man unsuccessfully sought an injunction preventing his wife from having an abortion (Paton versus trustees of British Pregnancy Advisory Services, 1979). This case was taken to the European Commission on Human Rights under Article 2 (right to life), but was rejected. The Court of Appeal's ruling on the case Re MB (1997) highlights not just issues of competence but also the legal status of the unborn child in relation to its mother's rights. In the judgement of the Court of Appeal, it was categorically stated that the right of a competent woman to agree to or refuse treatment takes precedence over the welfare of the fetus. In a subsequent case (Re S, 1992), the Court of Appeal concluded: 'Although human, and protected by the law in a number of different ways . . . an unborn child is not a separate person from its mother. Its need for medical assistance does not prevail over her rights. She is entitled not to be forced to submit to an invasion of her body against her will, whether her own life or that of her unborn child depends on it. Her right is not reduced or diminished merely because her decision to exercise it may appear morally repugnant.'

44.4 Voluntarily given consent

Consent will only be valid if given freely. The GMC starts the section entitled 'Ensuring voluntary decision making,' by stating, 'it is for the patient not the doctor, to determine what is in the patient's best interests' (GMC, 2008). However, it accepts that the doctor may want to recommend a particular treatment. This should be acceptable if evidence-based information is presented in a dispassionate manner. It is good practice to document the discussion.

The woman's partner and sometimes other relatives, any of whom may hold strong views about her management, often accompany the obstetric patient. When considering outside influence, 'The will of the patient and the relationship of the person trying to impose their will, must be considered' (Lord Donaldson, Re T 1992).

The same factors that may erode capacity may also undermine the woman's ability to withstand coercion (fatigue, pain, stress, etc.) Cultural factors characterising relationships between the sexes may also be a factor. In the not uncommon situation where a woman states, 'I will do as my husband decides,' it is important to try to establish the woman's wishes, preferably in the absence of the partner. The same may apply to parents, especially in the case of younger girls. In Re T, the Court of Appeal judge upheld the decision to allow a blood transfusion to a patient who was not a Jehovah's Witness but who declined blood, on the grounds that her mother, who was a Jehovah's Witness, had unduly influenced her.

It should be reiterated that no-one can consent to or refuse treatment on behalf of another adult, whether competent or not (unless they have power of attorney). Thus, the partner who says, 'my wife would have wanted/not have wanted a particular intervention,' has no right to impose his view. However, such a statement may alert the doctor to the existence of an advance directive that does have legal weight.

44.5 Who can obtain consent?

The person providing treatment is responsible for obtaining consent. The GMC guidance states that this task can be delegated, provided that the person to whom the task is delegated is suitably trained and qualified, obtains consent in an appropriate manner and has sufficient knowledge about the proposed procedure.

44.6 Summary

- Without basic consent, any physical contact with patients constitutes trespass and could result in a charge of battery or assault
- Doctors have a duty of care to ensure that their patients give informed consent to procedures; failure to do so may constitute negligence, especially if harm ensues
- Where informed consent cannot be obtained, doctors may legally provide care based on the principle of necessity, the basis of which is that the treatment is in the best interests of the patient
- While children under the age of 16 years may have the right to consent to treatment independently of their parents if they are deemed to have capacity ('Gillick competent'), they may not have the right to refuse treatment
- The fetus has no legal right to life; a pregnant or labouring woman's rights are paramount, even in the face of fetal demise
- Advance decisions, of which birth plans are examples, if valid, are legally binding
- In general, the obstetric population wants and requires more information to inform their treatment decisions

44.7 Further reading

Chan C, Tulloch E. Montgomery and informed consent: where are we now? *BMJ* 2017; 357: j2224.

GMC (General Medical Council). *Decision Making and Consent*. London: GMC, 2020. https://www.gmc-uk.org/ethical-guidance/ethical-guidance-for-doctors/decision-making-and-consent (last accessed January 2022).

RCOG (Royal College of Obstetricians and Gynaecologists). *Obtaining Valid Consent*. Clinical Governance Advice No. 6. London: RCOG, 2015.

References and further reading

CHAPTER 2

Knight M, Bunch K, Cairns A, et al. (eds), on behalf of MBRRACE-UK. *Saving Lives, Improving Mothers' Care Rapid Report: Learning from SARS-CoV-2-related and Associated Maternal Deaths in the UK March–May 2020*. Oxford: National Perinatal Epidemiology Unit, University of Oxford, 2020.

Knight M, Bunch K, Tuffnell D, et al. (eds), on behalf of MBRRACE-UK. *Saving Lives, Improving Mothers' Care – Lessons Learned to Inform Maternity Care from the UK and Ireland Confidential Enquiries into Maternal Deaths and Morbidity 2014–16*. Oxford: National Perinatal Epidemiology Unit, University of Oxford, 2018.

Knight M, Bunch K, Tuffnell D, et al. (eds), on behalf of MBRRACE-UK. *Saving Lives, Improving Mothers' Care – Lessons Learned to Inform Maternity Care from the UK and Ireland Confidential Enquiries into Maternal Deaths and Morbidity 2015–17*. Oxford: National Perinatal Epidemiology Unit, University of Oxford, 2019.

Knight M, Bunch K, Tuffnell D, et al. (eds), on behalf of MBRRACE-UK. *Saving Lives, Improving Mothers' Care – Lessons learned to Inform Maternity Care from the UK and Ireland Confidential Enquiries into Maternal Deaths and Morbidity 2016–18*. Oxford: National Perinatal Epidemiology Unit, University of Oxford, 2020.

CHAPTER 4

Flin R, O'Connor P, Crichton M. *Safety at the Sharp End: A guide to non-technical skills*. Abingdon: CRC Press, 2008.

Kohn LT, Corrigan JM, Donaldson MS (eds); Institute of Medicine (US) Committee on Quality of Health Care in American. *To Err is Human: Building a Safer Health System*. Washington DC: National Academies Press, 2010.

RCOG (Royal College of Obstetricians and Gynaecologists). 'Each Baby Counts' initiative. https://www.rcog.org.uk/en/guidelines-research-services/audit-quality-improvement/each-baby-counts/implementation/improving-human-factors/ (last accessed October 2020).

CHAPTER 5

Knight M, Bunch K, Tuffnell D, et al. (eds), on behalf of MBRRACE-UK. *Saving Lives, Improving Mothers' Care – Lessons Learned to Inform Maternity Care from the UK and Ireland Confidential Enquiries into Maternal Deaths and Morbidity 2015–17*. Oxford: National Perinatal Epidemiology Unit, University of Oxford, 2019.

Knight M, Bunch K, Tuffnell D, et al. (eds), on behalf of MBRRACE-UK. *Saving Lives, Improving Mothers' Care – Lessons learned to Inform Maternity Care from the UK and Ireland Confidential Enquiries into Maternal Deaths and Morbidity 2016–18*. Oxford: National Perinatal Epidemiology Unit, University of Oxford, 2020.

Managing Medical and Obstetric Emergencies and Trauma: A Practical Approach, Fourth Edition. Edited by Rosamunde Burns and Kara Dent.

Knight M, Kenyon S, Brocklehurst P, Neilson J, Shakespeare J, Kurinczuk (eds), on behalf of MBRRACE-UK. *Saving Lives, Improving Mothers' Care – Lessons Learned to Inform Maternity Care from the UK and Ireland Confidential Enquiries into Maternal Deaths and Morbidity 2009–12*. Oxford: National Perinatal Epidemiology Unit, University of Oxford, 2014.

RCP (Royal College of Physicians). *Acute Care Toolkit 15: Managing Acute Medical Problems in Pregnancy*. London: RCP, 2019.

CHAPTER 6

AAGBI (Association of Anaesthetists of Great Britain and Ireland). *Quick Reference Handbook 3-1 Anaphylaxis*, 2019. https://anaesthetists.org/Home/Resources-publications/Safety-alerts/Anaesthesia-emergencies/Quick-Reference-Handbook/PDF-version (last accessed October 2020).

Kemp HI, Thomas M, Cook TM, Harper NJN. UK anaesthetists' perspectives and experiences of severe perioperative anaphylaxis. *Br J Anaesth* 2017; 119: 132–9.

NAP (National Audit Project). *NAP6: Perioperative anaphylaxis*. https://www.nationalauditprojects.org.uk/NAP6home (last accessed September 2020).

CHAPTER 7

Knight M, Kenyon S, Brocklehurst P, Neilson J, Shakespeare J, Kurinczuk (eds), on behalf of MBRRACE-UK. *Saving Lives, Improving Mothers' Care – Lessons Learned to Inform Maternity Care from the UK and Ireland Confidential Enquiries into Maternal Deaths and Morbidity 2009–12*. Oxford: National Perinatal Epidemiology Unit, University of Oxford, 2014.

NICE (National Institute for Health and Care Excellence). *Sepsis: Recognition, Diagnosis and Early Management*. NG51. London: NICE, 2016.

Plant LA, Pacheco LD, Louis JM. Sepsis during pregnancy and the puerperium. SMFM Consult Series No. 47: *Am J Obstet Gynecol* 2019; 220(4): B2–B10.

Turner MJ. Maternal sepsis is an evolving challenge. *Int J Gynecol Obstet* 2019; 146: 39–42.

CHAPTER 8

NICE (National Institute for Health and Care Excellence). *Intraoperative Blood Cell Salvage in Obstetrics*. IPG144. London: NICE, 2005.

Sreelakshmi TR, Eldridge J. Acute hypotension associated with leucocyte depletion filters during cell salvaged blood transfusion. *Anaesthesia* 2010; 65: 742–4.

CHAPTER 9

Banerjee A, Begai I, Thorne S. Aortic dissection in pregnancy in England: an incidence study using linked national databases. *BMJ Open* 2015; 5: e008318.

Knight M, Bunch K, Cairns A, et al. (eds), on behalf of MBRRACE-UK. *Saving Lives, Improving Mothers' Care Rapid Report: Learning from SARS-CoV-2-related and Associated Maternal Deaths in the UK March–May 2020*. Oxford: National Perinatal Epidemiology Unit, University of Oxford, 2020.

Knight M, Bunch K, Tuffnell D, et al. (eds), on behalf of MBRRACE-UK. *Saving Lives, Improving Mothers' Care – Lessons Learned to Inform Maternity Care from the UK and Ireland Confidential Enquiries into Maternal Deaths and Morbidity 2015–17*. Oxford: National Perinatal Epidemiology Unit, University of Oxford, 2019.

RCP (Royal College of Physicians). *Acute Care Toolkit 15: Managing Acute Medical Problems in Pregnancy*. London: RCP, 2019.

RCUK (Resuscitation Council UK). *Advanced Life Support*. London: RCUK, 2021.

Regitz-Zagroskek V, Roos-Hesselink JW, Bauersachs J, et al. 2018 ESC guidelines for the management of cardiovascular diseases during pregnancy: the Task Force for the Management of Cardiovascular Diseases during Pregnancy of the European Society of Cardiology (ESC). *Eur Heart J* 2018; 39(34): 3165–241.

Souza JP, Tunçalp Ö, Vogel J, et al. Obstetric transition: the pathway towards ending preventable maternal deaths. *BJOG* 2014; 121: 1–4.

van Hagen IM, Cornette J, Johnson MR, Roos-Hesselink JW. Managing cardiac emergencies in pregnancy. *Heart* 2017; 103: 159–73.

CHAPTER 10

Cantwell R, Clutton-Brock T, Cooper G, et al. Saving Mothers' Lives: reviewing maternal deaths to make motherhood safer: 2006–2008. The Eighth Report of the Confidential Enquiries into Maternal Deaths in the United Kingdom. *BJOG* 2011; 118 (Suppl 1): 1–203.

OAA/DAS (Obstetric Anaesthetists' Association/Difficult Airway Society). *Guidelines for the Management of Difficult and Failed Intubation in Obstetrics – 2015*. https://das.uk.com/guidelines/obstetric_airway_guidelines_2015 (last accessed October 2020).

CHAPTER 11

Beckett V, Knight M, Sharpe P. The CAPS Study: incidence, management and outcomes of cardiac arrest in pregnancy in the UK: a prospective, descriptive study. *BJOG* 2017; 124(9): 1374–81.

CHAPTER 12

Cantwell R, Clutton-Brock T, Cooper G, et al. Saving Mothers' Lives: reviewing maternal deaths to make motherhood safer: 2006–2008. The Eighth Report of the Confidential Enquiries into Maternal Deaths in the United Kingdom. *BJOG* 2011; 118 (Suppl 1): 1–203.

Clark SL, Hankins GD, Dudley DA, et al. Amniotic fluid embolism: analysis of the national registry. *Am J Obstet Gynecol* 1995; 172: 1158–67.

Knight M, Bunch K, Tuffnell D, et al. (eds), on behalf of MBRRACE-UK. *Saving Lives, Improving Mothers' Care – Lessons Learned to Inform Maternity Care from the UK and Ireland Confidential Enquiries into Maternal Deaths and Morbidity 2016–18*. Oxford: National Perinatal Epidemiology Unit, University of Oxford, 2020.

Knight M, Nair M, Tuffnell D, Shakespeare J, Kenyon S, Kurinczuk JJ (eds), on behalf of MBRRACE-UK. *Saving Lives, Improving Mothers' Care – Lessons Learned to Inform Maternity Care from the UK and Ireland Confidential Enquiries into Maternal Deaths and Morbidity 2013–15*. Oxford: National Perinatal Epidemiology Unit, University of Oxford, 2017.

Knight M, Tuffnell D, Brocklehurst P, et al., on behalf of the UK Obstetric Surveillance System. Incidence and risk factors for amniotic-fluid embolism. *Obstet Gynecol* 2010; 115: 910–17.

Tuffnell DJ. United Kingdom amniotic fluid embolism register. *BJOG* 2005; 112: 1625–9.

CHAPTER 13

Khan F, Vaillancourt C, Bourjeily G. Diagnosis and management of deep vein thrombosis in pregnancy. *BMJ* 2017; 357 :j2344.

Greer IA. Thrombosis in pregnancy: updates in diagnosis and management. *Hematology Am Soc Hematol Educ Program* 2012; 2012: 203–7.

Guimicheva B, Czuprynska J, Arya R. The prevention of pregnancy-related venous thromboembolism. *Br J Haematol* 2015; 168: 163–74.

Martillotti G, Boehlen F, Robert-Ebadi H, Jastrow N, Righini M, Blondon M. Treatment options for severe pulmonary embolism during pregnancy and the postpartum period: a systematic review. *J Thromb Haemost* 2017; 15(10): 1942–50.

CHAPTER 14

Wyllie J, Ainsworth S, Tinnion R. *Guidelines: Resuscitation and Support of Transition of Babies at Birth*. London: Resuscitation Council UK, 2021.

CHAPTER 15

ACS (American College of Surgeons). *Advanced Trauma Life Support® Student Course Manual*, 10th edn. Chicago: ACS, 2018.

Battaloglu E, McDonnell D, Chu J, Lecky F, Porter K. Epidemiology and outcomes of pregnancy and obstetric complications in trauma in the United Kingdom. *Injury* 2016; 47: 184–7.

Battaloglu E, Porter K. Management of pregnancy and obstetric complications in prehospital trauma care: faculty of prehospital care consensus guidelines. *Emerg Med J* 2017; 34(5): 318–25.

Cameron PA, Gabbe BJ, Cooper DJ, Walker T, Judson R, McNeil J. A statewide system of trauma care in Victoria: effect on patient survival. *Med J Aust* 2008; 189(10): 546–50.

Celso B, Tepas J, Langland-Orban B, et al. A systematic review and meta-analysis comparing outcome of severely injured patients treated in trauma centers following the establishment of trauma systems. *J Trauma Acute Care Surg* 2006; 60(2): 371–8.

Findlay G, Martin IC, Carter S et al., on behalf of NCEPOD (National Confidential Enquiry into Patient Outcome and Death). *Trauma: Who Cares?* London: NCEPOD, 2007. www.ncepod.org.uk/2007report2/Downloads/SIP_report.pdf (last accessed October 2020).

Knight M, Bunch K, Tuffnell D, et al. (eds), on behalf of MBRRACE-UK. *Saving Lives, Improving Mothers' Care – Lessons Learned to Inform Maternity Care from the UK and Ireland Confidential Enquiries into Maternal Deaths and Morbidity 2015–17*. Oxford: National Perinatal Epidemiology Unit, University of Oxford, 2019.

Mercer SJ, Kingston EV, Jones CPL. The trauma call. *BMJ* 2018; 361: k2272.

Moran CG, Lecky F, Bouamra O, et al. Changing the system – major trauma patients and their outcomes in the NHS (England) 2008–2017. *EClinicalMedicine* 2018; 2: 13–21. https://doi.org/10.1016/j.eclinm.2018.07.001 (last accessed October 2020).

Nevin DG, Brohi K. Permissive hypotension for active haemorrhage in trauma. *Anaesthesia* 2017; 72: 1443–8.

NICE (National Institute for Health and Care Excellence). *Head Injury: Assessment and Early Management*. CG176. London: NICE, 2014 (updated September 2019).

NICE (National Institute for Health and Care Excellence). *Major Trauma: Assessment and Initial Management*. NG39. London: NICE, 2016.

Wiles MD. Blood pressure in trauma resuscitation: 'pop the clot' vs. 'drain the brain'? *Anaesthesia* 2017; 72: 1448–55.

CHAPTER 16

Home Office. *Definition of Domestic Violence and Abuse: Guide for Local Areas*. London: Home Office, 2013. https://www.gov.uk/government/publications/definition-of-domestic-violence-and-abuse-guide-for-local-areas (last accessed November 2020).

Knight M, Bunch K, Tuffnell D, et al. (eds), on behalf of MBRRACE-UK. *Saving Lives, Improving Mothers' Care – Lessons Learned to Inform Maternity Care from the UK and Ireland Confidential Enquiries into Maternal Deaths and Morbidity 2016–18*. Oxford: National Perinatal Epidemiology Unit, University of Oxford, 2020.

ONS (Office for National Statistics). *Domestic Abuse in England and Wales Overview: November 2021*. https://www.ons.gov.uk/peoplepopulationandcommunity/crimeandjustice/bulletins/domesticabuseinenglandandwalesoverview/november2021 (last accessed January 2022).

CHAPTER 17

ACS (American College of Surgeons) Committee on Trauma. Thoracic trauma. In: ACS Committee on Trauma. *Advanced Trauma Life Support® Student Course Manual*, 10th edn. Chicago: ACS, 2018: pp. 62–81.

Battaloglu E, McDonnell D, Chu J, Lecky F, Porter K. Epidemiology and outcomes of pregnancy and obstetric complications in trauma in the United Kingdom. *Injury* 2016; 47(1): 184–7.

Battaloglu E, Porter K. Management of pregnancy and obstetric complications in prehospital trauma care: faculty of prehospital care consensus guidelines. *Emerg Med J* 2017; 34(5): 318–25.

Havelock T, Teoh R, Laws D, Gleeson F, on behalf of the British Thoracic Society Pleural Disease Guideline Group. Pleural procedures and thoracic ultrasound: British Thoracic Society Pleural Disease Guideline 2010. *Thorax* 2010; 65 (Suppl 2): ii61–76.

NICE (National Institute for Health and Care Excellence). *Major Trauma: Assessment and Initial Management*. NG39. London: NICE, 2016.

CHAPTER 18

ACS (American College of Surgeons) Committee on Trauma. *Advanced Trauma Life Support® Student Course Manual*, 10th edn. Chicago: ACS, 2018.

Hayden B, Plaat F, Cox C. Managing trauma in the pregnant woman. *Br J Hosp Med* 2013; 74(6): 327–30.

Knight M, Bunch K, Tuffnell D, et al. (eds), on behalf of MBRRACE-UK. *Saving Lives, Improving Mothers' Care – Lessons Learned to Inform Maternity Care from the UK and Ireland Confidential Enquiries into Maternal Deaths and Morbidity 2015–17*. Oxford: National Perinatal Epidemiology Unit, University of Oxford, 2019.

Tran A, Yates J, Lau A, Lampron J, Matar M. Permissive hypotension versus conventional resuscitation strategies in adult trauma patients with hemorrhagic shock: a systematic review and meta-analysis of randomized controlled trials. *J Trauma Acute Care Surg* 2018; 84(5): 802–8.

CHAPTER 19

NICE (National Institute for Health and Social Care Excellence). *Head Injury: Assessment and Early Management*. CG176. London: NICE, 2014 (updated September 2019).

RCP (Royal College of Physicians). *National Early Warning Score (NEWS) 2: Standardising the Assessment of Acute-Illness Severity in the NHS. Updated Report of a Working Party*. London: RCP, 2017.

CHAPTER 20

NICE (National Institute for Health and Care Excellence). *Head Injury: Assessment and Early Management*. CG176. London: NICE, 2014 (updated September 2019).

NICE (National Institute for Health and Care Excellence). *Trauma*. QS166. London: NICE, 2018.

CHAPTER 21

Chavez LO, Leon M, Einav S, Varon J. Beyond muscle destruction: a systematic review of rhabdomyolysis for clinical practice. *Crit Care* 2016; 20: 135.

CHAPTER 22

British Burn Association. *National Standards for Provision and Outcomes in Adult and Paediatric Burn Care*. https://www.britishburnassociation.org/standards/ (last accessed October 2020).

Care of Burns in Scotland. www.cobis.scot.nhs.uk (last accessed October 2020).

CHAPTER 23

BMJ (British Medical Journal). *BMJ Best Practice. Assessment of Acute Abdomen*. London: BMJ, 2018 (updated July 2021). https://bestpractice.bmj.com/topics/en-gb/503 (last accessed January 2022).

Knight M, Bunch K, Tuffnell D, et al. (eds) on behalf of MBRRACE-UK. *Saving Lives, Improving Mothers' Care – Lessons Learned to Inform maternity care from the UK and Ireland Confidential Enquiries into Maternal Deaths and Morbidity 2016-18*. Oxford: National Perinatal Epidemiology Unit, University of Oxford, 2020.

O'Heaney JL, Barnett RE, MacSwan RM, Rasheed A. Acute and chronic pancreatitis in pregnancy. *Obstet Gynecol* 2021; 23(2): 89–93.

Taylor D. *Acute Abdomen and Pregnancy*. Medscape (updated 2020). http://emedicine.medscape.com/article/195976-overview (last accessed October 2020).

CHAPTER 24

Mohan M, Baagar KAM, Lindow S. Management of diabetic ketoacidosis in pregnancy. *Obstet Gynaecol* 2017; 19: 55–62.

NICE (National Institute for Health and Care Excellence). *Diabetes in Pregnancy: Management from Preconception to the Postnatal Period*. NG3. London: NICE, 2020.

CHAPTER 25

Ayanambakkam A, Owens KC, McIntosh JJ, Nester CM, George JN. (2017). A postpartum perfect storm. *Am J Hematol* ***2017***; 92(10), 1105–1110.

Friedman DI. A practical approach to intracranial hypertension. *Headache Curr* 2005; 2(1): 1–10.

Ho P, Khan S, Crompton D, Hayes L. Extensive cerebral venous sinus thrombosis after romiplostim treatment for immune thrombocytopenia (ITP) despite severe thrombocytopenia. *Intern Med J* 2015; 45(6): 682–3.

Knight M, Bunch K, Tuffnell D, et al. (eds), on behalf of MBRRACE-UK. *Saving Lives, Improving Mothers' Care – Lessons Learned to Inform M Maternity Care from the UK and Ireland Confidential Enquiries into Maternal Deaths and Morbidity 2016–18*. Oxford: National Perinatal Epidemiology Unit, University of Oxford, 2020.

Knight M, Bunch K, Tuffnell D, et al. (eds), on behalf of MBRRACE-UK. *Saving Lives, Improving Mothers' Care – Lessons Learned to Inform Maternity Care from the UK and Ireland Confidential Enquiries into Maternal Deaths and Morbidity 2017–19*. Oxford: National Perinatal Epidemiology Unit, University of Oxford, 2021.

Machner B, Neppert B, Paulsen M, et al. Pseudotumor cerebri as a reversible side effect of all-trans retinoic acid treatment in acute promyelocytic leukaemia. *Eur J Neurol* 2008; 15(7): e68–9.

Nelson-Piercy C. *Handbook of Obstetric Medicine*, 6th edn. Abingdon: CRC Press, 2020.

OAA (Obstetric Anaesthetists' Association). *Treatment of Obstetric Post-Dural Puncture Headache*. London: OAA, 2018.

RCP (Royal College of Physicians). *Acute Care Toolkit 15: Managing Acute Medical Problems in Pregnancy*. London: RCP, 2019.

RCOG (Royal College of Obstetrics and Gynaecologists). *Epilepsy in Pregnancy*. Green-top Guideline No. 68. London: RCOG, 2016.

Revell K, Morrish P. Headaches in pregnancy. *Obstet Gynaecol* 2014; 16: 179–84.

CHAPTER 26

NICE (National Institute for Health and Care Excellence). *Antenatal and Postnatal Mental Health: Clinical Management and Service Guidance*. CG192. London: NICE, 2014 (updated 2018).

RCOG (Royal College of Obstetricians and Gynaecologists). *Management of Women with Mental Health Issues during Pregnancy and the Postnatal Period*. Good Practice No. 14. London: RCOG, 2011.

CHAPTER 27

Knight M, Bunch K, Tuffnell D, et al. (eds), on behalf of MBRRACE-UK. *Saving Lives, Improving Mothers' Care – Lessons Learned to Inform Maternity Care from the UK and Ireland Confidential Enquiries into Maternal Deaths and Morbidity 2016–18*. Oxford: National Perinatal Epidemiology Unit, University of Oxford, 2020.

Magee LA, von Dadelszen P, Singer J, et al. The CHIPS randomized controlled trial (Control of Hypertension in Pregnancy study): is severe hypertension just an elevated blood pressure? *Hypertension* 2016; 68(5): 1153–9.

CHAPTER 28

B-Lynch C, Keith LG, Lalonde AB, Karoshi M (eds). *A Textbook of Postpartum Haemorrhage*. Duncow, Dumfriesshire: Sapiens Publishing, 2006.

Khan KS, Moore PAS, Wilson MJ, et al.; SALVO study group. Cell salvage and donor blood transfusion during caesarean section: a pragmatic, multicentre randomised controlled trial (SALVO). *PLoS Med* 2017; 14(12): e1002471.

Knight M, Bamber J, Lucas S, Paterson-Brown S, Tufnell D, on behalf of the MBRRACE-UK Haemorrhage Chapter Writing Group. Messages for prevention and treatment of morbidity from major obstetric haemorrhage. In: Knight M, Bunch K, Tuffnell D, et al. (eds), on behalf of MBRRACE-UK. *Saving Lives, Improving Mothers' Care – Lessons Learned to Inform Maternity Care from the UK and Ireland Confidential Enquiries into Maternal Deaths and Morbidity 2014–16*. Oxford: National Perinatal Epidemiology Unit, University of Oxford, 2018, pp. 23–33.

Knight M, Bunch K, Tuffnell D, et al. (eds) on behalf of MBRRACE-UK. *Saving Lives, Improving Mothers' Care – Lessons Learned to Inform Maternity Care from the UK and Ireland Confidential Enquiries into Maternal Deaths and Morbidity 2016-18*. Oxford: National Perinatal Epidemiology Unit, University of Oxford, 2020.

Lemmens HJM, Bernstein DP, Brodsky JB. Estimating blood volume in obese and morbidly obese patients. *Obes Surg* 2006; 16(6): 773–6.

RCOG (Royal College of Obstetricians and Gynaecologists). *Postpartum Haemorrhage, Prevention and Management*. Green-top Guideline No. 52. London: RCOG, 2016.

RCOG (Royal College of Obstetricians and Gynaecologists). *Antepartum Haemorrhage*. Green-top Guideline No. 63. London: RCOG, 2011 (updated December 2014).

RCS England (Royal College of Surgeons of England). *Caring for Patients who Refuse Blood – a Guide to Good Practice*. London: RCS England, 2016. https://www.rcseng.ac.uk/library-and-publications/rcs-publications/docs/caring-for-patients-who-refuse-blood/ (last accessed January 2022).

UKCSAG (UK Cell Salvage Action Group). *UKCSAG Intraoperative Cell Salvage Survey*. https://www.transfusionguidelines.org/transfusion-practice/uk-cell-salvage-action-group/ukcsag-intraoperative-cell-salvage-survey (last accessed January 2022).

CHAPTER 29

Boatin AA, Cullinane F, Torloni MR, Betrán AP. Audit and feedback using the Robson classification to reduce caesarean section rates: a systematic review. *BJOG* 2018; 125(1): 36–42.

Knight M, Nair M, Tuffnell D, Shakespeare J, Kenyon S, Kurinczuk JJ (eds), on behalf of MBRRACE-UK. *Saving Lives, Improving Mothers' Care – Lessons Learned to Inform Maternity Care from the UK and Ireland Confidential Enquiries into Maternal Deaths and Morbidity 2013–15*. Oxford: National Perinatal Epidemiology Unit, University of Oxford, 2017.

NICE (National Institute for Health and Care Excellence). *Caesarean Section Overview*. London: NICE (updated July 2017). http://pathways.nice.org.uk/pathways/caesarean-section (last accessed October 2020).

Olah KS. Reversal of the decision for casesarean section in the second stage of labour on the basis of consultant vaginal assessment. *J Obstet Gynaecol* 2005; 25: 115–16.

Porter S, Paterson-Brown S. Avoiding inadvertent laparoelytrotomy. *BJOG* 2003; 110: 91–2.

RCOG (Royal College of Obstetricians and Gynaecologists), Clinical Effectiveness Support Unit. *The National Sentinel Caesarean Section Audit Report*. London: RCOG, 2001.

RCOG (Royal College of Obstetricians and Gynaecologists). *Magnesium Sulphate to Prevent Cerebral Palsy following Preterm Birth*. Scientific Impact Paper No. 29. London: RCOG, 2011.

RCOG (Royal College of Obstetricians and Gynaecologists). *Placenta Praevia and Placenta Accreta. Diagnosis and Management*. Green-top Guideline No. 27a. London: RCOG, 2018.

CHAPTER 30

NICE (National Institute for Health and Care Excellence). *Intrapartum Care for Healthy Women and Babies*. CG190. London: NICE, 2014 (updated February 2017).

UKOSS (UK Obstetric Surveillance System). https://www.npeu.ox.ac.uk/ukoss (last accessed January 2022).

CHAPTER 31

Al-Zirqi I, Stray-Pedersen B, Forsén L, Vangen S. Uterine rupture after previous caesarean section. *BJOG* 2010; 117: 809–20.

Brar HS, Greenspoon JS, Platt LD, Paul RH. Acute puerperal uterine inversion. New approaches to management. *J Reprod Med* 1989; 34: 173–7.

Fitzpatrick KE, Kurinczuk JJ, Alfirevic Z, Spark P, Brocklehurst P, Knight M. Uterine rupture by intended mode of delivery in the UK: a national case control study. *PLoS Med* 2012; 9(3): e1001184.

Mwinyoglee J, Simelela N, Marivate M. Non-puerperal uterine inversions. A two case report and review of the literature. *Cent Afr J Med* 1997; 43: 268–72.

RCOG (Royal College of Obstetricians and Gynaecologists). *Birth after Previous Caesarean Section*. Green-top Guideline No. 45. London: RCOG, 2015.

Smith GC, Pell JP, Pasupathy D, Dobbie R. Factors predisposing to perinatal death related to uterine rupture during attempted vaginal birth after caesarean section: retrospective cohort study. *BMJ* 2004; 329: 375.

Watson P, Besch N, Bowes WA Jr. Management of acute and subacute puerperal inversion of the uterus. *Obstet Gynecol* 1980; 55: 12–16.

CHAPTER 32

NPEU (National Perinatal Epidemiology Unit), University of Oxford. *Surveillance of Uterine Rupture*. Oxford: NPEU, 2012. https://www.npeu.ox.ac.uk/research/projects/63-ukoss-uterine-rupture (last accessed January 2022).

CHAPTER 33

Attilakos G, Sibanda T, Winter C, et al. A randomised controlled trial of a new handheld vacuum extraction device. *BJOG* 2005; 112: 1510–15.

Bahl R, Murphy DJ, Strachan B. Qualitative analysis by interviews and video recordings to establish the components of a skilled low-cavity non-rotational vacuum delivery. *BJOG* 2009; 116: 319–26.

Bahl R, Murphy DJ, Strachan B. Non-technical skills for obstetricians conducting forceps and vacuum deliveries: qualitative analysis by interviews and video recordings. *Europ J Obstet Gynecol Reprod Biol* 2010; 150: 147–51.

Barata S, Cardoso E, Ferreira-Santo S, et al. Maternal and neonatal immediate effects of sequential delivery. *J Matern Fetal Neonatal Med* 2012; 25(7): 981–3.

Bird GC. The importance of flexion in vacuum extractor delivery. *BJOG* 1976; 83: 194–200.

Dupuis O, Decullier E, Clerc J, et al. Does forceps training in a birth simulator allow obstetricians to improve forceps blade placement? *Europ J Obstet Gynecol Reprod Biol* 2011; 159: 305–9.

Edozien LC. *Operative Vaginal Delivery*. Consent Advice No. 11. London: Royal College of Obstetricians and Gynaecologists, 2010.

Johanson RB, Menon V. Soft versus rigid vacuum extractor cups for assisted vaginal delivery. *Cochrane Database Syst Rev* 2004; Issue 2: CD000446.

Johanson RB, Menon V. Vacuum extraction versus forceps for assisted vaginal delivery. *Cochrane Database Syst Rev* 2004; Issue 2: CD000224.

Lewis EA, Barr C, Thomas K. The mode of delivery in women taken to theatre at full dilatation: does consultant presence make a difference? *J Obstet Gynaecol* 2011; 31(3): 229–31.

Malvasi A, Stark M, Ghi T, et al. Intrapartum sonography for fetal head asynclitism and transverse position: sonographic signs and comparison of diagnostic performance between transvaginal and digital examination. *J Matern Fetal Neonatal Med* 2012; 25(5): 508–12.

Murphy DJ, Macleod M, Bahl R, Strachan B. A cohort study of maternal and neonatal morbidity in relation to use of sequential instruments at operative vaginal delivery. *Eur J Obstet Gynaecol Reprod Biol* 2011; 156: 41–5.

O'Mahony F, Settatree R, Platt C, Johnson R. Review of singleton fetal and neonatal deaths associated with cranial trauma and cephalic delivery during a national intrapartum-related confidential enquiry. *BJOG* 2005; 112: 619–26.

RCOG (Royal College of Obstetricians and Gynaecologists). *Operative Vaginal Delivery*. Green-top Guideline No. 26. London: RCOG, 2011.

Suwannachat B, Laopaiboon M, Tonmat S, et al. Rapid versus stepwise application of negative pressure in vacuum extraction-assisted vaginal delivery: a multicentre randomised controlled non-inferiority trial. *BJOG* 2011; 118: 1247–52.

Unterscheider J, McMenamin M, Cullinane F. Rising rates of caesarean deliveries at full dilatation: a concerning trend. *Eur J Obstet Gynecol Reprod Biol* 2011; 157: 141–4.

Vacca A. The place of the vacuum extractor in modern obstetric practice. *Fetal Med Rev* 1990; 2: 103–22.

Yeo L, Romero R. Sonographic evaluation in the second stage of labor to improve the assessment of labor progress and its outcome [Editorial/opinion]. *Ultrasound Obstet Gynecol* 2009; 33: 253–8.

CHAPTER 34

Boekhuizen F, Washington J, Johnson F, Hamilton P. Vacuum extraction versus forceps delivery: indications and complications, 1979 to 1984. *Obstet Gynecol* 1987; 69: 338–42.

Cluver C, Hofmeyr GJ. Posterior axilla sling traction – a technique for intractable shoulder dystocia. *Obstet Gynecol* 2009; 113: 486–8.

Crofts JF, Fox R, Ellis D, et al. Observations from 450 shoulder dystocia simulations lessons for skills training. *Obstet Gynecol* 2008; 112: 906–12.

Draycott TJ, Crofts JF, Ash JP, et al. Improving neonatal outcome through practical shoulder dystocia training. *Obstet Gynecol* 2008; 112(1): 14–20.

Friesen CD, Miller AM, Rayburn WF. Influence of spontaneous labor on delivering macrosomic fetus. *Am J Perinatol* 1995; 12: 63–6.

Grimm MJ, Costello RE, Gonik B. Effect of clinician-applied maneuvers on brachial plexus stretch during a shoulder dystocia event: investigation using a computer simulation model. *Am J Obstet Gynecol* 2010; 203: 339.e1–5.

Gupta M, Hockley C, Quigley MA, et al. Antepartum and intrapartum prediction of shoulder dystocia. *Eur J Obstet Gynecol Reprod Biol* 2010; 150: 134–9.

Hartfield VJ. Symphysiotomy for shoulder dystocia. *Am J Obstet Gynecol* 1986; 155: 228.

Lerner H. *Shoulder Dystocia*. http://shoulderdystociainfo.com/index.htm (last accessed November 2020).

Lurie S, Ben-Arie, Hagay A. The ABC of shoulder dystocia management. *Asia Oceania J Obstet Gynaecol* 1994; 20: 195–7.

Magowan B. Shoulder dystocia: In: Magowan B. *Churchill's Pocketbook of Obstetrics and Gynaecology*, 2nd edn. Edinburgh: Churchill Livingstone, 2000: pp. 99–5.

Menticoglou S. A modified technique to deliver the posterior arm in severe shoulder dystocia. *Am J Obstet Gynecol* 2006; 108(30): 755–7.

O'Leary J. Cephalic replacement for shoulder dystocia: present status and future role of Zavanelli manoeuvre. *Obstet Gynecol* 1993; 82: 847–55.

Overland EA, Spydslaug A, Nielsen CS, Eskild A. Risk of shoulder dystocia in second delivery: does a history of shoulder dystocia matter? *Am J Obstet Gynecol* 2009; 200: 506.e1–6.

RCOG (Royal College of Obstetricians and Gynaecologists). *Shoulder Dystocia*, 2nd edn. Green-top Guideline No. 42. London: RCOG, 2012.

Resnik R. Management of shoulder girdle dystocia. *Clin Obstet Gynecol* 1980; 23: 559–64.

Sandmire HF, DeMott RK. Erb's palsy: concepts of causation. *Obstet Gynecol* 2000; 95: 941–2.

Wolf H, Hoeksma AF, Oei SL, Bleker OP. Obstetric brachial plexus injury: risk factors related to recovery. *Eur J Obstet Gynecol Reprod Biol* 2000; 88: 133–8.

CHAPTER 35

Chetty RM, Moodley J. Umbilical cord prolapse. *S Afr Med J* 1980; 57: 128–9.

RCOG (Royal College of Obstetricians and Gynaecologists). *Umbilical Cord Prolapse*. Green-top Guideline No. 50. London: RCOG, 2014.

Murphy DJ, MacKenzie IZ. The mortality and morbidity associated with umbilical cord prolapse. *BJOG* 1995; 102: 826–30.

Vago T. Prolapse of the umbilical cord. A method of management. *Am J Obstet Gynecol* 1970; 107: 967–9.

CHAPTER 36

Newman M, Beller U, Lavie O, et al. Intrapartum bimanual tocolytic-assisted reversal of face presentation: preliminary report. *Obstet Gynecol* 1994; 84: 146–52.

Shaffer BL, Cheng YW, Vargas JE, Laros RK, Caughey AB. et al. Face presentation: predictors and delivery route. *Am J Obstet Gynecol* (2006;) 194: ,e10–e12.

CHAPTER 37

External cephalic version

Cluver C, Hofmeyr GJ, Gyte GML, Sinclair M. Interventions for helping to turn term breech babies to head first presentation when using external cephalic version (review). *Cochrane Database Syst Rev* 2012; Issue 1: CD000184.

Hofmeyr GJ, Kulier R, West HM. External cephalic version for breech presentation at term. *Cochrane Database Syst Rev* 2015; Issue 4: CD000083.

Hutton EK, Hannah ME, Ross SJ, et al. The Early External Cephalic Version (ECV) 2 Trial: an international multicentre randomised controlled trial of timing of ECV for breech pregnancies. *BJOG* 2011; 118(5): 564–77.

Hutton EK, Hofmeyr GJ, Dowswell T. External cephalic version for breech presentation before term. *Cochrane Database Syst Rev* 2015; Issue 7: CD000084.

RCOG (Royal College of Obstetricians and Gynaecologists). *External Cephalic Version and Reducing the Incidence of Term Breech Presentation*. Green-top Guideline No. 20a. London: RCOG, 2017.

Term breech delivery

Goffine F, Carayol M, Foidart J-M, et al., for the PREMODA Study Group. Is planned vaginal delivery for breech presentation at term still an option? Results of an observational prospective survey in France and Belgium. *Am J Obstet Gynecol* 2006; 194(4): 1002–11.

Hannah ME, Hannah WJ, Hewson SA, et al., for the TBT Group planned caesarean section versus planned vaginal birth for breech presentation at term: a randomised multicentre trial. *Lancet* 2000; 356: 1375–83.

Schutt JM, Steegers EA, Santema JG, et al. Maternal deaths after elective caesarean section for breech presentation in the Netherlands. *Acta Obstet Gynecol Scand* 2007; 86: 240–3.

Verhoven AT, de Leeuw JP, Bruinse HW. Breech presentation at term: elective caesarean section is the wrong choice as a standard treatment because of too high risks for the mother and her future children. *Ned Tijdschr Geneeskd* 2005; 149: 2207–10.

Preterm breech delivery

Alfirevic Z, Milan SJ, Livio S. Caesarean section versus vaginal delivery for preterm birth in singletons. *Cochrane Database Syst Rev* 2013; Issue 9: CD000078.

Fumio Suyama, Kohei Ogawa, Yukiko Tazaki, et al. The outcomes and risk factors of fetal bradycardia associated with external cephalic version. *J Matern Fetal Neonatal Med* 2019; 32(6): 922–6.

Lorthe E, Sentilhes L, Quere M, et al., for the EPIPAGE-2 Obstetric Writing Group. Planned delivery route of preterm breech singletons, and neonatal and 2-year outcomes: a population-based cohort study. *BJOG* 2019; 126: 73–82.

Breech delivery technique

Chan LY, Leung TY, Fok WY, et al. Prediction of successful vaginal delivery in women undergoing external cephalic version at term for breech presentation. *Eur J Obstet Gynecol Reprod Biol* 2004; 116: 39–42.

Chan LY, Tang JL, Tsoi KF, et al. Intrapartum caesarean delivery after successful external cephalic version: a meta-analysis. *Obstet Gynecol* 2004; 104: 155–60.

Impey L, Pandit M. Tocolysis for repeat external cephalic version in breech presentation at term: a randomised, double-blinded, placebo-controlled trial. *BJOG* 2005; 112: 627–31.

Løvset, J. Shoulder delivery by breech presentation. *J Obstet Gynaecol Brit Empire* 1937; 44(5): 696–704.

RCOG (Royal College of Obstetricians and Gynaecologists). *Management of Breech Presentation*. Green-top Guideline No. 20b. London: RCOG, 2017.

CHAPTER 38

Barrett J, Aztalos E, Wilan A, et al. The Twin Birth Study: a multicenter RCT of planned cesarean section (CS) and planned vaginal birth (VB) for twin pregnancies 320 to 386/7 weeks. *Am J Obstet Gynaecol* 2013; 208: S4–5.

Crowther CA. Caesarean delivery for the second twin. *Cochrane Database Syst Rev* 2000; Issue 2: CD000047.

Feng TI, Swindle REJ, Huddleston JF. A lack of adverse effect of prolonged delivery interval between twins. *J Matern Fetal Investig* 1995; 5: 222–5.

Leung TY, Tam WH, Leung TN, et al. Effect of twin to twin delivery interval on umbilical cord blood gas in the second twins. *BJOG* 2002; 109: 63–7.

Rabinovici J, Barkai G, Richman B, et al. Internal podalic version with unruptured membranes for the second twin in transverse lie. *Obstet Gynecol* 1988; 71: 4280–300.

Tchabo JG, Tomai T. Selected intrapartum external cephalic version of the second twin. *Obstet Gynecol* 1992; 79: 421–3.

NICE (National Institute for Health and Care Excellence). *Twin and Triplet Pregnancy*. NG137. London: NICE, 2019.

RCOG (Royal College of Obstetricians and Gynaecologists). *Management of Monochorionic Twin Pregnancy*. Green-top Guideline No. 51. London: RCOG, 2016.

CHAPTER 39

Andrews V, Sultan AH, Thakar R, Jones PW. Occult anal sphincter injuries – myth or reality. *BJOG* 2006; 113: 195–200.

Andrews V, Thakar R, Sultan AH. Structured hands-on training in repair of obstetric anal sphincter injuries (OASIS): an audit of clinical practice. *Int Urogynecol J Pelvic Floor Dysfunct* 2009; 20: 193–9.

Andrews V, Thakar R, Sultan AH, Jones PW. Are mediolateral episiotomies actually mediolateral? *BJOG* 2005; 112: 1156–8.

Carroli G, Mignini L. Episiotomy for vaginal birth. *Cochrane Database Syst Rev* 2009; Issue 1: CD000081.

Fernando RJ, Sultan AH, Kettle C, Thakar R. Methods of repair for obstetric anal sphincter injury. *Cochrane Database Syst Rev* 2013; 12: CD002866.

Kettle C, Dowswell T, Ismail KMK. Absorbable suture materials for primary repair of episiotomy and second degree tears. *Cochrane Database Syst Rev* 2010; Issue 6: CD000006.

Koelbl H, Igawa T, Salvatore S, et al. Pathophysiology of urinary incontinence, faecal incontinence and pelvic organ prolapse. In: Abrams P, Cardozo L, Khoury S, Wein A (eds). *Incontinence*, 5th edn. Arnhem: ICUD-EAU, 2013: pp. 261–359.

Mahony R, Behan M, Daly L, Kirwan C, O'Herlihy C, O'Connell PR. Internal anal sphincter defect influences continence outcome following obstetric anal sphincter injury. *Am J Obstet Gynecol* 2007; 196: 217.e1–5.

RCOG (Royal College of Obstetricians and Gynaecologists). *Third- and Fourth-Degree Perineal Tears, Management*. Green-top Guideline No. 29. London: RCOG, 2015.

Roos A-M, Thakar R, Sultan AH. Outcome of primary repair of obstetric anal sphincter injuries (OASIS): does the grade of tear matter? *Ultrasound Obstet Gynecol* 2010: 36(3): 368–74.

Sultan AH, Thakar R, Fenner D. *Perineal and Anal Sphincter Trauma*. London: Springer, 2007.

CHAPTER 40

Symphysiotomy

Björklund K. Minimally invasive surgery for obstructed labour: a review of symphysiotomy during the twentieth century (including 5000 cases). *BJOG* 2002; 109: 236–48.

Hartfield VJ. Subcutaneous symphysiotomy: time for a reappraisal? *Aust NZ J Obstet Gynaecol* 1973; 13: 147–52.

Hartfield VJ. Late effects of symphysiotomy. *Trop Doct* 1975; 5: 76–8.

Menticoglou SM. Symphysiotomy for the trapped aftercoming parts of the breech: a review of the literature and a plea for its use. *Aust NZ J Obstet Gynaecol* 1990; 30: 1–9.

Pape GL. 27 Symphysiotomies. *Trop Doct* 1999; 29: 248–9.

Payne G. Ireland orders enquiry into barbaric obstetric practices. *BMJ* 2001; 322: 1200.

Van Roosmalen J. Symphysiotomy as an alternative to caesarean section. *Int J Gynecol Obstet* 1987; 25: 451–8.

Van Roosmalen J. Safe motherhood: cesarean section or symphysiotomy? *Am J Obstet Gynecol* 1990; 163: 1–4.

Verkuyl DAA. Symphysiotomies are an important option in the developed world. *BMJ* 2001: 323: 809.

Destructive procedures

Amo-Mensah S, Elkins T, Ghosh T, et al. Obstetric destructive procedures. *Int J Gynaecol Obstet* 1996; 54: 167–8.

Arora M, Rajaram P, Oumachigui A, Parveena P. Destructive operations in modern obstetrics in a developing country at tertiary level. *BJOG* 1993; 100: 967–8.

Ekwempu CC. Embryotomy versus caesarean section. *Trop Doct* 1978; 8: 195–7.

Giwa-Osaigie O, Azzan B. Destructive operations. In: Studd J (ed.). *Progress in Obstetrics and Gynaecology Volume 6*. Edinburgh: Churchill Livingstone, 1987: pp. 211–21.

Gogoi MP. Maternal mortality from caesarean section in infected cases. *J Obstet Gynaecol Br Empire* 1971; 78: 373–6.

Gupta U, Chitra R. Destructive operations still have a place in developing countries. *Int J Gynaecol Obstet* 1994; 44(1): 15–19.

Hudson CN. Obstructed labour and its sequelae. In: Lawson JB, Harrison KA, Berström S (eds). *Maternity Care in Developing Countries*. London: RCOG Press, 2001: pp. 201–14.

Konje JC, Obisesan KA, Ladipo OA. Obstructed labour in Ibadan. *Int J Gynaecol Obstet* 1992; 39: 17–21.

Lawson J. Embryotomy for obstructed labour. *Trop Doct* 1974; 4: 188–91.

Maharaj D, Moodley J. Symphysiotomy and fetal destructive operations. *Best Pract Res Clin Obstet Gynaecol* 2002; 16: 117–31.

Marsden DE, Chang AS, Shin KS. Decapitation and vaginal delivery for impacted transverse lie in late labour: reports of 4 cases. *Aust NZ J Obstet Gynaecol* 1982; 22: 46–9.

Mitra KN, John MP. Decapitation by thread saw. *J Obstet Gynaecol India* 1950; 1: 65–73.

Moir C, Myerscough P. *Munro Kerr's Operative Obstetrics*, 8th edn. London: Ballière Tindall and Cassell, 1971.

CHAPTER 41

Fettes PDW, Jansson J-R, Wildsmith JAW. Failed spinal anaesthesia: mechanisms, management, and prevention. *Br J Anaesth* 2009; 102(6): 739–48.

Kinsella SM, Winton AL, Mushambi MC, et al. Failed tracheal intubation during obstetric general anaesthesia: a literature review. *Int J Obstet Anesth* 2015; 24(4): 356–74.

Pan PH, Bogard TD, Owen MD. Incidence and characteristics of failures in obstetric neuraxial analgesia and anesthesia: a retrospective analysis of 19,259 deliveries. *Int J Obstet Anesth* 2004; 13(4): 227–33.

RCoA (Royal College of Anaesthetists). Complications after obstetric CNB. In: *NAP3. The 3rd National Audit Project. Major Complications of Central Neuraxial Block in the United Kingdom. Report and Findings January 2009*. London: RCoA, 2009: pp. 117–24.

RCoA (Royal College of Anaesthetists). Obstetrics. In: *NAP4. 4th National Audit Project. Major Complications of Airway Management in the United Kingdom. Report and Findings March 2011*. London: RCoA, 2011: pp. 181–6.

RCoA (Royal College of Anaesthetists). AAGA in obstetric anaesthesia. In: *NAP5. 5th National Audit Project. Accidental Awareness during General Anaesthesia in the United Kingdom and Ireland. Report and Findings September 2014*. London: RCoA, 2014: pp. 133–43.

RCOG (Royal College of Obstetricians and Gynaecologists). Thematic analysis 2. In: *Each Baby Counts. 2018 Progress Report*. London: RCOG, 2018: pp. 31–42.

Ruppen W, Derry S, McQuay H, Moore RA. Incidence of epidural hematoma, infection, and neurologic injury in obstetric patients with epidural analgesia/anesthesia. *Anesthesiology* 2006; 105: 394–9.

Wong CA. Neurologic deficits and labor analgesia. *Reg Anesth Pain Med* 2004; 29: 341–51.

CHAPTER 42

ALSG (Advanced Life Support Group); Carley S, Mackway-Jones K (eds). *Major Incident Medical Management and Support: The Practical Approach in the Hospital*, 2nd edn. Oxford: Wiley Blackwell, 2018.

ALSG (Advanced Life Support Group); Mackway-Jones K, Marsden J, Windle J (eds). *Emergency Triage: Manchester Triage Group*, 3rd edn. Oxford: Wiley Blackwell, 2013.

Vassallo J, Smith JE, Wallis LA. Major incident triage and implementation of a new triage tool, the MPTT-24. *J Roy Army Med Corps* 2017; 164(2): 103–6.

CHAPTER 43

ALSG (Advanced Life Support Group); Foex B, Fortune PM, Lawn C (eds). *Neonatal, Adult and Paediatric Safe Transfer and Retrieval: A Practical Approach to Transfers*. Oxford: Wiley Blackwell, 2019.

Marlow N, Bennett C, Draper ES, Hennessy EM, Morgan AS, Costeloe KL. Perinatal outcomes for extremely preterm babies in relation to place of birth in England: the EPICure 2 study. *Arch Dis Child Fetal Neonatal Ed* 2014; 99(3): F181–8.

CHAPTER 44

DoH (Department of Health). *Reference Guide to Consent for Examination or Treatment*, 2nd edn. London: DoH, 2009.

Farnhill D, Inglis S. Patients' desire for information about anaesthesia: Australian attitudes. *Anaesthesia* 1993; 48: 162–4.

GMC (General Medical Council). *Consent: Patients and Doctors Making Decisions Together*. GMC 2008 (www.gmc-uk.org/guidance/ethical_guidance/consent_guidance_index.asp) (last accessed January 2022).

Hewson B. Why the Human Rights Act matters to doctors. *BMJ* 2000; 321: 780–1.

Inglis S, Farnhill D. The effects of providing preoperative statistical anaesthetic risk information. *Anesth Intensive Care* 1993; 21: 799–805.

Kelly GD, Blunt C, Moore PAS, Lewis M. Consent for regional anaesthesia in the United Kingdom: what is material risk? *Int J Obstet Anesth* 2004; 13: 71–4.

Lewis G (ed.). *Why Mothers Die 2000–2002. Sixth Report of the Confidential Enquiries into Maternal Deaths in the United Kingdom*. London: RCOG Press, 2004.

Maybury M, Maybury J. *Consent in Clinical Practice*. Oxford: Radcliffe Medical Press, 2003.

NHSLA (NHS Litigation Authority). *NHSLA Risk Alert, Issue 4*. November 2004.

Pattee C, Ballantyne M, Milne B. Epidural analgesia for labour and delivery: informed consent issues. *Can J Anaesth* 1997; 44: 918–23.

Plaat F, McGlennan A. Women in the 21st century deserve more information: disclosure of material risk in obstetric anaesthesia. *Int J Obstet Anesth* 2004; 13: 69–70.

RCOG (Royal College of Obstetrics and Gynaecology) Clinical Effectiveness Support Unit. *The National Sentinel Caesarean Section Audit: Report*. London: RCOG, 2001.

Sedgwick P, Hall A. Teaching medical students and doctors how to communicate risk. *BMJ* 2003; 327: 694–5.

Switankowsky IS. *A New Paradigm for Informed Consent*. Lanham, MD: University Press of America, 1998.

Webber D, Higgins L, Baker V. Enhancing recall of information from a patient education booklet: a trial using cardiomyopathy patients. *Patient Educ Couns* 2001; 44: 263–70.

Yentis SM, Hartle AJ, Barker IR, et al. AAGBI: consent for anaesthesia 2017: Association of Anaesthetists of Great Britain and Ireland. *Anaesthesia* 2017; 72: 93–105.

Rulings

Bolam versus Friern Hospital Management Committee 1957.

Bolitho versus City & Hackney Health Authority 1997.

Chester versus Afshar [2004] UKHL 41.

Montgomery versus Lanarkshire Health Board (2015)SC 11(2015) 1 AC 1430.

Norfolk and Norwich NHS Trust versus W 1996.

Paton versus trustees of British Pregnancy Advisory Services 1979.

Pearce versus United Bristol Healthcare Trust 1999.

Re C (Adult: Refusal of treatment) 1994.

Re MB (Adult medical treatment) 1997.

Re S (Adult refusal of treatment) 1992.

Re T (Adult: Refusal of treatment) 1992.

Rochdale NHS Trust versus C 1997.

Rogers versus Whitaker 1992.

Sidaway versus Board of Governors of Bethlehem Royal Hospital 1985 AC 871.

Sidaway versus Board of Governors of the Bethlehem Royal Hospital and Maudsley Hospital and others [1965] AC 871, HL at 871.

Tameside and Glossop Acute Services Trust versus CH.

Index

Managing Medical and Obstetric Emergencies and Trauma: A Practical Approach, Fourth Edition. Edited by Rosamunde Burns and Kara Dent.